Infection in Knee Replacement

Umile Giuseppe Longo
Nicolaas C. Budhiparama
Sébastien Lustig
Roland Becker
João Espregueira-Mendes
Editors

Infection in Knee Replacement

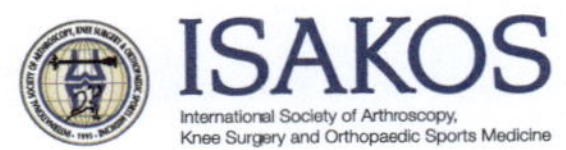

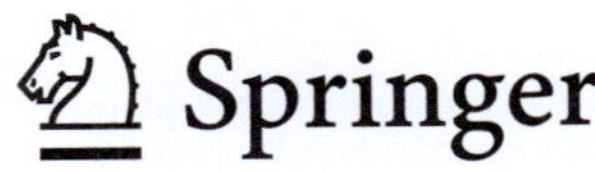

Editors
Umile Giuseppe Longo
Università Campus Bio-Medico
di Roma
Rome, Italy

Sébastien Lustig
Département de Chirurgie Ortopédique
Hôpital de la Croix-Rousse
Lyon, France

João Espregueira-Mendes
Clínica Espregueira -
FIFA Medical Centre of Excellence
Porto, Portugal

Nicolaas C. Budhiparama
Arthroplasty & Sports Medicine
Nicolaas Institute of Constructive
Orthopedic Research
Jakarta, Indonesia

Roland Becker
Department of Orthopaedics
and Traumatology
Center of Joint Replacement
Medical Director of the
University Hospital
University of Brandenburg an der Havel
Brandenburg, Germany

ISBN 978-3-030-81555-4   ISBN 978-3-030-81553-0   (eBook)
https://doi.org/10.1007/978-3-030-81553-0

This Springer imprint is published by the registered company Springer Nature Switzerland AG
The registered company address is: Gewerbestrasse 11, 6330 Cham, Switzerland

Foreword

It is an honor to write a preface for an excellent international text on Infection in Total Knee Arthroplasty (TKA). While knee arthroplasty can be traced back to 1863 when membrane interposition, including pig bladders, was used to resurface the arthritic knee joint. The modern history of TKA surface replacements began circa 1970 [1]. The first internationally recorded and widely used surface replacement designs were the Polycentric (Gunston 1969) and the Geomedic (aka Geometric 1970 USA). These anterior (ACL) and posterior cruciate (PCL) retention designs laid the foundation for an international frenzy to develop the science of non-hinged knee arthroplasty.

It is interesting to remember that the polycentric prosthesis was initially two independent femoral and tibial components which laid the groundwork for the now popular uni-compartment replacements. While the focus of the early designs was on the retention of both the ACL and PCL, John Insall and others at the Hospital for Special Surgery in New York felt that an entire ACL and PCL cruciate sacrificing prosthesis, with the first patellar replacement (Total Condylar 1974) [2], would be a better alternative. Within a few years, this cruciate-sacrificing design was modified and improved by adding the design change of an intercondylar femoral "cam" and tibial post to enhance the patient's range of motion and in addition, intercondylar coronal and sagittal stability. This Insall Burstein Posterior Stabilized Prosthesis of 1977 was modified further in the following decades and in 2021, the cruciate-substituting design is currently used in more than 50% of all total knee procedures in the USA.

In the first edition of *Surgery of the Knee*, 1984 [3], there were 26 chapters on all aspects of knee diseases requiring arthroplasty but no chapters on infection. In fact, to the best of our knowledge, the first significant text dealing with the infected Knee Arthroplasty was in 1992, *The Knee* [1]. Well, time has certainly brought about huge changes as evidenced by the abundance of articles, texts, and conferences devoted to the infected knee arthroplasty since 1984. This book, *Infection in Knee Replacement*, is a most welcome international update.

It is important to recognize that for the first 2–3 decades in the development of knee arthroplasty the patient was very different from our present population of surgical candidates. Circa 1970–1995, the primary pathological pathway for the development of severe destructive disease was inflammatory arthritis, primarily rheumatoid. These patients typically had severe biplanar deformities with similar complicating pathology often present in the ipsilateral and/or contralateral hip, foot, and ankle. Due to the massive amounts of steroids required for the treatment of these patients, their skin was frequently very attenuated and ulcerated, and wound closure often required skin grafting, muscle transfers, and tissue expanders [4]. The patient's deficient immune system often led to the necessity for multiple types of antibiotics with subsequent problems. Thank God for the DMARDS!

The worldwide variable operating theaters presented, in retrospect, very difficult sterility issues. These rooms were almost never dedicated to "clean cases." Sterilization procedures likewise had little resemblance to today's approaches. The surgical procedures were additionally often compromised by limited prosthetic sizes resulting in unnecessarily tight or excessive joint spaces as well as inadequate fixation which resulted in non-physiological component motion and instability. Hematomas developed and infection often followed.

This new text *Infection in Knee Replacement* is a compendium of the tremendous improvements in the treatment of one of the most dreadful complications in Knee Arthroplasty. The science attendant to the treatment of infection in Knee Replacement is extensively detailed by all the contributors in this book. Prosthetic joint infection (PJI) is, and unfortunately always will be, a very challenging therapeutic problem. It is especially apparent that when we consider that in the USA alone, the present estimate of annual knee replacements is 600,000 cases [5]. In 2030, there is a growth projection of 673% for a total number of 4,638,000 cases per annum (USA). In the world, the present projection of knee replacement cases is 1,234,000. Using the same rate of growth to 2030, the annual number of cases would be 10,234,520 in 2030. With infection rates presently ranging from 1 to 2% (primary and revision), we might anticipate upwards of 200,000 infected knee replacements per year in 2030. These are daunting numbers and require strict and updated attention to detail, in order to minimize the problem as best we can. The editors of this book accomplish this goal.

This book, *Infection in Knee Replacement*, is thorough in evaluating all the parameters that must be constantly evaluated and reassessed in minimizing TKR infections. Risk factors and prevention are a start. The patient's health must be maximized prior to surgery. Just giving prophylactic antibiotics is not enough. Each patient is somewhat different and these accomplished authors address that issue.

The diagnosis of an infected TKA is not necessarily as easy as one would expect. Precise periprosthetic joint infection (PJI) diagnosis has proven to be difficult throughout the years. The Musculoskeletal Infection Society (MSIS) has taken a worldwide leadership role in developing criteria required to establish a PJI. These criteria are identified clearly and further augmented by several critical points including a detailed and accepted identification of the pathogen. These exhaustive chapters are written by international experts who, in the past, helped to develop and currently continue to reassess the multiple complex criteria required for a PJI diagnosis. Treatment modalities from innovative pharmacological strategies are constantly changing for the better and the authors thoroughly explain the rationale.

In this text, all surgical options from Debridement, Antibiotics, and Implant Retention (DAIR), staged procedures, the use of static or dynamic spacers, arthrodesis, and unfortunately the extremely rare amputation are discussed in detail. This is a comprehensive book that will thoroughly educate the surgeon, medical physicians, and paraprofessionals who are all so crucial to the successful treatment of the PJI. The patient will be the winner thanks to the efforts of all these authors and editors who have done a tremendous service by advancing our knowledge in the prevention and treatment of the PJI.

Congratulations to the Editors, Umile Giuseppe Longo, Nicolaas C. Budhiparama, Sébastien Lustig, Roland Becker, and Joao Espregueira-Mendes, for invaluable, current, and an international perspective on a prevalent and difficult problem.

W. Norman Scott

Orthopedic Surgery, NYU Langone Orthopedic Hospital

New York, NY, USA

International Congress for Joint Reconstruction (ICJR)

New York, NY, USA

Insall Traveling Fellowship (ITF), New York, NY, USA

References

1. Scott WN. The knee, chap. 58. In: The evolution of total knee arthroplasty. St. Louis: Mosby; 1994.
2. Insall J, Scott WN, Ranawat CS. The total condylar knee prosthesis: a report of two hundred twenty cases. J Bone Joint Surg. 1979;61:173–80.
3. Insall JN. Surgery of the knee. London: Churchill Livingston; 1984.
4. Scott WN. Insall and Scott surgery of the knee. 5th ed.; chapters 78,79 Susan Craig Scott; 2006.
5. Kurtz SM, Ong KL, Edmund L, Widmer M, Maravic M, Gomez-Barrena E, de Fatima de Pina M, Manno V, Torre M, Walter WL, de Steiger R, Geesink, Geesink RGT, Peltola M, Roder C. International survey of primary and revision total knee replacement. International Orthopedics (SCIOT). 2011;35:1783–9.

Foreword

Knee replacement has evolved over decades to become one of the most successful interventions in orthopedic surgery. Many of the challenges that have been encountered over this time in the development of knee replacement have been addressed to a great extent. Improvements in implant materials have seen a reduction in revision surgery due to polyethylene wear, and implant design has continued to evolve to provide surgeons with consistent, reliable designs to address different severities and patterns of arthritis. New technologies such as computer navigation and robotics have allowed surgeons to perform surgery very precisely and reduce the risk of malalignment, and both cemented and cementless fixation are very reliable, with the risk of revision for loosening due to fixation failure very low. Multiple national joint registries have also assisted in informing surgeons and industry in a very objective, independent fashion about the many variables in implant design and technique that may influence outcome, particularly the risk of revision.

Prosthetic joint infection, however, remains a major challenge that is yet to be resolved and continues to be a major contributor to prosthetic revision and patient dissatisfaction. The exponential growth in the number of knee replacements performed annually across the world, coupled with the emergence of increasing numbers of resistant strains of bacteria, means that prosthetic joint infection remains a major burden for the health care community and a major challenge for orthopedic surgeons. There is a clear concern, with increasing antibiotic resistance, that infection will continue to increase in prevalence as a cause of knee replacement failure and will compromise the gains made in other areas of knee replacement technology. There is understandably great concern that, while all other areas of knee replacement surgery continue to advance, the morbidity associated with prosthetic knee joint infection may actually increase.

Infection accounts for nearly one quarter of all first revisions on the Australian National Registry, has a high rate of second revision, and is responsible for one quarter of all second revisions. Over one million knee replacements are now performed worldwide, with approximately 600,000 in the USA alone. A very conservative estimate of an infection incidence of 1% would result in 60,000 knee replacement infections requiring treatment annually in the USA alone. Prevention of primary infection is therefore of paramount importance and ideally could be achieved in over 99% of patients, reducing this burden. However, even with a reduced incidence of infection, there will still be a considerable number of infected prostheses requiring management, and surgeons therefore require clear guidelines for managing prosthetic infection. Early, accurate diagnosis and the application of timely, evidence-based management for each individual scenario are critical to optimize the outcome for these patients and to reduce the likelihood of second revision.

The timely publication of this excellent, comprehensive book on *Infection in Knee Replacement* provides a valuable resource for the orthopedic surgeon performing knee replacement surgery, clearly informing about the latest evidence for prevention, diagnosis, and management of prosthetic joint infection. Each chapter has been methodically researched to provide an evidence-based approach, coupled with the wisdom of the experience of orthopedic surgeons renowned for their expertise in this area. The result is a reference that surgeons can turn to for the most current and valid information to guide their practice in this area. I am honored to write this foreword, and I commend the editors and their team of authors for this fine work, which is a significant contribution to the ongoing fight against prosthetic knee joint infection.

David A. Parker
ISAKOS
Sydney, Australia

Preface

The number of total knee arthroplasty (TKA) has dramatically increased over the last few years. Due to the increasing number of primary surgery, we are facing an increase in revision surgery at the same time. The infection rate after TKA is currently about 0.7%. Infection in TKA, regardless of the early or late stage, is the most devastating situation for both patients and orthopedic surgeons. Due to the aging population, comorbidities are more likely and thus increase the risk of infection. We are dealing with a new microorganism often multiresistant and difficult to treat.

Patients require long-lasting treatment and sometimes weeks of hospitalization. The treatment of infected TKA is one of the most challenging works for the Orthopedic Surgeon. It requires aggressive treatment but often surgeons the management of knee infections requires aggressive treatments, and surgeons are usually scared for the complications is sometimes very difficult. Every painful knee after TKA should be considered for being infected until the tentative diagnosis is rejected. Finding new methods that can accurately detect an early infection is essential for rapid diagnosis and a therapeutic algorithm design. With new technologies, it is now possible to achieve a timely diagnosis and appropriate treatment, with clinical outcomes previously only imaginable.

The treatment of infected TKA is complex and requires a good team work, including the infection specialist, microbiologist, plastic surgeon, internist, and sometimes even the psychologist in order to provide the best care for these patients.

This book aims to collect the most up-to-date information regarding the optimal management of infected TKA, with the guidance of experts from all over the world.

We hope that readers will find the data they need, improving patient treatment management and allowing patients to recover "normal" knee function.

<table>
<tr><td>Rome, Italy</td><td>Umile Giuseppe Longo</td></tr>
<tr><td>Jakarta, Indonesia</td><td>Nicolaas C. Budhiparama</td></tr>
<tr><td>Lyon, France</td><td>Sébastien Lustig</td></tr>
<tr><td>Brandenburg, Germany</td><td>Roland Becker</td></tr>
<tr><td>Braga, Portugal</td><td>João Espregueira-Mendes</td></tr>
</table>

Contents

Part V Treatment of Knee Replacement Infections

Part I

Introduction

Epidemiology and Socioeconomic Impact of Infections in Knee Replacement

Laura Risi Ambrogioni, Calogero Di Naro,
Vincenzo Candela, Carlo Casciaro,
Umile Giuseppe Longo, and Vincenzo Denaro

1.1 Introduction

Periprosthetic joint infection (PJI) after total joint replacement is the most serious and feared complication [1]. While more commonly observed in the postoperative period, PJIs may occur throughout life with negative physical and psychological repercussions on the patient, leading to potentially fatal consequences [2–4]. A recent meta-analysis based on a cohort of 20,719 patients who received a two-stage revision for PJI after TKA observed that the 1-year mortality rate was 4.33% and the 5-year mortality rate was 21.64% [5]. Recent studies demonstrate that PJI is the third most common indication for revision hip arthroplasty (14.7% of cases) and the leading cause for failure of total knee arthroplasty (TKA) (25.2% of cases) [6–8]. Boddapati et al. conducted a study of the American College of Surgeons National Surgical Quality Improvement Program from 2005 to 2015. During this study period, 162,981 primary TKAs and 12,780 revision TKAs were recorded, of which 17.2% were performed as a result of PJI. Apart from being the primary cause of TKA revision, PJIs are more frequently responsible for non-household resignations, readmissions and length of stay compared to other non-infectious causes of TKA revision [9]. Male gender, advanced age, high body mass index, comorbidities and immunosuppression, prolonged operative time (>90′) and tourniquet time (>60′) have been identified as significant contributors to the development of PJI following total joint arthroplasty. Genetic predisposition has not been excluded with possible risk factor for the onset of PJIs [8, 10, 11].

Significant rise in the number of total joint arthroplasty procedures has been recorded in the USA over the years [1]. The frequency of joint replacement is estimated to grow in all countries, implying an increased risk of PJIs [12–14]. Approximately 3.5 million primary hip and knee arthroplasties will be performed in the USA alone by the year 2030 [15–18]. Similar forecasts are expected for England and Wales [19]. Moreover, future projections indicate that PJIs, compared to other causes of failure, will account for 60% of all revisions over the next two decades [20].

The treatment of PJIs commonly comprises one or two stages of surgical revision. The first approach consists of a single major surgical procedure whereby the prosthesis and infected tissues are removed while a second implant is replaced. Conversely, in the two-stage revision treatment, the replacement of a new prosthesis is performed in a second surgery. Between these two procedures, antibiotic-impregnated cement spacer is administered. Although the latter

L. Risi Ambrogioni · C. Di Naro · V. Candela
C. Casciaro · U. G. Longo (✉) · V. Denaro
Department of Orthopaedic and Trauma Surgery,
Campus Bio-Medico University, Rome, Italy
e-mail: g.longo@unicampus.it

© ISAKOS 2022
U. G. Longo et al. (eds.), *Infection in Knee Replacement*,
https://doi.org/10.1007/978-3-030-81553-0_1

treatment option is preferred, it is more expensive compared to one-stage revision [21]. The use of antibiotics has been implemented in the surgical procedure to reduce the rate of PJIs. In particular, a retrospective study conducted on 15,972 US veterans showed that the use of antibiotic-laden bone cement in primary TKA is related to a lower revision rate for PJI [22, 23]. As S. Aureus is the primary bacterial pathogen involved in the development of PJIs, a retrospective study on 400 patients showed that a decolonization protocol based on mupirocin nasal ointment and chlorhexidine soap reduced the onset of PJI [24].

Conversely, a national joint registry study conducted on 258 consecutive primary hip and knee arthroplasties showed that the use of gentamycin-loaded bone cement at primary surgery could increase Staphylococcal resistance to gentamycin and methicillin at revision for PJI [25]. Recent evidence has suggested a possible role of anaesthesia in PJI development. In particular, it was observed that out of 3909 procedures, of which 42% were performed under general anaesthesia and 58% under spinal anaesthesia, early PJI occurred more frequently in the general anaesthesia group [26].

Therefore, it appears crucial to define the optimal prevention and treatment protocols for PJIs to reduce the socioeconomic burden across all countries.

1.2 Epidemiology and Socioeconomic Burden of PJIs in TKA

The incidence and prevalence rates of PJIs after TKA remain controversial. To date, most of the data available on PJIs are reported from monocentric studies or studies conducted in few centres [3, 27–29]. Moreover, the sample population is often small and limited to a geographical region that may not be representative of the general population, since a considerable influence of geographic variability on the risk of PJI development has been described [28].

The advent of National Joint Registry data has opened up the potential for dataset linkage, vastly expanding the number of cases available to design prophylactic and therapeutic management strategies [30]. To date, comparisons can be conducted across five nation-wide total joint registries: the Swedish Knee Arthroplasty Register [27], the New Zealand Joint Registry [3], the National Joint Registry of England, Wales, Northern Ireland, and the Isle of Man [31], the Australian Orthopaedic Association National Joint Replacement Registry [32] and the National Inpatient Sample (NIS) database (USA) [7].

The oldest nation-wide registry study was conducted by Knutson et al. in Sweden from 1976 to 1992 on 30,003 knees, showing a steady increase in the number of TKA [27]. The incidence and prevalence rates reported in this study were calculated over a relatively distant study period. Due to the lengthening of the average life expectancy, the improvement in diagnosis and the growth in surgical procedures, it is not possible to calculate statistical inference by generalizing these rates to the overall population.

Koh et al. conducted a retrospective study on the New Zealand Joint Registry from 2000 to 2015. PJI was the most common reason for TKA revision in patients with an average age of 65 years, accounting for up to 45% of all causes of failure. The peak of incidence was observed during the first 2 years (1%), while it diminished to less than 0.2% after 5 years from the primary intervention [3, 33]. The time after surgery in which complications occurred has been widely noted. The observation that the peak of PJIs was found in the first 2 years in this national registry study is following the evidence available in the literature that ascribes 18–27% of early revisions to PJIs.

Lenguerrand et al. recorded revision knee replacements due to PJI from the National Joint Registry of England, Wales, Northern Ireland and the Isle of Man during the study period 2003–2014. The three postoperative months were identified as the most sensitive period for PJI development after TKA. Interestingly, a significantly higher rate of PJIs was observed after aseptic knee revision compared to primary knee replacement [31].

Ackerman et al. obtained data of TKA from the Australian Orthopaedic Association National

Joint Replacement Registry during 2003–2013. 350,994 TKA procedures were performed on 279,453 patients in 10 years. Even though a continuous growth in procedure rates was observed for all age groups, a significant peak was recorded in patients between 40 and 69 years of age. Furthermore, it has been reported that the costs associated with the procedure were almost doubled in 2013 compared to 2003 [32].

Kamath et al. identified the TKA revision procedures due to PJIs from the National Inpatient Sample (NIS) database (USA) during 2005–2010. The highest number of revisions for PJI was performed in white patients aged 65–69 years. The average length of stay following the revision was 7.5 days (3.5 days longer than an uninfected procedure) with a total cost of $25,692 per patient. As found in the Australian registry study, the annual cost of a TKA revision has nearly doubled from $320 million in 2005 to $566 million in 2010 [7].

Although one or more organisms may be responsible for PJI, the bacterial infections are the most widespread. Fungal PJI after TKA is rare and is estimated to account for nearly 1% of all PJIs. The bacteria most frequently isolated is Staphylococcus Aureus accounting for 72% of all cases, whereas Gram-negative bacteria of the substantial amount ranging from 5 to 23% [19]. S. Aureus is a commensal bacterium of the human body that colonizes the anterior nares and extra nasal skin surfaces in approximately one-third of the population. It has been shown that being a carrier of S. Aureus is a risk factor for the development of PJIs. Conversely, streptococcal infections are responsible for 4–16% of all PJI and related to a poor outcome. They generally occur through haematogenic spread from infected sites such as oral cavity, heart valves, skin and soft tissue, intestinal or genitourinary tract. Despite the high sensitivity to antibiotics, total eradication is difficult in the presence of a foreign body such as a prosthesis. However, long-term oral treatment with antibiotics has been associated with a significantly better outcome in PJIs management [34].

Moreover, wide variability in the distribution of methicillin-resistant S. aureus (MRSA) strains has been described, ranging from 13% in Europe to 48% in the USA [35]. Furthermore, it was observed that MRSA infections acquired in the community increased compared to those developed in the hospital. Regardless of how the microorganism is received, the PJI caused by MRSA had the highest failure rates. Besides, the increased length of stay, readmissions and reduced joint function have been associated with PJIs caused by MRSA compared to methicillin-sensitive PJIs, resulting in additional costs related to the management of methicillin-resistant PJIs [17]. The treatment of PJI does not depend on pathogen sensitivity to antibiotic therapy. However, whether the aetiological agent is atypical or not detected at culture, then a consult with an infectious disease specialist should be considered. Current guidelines provide that systemic therapy should not be discontinued until infection remission, normalization of serum markers and culture negation at least 2 weeks after cessation of antimicrobials. If laboratory data remain positive, consultation with an infectious disease specialist is required. Parvizi et al. have shown that the additional cost for the treatment of methicillin-resistant cases compared to sensitive cases was about $20,000 [17]. Generally, it has been estimated that compared to PJI caused by microorganisms sensitive to antibiotic therapy, the costs of PJI caused by MRSA increase by about 60%. Preventive S. Aureus decolonization in patients undergoing TKA could be a therapeutic option to reduce the risk of PJI. According to recent evidence, the risk of PJI may also depend on the type of prosthetic material, in particular, polymethylmethacrylate cement. A cost analysis should be performed to evaluate the potential benefits of adding antibiotic-loaded polymethylmethacrylate to the primary TKA protocol in advance [36].

1.3 The Psychological Impact of PJIs

Quality of life and fear of the disease in patients with PJIs are comparable to those of oncology patients [37]. Routine screening should be conducted to identify affected patients early for appropriate treatment, improving long-term outcomes.

Patients with PJI should be followed by psychologists to maintain long-term quality of life [37]. PJIs are life-changing complications for patients. Loss of joint function, prolonged hospitalization and follow-up visits impact not only on the patient's life but also on those around him. To date, few studies on the psychological effects of PJIs are available. The inability to fulfil daily life activities in which the identity of the person is determined, the increasing dependence on relatives, depression and anxiety, as well as uncertainty about the future are the main psychological consequences of PJIs [38, 39]. The patient's psychology may affect the perception and management of pain that could affect the outcome. Recent evidence suggests that patients who received a preoperative education for TKA have a statistically reduced hospital stay of almost 2 days [40].

1.4 Conclusion

PJI after TKA is the most common, severe and feared complication with a 1-year mortality rate of 4.33% and a 5-year mortality rate of 21.64%. Several modifiable and unmodifiable risk factors have been identified, but their treatment has not yet been implemented in PJIs prevention protocols. Given the relentless increase in TKA procedures all over the world, more than half of the TKA revisions in the next two decades will be due to the occurrence of PJIs. The primary pathogen responsible for the development of PJIs is S. Aureus, while the family of gram-negative bacteria determines up to 20% of PJIs. Due to the spread of antibiotic resistance of S. Aureus, ranging from 13% in Europe to 48% in the USA, the management of PJIs is more challenging. The economic burden on national health systems for total joint replacement interventions is significant and continuously increasing. PJIs are responsible for economic overburdening due to non-household resignations, readmissions, length of stay and, eventually, drug therapy of methicillin-resistant infections. However, PJIs cannot be defined only as postoperative complications. They represent real aggression to the patients'

self-awareness and the course of their lives. The need to find preventive strategies for PJIs can no longer be postponed since the socioeconomic implications of the PJI after TKA remain overwhelming.

References

1. Kurtz SM, Ong KL, Schmier J, Zhao K, Mowat F, Lau E. Primary and revision arthroplasty surgery caseloads in the United States from 1990 to 2004. J Arthroplast. 2009;24(2):195–203.
2. Kurtz SM, Lau EC, Son MS, Chang ET, Zimmerli W, Parvizi J. Are we winning or losing the battle with periprosthetic joint infection: trends in periprosthetic joint infection and mortality risk for the medicare population. J Arthroplast. 2018;33(10):3238–45.
3. Koh CK, Zeng I, Ravi S, Zhu M, Vince KG, Young SW. Periprosthetic joint infection is the main cause of failure for modern knee arthroplasty: an analysis of 11,134 knees. Clin Orthop Relat Res. 2017;475(9):2194–201.
4. Jaekel DJ, Day JS, Klein GR, Levine H, Parvizi J, Kurtz SM. Do dynamic cement-on-cement knee spacers provide better function and activity during two-stage exchange? Clin Orthop Relat Res. 2012;470(9):2599–604.
5. Lum ZC, Natsuhara KM, Shelton TJ, Giordani M, Pereira GC, Meehan JP. Mortality during total knee periprosthetic joint infection. J Arthroplast. 2018;33(12):3783–8.
6. Bozic KJ, Ries MD. The impact of infection after total hip arthroplasty on hospital and surgeon resource utilization. J Bone Joint Surg Am. 2005;87(8):1746–51.
7. Kamath AF, Ong KL, Lau E, Chan V, Vail TP, Rubash HE, et al. Quantifying the burden of revision total joint arthroplasty for periprosthetic infection. J Arthroplast. 2015;30(9):1492–7.
8. Papalia R, Vespasiani-Gentilucci U, Longo UG, Esposito C, Zampogna B, Antonelli Incalzi R, et al. Advances in management of periprosthetic joint infections: an historical prospective study. Eur Rev Med Pharmacol Sci. 2019;23(2 Suppl):129–38.
9. Boddapati V, Fu MC, Mayman DJ, Su EP, Sculco PK, McLawhorn AS. Revision total knee arthroplasty for periprosthetic joint infection is associated with increased postoperative morbidity and mortality relative to noninfectious revisions. J Arthroplast. 2018;33(2):521–6.
10. Zmistowski B, Karam JA, Durinka JB, Casper DS, Parvizi J. Periprosthetic joint infection increases the risk of one-year mortality. J Bone Joint Surg Am. 2013;95(24):2177–84.
11. Blanco JF, Díaz A, Melchor FR, da Casa C, Pescador D. Risk factors for periprosthetic joint infection after

total knee arthroplasty. Arch Orthop Trauma Surg. 2020;140(2):239–45.

12. Kurtz SM, Lau E, Watson H, Schmier JK, Parvizi J. Economic burden of periprosthetic joint infection in the United States. J Arthroplasty. 2012;27(8 Suppl):61–5.e1.

13. Longo UG, Loppini M, Trovato U, Rizzello G, Maffulli N, Denaro V. No difference between unicompartmental versus total knee arthroplasty for the management of medial osteoarthtritis of the knee in the same patient: a systematic review and pooling data analysis. Br Med Bull. 2015;114(1):65–73.

14. Longo UG, Ciuffreda M, D'Andrea V, Mannering N, Locher J, Denaro V. All-polyethylene versus metal-backed tibial component in total knee arthroplasty. Knee Surg Sports Traumatol Arthrosc. 2017;25(11):3620–36.

15. Kurtz SM, Ong KL, Lau E, Bozic KJ. Impact of the economic downturn on total joint replacement demand in the United States: updated projections to 2021. J Bone Joint Surg Am. 2014;96(8):624–30.

16. Kurtz SM, Ong KL, Schmier J, Mowat F, Saleh K, Dybvik E, et al. Future clinical and economic impact of revision total hip and knee arthroplasty. J Bone Joint Surg Am. 2007;89(Suppl 3):144–51.

17. Parvizi J, Pawasarat IM, Azzam KA, Joshi A, Hansen EN, Bozic KJ. Periprosthetic joint infection: the economic impact of methicillin-resistant infections. J Arthroplast. 2010;25(6 Suppl):103–7.

18. Kurtz S, Ong K, Lau E, Mowat F, Halpern M. Projections of primary and revision hip and knee arthroplasty in the United States from 2005 to 2030. J Bone Joint Surg Am. 2007;89(4):780–5.

19. Holleyman RJ, Baker P, Charlett A, Gould K, Deehan DJ. Microorganisms responsible for periprosthetic knee infections in England and Wales. Knee Surg Sports Traumatol Arthrosc. 2016;24(10):3080–7.

20. Kurtz SM, Lau E, Schmier J, Ong KL, Zhao K, Parvizi J. Infection burden for hip and knee arthroplasty in the United States. J Arthroplast. 2008;23(7):984–91.

21. Mallon CM, Gooberman-Hill R, Moore AJ. Infection after knee replacement: a qualitative study of impact of periprosthetic knee infection. BMC Musculoskelet Disord. 2018;19(1):352.

22. Bendich I, Zhang N, Barry JJ, Ward DT, Whooley MA, Kuo AC. Antibiotic-laden bone cement use and revision risk after primary total knee arthroplasty in U.S. veterans. J Bone Joint Surg Am. 2020;102:1939–47.

23. Longo UG, Ciuffreda M, Mannering N, D'Andrea V, Locher J, Salvatore G, et al. Outcomes of posterior-stabilized compared with cruciate-retaining total knee arthroplasty. J Knee Surg. 2018;31(4):321–40.

24. Pelfort X, Romero A, Brugués M, García A, Gil S, Marrón A. Reduction of periprosthetic Staphylococcus aureus infection by preoperative screening and decolonization of nasal carriers undergoing total knee arthroplasty. Acta Orthop Traumatol Turc. 2019;53(6):426–31.

25. Holleyman RJ, Deehan DJ, Walker L, Charlett A, Samuel J, Shirley MDF, et al. Staphylococcal resistance profiles in deep infection following primary hip and knee arthroplasty: a study using the NJR dataset. Arch Orthop Trauma Surg. 2019;139(9):1209–15.

26. Scholten R, Leijtens B, Hannink G, Kamphuis ET, Somford MP, van Susante JLC. General anesthesia might be associated with early periprosthetic joint infection: an observational study of 3,909 arthroplasties. Acta Orthop. 2019;90(6):554–8.

27. Knutson K, Lewold S, Robertsson O, Lidgren L. The Swedish knee arthroplasty register. A nation-wide study of 30,003 knees 1976-1992. Acta Orthop Scand. 1994;65(4):375–86.

28. Foster C, Posada C, Pack B, Hallstrom BR, Hughes RE. Summary of knee implant one, three, five, and 10-year revision risk reported by national and regional arthroplasty registries: a valuable source of evidence for clinical decision-making. EFORT Open Rev. 2020;5(5):268–72.

29. Longo UG, Maffulli N, Denaro V. Minimally invasive total knee arthroplasty. N Engl J Med. 2009;361(6):633–4; author reply 4.

30. Baker P, Petheram TG, Kurtz S, Konttinen YT, Gregg P, Deehan D. Patient reported outcome measures after revision of the infected TKR: comparison of single versus two-stage revision. Knee Surg Sports Traumatol Arthrosc. 2013;21(12):2713–20.

31. Lenguerrand E, Whitehouse MR, Beswick AD, Toms AD, Porter ML, Blom AW, et al. Description of the rates, trends and surgical burden associated with revision for prosthetic joint infection following primary and revision knee replacements in England and Wales: an analysis of the National Joint Registry for England, Wales, Northern Ireland and the Isle of Man. BMJ Open. 2017;7(7):e014056.

32. Ackerman IN, Bohensky MA, Zomer E, Tacey M, Gorelik A, Brand CA, et al. The projected burden of primary total knee and hip replacement for osteoarthritis in Australia to the year 2030. BMC Musculoskelet Disord. 2019;20(1):90.

33. Longo UG, Candela V, Pirato F, Hirschmann MT, Becker R, Denaro V. Midflexion instability in total knee arthroplasty: a systematic review. Knee Surg Sports Traumatol Arthrosc. 2021;29:370.

34. Renz N, Rakow A, Müller M, Perka C, Trampuz A. Long-term antimicrobial suppression prevents treatment failure of streptococcal periprosthetic joint infection. J Infect. 2019;79(3):236–44.

35. Aggarwal VK, Bakhshi H, Ecker NU, Parvizi J, Gehrke T, Kendoff D. Organism profile in periprosthetic joint infection: pathogens differ at two arthroplasty infection referral centers in Europe and in the United States. J Knee Surg. 2014;27(5):399–406.

36. Gutowski CJ, Zmistowski BM, Clyde CT, Parvizi J. The economics of using prophylactic antibiotic-loaded bone cement in total knee replacement. Bone Joint J. 2014;96-B(1):65–9.

37. Knebel C, Menzemer J, Pohlig F, Herschbach P, Burgkart R, Obermeier A, et al. Peri-prosthetic joint infection of the knee causes high levels of psychosocial distress: a prospective cohort study. Surg Infect. 2020;21:877–83.

38. Bury M. Chronic illness as biographical disruption. Sociol Health Illn. 1982;4(2):167–82.

39. Lueck E, Schlaepfer TE, Schildberg FA, Randau TM, Hischebeth GT, Jaenisch M, et al. The psychological burden of a two-stage exchange of infected total hip and knee arthroplasties. J Health Psychol. 2020:1359105320948583.

40. McDonald S, Page MJ, Beringer K, Wasiak J, Sprowson A. Preoperative education for hip or knee replacement. Cochrane Database Syst Rev. 2014;(5):CD003526.

Etiology and Pathogenesis of Knee Replacement Infections

2

Tristan Ferry, Anne Conrad, Jérôme Josse,
Claire Triffault-Fillit, Agathe Becker,
Pierre Chauvelot, Cécile Batailler, Sophie Brosset,
Alexis Trecourt, Elliot Sappey-Marinier,
Frédéric Laurent, Sébastien Lustig, Florent Valour,
and on behalf of the Lyon BJI Study Group

on behalf of the Lyon BJI Study Group

T. Ferry (✉) · A. Conrad · F. Valour
Service des maladies infectieuses et tropicales,
Hospices Civils de Lyon, Hôpital de la Croix-Rousse,
Lyon, France

Université Claude Bernard Lyon 1,
Villeurbanne, France

Centre interrégional de référence pour la prise en
charge des infections ostéo-articulaires complexes
(CRIOAc Lyon), Hôpital de la Croix-Rousse,
Lyon, France

CIRI – Centre International de Recherche en
Infectiologie, Inserm, U1111, Université Claude
Bernard Lyon 1, CNRS, UMR5308, Ecole Normale
Supérieure de Lyon, Univ Lyon, Lyon, France
e-mail: tristan.ferry@univ-lyon1.fr

J. Josse · F. Laurent
Université Claude Bernard Lyon 1,
Villeurbanne, France

Centre interrégional de référence pour la prise en
charge des infections ostéo-articulaires complexes
(CRIOAc Lyon), Hôpital de la Croix-Rousse,
Lyon, France

CIRI – Centre International de Recherche en
Infectiologie, Inserm, U1111, Université Claude
Bernard Lyon 1, CNRS, UMR5308, Ecole Normale
Supérieure de Lyon, Univ Lyon, Lyon, France

Institut des agents infectieux, Laboratoire de
bactériologie, Centre National de référence des
staphylocoques, Hôpital de la Croix-Rousse,
Lyon, France

C. Triffault-Fillit · A. Becker · P. Chauvelot
Service des maladies infectieuses et tropicales,
Hospices Civils de Lyon, Hôpital de la Croix-Rousse,
Lyon, France

Centre interrégional de référence pour la prise en
charge des infections ostéo-articulaires complexes
(CRIOAc Lyon), Hôpital de la Croix-Rousse,
Lyon, France

C. Batailler · E. Sappey-Marinier · S. Lustig
Université Claude Bernard Lyon 1,
Villeurbanne, France

Centre interrégional de référence pour la prise en
charge des infections ostéo-articulaires complexes
(CRIOAc Lyon), Hôpital de la Croix-Rousse,
Lyon, France

Service de chirurgie orthopédique, Hôpital de la
Croix-Rousse, Lyon, France

S. Brosset
Université Claude Bernard Lyon 1, Villeurbanne, France

Centre interrégional de référence pour la prise en
charge des infections ostéo-articulaires complexes
(CRIOAc Lyon), Hôpital de la Croix-Rousse,
Lyon, France

Service de chirurgie plastique et reconstructrice,
Hôpital de la Croix-Rousse, Lyon, France

A. Trecourt
Université Claude Bernard Lyon 1, Villeurbanne, France

Centre interrégional de référence pour la prise en
charge des infections ostéo-articulaires complexes
(CRIOAc Lyon), Hôpital de la Croix-Rousse,
Lyon, France

© ISAKOS 2022
U. G. Longo et al. (eds.), *Infection in Knee Replacement*,
https://doi.org/10.1007/978-3-030-81553-0_2

2.1 Introduction

Prosthetic joint infection (PJI) is the most dramatic complication after arthroplasty [1, 2]. Its relative incidence ranged from 1 to 5%, but can reach 50% depending on the patient comorbidity, the smoking status, and the number of prior procedures [1–6]. With the aging of the population, the absolute number of arthroplasty never stops to increase during the last decades, resulting in an ever increasing absolute number of PJI [7]. PJI is considered to be one of the most difficult-to-treat bacterial diseases, with a significant morbidity, cost, risk of relapse, and loss of function [1–5].

S. aureus is one the most frequent pathogen involved in PJI and is particularly associated with persistence and relapse [8–11]. In the USA, the annual cost of infected revisions to hospitals increased from $320 million to $566 million from 2001 to 2009 and was projected to exceed $1.62 billion in 2020 [7].

As a consequence, prevent, diagnose, and treat PJI accordingly are essential. For that purpose, a better understanding of its etiology and pathogenesis is the first step.

We propose in this chapter to describe the different ways that have the bacteria to contaminate the prosthesis. It is of crucial importance, as depending on the age of the infection, the bacteria could have the opportunity to develop different mechanisms of persistence. We also plan to describe the variability of the microbiological epidemiology, especially depending on the time to PJI-onset, in the context of worldwide spread of antimicrobial resistance. Finally, we will decipher the different mechanisms involved in the bacterial persistence, such as the biofilm production and the intracellular persistence in bone cells, to finally conclude on what can bring the best knowledge of the pathophysiology in the management of PJI.

2.2 The Different Ways to Infect a Prosthetic Joint

To reach the prosthesis surface, bacteria use three main ways: (a) the inoculation could occur at the time of surgery, or during any invasive procedure that concerns the prosthetic joint; (b) the inoculation could take as origin a contiguous infection from a nearby site that spreads gradually until the prosthesis; (c) the inoculation could occur during a bacteremia, with hematogenous seeding from a separate infectious site that could be clinically obvious or occult (Fig. 2.1) [1, 2, 12].

2.2.1 Direct Inoculation During Invasive Procedures

It is largely considered that a PJI occurring in the year following the implantation is generally associated with an intraoperative inoculation. This inoculation may come from fallout of aerosolized bacteria or from direct contamination of the operating site by bacteria on the instruments, the gloves, or the patient's own skin [1, 12]. Despite considerable progress in preoperative and intraoperative antiseptic measures, completely sterilizing the skin at the operating site remains illusory [13, 14]. It was found that skin of the incisal edges was recolonized with bacteria within 30–180 min after the antiseptic procedures [13, 14]. In addition, airborne bacteria can never be completely eliminated from operating rooms since microorganisms could not be eradicated from the skin, hair, nose, and mouth of patients and staff of the operating room [14, 15]. This inoculation could occur at the time of implantation and also during revision with a gradual increased risk depending on the number of procedures and the implant's surface. In fact, the "perioperative" inoculation also includes inoculation that could also occur in the days following the surgery, especially as the scar is not fully waterproofed and could be soiled.

2.2.2 Inoculation by Contiguous Spread

A superficial post-operative infection of the scar could occur few days after the surgery, due to the recolonization of the skin by bacteria that can then gain depth step by step, until the articular space through the tissues that are incompletely

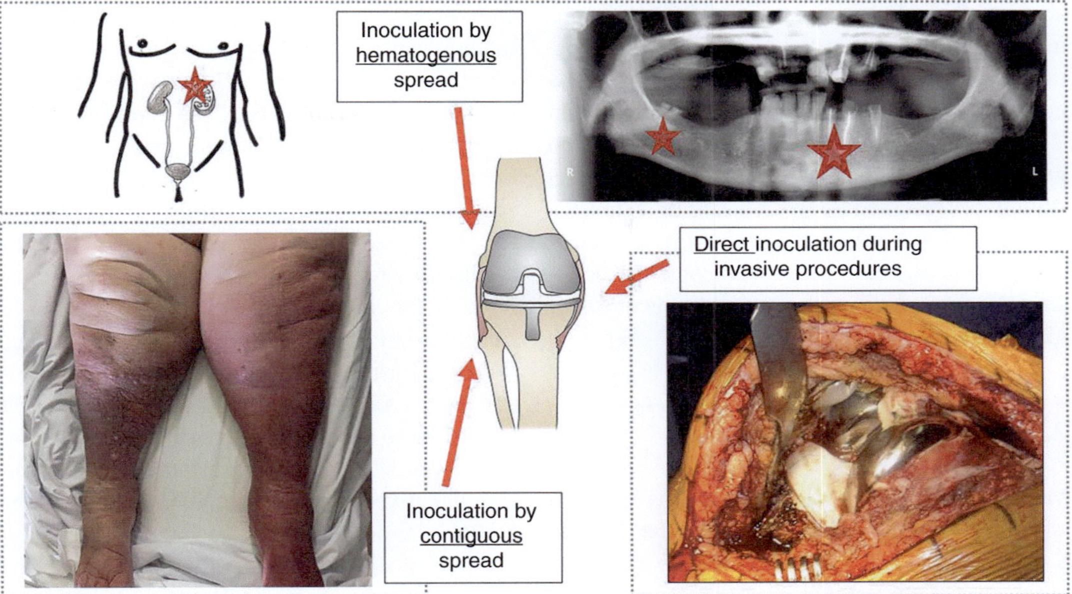

Fig. 2.1 The three different ways to infect a knee prosthesis: The most frequent way of inoculation of a knee prosthesis is a direct inoculation during invasive procedure, such as surgery, despite all the preventive measures that are usually implemented to reduce this risk. PJI could also occur by contiguous spread of a bacterial disease, which reaches the prosthesis as during erysipelas. Finally, an acute or chronic focus of infection could be responsible for clinically obvious or occult bacteremia with secondary seeding to the prosthetic joint

healed. This is the second mechanism of inoculation that results from the contiguous spread of an adjacent infection [1, 2]. This mechanism could also occur years after the prosthesis implantation, if the patient experienced an erysipela or another skin and soft tissue infection of the index limb [16]. The typical clinical situation is the patient with a knee prosthesis, who develops extensive erysipelas (Fig. 2.1).

2.2.3 Inoculation by Hematogenous Spread

The final way of prosthesis bacterial inoculation concerns inoculation by hematogenous spread that occurs usually years after prosthesis implantation [12, 17–20]. Bacteria could enter the bloodstream from a distant infectious focus or during transient bacteremia of dental, urogenital, or gastrointestinal origin (Fig. 2.1). Few studies focused on the rates of PJI in patients with a prosthetic joint after bacteremia. This risk seems to be extremely variable (6–40%), depending on the clinical presentation and the pathogen involved. *S. aureus* seems to be clearly associated with a high risk of hematogenous contamination of a joint prosthesis, in comparison with other bacteria [12, 17–20]. Even if the risk of PJI from a dental site of infection is considered to be low, this risk exists as: (a) occult bacteremia with odontogenic bacteria could occur in patients with chronic dental foci of infection, during surgical dental procedures, but even also during tooth brushing [21]; (b) some patients with chronic dental foci of infection can develop PJI several years after the prosthesis implantation due to typical odontogenic bacteria [22]. However, several studies concluded that given routine dental antibiotic prophylaxis prior to dental procedures for non-infected causes does not reduce the rate of PJI [23–26]. Patients with clear suppurative dental infection have to receive antimicrobial therapy for the local infection, but it has not been demonstrated if it can prevent a hematogenous location on the prosthesis. In the absence of evidence supporting the role of anti-microbial prophylaxis for patients with a prosthetic joint undergoing dental procedure for a non-infectious cause, the International Consensus Meeting (ICM2018) and Dutch guidelines recommended that prophylaxis should be reserved to patients with extensive comorbidities in whom the probability of developing PJI is higher or those with complex reconstructive procedure in whom development of PJI may have more dire consequences [27–29].

2.3 Epidemiology

Microbiological epidemiology depends on time and way of infection. Staphylococci, that include *S. aureus* and also coagulase-negative staphylococci, are the most common pathogen involved in PJI, as they are responsible for about 60% of all PJI [30–34]. Other gram-positive pathogens (streptococci, enterococci) represent about 10–20% of PJI and gram-negative rods, 5–20% [30–34]. Beyond this global distribution, there are some important differences that have to be pointed out.

2.3.1 Knee vs. Hip Location

Most of the available data show results for pooled microbiology from knee and hip arthroplasties. However, some differences have been reported in large cohort studies. For example, the rate of *S. aureus* infection seems to be higher in the knee location, in comparison with the hip. On the contrary, a lower rate of *C. acnes* is described in prosthetic-knee infections. Finally, polymicrobial infection seems to be more represented in the hip location. These differences might be explained by a diversity of the microbial flora, which can vary according to the sites and according to the kind of surgical approach [35, 36].

2.3.2 Antimicrobial Resistance

Antimicrobial resistance is considered as a worldwide health issue, as it is considered as a

slow motion tsunami [37]. Antimicrobial resistance is particularly a key issue in the management of patients with PJI, as it impacts the antimicrobial prophylaxis, the type of antimicrobial used for the treatment (mainly intravenous), the cost, and the outcome [8, 38–43]. Antimicrobial resistance differs a lot according to the geographic area. For example, methicillin-resistant *S. aureus* represent almost 50% of the strains in the USA, while 12% in Europe (but with large differences between West vs. East, as vs. North vs. South countries) and has a range between 2 and 5% to 39% according to different countries in Asia [40, 44, 45]. Even if methicillin resistance in coagulase-negative staphylococci is less studied, the global rate of methicillin resistance in staphyloccoci is significant worldwide, making the prescription of a broad spectrum anti-gram positive agent (vancomycin, teicoplanin, daptomycin, or linezolid) essential as empirical antimicrobial therapy [30–32, 34, 40]. However, as these antibiotics are not active on gram-negative rods, they have to be combined with another antibiotic (usually a broad spectrum β-lactam) to complete the spectrum of activity. Resistance in gram-negative rods is clearly emergent, especially concerning Enterobacteriaceae, *P. aeruginosa*, and *Acinetobacter spp.* Indeed, multidrug- and extensively drug-resistance are increasing rapidly worldwide in such species (especially extended spectrum β-lactamases or carbapenemase in *E. coli* and *K. pneumoniae* and extensively drug resistance in *P. aeruginosa*), and these bacteria are currently not covered by usual antimicrobial prophylaxis [40, 42, 43].

2.3.3 Time to PJI-Onset

In fact, the PJI bacterial epidemiology mainly depends on the time and way of infection. For that purpose, multiple classifications have been previously described and used. The most common one classifies PJI according to the time between the prosthesis implantation and the symptoms occurrence [4, 46]:

- "Early," if the PJI occurred in the first 3 months after arthroplasty;
- "Delayed," if the PJI occurred between 3 months and 1 year (some suggest 2 years) after arthroplasty;
- "Late," if the PJI occurred after 1 year (some suggest 2 years) after arthroplasty.
- Nevertheless, it's more clinically relevant to classify the PJI according to the time of symptoms duration. In this way, a PJI can be called as [1, 47]:
- "Post-operative," when symptom occurs within a month following the surgery. Usually, the inoculation suspected way is per-operative or due to healing trouble;
- "Acute" when symptoms last for less than 3 weeks;
- "Chronic," when symptoms last for more than 3 weeks.

This latter classification guides the physician in the PJI management: an acute PJI can be managed with a "debridement antibiotic and implant retention" (DAIR) procedure, while a chronic one needs a prosthesis replacement. However, this classification is independent of the time of prosthesis implantation. For example, in a PJI occurring by a hematogenous way, clinical picture will be "acute," with frequently fever, pain, and clinical signs of septic arthritis and will be managed by a DAIR strategy, even if it occurs over a year after the prosthesis implantation. That makes sense, especially as the inoculation of the bacteria on the prosthesis is recent, and as it did not usually have significant time to develop the mechanisms of persistence like the biofilm (see below). The primary bacterial focus of infection that secondary spreads to the prosthesis is most often evident clinically, and blood cultures are usually positive, especially if the primary source of infection comes from a urinary tract infection or a catheter-related infection. However, some patients develop acute clinical presentation, late after the prosthesis implantation, but there is clinically no detectable focus of primary infection. These latter patients with "late acute" PJI probably have potentially and inoculation at the time of surgery that was asymptomatic, with set up of

microbial persistence and dormant mechanism (see the pathophysiology of PJI below), until sudden appearance of clinical symptoms a long time after the implantation. Staphylococci, that are associated with a low success rate in this clinical setting, seemed to be particularly involved in such clinical presentation [11]. In clinical practice, the physician has to be stubborn in the research for the pathogen inoculation way in, and when he cannot find it, which is more frequent than we would like, he has to ask himself the question: Is it an acute presentation of an acute PJI? Or an acute presentation of a suddenly woke up of an old sleeping pathogen, with dispersal of the biofilm? Answering this question is crucial for "late acute" PJI, as if the inoculation occurred at the time of surgery, the treatment would be prosthesis exchange, or DAIR followed by suppressive antimicrobial therapy, as DAIR is not able to eradicate the biofilm. We developed in our center an algorithm, called CRIOAc Lyon's PJI treatment algorithm, that combines clinical symptoms, the delay from the implantation, and a potential prosthesis loosening to integrate the suspected pathophysiology and the time of inoculation in the patient's management (Fig. 2.2).

2.3.4 Main Pathogens Involved

S. aureus: Because combining virulent and persistence factors, *S. aureus* is one of the most involved pathogens in PJI. From the virulence results frequently acute presentations with fever, pain, and clinical signs of septic arthritis, while the persistence factors concern adherence proteins, intracellular persistence, and production of biofilm (see below). With this pathogen, it is noteworthy that the PJI can occur at any time from the implantation. The most well-known side of *S. aureus* is the virulent presentation, with an over-representation in post-operative and acute PJI [1, 2, 8, 34, 40, 42, 48–50]. However, it has also been described in chronic PJI, with indolent clinical signs of infection, probably by setting up only mechanisms of persistence in vivo [51].

Coagulase-negative staphylococci: The most represented pathogen of this group is *S. epider-*

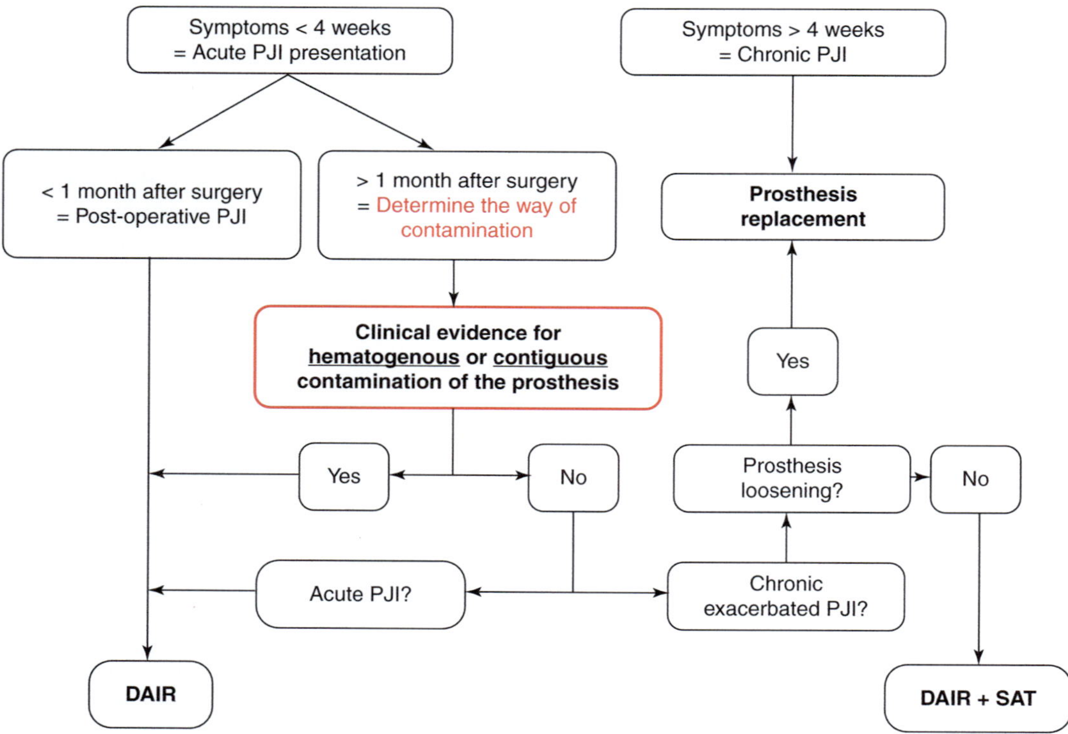

Fig. 2.2 Pathophysiology-based CRIOAc Lyon's PJI treatment algorithm: The clinical management of patients with acute post-operative PJI, or with chronic PJI with prosthesis loosening is clear: A "debridement antibiotics and implant retention" (DAIR) procedure or a prosthesis exchange has to be, respectively, done. The clinical inves-tigation, by determining the mechanism of prosthesis inoculation, is essential in patients with acute symptoms but occurring >1 month after the implantation. Depending on the clinical presentation, the appropriate medicosurgical could be a DAIR, a prosthesis exchange, or a DAIR followed by suppressive antimicrobial therapy (SAT)

midis, that is a commensal bacterial of human skin. Coagulase-negative staphylococci are classically considered as low-virulent pathogens with insidious clinical presentations and pain that is the main if not the only one symptom in chronic PJI. But they can also be responsible, and especially *S. lugdunensis*, of early-onset PJI with acute clinical picture. *S. lugdunensis* is particular coagulase-negative staphylococci that acts in many points with *S. aureus* and can also lead to invasive infections. Main differences are observed concerning the antimicrobial resistance profile. Indeed, a methicillin resistance rate around 50–60% is described for coagulase-negative staphylococci, but *S. lugdunensis* is reported to be almost all the time methicillin susceptible [34, 40, 44, 52, 53]. Moreover, 50–75% of the *S. lug-dunensis* strains do even not produce any

β-lactamase, making it in those cases, susceptible to penicillin G [53, 54].

Other gram-positive pathogens: streptococci and enterococci. Those two species together represent about 10–20% of PJI, regardless of the time or way of infection. Streptococci are more represented in acute PJI, and more frequently in polymicrobial infections if occurring in a post-operative or early timing. They are in contrary more responsible for monomicrobial infection when involved in acute hematogenous PJI. Streptococci represent a wide range of pathogens with multiple human habitats: oral streptococci, digestive streptococci, or cutaneous streptococci, with here again the need to look for the way in (neoplasia, dental abscess, post-digestive procedures, etc. Enterococci are considered as less virulent agents, with a digestive location, and can be involved in acute, or chronic presentation, but are considered to be difficult to treat [34, 35, 40].

Gram-negative rods: This group involved various species, with very different virulent characteristics. By order of frequency, *E. coli* and *P. aeruginosa* are the main encountered pathogens. They are mainly involved in acute PJI, whether in post-operative/early-onset or in late-onset by a hematogenous way [34, 40, 41, 55]. Enterobacteriaceae are usually not associated with chronic PJI, probably due to a less capacity, in comparison with staphylococci, to survive and set up mechanisms of persistence in vivo. *P. aeruginosa* must be separately classified. It is a non-fermenting pathogen, not very frequently involved in PJI but with persistence and adhesive factors, who makes it very difficult to treat. Mainly found in early PJI, it can also sometimes be responsible for chronic PJI, occurring lately [34].

Anaerobes: *C. acnes* is the most common pathogen in this group, even if less involved in TKA infection than in hip or shoulder prosthesis [36, 56]. *C. acnes*, a commensal bacterium of the human skin, is a typically low-virulent pathogens, responsible for indolent and chronic infection, which can become symptomatic years after the inoculation and the bacterial inoculation. Because they have a slow growth which usually needed an extended incubation time or at least a supplemented growth culture media, they are often under-diagnosed and involved in many failure management [56–58]. Other anaerobes could be involved, especially anaerobes from the gastrointestinal tracts, and they are frequently associated with other pathogens, leading to polymicrobial PJI [30, 34, 42, 51].

Polymicrobial PJI: It occurs in 15% of all the PJI. They are more frequently found in post-operative and early PJI, especially in knee PJI where difficulties of coverage with skin necrosis occurred after surgery. Some authors reported that multiple pathogens are more frequent in hip PJI in comparison with the knee PJI, probably as the hip location, in comparison with the knee, is closer to the perineum [30, 34, 42, 51]. Another reported risk factor for polymicrobial infection is obesity, with a polymicrobial infection rate reaching 60% in this specific population [59].

Negative cultures: Sometimes, besides history, clinical presentation, and per-operative findings which make the physician convinced of the PJI, cultures will remain sterile. This is often the case when a prior antimicrobial therapy is used before surgery. This can also be due to very fastidious growth bacteria. That reminds us the importance of the free antimicrobial therapy period before surgery, classically 15 days for patients with chronic PJI, and the need of multiple microbiologic samples with extended cultures (14 days). In those cases, pathology and molecular microbiology could be very helpful [60, 61].

2.4 The Pathophysiology of Chronic PJI

The pathogenesis of PJI involves interactions between the bacteria, the implant, and the host's immune system [62]. Very few numbers of microbes are needed to infect the prosthesis. Such organisms firstly adhere to the prosthesis surface at the bone–implant interface (stem) and/ or into the joint cavity. In the latter, microbes frequently replicate themselves as planktonic bacteria that are bacteria in "optimal" environmental conditions to growth (i.e. with a lot of nutriments), leading to recruitment of polymorphonuclear cells (PMNs), and clinical signs of septic arthritis (Fig. 2.3). PMNs are major actors of inflammation that try to control the bacterial multiplication and could result in the formation of pus that is composed by bacterial and PMNs remnants. At the surface of the implant, most of the bacteria have the ability to modify their phenotype and to develop biofilm, after adhering to the surface. Once the biofilm is made, it is inseparable from the implant surface and tolerant to the immune system. It is indeed quite impossible for PMNs to eradicate the biofilm, and other components of the immune system cannot penetrate the biofilm that mainly contain dormant bacterial cells, with low replication process. Different types of biofilm exist, which form themselves at different speeds, depending on the pathogen involved in the PJI. Bacteria can persist for decades in biofilm, and the interaction between the surface of the biofilm and the host cells could lead to prosthesis loosening, by persistent local activation of immune cells. Intracellular penetration and survival are another mechanism of persistence that particular pathogen could combine with biofilm formation.

2.4.1 Biofilm in TKA Infection

PJI is often described as typical biofilm-associated infections, especially the chronic and persistent ones. Biofilm is "a protected mode of growth that allows survival in a hostile environment" as defined by Bill Costerton, a pioneer in biofilm research [63]. Biofilm is defined as a bacterial community which is metabolically heterogeneous and embedded in a self-produced extracellular matrix, a kind of glue that defini-

tively attached the bacterial community to the prosthesis. To note, all bacteria incriminated in PJI can virtually form biofilm. However, the ability to form biofilm in vivo, in patients with an arthroplasty, can vary from a strain to another in the same species. Biofilm formation is classically described as a succession of several stages that are mostly conserved in all the bacterial species: (a) attachment, (b) accumulation/maturation, and (c) detachment/dispersal (Fig. 2.3) [64, 65].

2.4.2 Attachment

First, free bacteria (called planktonic bacteria, with usual multiplication process) attach to abiotic (metallic or polyethylene components of the prosthesis) or biotic (soft tissues, bone, or prothesis surfaces covered by host proteins), into the joint or at the bone/implant interface. Bacteria use their adhesin to adhere to the surfaces. In *S. aureus*, initial attachment is made through pro-

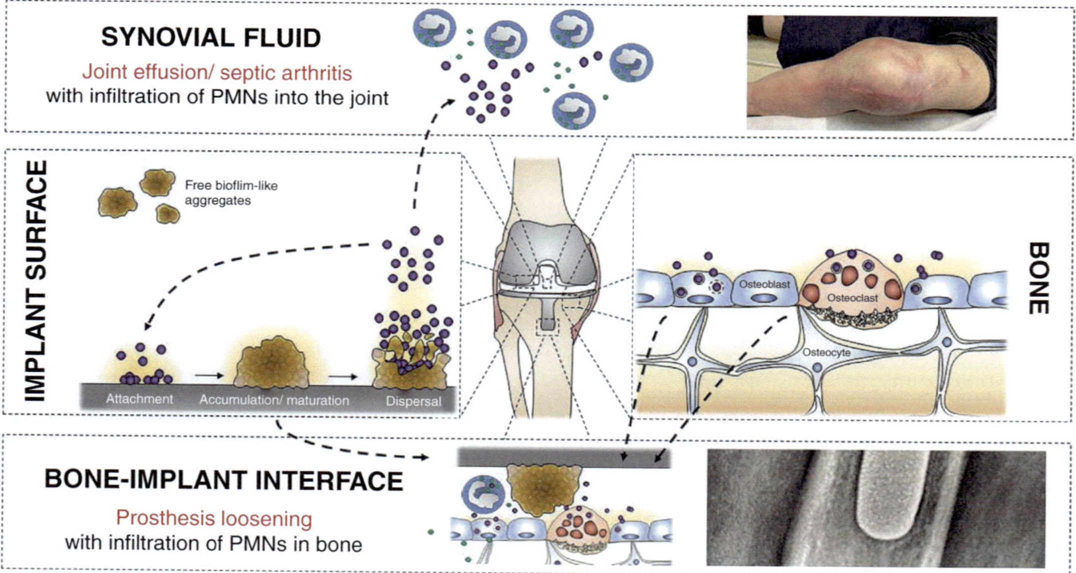

Fig. 2.3 Pathophysiology of chronic prosthetic-knee infection with set up of antimicrobial persistence mechanisms and host response: At the implant surface, the bacteria firstly adhere and then produce a biofilm that can release planktonic bacteria, especially in the synovial fluid, leading to a joint effusion with infiltration of polymorphonuclear cells (PMNs) into the joint synovial fluid. The second mechanism of persistence, mainly described for *S. aureus*, concerns the intracellular persistence in bone cells such as osteoblast and osteoclasts, with activation of osteoclasts and induction of osteolysis. Finally, both mechanisms of persistence (biofilm and intracellular persistence) lead to inflammation and infiltration of PMNs at the bone–implant interface, leading to prosthesis loosening

teins belonging to the group of microbial surface components recognizing adhesive matrix molecules (MSCRAMMs). These adhesins can attach to various host matrix components such as collagen, fibronectin, or fibrinogen that quickly coat the surface of the prosthesis [65]. Similar mechanisms, involving adhesins that can bind to host matrix components, were described in *S. epidermidis* and *S. lugdunensis* [66, 67]. In *S. epidermidis*, the giant extracellular matrix-binding protein (Embp) mediates attachment to fibronectin [68]. Concerning primary attachment to abiotic surfaces (nude surface of the prosthesis components), it may be due to electrostatic or hydrophobic interactions with the help of autolysin (AtlA in *S. aureus*, AtlE in *S. epidermidis*, and AtlL in *S. lugdunensis*) that can induce modifications in bacterial surface hydrophobicity [65, 67, 69]. In *P. aeruginosa*, the flagellum, type IV pili and surface adhesion are required for biofilm attachment [70].

2.4.3 Accumulation/Maturation

The second stage called "accumulation/maturation" is characterized by the formation of intercellular bindings and production of the extracellular biofilm matrix. This stage leads to the development of the typical biofilm architecture. The principle components of the biofilm matrix are polysaccharides, proteins, lipids, and extracellular DNA. In staphylococci, the polysaccharide intercellular adhesin (PIA) coded by the operon *ica*ADBC was the first described molecule of the biofilm matrix. It favors cell aggregation in *S. aureus* and *S. epidermidis* [71, 72]. Its importance in biofilm accumulation is species and strain dependent. It was notably reported for *S. aureus* that biofilm formation by methicillin-susceptible *S. aureus* (MSSA) are more dependent to PIA than the one by methicillin-resistant *S. aureus* (MRSA) [73]. Moreover, Frank and Patel observed that PIA is not a major component of extracellular matrix in biofilms formed by *S. lugdunensis* [74]. Proteins and extracellular DNA (eDNA) are also components of extracellular matrix of staphylococcal biofilms [65, 67, 75].

These two types of molecules come from the bacteria themselves. Indeed, lysis of bacteria allows the release of eDNA and cytoplasmic proteins [76, 77]. Proteins and eDNA can interact together to form a kind of network that keeps biofilm tight [78]. Interaction between PIA and eDNA has also been reported in *S. aureus* [79]. To note, proteins that are involved in primary attachment are also involved in biofilm accumulation, such as fibronectin-binding proteins (FnBP) in *S. aureus* or Embp in *S. epidermidis* [68, 80]. In *P. aeruginosa*, the matrix is composed of at least three types of exopolysaccharides (Pls, Pel, and alginate) and contains eDNA [81].

2.4.4 Detachment/Dispersal

The last stage is the dispersal of the biofilm, allowing the propagation of the infection to other surfaces or tissues. This mechanism could be involved in "late acute" PJI, in patients without evidence of hematogenous spreading of a distant site of infection. In *S. aureus*, dispersal is controlled by quorum sensing through the activity of the accessory genre regulator *agr* [65]. It promotes the degradation of the protein inside the biofilms through the production of proteases such as metalloprotease aureolysin and serine proteases splABCDEF [82]. Phenol soluble modulins (PSM), also controlled by *agr*, can play a role in biofilm dispersal. These toxins, notably known for their cytotoxic effects [83, 84], could disrupt biofilm structure thanks to their surfactant properties [85]. Similar properties of PSM in biofilm dispersal have been reported for *S. epidermidis* [86]. A role in biofilm stabilization was also suggested for PSMs through the formation of amyloid fibers but this possibility is debated [87–90].

To note, it is important to keep in mind that most of the current data about biofilm were obtained from in vitro models that are not representative of in vivo biofilms found in chronic infections. Indeed, in vivo biofilms are smaller, they are not shaped in mushroom-like structures, incorporate host components, and are continuously challenged by the host immune system [91].

Two major properties, tolerance to antibiotics and the hijacking of host immunity, confer to biofilm-associated infection its "difficult-to-treat" character.

The tolerance to antibiotics corresponds to a transient loss of susceptibility to antibiotics that can be restored when bacteria in biofilms switch back to a planktonic phenotype. In opposite to resistance, there is no impact on the minimal inhibitory concentration (MIC) [92]. This property is mostly due to the metabolic status of bacteria inside the biofilm. Indeed, they are deprived of oxygen and nutrient and lower their metabolic activity to survive in these conditions. In consequence, bacteria in biofilm are less susceptible to antibiotics as antibiotics are mostly efficient on metabolically active bacteria [93]. To eradicate biofilms, antibiotic concentrations have to be 10 to 1000-fold superior to the MIC determined for planktonic bacteria. This tolerance property is shared by most of the bacterial species. Regarding antibiotics that can be used for treating biofilm-related PJIs, rifampicin is considered as the "anti-biofilm" antibiotics [94].

Another important property of biofilm is its ability to interact with the immune cells and to hijack the normal immune response. In the course of an infection, the first responders are the PMNs. Even if PMNs can attack and phagocyte biofilms by staphylococci, meaning that biofilms are not protected from immune cells, it is reduced compared to what is observed with planktonic bacteria [95–97]. Moreover, PMNs can favor the bone resorption through the release of IL-8 and the activation of osteoclasts [98]. PMNs infiltrations in the synovial fluid or in bone tissue at the interface of the prosthesis are major pathology criteria for a PJI. Biofilm can also interact with macrophages and hijacking their inflammatory properties. Instead of eliciting pro-inflammatory properties with high phagocytosis and the production of pro-inflammatory cytokines and chemokines (defined as M1 phenotype), macrophages interacting with biofilm display a low capacity of phagocytosis and gene patterns relative to anti-inflammatory properties, revealing a polarization to M2 phenotype [99, 100]. Macrophage infiltration is however non-specific, as mechanical prosthesis loosening could also be associated with such infiltration, as these cells participated in the phagocytic process of the released microparticles [62]. Biofilm-related PJIs are also associated with the presence of myeloid-derived suppressor cells (MDSC). These immature cells are involved in the regulation of inflammation and the immunosuppression. They inhibit the T cell proliferation and prevent the pro-inflammatory activity of macrophages, especially through the release of IL-10 [101, 102]. MDSC infiltrates were also observed in periprosthetic tissues from PJI patients whereas they were not observed in tissues from patients with aseptic loosening [103]. The presence and role of T lymphocytes in biofilm-associated PJI are still unclear. The few studies on this subject reported a reduced T cell proliferation (in accordance with the high presence of MDSCs) with a pro-inflammatory Th1/Th17 profile [104]. Finally, infiltration of plasma cells could participate in the immune response in patients with PJI. Plasma cells are the final step in maturation of B cell line, they are part of adaptive immunity, and classically, it has been described that acute inflammation can evolve into prolonged subacute and chronic inflammation when the initial cause of inflammation persists in tissues [105–107]. Few data are available about the description of plasma cell infiltration in patients with PJI, but such infiltration has to be investigated as a potential pathology marker of chronic PJI [108, 109].

Regarding the localization of biofilm in knee prosthesis environment, it can first attach and develop onto the metallic, ceramic, or polyethylene components of the biofilm. Studying the components from total hip prosthesis, Lass et al. reported that a higher bacterial load was present on the polyethylene liner than on the metal components [104]. Similar results were observed for biofilm by *S. aureus, S. epidermidis, E. coli, K. pneumoniae,* and *P. aeruginosa* [110]. Biofilm can also form biofilm-like aggregates in synovial fluid for *S. aureus* and *S. epidermidis* [111, 112]. The formation of these aggregates is mostly due to the presence of fibrin in synovial fluid. However, surprisingly, in vitro experiments showed that synovial fluid reduced the ability of biofilm-like aggregates to adhere to various surfaces [113]. Abscesses are sometimes described as a type of biofilm [114]. However, this definition is controversial. Indeed, Cheng et al. strictly affirmed that abscess formation "should not be mistaken for biofilm growth" [115]. Finally, invasion of osteocyte-lacuno canalicular network by bacteria was also proposed as a new type of biofilm [114, 116]. It was reported that *S. aureus* can invade the lacuna left empty by osteocytes after their death [117]. However, even if this new mechanism must be taken into account to fully understand PJI pathogenesis, formation of extracellular matrix was not investigated in this case, questioning the "biofilm" appellation.

2.4.5 Bacterial Interactions with Bone Cells

Despite no existing data specifically regarding knee prosthesis infection, the ability of bacteria to invade and persist within bone cells has been proposed as another mechanism of host immune system subversion, constituting a reservoir that might lead to infection chronicity and relapse (Fig. 2.3) [118, 119]. The interaction of *S. aureus* with osteoblast—the non-professional phagocytes specialized in bone apposition—has been extensively described in vitro, mostly in gentamicin- or lysostaphin-protection assays. The internalization of *S. aureus* within osteoblasts is mainly driven by the interaction of staphylococcal fibronectin-binding proteins (FnBP) with host fibronectin that acts as a bridge with the cellular $\alpha5\beta1$ integrin to prompted bacterial endocytosis by an active cellular process akin to phagocytosis [120–122]. After cell invasion, *S. aureus* can persist within vacuoles or escape to the cytosol, through complex mechanisms (Fig. 2.3). First, staphylococcal membrane-damaging factors and toxins, including phenol soluble modulins, are involved in vesicular escape and cytotoxicity [83, 123]. Second, *S. aureus* has been shown to subvert the autophagy process, a highly conserved eukaryote cellular process allowing cellular component destruction and recycling. This mechanism is also

part of the innate immune response, leading to the formation of a double-membrane compartment that encapsulates intracellular bacteria (phagosome) that merges with lysosome to create a phagolysosome, a digestive hybrid organelle with an acidic environment base of intracellular bacteria eradication [124, 125]. *S. aureus* has been shown to activate autophagosome formation while inhibiting the autophagic flux and especially the fusion of autophagosomes with lysosomes, then promoting its intracellular persistence [126, 127]. Finally, the intracellular conversion to a slow-growing phenotype called small-colony variants (SCVs) facilitates intracellular survival and resistance to antimicrobial therapy [128, 129]. The impact of *S. aureus* persistence within osteoblast in vivo has not been well established and is still controversial. Some electronic microscopy observations revealed the presence of *S. aureus* within bone cells during the course of chronic osteomyelitis [130]. Additionally, some cohort studies showed a correlation between infection chronicity and the ability of *S. aureus* to invade osteoblasts [83, 131].

The ability of other bacteria to invade and persist within bone cells has been less investigated. In a study screening 15 different coagulase-negative staphylococci species, only *S. pseudintermedius* appeared to be able to invade osteoblastic cells in a comparable way to *S. aureus*, but is not a common etiological agent of BJI [132]. *S. delphini*, a recently described invasive staphylococci species, also seem to be able to invade osteoblasts, following a FnBP-like protein pathway [133]. This mechanism seems less important for *S. epidermidis*, the most commonly involved coagulase-negative staphylococci in PJI, even if this point is still controversial [134–136]. Streptococcal invasion of eukaryotic host cells has been assessed for *S. pyogenes* [137]. Turning especially to bone cells, interaction of oral streptococci with osteoblasts has been studied, for a better understanding of osteo-dental pathology: *S. gordonii* is internalized in osteoblast via a process similar to *S. aureus*, triggering an inflammatory response that promotes bone resorption, but its intracellular survival is shorter than *S. aureus* [138]. Invasion of human cell has been described as a major feature for Enterobacteriaceae pathogeny in other clinical settings, including internalization in intestinal epithelial cells to cross the intestinal barrier during *Salmonella* infections [139–141]. However, few authors studied the interaction of Enterobacteriaceae with bone cells. Using clinical isolates responsible for PJI, Crémet et al. showed that *E. coli* was unable to invade osteoblastic cells in gentamicin protection assay and elicited a high cytotoxicity [142]. Regarding non-fermenting gram-negative bacteria, *P. aeruginosa* invades various epithelial cells (as proven by electronic microscopy and gentamicin protection assays) via complex mechanisms, probably dependent of the type of infected cells [143–146]. However, the invasive ability of *P. aeruginosa* within osteoblasts remains to be confirmed [142]. Among anaerobic bacteria, *C. acnes* is probably the most frequent and better-characterized pathogen in bone and joint infection—especially device-associated chronic infections—and has been shown to be able to invade osteoblasts [147]. Finally, corynebacteria, mostly implicated in knee infections after major trauma, displayed strain-dependent capacities of osteoblastic internalization, via a fibronectin-dependent pathway similar to *S. aureus*, which seems implicated in chronicity [148].

The interaction of *S. aureus* with osteoclasts has also been studied, leading to bone resorption and consequently potentially involved in prosthesis loosening (Fig. 2.3). In particular, an in vitro model of osteoclasts infection at different maturations stages provided insight into this complex mechanism [149]. The infection of osteoclast precursors inhibits osteoclastogenesis but leads to pro-inflammatory cytokine secretion that enhances bone resorption by mature osteoclasts. Conversely, infection of mature osteoclasts directly increases their bone resorption ability. In addition, the infection of surrounding osteoblasts can lead to a direct decreased bone formation, and a secretion of RANK-L that stimulates osteoclast activities [118]. With the exception of *C. acnes*, for which the inhibitory effect on osteoclastogenesis has been suggested in one study [147], there is no data regarding the interactions of other bacterial species with osteoclasts.

Unlike the "antibiofilm" activity of antimicrobials, their ability of eradicating the intracellular bacterial reservoir is currently not taken into account in the choice of treatment strategies for PJI. However, intraosteoblastic persisting *S. aureus* demonstrate heterogeneous antimicrobial susceptibility [150]. This intracellular activity is difficult to predict and relies on: (a) intracellular penetrations of the molecules and their distribution in the subcellular location of *S. aureus*; (b) intracellular bacterial wall modifications [151] and reduced metabolism [152]; and (c) drug inactivation by the acidic pH of intracellular organelles [153, 154]. Consequently, some antimicrobials with a low cellular accumulation can have a surprisingly high activity due to local chemical conditions, such as β-lactams of which activity is even restored intracellularly against methicillin-resistant staphylococci [153]. In final, the most active molecules against intraosteoblastic *S. aureus* remain clindamycin, fluoroquinolones, and rifamycins [150, 155]. The intraosteoblastic activity of antimicrobials against other bacterial species implicated in PJI is unknown.

2.5 Conclusion

Understanding the etiology and pathogenesis of knee replacement infections is crucial to prevent, diagnose, and treat such catastrophic complication. Physicians have to be aware about the different ways that has a bacteria to contaminate the prosthesis, to precise the date of inoculation in each individual patient. Moreover, depending on different factors, the bacterial epidemiology, and the resistance profile of the bacteria involved are heterogenous, leading to discuss the empirical antimicrobial also individually. Finally, the different involved bacteria have various capacities to persist in vivo. The two main mechanisms of persistence are the biofilm and the intracellular persistence, especially for *S. aureus* in osteoblast and osteoclast cells. If these mechanisms have been set up in a patient with PJI, eradication is considered as impossible, and the patient has to be managed by prosthesis exchange. However, a conservative approach is sometimes performed, especially in patients with revision prosthesis without loosening, but these patients have to receive a suppressive antimicrobial therapy to keep the bacteria asleep and prevent biofilm growing, bacterial multiplication, and prosthesis loosening. The pathophysiology of the infection directly affects the clinical management of PJI, and bacterial mechanisms of persistence have to be targeted by innovative therapeutic approaches.

Acknowledgments Lyon bone and joint study group (list of collaborators)

Coordinator: *Tristan Ferry*; **Infectious diseases specialists:** *Tristan Ferry, Florent Valour, Thomas Perpoint, Patrick Miailhes, Florence Ader, Sandrine Roux, Agathe Becker, Claire Triffault-Fillit, Anne Conrad, Cécile Pouderoux, Nicolas Benech, Pierre Chauvelot, Marielle Perry, Fatiha Daoud, Johanna Lippman, Evelyne Braun, Christian Chidiac;* **Surgeons:** *Elvire Servien, Cécile Batailler, Stanislas Gunst, Axel Schmidt, Matthieu Malatray, Elliot Sappey-Marinier, Michel-Henry Fessy, Anthony Viste, Jean-Luc Besse, Philippe Chaudier, Lucie Louboutin, Quentin Ode, Adrien Van Haecke, Marcelle Mercier, Vincent Belgaid, Arnaud Walch, Sébastien Martres, Franck Trouillet, Cédric Barrey, Ali Mojallal, Sophie Brosset, Camille Hanriat, Hélène Person, Nicolas Sigaux, Philippe Céruse, Carine Fuchsmann;* **Anesthesiologists:** *Frédéric Aubrun, Mikhail Dziadzko, Caroline Macabéo;* **Microbiologists:** *Frédéric Laurent, Laetitia Beraud, Tiphaine Roussel-Gaillard, Céline Dupieux, Camille Kolenda, Jérôme Josse;* **Pathology:** *Marie Brevet, Alexis Trecourt;* **Imaging:** *Fabien Craighero, Loic Boussel, Jean-Baptiste Pialat, Isabelle Morelec;* **PK/PD specialists:** *Michel Tod, Marie-Claude Gagnieu, Sylvain Goutelle;* **Clinical research assistant and database manager:** *Eugénie Mabrut.*

References

1. Tande AJ, Patel R. Prosthetic joint infection. Clin Microbiol Rev. 2014;27(2):302–45.
2. Del Pozo JL, Patel R. Clinical practice. Infection associated with prosthetic joints. N Engl J Med. 2009;361(8):787–94.
3. Société de Pathologie Infectieuse de Langue Française (SPILF), Collège des Universitaires de Maladies Infectieuses et Tropicales (CMIT), Groupe de Pathologie Infectieuse Pédiatrique (GPIP), Société Française d'Anesthésie et de Réanimation (SFAR), Société Française de Chirurgie Orthopédique et Traumatologique (SOFCOT), Société Française d'Hygiène Hospitalière (SFHH), et al. Recommendations for bone and joint prosthetic device infections in clinical practice (prosthe- sis, implants, osteosynthesis). Société de Pathologie Infectieuse de Langue Française. Med Mal Infect. 2010;40(4):185–211.
4. Osmon DR, Berbari EF, Berendt AR, Lew D, Zimmerli W, Steckelberg JM, et al. Diagnosis and management of prosthetic joint infection: clinical practice guidelines by the Infectious Diseases Society of America. Clin Infect Dis. 2013;56(1):e1–25.
5. Ariza J, Cobo J, Baraia-Etxaburu J, Benito N, Bori G, Cabo J, et al. Executive summary of management of prosthetic joint infections. Clinical practice guide- lines by the Spanish Society of Infectious Diseases and Clinical Microbiology (SEIMC). Enferm Infecc Microbiol Clin. 2017;35(3):189–95.
6. Kheir MM, Tan TL, George J, Higuera CA, Maltenfort MG, Parvizi J. Development and evalua- tion of a prognostic calculator for the surgical treat- ment of periprosthetic joint infection. J Arthroplasty. 2018;33(9):2986–2992.e1.
7. Kurtz SM, Lau E, Watson H, Schmier JK, Parvizi J. Economic burden of periprosthetic joint infec- tion in the United States. J Arthroplasty. 2012;27(8 Suppl):61–65.e1.
8. Lora-Tamayo J, Murillo O, Iribarren JA, Soriano A, Sánchez-Somolinos M, Baraia-Etxaburu JM, et al. A large multicenter study of methicillin-susceptible and methicillin-resistant Staphylococcus aureus prosthetic joint infections managed with implant retention. Clin Infect Dis. 2013;56(2):182–94.
9. Byren I, Bejon P, Atkins BL, Angus B, Masters S, McLardy-Smith P, et al. One hundred and twelve infected arthroplasties treated with "DAIR" (debride- ment, antibiotics and implant retention): antibiotic duration and outcome. J Antimicrob Chemother. 2009;63(6):1264–71.
10. Lesens O, Ferry T, Forestier E, Botelho-Nevers E, Pavese P, Piet E, et al. Should we expand the indica- tions for the DAIR (debridement, antibiotic therapy, and implant retention) procedure for Staphylococcus aureus prosthetic joint infections? A multicenter retrospective study. Eur J Clin Microbiol Infect Dis. 2018;37(10):1949–56.
11. Wouthuyzen-Bakker M, Sebillotte M, Huotari K, Escudero Sánchez R, Benavent E, Parvizi J, et al. Lower success rate of débridement and implant retention in late acute versus early acute peripros- thetic joint infection caused by Staphylococcus spp. Results from a Matched Cohort Study. Clin Orthop Relat Res. 2020;478(6):1348–55.
12. Gallo J, Kolár M, Novotný R, Riháková P, Tichá V. Pathogenesis of prosthesis-related infection. Biomed Pap Med Fac Univ Palacky Olomouc Czech Repub. 2003;147(1):27–35.
13. Johnston DH, Fairclough JA, Brown EM, Morris R. Rate of bacterial recolonization of the skin after preparation: four methods compared. Br J Surg. 1987;74(1):64.
14. Ritter MA. Operating room environment. Clin Orthop Relat Res. 1999;369:103–9.

15. Hughes SP, Anderson FM. Infection in the operating room. J Bone Joint Surg Br. 1999;81(5):754–5.

16. Wouthuyzen-Bakker M, Lora-Tamayo J, Senneville E, Scarbourough M, Ferry T, Uçkay I, et al. Erysipelas or cellulitis with a prosthetic joint in situ. J Bone Joint Infect. 2018;3(4):222–5.

17. Dufour S, Piroth L, Chirouze C, Tattevin P, Becker A, Braquet P, et al. Staphylococcus aureus bloodstream infection in patients with prosthetic joints in the prospective VIRSTA Cohort Study: frequency and time of occurrence of periprosthetic joint infection. Open Forum Infect Dis. 2019;6(12):ofz515.

18. Sendi P, Banderet F, Graber P, Zimmerli W. Periprosthetic joint infection following Staphylococcus aureus bacteremia. J Infect. 2011;63(1):17–22.

19. Honkanen M, Jämsen E, Karppelin M, Huttunen R, Eskelinen A, Syrjänen J. Periprosthetic joint infections as a consequence of bacteremia. Open Forum Infect Dis. 2019;6(6):ofz218.

20. Schmalzried TP, Amstutz HC, Au MK, Dorey FJ. Etiology of deep sepsis in total hip arthroplasty. The significance of hematogenous and recurrent infections. Clin Orthop Relat Res. 1992;280:200–7.

21. Lockhart PB, Brennan MT, Sasser HC, Fox PC, Paster BJ, Bahrani-Mougeot FK. Bacteremia associated with toothbrushing and dental extraction. Circulation. 2008;117(24):3118–25.

22. Renz N, Chevaux F, Borens O, Trampuz A. Successful treatment of periprosthetic joint infection caused by Granulicatella para-adiacens with prosthesis retention: a case report. BMC Musculoskelet Disord. 2016;17:156.

23. Kotzé MJ. Prosthetic joint infection, dental treatment and antibiotic prophylaxis. Orthop Rev (Pavia). 2009;1(1):e7.

24. Berbari EF, Osmon DR, Carr A, Hanssen AD, Baddour LM, Greene D, et al. Dental procedures as risk factors for prosthetic hip or knee infection: a hospital-based prospective case-control study. Clin Infect Dis. 2010;50(1):8–16.

25. Kao F-C, Hsu Y-C, Chen W-H, Lin J-N, Lo Y-Y, Tu Y-K. Prosthetic joint infection following invasive dental procedures and antibiotic prophylaxis in patients with hip or knee arthroplasty. Infect Control Hosp Epidemiol. 2017;38(2):154–61.

26. Moreira AI, Mendes L, Pereira JA. Is there scientific evidence to support antibiotic prophylaxis in patients with periodontal disease as a means to decrease the risk of prosthetic joint infections? A systematic review. Int Orthop. 2020;44(2):231–6.

27. Slullitel PA, Oñativia JI, Piuzzi NS, Higuera-Rueda C, Parvizi J, Buttaro MA. Is there a role for antibiotic prophylaxis prior to dental procedures in patients with total joint arthroplasty? A systematic review of the literature. J Bone Joint Infect. 2020;5(1):7–15.

28. Arnold WV, Bari AK, Buttaro M, Huang R, Mirez JP, Neira I, et al. General assembly, prevention, postoperative factors: proceedings of International Consensus on Orthopedic Infections. J Arthroplasty. 2019;34(2S):S169–74.

29. Rademacher WMH, Walenkamp GHIM, Moojen DJF, Hendriks JGE, Goedendorp TA, Rozema FR. Antibiotic prophylaxis is not indicated prior to dental procedures for prevention of periprosthetic joint infections. Acta Orthop. 2017;88(5):568–74.

30. Moran E, Masters S, Berendt AR, McLardy-Smith P, Byren I, Atkins BL. Guiding empirical antibiotic therapy in orthopaedics: the microbiology of prosthetic joint infection managed by debridement, irrigation and prosthesis retention. J Infect. 2007;55(1):1–7.

31. Benito N, Franco M, Ribera A, Soriano A, Rodriguez-Pardo D, Sorlí L, et al. Time trends in the aetiology of prosthetic joint infections: a multicentre cohort study. Clin Microbiol Infect. 2016;22(8):732.e1–8.

32. Rosteius T, Jansen O, Fehmer T, Baecker H, Citak M, Schildhauer TA, et al. Evaluating the microbial pattern of periprosthetic joint infections of the hip and knee. J Med Microbiol. 2018;67(11):1608–13.

33. Manning L, Metcalf S, Clark B, Robinson JO, Huggan P, Luey C, et al. Clinical characteristics, etiology, and initial management strategy of newly diagnosed periprosthetic joint infection: a multicenter, prospective observational cohort study of 783 patients. Open Forum Infect Dis. 2020;7(5):ofaa068.

34. Triffault-Fillit C, Ferry T, Laurent F, Pradat P, Dupieux C, Conrad A, et al. Microbiologic epidemiology depending on time to occurrence of prosthetic joint infection: a prospective cohort study. Clin Microbiol Infect. 2019;25(3):353–8.

35. Flurin L, Greenwood-Quaintance KE, Patel R. Microbiology of polymicrobial prosthetic joint infection. Diagn Microbiol Infect Dis. 2019;94(3):255–9.

36. Tsai Y, Chang C-H, Lin Y-C, Lee S-H, Hsieh P-H, Chang Y. Different microbiological profiles between hip and knee prosthetic joint infections. J Orthop Surg (Hong Kong). 2019;27(2):2309499019847768.

37. O'Neill J. Tackling drug-resistant infections globally: final report and recommendations—the review on antimicrobial resistance. [Internet]. 2016. https://amr-review.org/sites/default/files/160525_Final%20paper_with%20cover.pdf.

38. Parvizi J, Pawasarat IM, Azzam KA, Joshi A, Hansen EN, Bozic KJ. Periprosthetic joint infection: the economic impact of methicillin-resistant infections. J Arthroplasty. 2010;25(6 Suppl):103–7.

39. Peel TN, Cheng AC, Lorenzo YP, Kong DCM, Buising KL, Choong PFM. Factors influencing the cost of prosthetic joint infection treatment. J Hosp Infect. 2013;85(3):213–9.

40. Murillo O, Grau I, Lora-Tamayo J, Gomez-Junyent J, Ribera A, Tubau F, et al. The changing epidemiology of bacteraemic osteoarticular infections in the early 21st century. Clin Microbiol Infect. 2015;21(3):254.e1–8.

41. Rodríguez-Pardo D, Pigrau C, Lora-Tamayo J, Soriano A, del Toro MD, Cobo J, et al. Gram-negative prosthetic joint infection: outcome of a debridement, antibiotics and implant retention approach. A large multicentre study. Clin Microbiol Infect. 2014;20(11):O911–9.

42. Peel TN, Cheng AC, Buising KL, Choong PFM. Microbiological aetiology, epidemiology, and clinical profile of prosthetic joint infections: are current antibiotic prophylaxis guidelines effective? Antimicrob Agents Chemother. 2012;56(5):2386–91.

43. Papadopoulos A, Ribera A, Mavrogenis AF, Rodriguez-Pardo D, Bonnet E, Salles MJ, et al. Multidrug-resistant and extensively drug-resistant Gram-negative prosthetic joint infections: role of surgery and impact of colistin administration. Int J Antimicrob Agents. 2019;53(3):294–301.

44. Aggarwal VK, Bakhshi H, Ecker NU, Parvizi J, Gehrke T, Kendoff D. Organism profile in periprosthetic joint infection: pathogens differ at two arthroplasty infection referral centers in Europe and in the United States. J Knee Surg. 2014;27(5):399–406.

45. Chuang Y-Y, Huang Y-C. Molecular epidemiology of community-associated meticillin-resistant Staphylococcus aureus in Asia. Lancet Infect Dis. 2013;13(8):698–708.

46. Zimmerli W, Trampuz A, Ochsner PE. Prosthetic-jointinfections.NEnglJMed.2004;351(16):1645–54.

47. Tsukayama DT, Estrada R, Gustilo RB. Infection after total hip arthroplasty. A study of the treatment of one hundred and six infections. J Bone Joint Surg Am. 1996;78(4):512–23.

48. Ferry T, Perpoint T, Vandenesch F, Etienne J. Virulence determinants in Staphylococcus aureus and their involvement in clinical syndromes. Curr Infect Dis Rep. 2005;7(6):420–8.

49. Ascione T, Pagliano P, Mariconda M, Rotondo R, Balato G, Toro A, et al. Factors related to outcome of early and delayed prosthetic joint infections. J Infect. 2015;70(1):30–6.

50. Rodríguez D, Pigrau C, Euba G, Cobo J, García-Lechuz J, Palomino J, et al. Acute haematogenous prosthetic joint infection: prospective evaluation of medical and surgical management. Clin Microbiol Infect. 2010;16(12):1789–95.

51. Tande AJ, Osmon DR, Greenwood-Quaintance KE, Mabry TM, Hanssen AD, Patel R. Clinical characteristics and outcomes of prosthetic joint infection caused by small colony variant staphylococci. mBio. 2014;5(5):e01910–4.

52. Shah NB, Osmon DR, Fadel H, Patel R, Kohner PC, Steckelberg JM, et al. Laboratory and clinical characteristics of Staphylococcus lugdunensis prosthetic joint infections. J Clin Microbiol. 2010;48(5):1600–3.

53. Lourtet-Hascoët J, Bicart-See A, Félicé MP, Giordano G, Bonnet E. Staphylococcus lugdunensis, a serious pathogen in periprosthetic joint infections: comparison to Staphylococcus aureus and Staphylococcus epidermidis. Int J Infect Dis. 2016;51:56–61.

54. Mohamad M, Uçkay I, Hannouche D, Miozzari H. Particularities of Staphylococcus Lugdunensis in orthopaedic infections. Infect Dis (Lond). 2018;50(3):223–5.

55. Aboltins CA, Dowsey MM, Buising KL, Peel TN, Daffy JR, Choong PFM, et al. Gram-negative prosthetic joint infection treated with debridement, prosthesis retention and antibiotic regimens including a fluoroquinolone. Clin Microbiol Infect. 2011;17(6):862–7.

56. Boisrenoult P. Cutibacterium acnes prosthetic joint infection: diagnosis and treatment. Orthop Traumatol Surg Res. 2018;104(1S):S19–24.

57. Schäfer P, Fink B, Sandow D, Margull A, Berger I, Frommelt L. Prolonged bacterial culture to identify late periprosthetic joint infection: a promising strategy. Clin Infect Dis. 2008;47(11):1403–9.

58. Rieber H, Frontzek A, Jerosch J, Alefeld M, Strohecker T, Ulatowski M, et al. Periprosthetic joint infection caused by anaerobes. Retrospective analysis reveals no need for prolonged cultivation time if sensitive supplemented growth media are used. Anaerobe. 2018;50:12–8.

59. Löwik CAM, Zijlstra WP, Knobben BAS, Ploegmakers JJW, Dijkstra B, de Vries AJ, et al. Obese patients have higher rates of polymicrobial and Gram-negative early periprosthetic joint infections of the hip than non-obese patients. PLoS One. 2019;14(4):e0215035.

60. Berbari EF, Marculescu C, Sia I, Lahr BD, Hanssen AD, Steckelberg JM, et al. Culture-negative prosthetic joint infection. Clin Infect Dis. 2007;45(9):1113–9.

61. Malekzadeh D, Osmon DR, Lahr BD, Hanssen AD, Berbari EF. Prior use of antimicrobial therapy is a risk factor for culture-negative prosthetic joint infection. Clin Orthop Relat Res. 2010;468(8):2039–45.

62. Josse J, Valour F, Maali Y, Diot A, Batailler C, Ferry T, et al. Interaction between Staphylococcal biofilm and bone: how does the presence of biofilm promote prosthesis loosening? Front Microbiol. 2019;10:1602.

63. Costerton JW, Stewart PS, Greenberg EP. Bacterial biofilms: a common cause of persistent infections. Science. 1999;284(5418):1318–22.

64. Hall-Stoodley L, Costerton JW, Stoodley P. Bacterial biofilms: from the natural environment to infectious diseases. Nat Rev Microbiol. 2004;2(2):95–108.

65. Moormeier DE, Bayles KW. Staphylococcus aureus biofilm: a complex developmental organism. Mol Microbiol. 2017;104(3):365–76.

66. Geoghegan JA, Ganesh VK, Smeds E, Liang X, Höök M, Foster TJ. Molecular characterization of the interaction of staphylococcal microbial surface components recognizing adhesive matrix molecules (MSCRAMM) ClfA and Fbl with fibrinogen. J Biol Chem. 2010;285(9):6208–16.

67. Büttner H, Mack D, Rohde H. Structural basis of Staphylococcus epidermidis biofilm formation: mechanisms and molecular interactions. Front Cell Infect Microbiol. 2015;5:14.

68. Christner M, Franke GC, Schommer NN, Wendt U, Wegert K, Pehle P, et al. The giant extracellular matrix-binding protein of Staphylococcus epidermidis mediates biofilm accumulation and attachment to fibronectin. Mol Microbiol. 2010;75(1):187–207.

69. Hussain M, Steinbacher T, Peters G, Heilmann C, Becker K. The adhesive properties of the Staphylococcus lugdunensis multifunctional autolysin AtlL and its role in biofilm formation and internalization. Int J Med Microbiol. 2015;305(1):129–39.

70. Olivares E, Badel-Berchoux S, Provot C, Prévost G, Bernardi T, Jehl F. Clinical impact of antibiotics for the treatment of Pseudomonas aeruginosa biofilm infections. Front Microbiol. 2019;10:2894.

71. Mack D, Fischer W, Krokotsch A, Leopold K, Hartmann R, Egge H, et al. The intercellular adhesin involved in biofilm accumulation of Staphylococcus epidermidis is a linear beta-1,6-linked glucosaminoglycan: purification and structural analysis. J Bacteriol. 1996;178(1):175–83.

72. Cramton SE, Gerke C, Schnell NF, Nichols WW, Götz F. The intercellular adhesion (ica) locus is present in Staphylococcus aureus and is required for biofilm formation. Infect Immun. 1999;67(10):5427–33.

73. McCarthy H, Rudkin JK, Black NS, Gallagher L, O'Neill E, O'Gara JP. Methicillin resistance and the biofilm phenotype in Staphylococcus aureus. Front Cell Infect Microbiol. 2015;5:1.

74. Frank KL, Patel R. Poly-N-acetylglucosamine is not a major component of the extracellular matrix in biofilms formed by icaADBC-positive Staphylococcus lugdunensis isolates. Infect Immun. 2007;75(10):4728–42.

75. Ravaioli S, Campoccia D, Speziale P, Pietrocola G, Zatorska B, Maso A, et al. Various biofilm matrices of the emerging pathogen Staphylococcus lugdunensis: exopolysaccharides, proteins, eDNA and their correlation with biofilm mass. Biofouling. 2020;36(1):86–100.

76. Mann EE, Rice KC, Boles BR, Endres JL, Ranjit D, Chandramohan L, et al. Modulation of eDNA release and degradation affects Staphylococcus aureus biofilm maturation. PLoS One. 2009;4(6):e5822.

77. Foulston L, Elsholz AKW, DeFrancesco AS, Losick R. The extracellular matrix of Staphylococcus aureus biofilms comprises cytoplasmic proteins that associate with the cell surface in response to decreasing pH. mBio. 2014;5(5):e01667–14.

78. Dengler V, Foulston L, DeFrancesco AS, Losick R. An electrostatic net model for the role of extracellular DNA in biofilm formation by Staphylococcus aureus. J Bacteriol. 2015;197(24):3779–87.

79. Mlynek KD, Bulock LL, Stone CJ, Curran LJ, Sadykov MR, Bayles KW, et al. Genetic and biochemical analysis of CodY-mediated cell aggregation in Staphylococcus aureus reveals an interaction between extracellular DNA and polysaccharide in the extracellular matrix. J Bacteriol. 2020;202(8):e00593.

80. O'Neill E, Pozzi C, Houston P, Humphreys H, Robinson DA, Loughman A, et al. A novel Staphylococcus aureus biofilm phenotype mediated by the fibronectin-binding proteins, FnBPA and FnBPB. J Bacteriol. 2008;190(11):3835–50.

81. Ma L, Conover M, Lu H, Parsek MR, Bayles K, Wozniak DJ. Assembly and development of the Pseudomonas aeruginosa biofilm matrix. PLoS Pathog. 2009;5(3):e1000354.

82. Boles BR, Horswill AR. Agr-mediated dispersal of Staphylococcus aureus biofilms. PLoS Pathog. 2008;4(4):e1000052.

83. Rasigade J-P, Trouillet-Assant S, Ferry T, Diep BA, Sapin A, Lhoste Y, et al. PSMs of hypervirulent Staphylococcus aureus act as intracellular toxins that kill infected osteoblasts. PLoS One. 2013;8(5):e63176.

84. Surewaard BGJ, de Haas CJC, Vervoort F, Rigby KM, DeLeo FR, Otto M, et al. Staphylococcal alpha-phenol soluble modulins contribute to neutrophil lysis after phagocytosis. Cell Microbiol. 2013;15(8):1427–37.

85. Periasamy S, Joo H-S, Duong AC, Bach T-HL, Tan VY, Chatterjee SS, et al. How Staphylococcus aureus biofilms develop their characteristic structure. Proc Natl Acad Sci U S A. 2012;109(4):1281–6.

86. Wang R, Khan BA, Cheung GYC, Bach T-HL, Jameson-Lee M, Kong K-F, et al. Staphylococcus epidermidis surfactant peptides promote biofilm maturation and dissemination of biofilm-associated infection in mice. J Clin Invest. 2011;121(1):238–48.

87. Schwartz K, Syed AK, Stephenson RE, Rickard AH, Boles BR. Functional amyloids composed of phenol soluble modulins stabilize Staphylococcus aureus biofilms. PLoS Pathog. 2012;8(6):e1002744.

88. Schwartz K, Ganesan M, Payne DE, Solomon MJ, Boles BR. Extracellular DNA facilitates the formation of functional amyloids in Staphylococcus aureus biofilms. Mol Microbiol. 2016;99(1):123–34.

89. Zheng Y, Joo H-S, Nair V, Le KY, Otto M. Do amyloid structures formed by Staphylococcus aureus phenol-soluble modulins have a biological function? Int J Med Microbiol. 2018;308(6):675–82.

90. Le KY, Villaruz AE, Zheng Y, He L, Fisher EL, Nguyen TH, et al. Role of phenol-soluble modulins in Staphylococcus epidermidis biofilm formation and infection of indwelling medical devices. J Mol Biol. 2019;431(16):3015–27.

91. Bjarnsholt T, Alhede M, Alhede M, Eickhardt-Sørensen SR, Moser C, Kühl M, et al. The in vivo biofilm. Trends Microbiol. 2013;21(9):466–74.

92. Brauner A, Fridman O, Gefen O, Balaban NQ. Distinguishing between resistance, tolerance and persistence to antibiotic treatment. Nat Rev Microbiol. 2016;14(5):320–30.

93. Crabbé A, Jensen PØ, Bjarnsholt T, Coenye T. Antimicrobial tolerance and metabolic adaptations in microbial biofilms. Trends Microbiol. 2019;27(10):850–63.

94. Jacqueline C, Caillon J. Impact of bacterial biofilm on the treatment of prosthetic joint infections. J Antimicrob Chemother. 2014;69(Suppl 1):i37–40.

95. Vuong C, Voyich JM, Fischer ER, Braughton KR, Whitney AR, DeLeo FR, et al. Polysaccharide intercellular adhesin (PIA) protects Staphylococcus epidermidis against major components of the human innate immune system. Cell Microbiol. 2004;6(3):269–75.

96. Kristian SA, Birkenstock TA, Sauder U, Mack D, Götz F, Landmann R. Biofilm formation induces C3a release and protects Staphylococcus epidermidis from IgG and complement deposition and from neutrophil-dependent killing. J Infect Dis. 2008;197(7):1028–35.

97. Meyle E, Stroh P, Günther F, Hoppy-Tichy T, Wagner C, Hänsch GM. Destruction of bacterial biofilms by polymorphonuclear neutrophils: relative contribution of phagocytosis, DNA release, and degranulation. Int J Artif Organs. 2010;33(9):608–20.

98. Gaida MM, Mayer B, Stegmaier S, Schirmacher P, Wagner C, Hänsch GM. Polymorphonuclear neutrophils in osteomyelitis: link to osteoclast generation and bone resorption. Eur J Inflamm. 2012;10(3):413–26.

99. Thurlow LR, Hanke ML, Fritz T, Angle A, Aldrich A, Williams SH, et al. Staphylococcus aureus biofilms prevent macrophage phagocytosis and attenuate inflammation in vivo. J Immunol. 2011;186(11):6585–96.

100. Hanke ML, Angle A, Kielian T. MyD88-dependent signaling influences fibrosis and alternative macrophage activation during Staphylococcus aureus biofilm infection. PLoS One. 2012;7(8):e42476.

101. Heim CE, Vidlak D, Scherr TD, Kozel JA, Holzapfel M, Muirhead DE, et al. Myeloid-derived suppressor cells contribute to Staphylococcus aureus orthopedic biofilm infection. J Immunol. 2014;192(8):3778–92.

102. Heim CE, Vidlak D, Kielian T. Interleukin-10 production by myeloid-derived suppressor cells contributes to bacterial persistence during Staphylococcus aureus orthopedic biofilm infection. J Leukoc Biol. 2015;98(6):1003–13.

103. Heim CE, Vidlak D, Odvody J, Hartman CW, Garvin KL, Kielian T. Human prosthetic joint infections are associated with myeloid-derived suppressor cells (MDSCs): implications for infection persistence. J Orthop Res. 2018;36(6):1605–13.

104. Lass R, Giurea A, Kubista B, Hirschl AM, Graninger W, Presterl E, et al. Bacterial adherence to different components of total hip prosthesis in patients with prosthetic joint infection. Int Orthop. 2014;38(8):1597–602.

105. Klein M, Bonar S, Freemont T. Infectious and inflammatory diseases. In: AFIP atlas of nontumor pathology non-neoplastic diseases of bones and joints. Washington, DC: AFIP; 2011. p. 411–543.

106. Ribatti D. The discovery of plasma cells: an historical note. Immunol Lett. 2017;188:64–7.

107. Manzo A, Bugatti S, Caporali R, Montecucco C. Histopathology of the synovial tissue: perspectives for biomarker development in chronic inflammatory arthritides. Reumatismo. 2018;3:121–32.

108. Ferry T, Trecourt A, Batailler C, Brevet M. Plasma cell infiltration in a 28-year-old patient with chronic indolent fracture-related tibial infection due to Cutibacterium acnes. BMJ Case Rep. 2019;12(12):e232345.

109. Trecourt A. Plasma cell infiltration on histopathological samples of chronic bone and joint infection due to Cutibacterium acnes: a series of 25 cases. 2020; In Press.

110. Malhotra R, Dhawan B, Garg B, Shankar V, Nag TC. A comparison of bacterial adhesion and biofilm formation on commonly used orthopaedic metal implant materials: an in vitro study. Indian J Orthop. 2019;53(1):148–53.

111. Dastgheyb S, Parvizi J, Shapiro IM, Hickok NJ, Otto M. Effect of biofilms on recalcitrance of staphylococcal joint infection to antibiotic treatment. J Infect Dis. 2015;211(4):641–50.

112. Perez K, Patel R. Biofilm-like aggregation of Staphylococcus epidermidis in synovial fluid. J Infect Dis. 2015;212(2):335–6.

113. Pestrak MJ, Gupta TT, Dusane DH, Guzior DV, Staats A, Harro J, et al. Investigation of synovial fluid induced Staphylococcus aureus aggregate development and its impact on surface attachment and biofilm formation. PLoS One. 2020;15(4):e0231791.

114. Masters EA, Trombetta RP, de Mesy Bentley KL, Boyce BF, Gill AL, Gill SR, et al. Evolving concepts in bone infection: redefining "biofilm", "acute vs. chronic osteomyelitis", "the immune proteome" and "local antibiotic therapy". Bone Res. 2019;7:20.

115. Cheng AG, Kim HK, Burts ML, Krausz T, Schneewind O, Missiakas DM. Genetic requirements for Staphylococcus aureus abscess formation and persistence in host tissues. FASEB J. 2009;23(10):3393–404.

116. Schwarz EM, McLaren AC, Sculco TP, Brause B, Bostrom M, Kates SL, et al. Adjuvant antibiotic-loaded bone cement: concerns with current use and research to make it work. J Orthop Res 2020.

117. de Mesy Bentley KL, Trombetta R, Nishitani K, Bello-Irizarry SN, Ninomiya M, Zhang L, et al. Evidence of Staphylococcus Aureus deformation, proliferation, and migration in canaliculi of live cortical bone in murine models of osteomyelitis. J Bone Miner Res. 2017;32(5):985–90.

118. Josse J, Velard F, Gangloff SC. Staphylococcus aureus vs. osteoblast: relationship and consequences in osteomyelitis. Front Cell Infect Microbiol. 2015;5:85.

119. Wright JA, Nair SP. Interaction of staphylococci with bone. Int J Med Microbiol. 2010;300(2–3):193–204.

120. Ellington JK, Reilly SS, Ramp WK, Smeltzer MS, Kellam JF, Hudson MC. Mechanisms of Staphylococcus aureus invasion of cultured osteoblasts. Microb Pathog. 1999;26(6):317–23.

121. Sinha B, François PP, Nüsse O, Foti M, Hartford OM, Vaudaux P, et al. Fibronectin-binding protein acts as Staphylococcus aureus invasin via fibronectin bridging to integrin alpha5beta1. Cell Microbiol. 1999;1(2):101–17.

122. Josse J, Laurent F, Diot A. Staphylococcal adhesion and host cell invasion: fibronectin-binding and other mechanisms. Front Microbiol. 2017;8:2433.

123. Giese B, Glowinski F, Paprotka K, Dittmann S, Steiner T, Sinha B, et al. Expression of δ-toxin by Staphylococcus aureus mediates escape from phago-endosomes of human epithelial and endothelial cells in the presence of β-toxin. Cell Microbiol. 2011;13(2):316–29.

124. Sokolovska A, Becker CE, Ip WKE, Rathinam VAK, Brudner M, Paquette N, et al. Activation of caspase-1 by the NLRP3 inflammasome regulates the NADPH oxidase NOX2 to control phagosome function. Nat Immunol. 2013;14(6):543–53.

125. Dikic I, Elazar Z. Mechanism and medical implications of mammalian autophagy. Nat Rev Mol Cell Biol. 2018;19(6):349–64.

126. Horn J, Stelzner K, Rudel T, Fraunholz M. Inside job: Staphylococcus aureus host-pathogen interactions. Int J Med Microbiol. 2018;308(6):607–24.

127. Wang H, Zhou Y, Zhu Q, Zang H, Cai J, Wang J, et al. Staphylococcus aureus induces autophagy in bovine mammary epithelial cells and the formation of autophagosomes facilitates intracellular replication of Staph. aureus. J Dairy Sci. 2019;102(9):8264–72.

128. Tuchscherr L, Heitmann V, Hussain M, Viemann D, Roth J, von Eiff C, et al. Staphylococcus aureus small-colony variants are adapted phenotypes for intracellular persistence. J Infect Dis. 2010;202(7):1031–40.

129. Tuchscherr L, Medina E, Hussain M, Völker W, Heitmann V, Niemann S, et al. Staphylococcus aureus phenotype switching: an effective bacterial strategy to escape host immune response and establish a chronic infection. EMBO Mol Med. 2011;3(3):129–41.

130. Bosse MJ, Gruber HE, Ramp WK. Internalization of bacteria by osteoblasts in a patient with recurrent, long-term osteomyelitis. A case report. J Bone Joint Surg Am. 2005;87(6):1343–7.

131. Valour F, Rasigade J-P, Trouillet-Assant S, Gagnaire J, Bouaziz A, Karsenty J, et al. Delta-toxin production deficiency in Staphylococcus aureus: a diagnostic marker of bone and joint infection chronicity linked with osteoblast invasion and biofilm formation. Clin Microbiol Infect. 2015;21(6):568.e1–11.

132. Maali Y, Martins-Simões P, Valour F, Bouvard D, Rasigade J-P, Bes M, et al. Pathophysiological mechanisms of Staphylococcus non-aureus bone and joint infection: interspecies homogeneity and

133. Maali Y, Diot A, Martins-Simões P, Bes M, Bouvard D, Vandenesch F, et al. Identification and characterization of Staphylococcus delphini internalization pathway in nonprofessional phagocytic cells. Infect Immunol. 2020;88(5):e00002.

134. Valour F, Trouillet-Assant S, Rasigade J-P, Lustig S, Chanard E, Meugnier H, et al. Staphylococcus epidermidis in orthopedic device infections: the role of bacterial internalization in human osteoblasts and biofilm formation. PLoS One. 2013;8(6):e67240.

135. Campoccia D, Testoni F, Ravaioli S, Cangini I, Maso A, Speziale P, et al. Orthopedic implant infections: incompetence of Staphylococcus epidermidis, Staphylococcus lugdunensis, and Enterococcus faecalis to invade osteoblasts. J Biomed Mater Res A. 2016;104(3):788–801.

136. Khalil H, Williams RJ, Stenbeck G, Henderson B, Meghji S, Nair SP. Invasion of bone cells by Staphylococcus epidermidis. Microbes Infect. 2007;9(4):460–5.

137. Wang B, Cleary PP. Intracellular invasion by Streptococcus pyogenes: invasins, host receptors, and relevance to human disease. Microbiol Spectr. 2019;7(4).

138. Jauregui CE, Mansell JP, Jepson MA, Jenkinson HF. Differential interactions of Streptococcus gordonii and Staphylococcus aureus with cultured osteoblasts. Mol Oral Microbiol. 2013;28(4):250–66.

139. Francis CL, Ryan TA, Jones BD, Smith SJ, Falkow S. Ruffles induced by Salmonella and other stimuli direct macropinocytosis of bacteria. Nature. 1993;364(6438):639–42.

140. Finlay BB, Falkow S. Comparison of the invasion strategies used by Salmonella cholerae-suis, Shigella flexneri and Yersinia enterocolitica to enter cultured animal cells: endosome acidification is not required for bacterial invasion or intracellular replication. Biochimie. 1988;70(8):1089–99.

141. Garcia-del Portillo F, Finlay BB. Salmonella invasion of nonphagocytic cells induces formation of macropinosomes in the host cell. Infect Immun. 1994;62(10):4641–5.

142. Crémet L, Broquet A, Brulin B, Jacqueline C, Dauvergne S, Brion R, et al. Pathogenic potential of Escherichia coli clinical strains from orthopedic implant infections towards human osteoblastic cells. Pathog Dis. 2015;73(8):ftv065.

143. Fleiszig SM, Zaidi TS, Fletcher EL, Preston MJ, Pier GB. Pseudomonas aeruginosa invades corneal epithelial cells during experimental infection. Infect Immun. 1994;62(8):3485–93.

144. Ha U, Jin S. Growth phase-dependent invasion of Pseudomonas aeruginosa and its survival within HeLa cells. Infect Immun. 2001;69(7):4398–406.

145. Pier GB, Grout M, Zaidi TS, Olsen JC, Johnson LG, Yankaskas JR, et al. Role of mutant CFTR in hyper-

susceptibility of cystic fibrosis patients to lung infections. Science. 1996;271(5245):64–7.

146. Sana TG, Baumann C, Merdes A, Soscia C, Rattei T, Hachani A, et al. Internalization of Pseudomonas aeruginosa strain PAO1 into epithelial cells is promoted by interaction of a T6SS effector with the microtubule network. mBio. 2015;6(3):e00712.

147. Aubin GG, Baud'huin M, Lavigne J-P, Brion R, Gouin F, Lepelletier D, et al. Interaction of Cutibacterium (formerly Propionibacterium) acnes with bone cells: a step toward understanding bone and joint infection development. Sci Rep. 2017;7:42918.

148. Chauvelot P. Invasion of osteoblasts by corynebacterium via the cellular integrin beta1 leads to bone and joint infection chronicity. CONGRES ECCMID; 2018.

149. Trouillet-Assant S, Gallet M, Nauroy P, Rasigade J-P, Flammier S, Parroche P, et al. Dual impact of live Staphylococcus aureus on the osteoclast lineage, leading to increased bone resorption. J Infect Dis. 2015;211(4):571–81.

150. Valour F, Trouillet-Assant S, Riffard N, Tasse J, Flammier S, Rasigade J-P, et al. Antimicrobial activity against intraosteoblastic Staphylococcus aureus. Antimicrob Agents Chemother. 2015;59(4):2029–36.

151. Ellington JK, Harris M, Hudson MC, Vishin S, Webb LX, Sherertz R. Intracellular Staphylococcus aureus and antibiotic resistance: implications for treatment of staphylococcal osteomyelitis. J Orthop Res. 2006;24(1):87–93.

152. Tuchscherr L, Kreis CA, Hoerr V, Flint L, Hachmeister M, Geraci J, et al. Staphylococcus aureus develops increased resistance to antibiotics by forming dynamic small colony variants during chronic osteomyelitis. J Antimicrob Chemother. 2016;71(2):438–48.

153. Dupieux C, Trouillet-Assant S, Camus C, Abad L, Bes M, Benito Y, et al. Intraosteoblastic activity of daptomycin in combination with oxacillin and ceftaroline against MSSA and MRSA. J Antimicrob Chemother. 2017;72(12):3353–6.

154. Baudoux P, Bles N, Lemaire S, Mingeot-Leclercq M-P, Tulkens PM, Van Bambeke F. Combined effect of pH and concentration on the activities of gentamicin and oxacillin against Staphylococcus aureus in pharmacodynamic models of extracellular and intracellular infections. J Antimicrob Chemother. 2007;59(2):246–53.

155. Abad L, Josse J, Tasse J, Lustig S, Ferry T, Diot A, et al. Antibiofilm and intraosteoblastic activities of rifamycins against Staphylococcus aureus: promising in vitro profile of rifabutin. J Antimicrob Chemother. 2020;75(6):1466–73.

Part II

Biomaterials in Artificial Joint Replacements

The Role of the Surface on Bacteria-Implant Interactions

Chuan-Jiang Xie, Chao-Chao Fan, and Yan Xiong

3.1 Introduction

TKA prostheses postoperative infection (periprosthetic be infection, PJI) is the most terrible complications, the most serious in TKA can have disastrous consequences [1–4]. As the population ages and the demand for TKA continues to rise, the incidence of PJI is also increasing. The main reason for treatment failure is the formation of bacterial biofilm on the surface of the implant and the adhesion of bacterial biofilm in the surrounding tissues and bones. Biofilm is a barrier to protect bacterial cells and has many unique properties leading to antibiotic resistance [4]. The first step in clinical PJI treatment is to find the pathogenic microorganisms. However, in clinical microbial culture, the result of culture test is negative because the bacteria are wrapped in biofilm, which makes microbial diagnosis difficult [5]. Moreover, because biofilms can protect pathogenic bacteria from antibiotics and host defense, PJI after total knee replacement (TKA) is difficult to treat. This chapter will elaborate the formation mechanism of the implant biofilm and the mechanism of antibiotic resistance in the biofilm as well as the detection and treatment of the biofilm.

C.-J. Xie · C.-C. Fan · Y. Xiong (✉)
Department of Orthopedics, Daping Hospital, Army Medical University (Third Military Medical University), Chongqing, China

3.2 Mechanism of Implant Biofilm Formation

Biofilm studies of microorganisms are getting more and more attention. Biofilms are common in natural industry and clinical environment, but it is difficult to eradicate them. The main difficulty of PJI treatment after KTA is the biofilm formation of pathogenic bacteria. Bacterial cells in the surface of the orthopaedic material have very high affinity, the most commonly used material in modern orthopedic surgery including titanium (and its alloys), cobalt chromium stainless steel, and various polymers, including ultra-high molecular weight polyethylene (UHMWPE) silicone polyether ketone all kinds of ceramic and hydroxyapatite and polymethyl methacrylate (PMMA) cement are vulnerable to biofilm formation of bacteria to colonize [6]. Bacterial biofilms have been reported to form after placement for 16 h [7]. The National Institutes of Health estimates that about 65 percent of infections are caused by bacterial biofilms, biofilm pathogens include gram-positive bacteria (Staphylococcus aureus, Staphylococcus epidermococcus, Streptococcus enterococcus) or gram-negative bacteria (E. coli, K. pneumoniae, Pseudomonas aeruginosa) [8]. Propionibacterium acneum is a gram-positive facultative anaerobe and a conditioned pathogen capable of forming biofilms [9]. The most common biofilm bacteria in PJI in TKA are Staphylococcus aureus, especially

U. G. Longo et al. (eds.), *Infection in Knee Replacement*,
https://doi.org/10.1007/978-3-030-81553-0_3

Staphylococcus aureus and Staphylococcus epidermidis, which account for nearly 50–60% of culture infections [10]. Zimmerli et al. [11] reported that it only takes 100 colony forming units to cause PJI. Once the bacteria adhesion together, they gathered in the community and produce extracellular polymer matrix (extra polysaccharide matrix, EPS), EPS by extracellular polysaccharide protein cell DNA (extracellular DNA, eDNA) lipid composition, called biofilms [12, 13]. Biofilm is adhered on the surface of the bacterial cell, it is composed of 10% of the cells and 90% of EPS, EPS provides the mechanical stability of the biofilm, mediated and surface adhesion, and form a tight three-dimensional polymer network, make the mutual connection and temporarily fixed biofilm cells, has a defense mechanism that can effectively protect bacteria against their antibiotic treatment [14, 15]. According to Gilbert et al. [16], biofilms have the ability to protect bacteria in the membrane against antibiotic treatment. Compared with planktonic bacteria, mature biofilms can tolerate antibiotics with a concentration 100–1000 times higher. This makes them harder to detect

and eradicate with conventional therapies, increasing antibiotic resistance [4]. Arciola et al. [17] summarized the process of biofilm formation in four steps:(1) free floating (plankton-cell) adhesion; (2) colony formation; (3) mature; (4) separation. The first step in the formation of a biofilm is for free-floating bacteria to attach to the surface of an object. Staphylococcus epidermidis (Fig. 3.1) and Staphylococcus aureus specifically express proteins at this stage of growth that strongly interact with the host extracellular matrix (ECM). These proteins are thought to be key to the bacteria's attachment to foreign bodies, as the ECM wraps them up when they enter the body. Surgery can lead to tissue destruction and trauma caused by partial produce extracellular matrix (ECM) protein host (such as the fibrous connections to the implant surface protein and collagen), the mechanism of extracellular protein deposition enhances bacterial colonization ability, let host bacteria on the surface of protein and protein matrix combination, more easily in the kind of anchor implant surface [13]. In addition, surgical trauma also leads to tissue ischemia and local immunosuppression, which further pro-

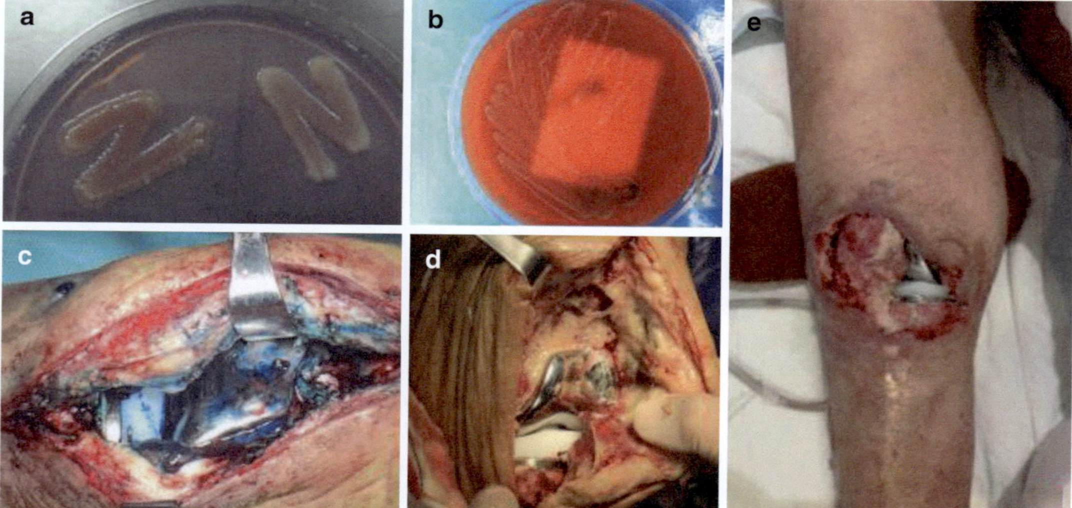

Fig. 3.1 (**a**) Observation of polysaccharide secretion by Staphylococcus epidermidis in PJI Congo red medium after TKA operation (the picture is a gift from doctor Chen peng of Guizhou Provincial Pople's Hospital), (**b**) culture observation of Streptococcus agalactiae of PJI after TKA operation, (**c**) after TKA, chronic PJI infection was demonstrated by injection of sterile meilan through the sinus tract, (**d**) knee cavity abscess of PJI after TKA operation, (**e**) PJI prosthesis was exposed after TKA

motes the colonization of bacterial cells [18]. Extracellular DNA (eDNA) also accumulates during the attachment phase through bacterial autolysis. Although the role of extracellular DNA (eDNA) in biofilm formation is not fully understood, it is thought to contribute to the stability of biofilms and may be an intercellular adhesin. This is followed by irreversible attachment to the surface and loss of movement. The new plankton-bacteria can interact with the bacteria attached to the surface to form bacterial microcolonies [19]. In addition to population expansion, bacteria also produce extracellular compounds called self-inducers during the entire attachment growth phase [20, 21]. These automatic inducers act as signals between and within bacteria, specifically to convey the local density of bacterial populations [19]. With the aggregation of bacteria, the production of extracellular polymer matrix (EPS) was upregulated and embedded into the EPS matrix. In this screened environment, the biofilms begin to mature and thicken as bacterial cells multiply to form multilayer colonies [22]. In the mature stage of biofilm, bacteria are constantly multiplying. When the critical threshold is reached, the bacteria in the biofilm will undergo densi-related changes. This process is described as quorum sensing. Quorum sensing mechanism is the basic chemical signal means for bacterial population to communicate, coordinate, and cooperate [19]. Quorum sensing is a complex internal network that connects colonies in a biofilm microenvironment. Bacterial cells use quorum sensing to communicate with one another through cellular signals, exchanging nutrients and promoting resistance to antibiotics and avoiding the immune system's toxic genes [23]. The different stages of bacterial biofilm formation are closely related to quorum sensing. Besides the formation of biofilm, quorum sensing also regulates the production of bioluminescent sporogenic antibiotics and the secretion of virulence factors [24]. Biofilm separation requires a protease to separate the bacterial cells, helping the plankton-bacteria to release from the biofilm, spread again and cause further infection [4]. The maturation time of the biofilm of different bacteria was not consistent, and the

time of Staphylococcus epidermidis was 24 h [25, 26],

Staphylococcus aureus for 24 h [27, 28], Pseudomonas aeruginosa for 72 h [29]. At present, PJI infection can be divided into acute phase and chronic phase according to the maturity of biofilms. In acute PJI, microorganisms do not form biofilms, while in chronic PJI, microorganisms have formed mature biofilms. Therefore, the treatment methods for different infections are different [30].

3.3 Mechanisms of Antibiotic Resistance in Biofilms

Under the protection of the biofilm, the bacteria developed drug resistance by increasing the minimum antibiotic inhibition concentration required for infection control [16]. Lazăr [31] pointed out that resistance to antibiotics of biological membrane has four main mechanisms: (1) due to the existence of the biofilm matrix, antibiotics cannot infiltrate into the depths of the mature biofilm; (2) accumulation of high levels of antibiotic degrading enzymes; (3) in the depths of the biofilm, bacterial cells are experiencing nutrient restriction and entering a state of slow growth or starvation; slow-growing or non-growing bacterial cells are not sensitive to antimicrobial agents, which can be amplified by phenotypic variation or the presence of permanent cells. Moreover, biofilm bacteria can turn on stress response genes and convert to a more drug-resistant phenotype when exposed to environmental stress. (4) Genetic changes may be selected by different stress conditions, such as mutations and gene transfer may occur in the biofilm. Akanda et al. [4] proposed three main factors of antibiotic resistance mechanism in biofilms: (1) physical barrier against host defense and antibiotic penetration; (2) reduce the metabolic activity of bacterial cells; (3) quorum sensing promotes the communication of antibiotic resistance genes. In order for antibiotics to have a bactericidal effect on the bacteria in the biofilm in the treatment of PJI, the antibiotics used must be able to penetrate the EPS matrix. Singh, etc. [32] discussed the various antibiotics on Staphylococcus aureus and epidermis Staphylococcus aureus biological membrane permeability, the results confirmed that the benzene azole Westwood cefotaxime (beta lactam type) and vancomycin (sugar peptide) on Staphylococcus aureus and epidermis Staphylococcus aureus biofilm osmosis are decreased obviously, and aminoglycoside drug amikacin ciprofloxacin and fluoroquinolone drugs of osmosis are not affected.

Biofilm the physical structure of the antibiotic produced a concentration gradient, internal bacterial biofilm to accept less than planktonic bacteria antibiotic concentration, which resulted in increased the risk of resistance, but the bacteria in the biofilm mutations faster, this phenomenon is associated with increased oxidative stress in biofilm environment, this kind of oxidative stress are both endogenous and caused by the antibiotics [33]. Adaptive stress response in biofilms is an active process mediated by quorum sensing, which promotes the expression of genes and signaling molecules that contribute to antibiotic resistance, and the production of enzymes and effervescent pumps that put cells into a dormant state or inactivate antibiotics, depending on the strain [34]. Donlan et al. [35] proposed another hypothesis that antibiotic resistance was related to the weakened growth state of microorganisms in the biofilm and found that the deep biofilm microorganisms with nutrient deficiency showed lower metabolic activity and slower growth rate. Studies have shown a correlation between slow-growing microbes and reduced antibiotic sensitivity to the microbes. Antibiotics depend on interfering with cell metabolism to regulate their bactericidal action, so they need to actively proliferate cells to kill them [36]. In biofilms, groups of cells that remain after antibiotic treatment are called permanent cells and these permanent cells can regenerate after antibiotic treatment, making it very difficult to get rid of all the biofilms that are embedded in the infection [31, 37]. Permanent cells are highly antibiotic resistant, metabolically dormant non-dividing bacteria that acquire this phenotype in the presence of antibiotics; once the antibiotics are removed, they resume metabolic activity and because drug-resistant cells are a

source of recurrent chronic infections, they play an important role in the challenge of treating biofilms with antibiotics [36]. Environments such as pH metabolites and oxygen levels in the biofilm can alter the efficacy of antibiotics [38]. Ernest et al. [39] found that biofilms could survive slight changes in pH and could only partially eradicate the biofilms of Staphylococcus aureus in common topical adjuvant therapies (such as povidone-iodohypochlorite or hydrogen peroxide).

3.4 Microbiology of Periprosthetic Infection (PJI)

Infection control after total knee arthroplasty (TKA) is difficult, mainly because biofilm formation effectively protects pathogenic bacteria from antibiotics and host defense. For PJI biofilms, there is still a lack of adequate prevention, diagnosis, and treatment. There are new chemical and mechanical approaches to the treatment of biofilm infection, which will be important for the eradication of orthopedic infections in the future. Biofilms have been studied using topical and systemic antibiotics. Strategies for the prevention and treatment of biofilms include the use of surface coatings (including surface reserved antibiotic and metal oxide nanoparticle coatings) and the destruction of established biofilms by mechanical or pharmacological means. It has been reported that the most common pathogens of PJI in the USA are Staphylococcus aureus and Staphylococcus epidermidis, while the most common pathogens in Europe are thrombin negative Staphylococcus aureus and Staphylococcus enterococcus, followed by Staphylococcus aureus and Staphylococcus enterococcus [40]. Benito et al. [41] collected 2288 cases (hip and knee joint) for microbiological diagnosis in 15 years, and the result was that the gram-positive bacteria accounted for 78% (mainly Staphylococcus), gram-negative bacteria accounted for 28%, and anaerobe bacteria accounted for 7%. Methicillin-resistant Staphylococcus aureus (MRSA) is a tricky problem, leading to more complications in postoperative functional recovery and reoperation rates than other pathogens [42]. M. tuberculosis is also a pathogen leading to artificial joint infection. In 2013, Kim et al. [43] reported a systematic evaluation of mycobacterium tuberculosis infection. Jakobs et al. [44] found that candida accounted for about 80% of fungal PJIs (36 out of 45 cases). PJI caused by mycoplasma is extremely rare in clinical practice. Qiu et al. [45] reported 1 case of mycoplasma infection after TKA.

3.5 Methods for the Detection of Biofilms

Recent studies have focused on the detection of the formation and destruction of biofilms. The improvement of the detection method of biofilm bacteria is usually based on the growth of culture. The presence of biofilm leads to negative culture of bacteria, which increases the difficulty of diagnosis. Parvizi et al. [46] proposed the latest diagnostic criteria for infection around joint prosthesis in 2018: the main criteria and diagnostic method for infection around joint prosthesis are the presence of positive culture or sinus tract for two or more times. Serum c-reactive protein (>10 mg/L), D-dimer (>860 living g/L), and serum erythrocyte sedimentation rate (>30 mm/h) were 2, 2, and 1, respectively. In addition, elevated leukocyte count in the fluid (>3109/L), leucocyte esterase (++), leucocyte percentage (>80%), and syn c-reactive protein (>6.9 mg/L) scored 3, 3, 3, 2, and 1, respectively. Patients with a total score of 6 are considered to be infected, while patients with a score of 2–5 need intraoperative results to confirm the diagnosis. The results of positive histology, purulent, and single positive culture were 3, 3, and 2 points, respectively. Combined with preoperative scores, a total of 6 points were considered infected, 4–5 points were inconclusive, and 3 points were not infected. The diagnostic criteria were 97.7% sensitivity and 99.5% specificity as defined by the society for musculoskeletal infection (79.3%) and the international consensus meeting (86.9%). Despite the introduction of the new diagnostic criteria, there are still limitations. In some cases, patients who do not meet the diagnostic criteria may still be infected.

Therefore, other methods should be used to improve the diagnosis of PJI, especially those related to body recognition. PCR has been used to identify a variety of bacteria in biofilms [47] and has been shown to be more sensitive to tissue culture [48, 49]. Other methods for detecting biofilms include fluorescence in situ hybridization (FISH) and DNA microarrays [50–52]. FISH can identify bacteria in culture negative infection, reduce false positive by improving the recognition of environmental bacterial pollution, detect cross-reactivity with human tissues, and eliminate viable staining dead bacteria [52]. DNA microarrays, which can simultaneously evaluate the DNA of thousands of bacteria, are cheaper, faster, and more productive than PCR [52]. Biofilm imaging technology also includes confocal laser scanning microscopy [53] and scanning electron microscope. Confocal laser scanning microscopy can show live bacteria in biofilms and even culture of negative PJI, while scanning electron microscopy can see the aggregation of microbial cells [52]. However, limitations of these imaging techniques include cost of use and training requirements for obtaining the best images. Sonication refers to the use of ultrasound to degrade cell viruses, etc. It can also be used to detect PJI. It improves the sensitivity and specificity of culture to microbial detection, and even the samples obtained after antibiotic treatment can be used to detect bacteria [52].

3.6 The Treatment of PJI Biofilm After TKA

A number of new treatments are being developed, focusing on ways to improve bacterial clearance and destruction of biofilms, thereby reducing bacterial resistance to antibiotics and immune defenses. New antibiotic research can improve the penetration of bone and joint tissue, which may increase activity against biofilm bacteria. These antibiotics (such as tizolamide phosphate and oliban star) target gram-positive bacteria, including methicillin-resistant Staphylococcus aureus (MSSA), methicillin-resistant Staphylococcus aureus (MRSA), vancomycin-resistant Staphylococcus aureus, and methicillin-resistant coagulase-negative Staphylococcus [54, 55]. In clinical biology studies, it has been found that some drugs used for tumor chemotherapy can effectively combat biofilm activity. For example, cisplatin 5-fluorouracil and mitomycin C have been reported to be able to remove bacteria embedded in the biofilm. These chemotherapeutic drugs may be the subject of research in the emerging field in the future [56]. Currently, two antibiotics with anti-biofilm activity are commonly used: rifampicin (inhibition of transcription) and meropenem (inhibition of cell wall biosynthesis) [57, 58].

Antibiotic bone cement can be used to prevent biofilm formation, which is an evidence-based placement method to prevent biofilm formation [59], but there is growing evidence that a strategy based on the surface properties of the implant (containing some specific metals) may play a role in preventing biofilm formation. The surface properties of the implant affect the ability of the bacteria to adhere to and form biofilms [60]. Basic scientific research suggests that current implant materials, such as vitamin E hybrid ultra-high molecular weight polyethylene (ve-pe) and ceramics, may offer a degree of protection against the formation of biofilms [61–64]. Many researchers are now trying to develop an anti-biofilm coating on the surface of the implant, including changing the surface shape of the implant material using the material's inherent antibacterial properties (such as when coated with silver or copper) and placing antibiotics on the surface of the implant [65]. The surface of the implant can be modified to reduce the risk of PJI, with the aim of achieving a bactericidal coating that does not inhibit bone growth, is biocompatible and durable. For example, silver oxide, titanium oxide, copper oxide, iodine, and other nanoparticles have bactericidal effects on gram-positive and negative-positive bacteria, and silver oxide particles have been shown to inhibit the formation of biofilms on the catheter. Secinti et al. [66] studied in the rabbit model and concluded that nanometer silver ion coated implants were as safe as uncoated titanium screws, and nanometer silver ion

coated implants could prevent the formation and infection of biofilms. Silver-containing hydroxyapatite (Ag-HA) coating can reduce the formation of MRSA biofilm both in vivo and in vitro, which may be an effective method to reduce implant-related infections. Silver-containing hydroxyapatite (Ag-HA) coating can reduce the formation of MRSA biofilm both in vivo and in vitro, which may be an effective method to reduce implant-related infections [67]. Immunotherapy, especially monoclonal antibodies, can be used as an alternative and adjunct to antibiotic therapy, and multiple targets of antibody therapy can be studied in the preclinical stage [68]. Bacteriophages are another potential therapy for biofilm-related bacteria. Bacteriophages are naturally occurring viruses that target and kill bacteria and can destroy the biofilm matrix, potentially affecting metabolically active bacteria and persistent cells because bacteriophages remain active at low temperatures and in low nutrient status [4].

3.7 Conclusions

The main reason for the difficulty in treating PJI after TKA is the formation of biofilm by pathogenic microorganisms. Biofilms prevent antibiotics and host defense, promote bacterial nutrition, allow interactions between bacteria (quorum sensing), and allow the spread of drug resistance. While acute PJI can be identified by clinical and planktonic bacterial cultures, chronic PJI is associated with the production of biofilms by pathogens, significantly reducing the ability to prevent diagnosis and treat infection. Current biofilm treatment strategies include antibiotics and surgery, and other innovative treatment strategies, including new antibiotics with improved permeability, drug Immunotherapy against persistent bacteria, antimicrobial peptide nanoparticles and bacteriophage ultrasound, are also being improved.

Although some of these strategies are still in the early stages of research, the results of future studies may revolutionize the prevention and treatment of PJI.

References

1. Blanco JF, Díaz A, Melchor FR, et al. Risk factors for periprosthetic joint infection after total knee arthroplasty. Arch Orthop Trauma Surg. 2020;140(2):239–45. https://doi.org/10.1007/s00402-019-03304-6.
2. Ritter MA, Farris A. Outcome of infected total joint replacement. Orthopedics. 2010;33(3) https://doi.org/10.3928/01477447-20100129-09.
3. Lum ZC, Natsuhara KM, Shelton TJ, et al. Mortality during total knee periprosthetic joint infection. J Arthroplasty. 2018;33(12):3783–8. https://doi.org/10.1016/j.arth.2018.08.021.
4. Akanda ZZ, Taha M, Abdelbary H. Current review-the rise of bacteriophage as a unique therapeutic platform in treating peri-prosthetic joint infections. J. Orthop. Res. 2018;36(4):1051–60.
5. Oliva A, Pavone P, D'Abramo A, et al. Role of sonication in the microbiological diagnosis of implant-associated infections: beyond the orthopedic prosthesis. Adv Exp Med Biol. 2016;897:85–102. https://doi.org/10.1007/5584_2015_5007.
6. Rochford ETJ, Richards RG, Moriarty TF. Influence of material on the development of device-associated infections. Clin Microbiol Infect. 2012;18(12):1162–7. https://doi.org/10.1111/j.1469-0691.2012.04002.x.
7. He W, Wang D, Ye Z, et al. Application of a nanotechnology antimicrobial spray to prevent lower urinary tract infection: a multicenter urology trial. J Transl Med. 2012;10:S14. https://doi.org/10.1186/1479-5876-10-S1-S14.
8. Frei E, Hodgkiss-Harlow K, Rossi Peter J, et al. Microbial pathogenesis of bacterial biofilms: a causative factor of vascular surgical site infection. Vasc Endovascular Surg. 2011;45(8):688–96. https://doi.org/10.1177/1538574411419528.
9. Aubin GG, Portillo ME, Trampuz A, et al. Propionibacterium acnes, an emerging pathogen: from acne to implant-infections, from phylotype to resistance. Med Mal Infect. 2014;44(6):241–50. https://doi.org/10.1016/j.medmal.2014.02.004.
10. Tande AJ, Patel R. Prosthetic joint infection. Clin Microbiol Rev. 2014;27(2):302–45. https://doi.org/10.1128/CMR.00111-13.
11. Zimmerli W, Waldvogel FA, Vaudaux P, et al. Pathogenesis of foreign body infection: description and characteristics of an animal model. J Infect Dis. 1982;146(4):487–97. https://doi.org/10.1093/infdis/146.4.487.
12. Hall-Stoodley L, Costerton JW, Stoodley P. Bacterial biofilms: from the natural environment to infectious diseases. Nat Rev Microbiol. 2004;2(2):95–108. https://doi.org/10.1038/nrmicro821.
13. Gbejuade HO, Lovering AM, Webb JC. The role of microbial biofilms in prosthetic joint infections. Acta Orthop. 2015;86(2):147–58. https://doi.org/10.3109/17453674.2014.966290.
14. Thurlow LR, Hanke ML, Fritz T, et al. Staphylococcus aureus biofilms prevent macrophage phagocytosis and attenuate inflammation in vivo. J Immunol. 2011;186(11):6585–96. https://doi.org/10.4049/jimmunol.1002794.
15. Flemming HC, Wingender J. The biofilm matrix. Nat Rev Microbiol. 2010;8(9):623–33. https://doi.org/10.1038/nrmicro2415.
16. Gilbert P, Allison DG, McBain AJ. Biofilms in vitro and in vivo: do singular mechanisms imply cross-resistance? J Appl Microbiol. 2002;92:98S–110S. https://doi.org/10.1046/j.1365-2672.92.5s1.5.x.
17. Arciola CR, Campoccia D, Speziale P, et al. Biofilm formation in Staphylococcus implant infections. A review of molecular mechanisms and implications for biofilm-resistant materials. Biomaterials. 2012;33(26):5967–82. https://doi.org/10.1016/j.biomaterials.2012.05.031.
18. Campoccia D, Montanaro L, Arciola CR. The significance of infection related to orthopedic devices and issues of antibiotic resistance. Biomaterials. 2006;27(11):2331–9. https://doi.org/10.1016/j.biomaterials.2005.11.044.
19. Mooney JA, Pridgen EM, Manasherob R, et al. Periprosthetic bacterial biofilm and quorum sensing. JOrthop Res. 2018;36(9):2331–9. https://doi.org/10.1002/jor.24019.
20. Schaefer AL, Greenberg EP, Oliver CM, et al. A new class of homoserine lactone quorum-sensing signals. Nature. 2008;454(7204):595–9. https://doi.org/10.1038/nature07088.
21. Fuqua C, Parsek MR, Greenberg EP. Regulation of gene expression by cell-to-cell communication: acyl-homoserine lactone quorum sensing. Annu Rev Genet. 2001;35:439–68. https://doi.org/10.1146/annurev.genet.35.102401.090913.
22. Costerton JW, Stewart PS, Greenberg EP. Bacterial biofilms: a common cause of persistent infections. Science. 1999;284(5418):1318–22. https://doi.org/10.1126/science.284.5418.1318.
23. Høiby N, Bjarnsholt TS, Givskov M, et al. Antibiotic resistance of bacterial biofilms. Int J Antimicrob Agents. 2010;35(4):322–32. https://doi.org/10.1016/j.ijantimicag.2009.12.011.
24. Williams P, Cámara M. Quorum sensing and environmental adaptation in Pseudomonas aeruginosa: a tale of regulatory networks and multifunctional signal molecules. CurrOpin Microbiol. 2009;12(2):182–91. https://doi.org/10.1016/j.mib.2009.01.005.
25. Sharma M, Visai L, Bragheri F, et al. Toluidine blue-mediated photodynamic effects on staphylococcal biofilms. Antimicrob. Agents Chemother. 2008;52(1):299–305. https://doi.org/10.1128/AAC.00988-07.
26. Olwal CO, Ang'ienda PO, Onyango DM, et al. Susceptibility patterns and the role of extracellular DNA in Staphylococcus epidermidis biofilm resistance to physico-chemical stress exposure. BMC

Microbiol. 2018;18(1):40. https://doi.org/10.1186/s12866-018-1183-y₀ .

27. Kostenko V, Salek MM, Sattari P, et al. Staphylococcus aureus biofilm formation and tolerance to antibiotics in response to oscillatory shear stresses of physiological levels. FEMS Immunol Med Microbiol. 2010;59(3):421–31. https://doi.org/10.1111/j.1574-695X.2010.00694.x.

28. Gil C, Solano C, Burgui S, et al. Biofilm matrix exoproteins induce a protective immune response against Staphylococcus aureus biofilm infection. Infect Immun. 2014;82(3):1017–29. https://doi.org/10.1128/IAI.01419-13.

29. Harmsen M, Yang L, Pamp SJ, et al. An update on Pseudomonas aeruginosa biofilm formation, tolerance, and dispersal. FEMS Immunol Med Microbiol. 2010;59(3):253–68. https://doi.org/10.1111/j.1574-695X.2010.00690.x.

30. LI C, Renz N, Trampuz A. Management of periprosthetic joint infection. Hip Pelvis. 2018;30(3):138–46. https://doi.org/10.5371/hp.2018.30.3.138.

31. Lazăr V, Chifiriuc MC. Medical significance and new therapeutical strategies for biofilm associated infections. Roum Arch Microbiol Immunol. 2010;69(3):125–38.

32. Singh R, Ray P, Das A, et al. Penetration of antibiotics through Staphylococcus aureus and Staphylococcus epidermidis biofilms. J Antimicrob Chemother. 2010;65(9):1955–8. https://doi.org/10.1093/jac/dkq257.

33. Bjarnsholt T, Ciofu O, Molin S, et al. Applying insights from biofilm biology to drug development - can a new approach be developed? Nat Rev Drug Discov. 2013;12(10):791–808. https://doi.org/10.1038/nrd4000.

34. Fux CA, Costerton JW, Stewart PS, et al. Survival strategies of infectious biofilms. Trends Microbiol. 2005;13(1):34–40. https://doi.org/10.1016/j.tim.2004.11.010.

35. Donlan RM. Role of biofilms in antimicrobial resistance. ASAIO J. 2000;46(6):S47–52. https://doi.org/10.1097/00002480-200011000-00037.

36. Lewis K. Persister cells. Annu Rev Microbiol. 2010;64:357–72. https://doi.org/10.1146/annurev.micro.112408.134306.

37. Fauvart M, De GVN, Michiels J. Role of persister cells in chronic infections: clinical relevance and perspectives on anti-persister therapies. J Med Microbiol. 2011;60:699–709. https://doi.org/10.1099/jmm.0.030932-0.

38. Stewart PS, Costerton JW. Antibiotic resistance of bacteria in biofilms. Lancet. 2001;358(9276):135–8. https://doi.org/10.1016/s0140-6736(01)05321-1.

39. Ernest EP, Machi AS, Karolcik BA, et al. Topical adjuvants incompletely remove adherent Staphylococcus aureus from implant materials. J. Orthop. Res. 2018;36(6):1599–604. https://doi.org/10.1002/jor.23804.

40. Aggarwal VK, Bakhshi H, Ecker NU, et al. Organism profile in periprosthetic joint infection: pathogens differ at two arthroplasty infection referral centers in Europe and in the United States. J Knee Surg. 2014;27(5):399–405.

41. Benito N, Franco M, Ribera A, et al. Time trends in the aetiology of prosthetic joint infections: a multicentre cohort study. Clin Microbiol Infect. 2016;22:732.e1–8.

42. Laudermilch DJ, Fedorka CJ, Heyl A, Rao N, McGough RL. Outcomes of revision total knee arthroplasty after methicillin-resistant Staphylococcus aureus infection. Clin Orthop Relat Res. 2010;468:2067–73.

43. Kim SJ, Kim JH. Late onset Mycobacterium tuberculosis infection after total knee arthroplasty: a systematic review and pooled analysis. Scand J Infect Dis. 2013;45:907–14.

44. Jakobs O, Schoof B, Klatte TO, Schmidl S, Fensky F, Guenther D, et al. Fungal periprosthetic joint infection in total knee arthroplasty: a systematic review. Orthop Rev (Pavia). 2015;7:5623.

45. Qiu HJ, Lu WP, Li M, et al. The infection of Mycoplasma hominis after total knee replacement: case report and literature review. Chin J Traumatol. 2017;20(4):243–5.

46. Parvizi J, Tan TL, Goswami K, et al. The 2018 definition of periprosthetic hip and knee infection: an evidence-based and validated criteria. J Arthroplasty. 2018;33(5):1309–1314.e2.

47. Xu Y, Rudkjøbing VB, Simonsen O, et al. Bacterial diversity in suspected prosthetic joint infections: an exploratory study using 16S rRNA gene analysis. FEMS Immunol Med Microbiol. 2012;65(2):291–304. https://doi.org/10.1111/j.1574-695X.2012.00949.x.

48. Cazanave C, Greenwood-Quaintance KE, Hanssen AD, et al. Rapid molecular microbiologic diagnosis of prosthetic joint infection. J Clin Microbiol. 2013;51(7):2280–7. https://doi.org/10.1128/JCM.00335-13.

49. Bjerkan G, Witsø E, Nor A, et al. A comprehensive microbiological evaluation of fifty-four patients undergoing revision surgery due to prosthetic joint loosening. J Med Microbiol. 2012;61:572–81. https://doi.org/10.1099/jmm.0.036087-0.

50. Tzeng A, Tzeng TH, Vasdev S, et al. Treating periprosthetic joint infections as biofilms: key diagnosis and management strategies. Diagn Microbiol Infect Dis. 2015;81(3):192–200. https://doi.org/10.1016/j.diagmicrobio.2014.08.018.

51. McDowell A, Patrick S. Evaluation of nonculture methods for the detection of prosthetic hip biofilms. Clin Orthop Relat Res. 2005;(437):74–82. https://doi.org/10.1097/01.blo.0000175123.58428.93.

52. Shoji MM, Chen AF. Biofilms in periprosthetic joint infections: a review of diagnostic modalities, current treatments, and future directions. J Knee Surg. 2020;33(2):119–31. https://doi.org/10.1055/s-0040-1701214.

53. Stoodley P, Nistico L, Johnson S, et al. Direct demonstration of viable Staphylococcus aureus biofilms

in an infected total joint arthroplasty. A case report. J Bone Joint Surg Am. 2008;90(8):1751–8. https://doi.org/10.2106/JBJS.G.00838.

54. Crotty Matthew P, Tamara K, Burnham CA, et al. New Gram-positive agents: the next generation of oxazolidinones and lipoglycopeptides. J Clin Microbiol. 2016;54(9):2225–32. https://doi.org/10.1128/JCM.03395-15.

55. Brade KD, Rybak JM, Rybak MJ. Oritavancin: a new lipoglycopeptide antibiotic in the treatment of Gram-positive infections. Infect Dis Ther. 2016;5(1):1–15. https://doi.org/10.1007/s40121-016-0103-4.

56. McConoughey SJ, Howlin R, Granger JF, et al. Biofilms in periprosthetic orthopedic infections. Future Microbiol. 2014;9(8):987–1007. https://doi.org/10.2217/fmb.14.64.

57. Mihailescu R, Furustrand TU, Corvec S, et al. High activity of Fosfomycin and Rifampin against methicillin-resistant staphylococcus aureus biofilm in vitro and in an experimental foreign-body infection model. Antimicrob Agents Chemother. 2014;58(5):2547–53. https://doi.org/10.1128/AAC.02420-12.

58. Viganor L, Galdino ACM, Nunes APF, et al. Anti-Pseudomonas aeruginosa activity of 1,10-phenanthroline-based drugs against both planktonic- and biofilm-growing cells. J Antimicrob Chemother. 2016;71(1):128–34. https://doi.org/10.1093/jac/dkv292.

59. Peñalba AP, Furustrand TU, Bétrisey B, et al. Activity of bone cement loaded with daptomycin alone or in combination with gentamicin or PEG600 against Staphylococcus epidermidis biofilms. Injury. 2015;46(2):249–53. https://doi.org/10.1016/j.injury.2014.11.014.

60. Mitik DN, Wang J, Mocanasu RC, et al. Impact of nano-topography on bacterial attachment. Biotechnol J. 2008;3(4):536–44. https://doi.org/10.1002/biot.200700244.

61. Banche G, Allizond V, Bracco P, et al. Interplay between surface properties of standard, vitamin E blended and oxidised ultra high molecular weight polyethylene used in total joint replacement and adhesion of Staphylococcus aureus and Escherichia coli. Bone Joint J. 2014;(4):497–501. https://doi.org/10.1302/0301-620X.96B4/32895.

62. Mi K, Shobuike T, Moro T, et al. Prevention of bacterial adhesion and biofilm formation on a vitamin E-blended, cross-linked polyethylene surface with a poly(2-methacryloyloxyethyl phosphorylcholine) layer. Acta Biomater. 2015;24:24–34. https://doi.org/10.1016/j.actbio.2015.05.034.

63. Williams DL, Vinciguerra J, Lerdahl JM, et al. Does vitamin E-blended UHMWPE prevent biofilm formation? Clin Orthop Relat Res. 2015;473(3):928–35. https://doi.org/10.1007/s11999-014-3673-z.

64. Lass R, Giurea A, Kubista B, et al. Bacterial adherence to different components of total hip prosthesis in patients with prosthetic joint infection. Int Orthop. 2014;38(8):1597–602. https://doi.org/10.1007/s00264-014-2358-2.

65. Getzlaf MA, Lewallen EA, Kremers HM, et al. Multidisciplinary antimicrobial strategies for improving orthopaedic implants to prevent prosthetic joint infections in hip and knee. J Orthop Res. 2016;34(2):177–86. https://doi.org/10.1002/jor.23068.

66. Secinti KD, Özalp H, Attar A, et al. Nanoparticle silver ion coatings inhibit biofilm formation on titanium implants. J Clin Neurosci. 2011;18(3):391–5. https://doi.org/10.1016/j.jocn.2010.06.022.

67. Singh G, Hameister R, Feuerstein B, et al. Low-frequency sonication may alter surface topography of endoprosthetic components and damage articular cartilage without eradicating biofilms completely. J Biomed Mater Res Part B Appl Biomater. 2014;102:1835–46.

68. Raafat D, Otto M, Reppschläger K, et al. Fighting Staphylococcus aureus biofilms with monoclonal antibodies. Trends Microbiol. 2019;27(4):303–22. https://doi.org/10.1016/j.tim.2018.12.009.

69. Roe D, Karandikar B, Bonn SN, et al. Antimicrobial surface functionalization of plastic catheters by silver nanoparticles. J Antimicrob Chemother. 2008;61(4):869–76. https://doi.org/10.1093/jac/dkn034.

70. Ueno M, Miyamoto H, Tsukamoto M, et al. Staphylococcus aureus silver-containing hydroxyapatite coating reduces biofilm formation by methicillin-resistant in vitro and in vivo. Biomed Res Int. 2016;2016:8070597. https://doi.org/10.1155/2016/8070597.

In-Vitro and In-Vivo Models for the Study of Prosthetic Joint Infections

Nicholas Mannering [ID], Raj Narulla, and Benjamin Lenane

4.1 In-Vitro Models of PJI

In-vitro, from the Latin meaning "within the glass", refers to the study of processes taking place outside a living organism. This can take many forms and specific to the study of PJI involves assays developed to identify bacterial properties [1–3], biofilm formation [1, 4–9], and the response to antimicrobial agents [5, 10–16]. Moriarty et al. [17] outline several key areas for in-vitro modelling of PJI, including (1) bacterial species to be tested; (2) antimicrobial efficacy/activity; and (3) if the in-vitro study is deemed suitable to proceed to in-vivo testing.

4.1.1 Bacterial Adherence

Gram-positive bacteria demonstrate persistent adherence to prostheses, which has influenced prosthetic design. The adherence of *Staphylococcus epidermidis* strains to orthopaedic grade hydroxyapatite-coated stainless steel screws was examined in-vitro by Arciola et al.

[18]. Coated prostheses had significantly lower bacterial adherence compared with uncoated metal prostheses. An earlier in-vitro study also concluded that *S. aureus* colonized both metal prostheses and ultra-high molecular weight polyethylene (UHMWPE) more rapidly than *S. epidermidis* [19]. It was also shown that *S. aureus* had an affinity to metal, whereas *S. epidermidis* preferentially colonized UHMWPE. As a potential therapeutic option, vitamin E impregnated UHMWPE is associated with reduced bacterial adherence of *S. aureus* and *S. epidermidis* strains [20], in addition to providing oxidative protection and lower wear rates [21–24].

4.1.2 Biofilm

The ability to form biofilm plays a crucial role in the pathogenesis of PJI, for both gram-positive and gram-negative bacteria [25, 26]. This has major implications for in-vitro studies, which have assessed the structural and protective qualities of the polymeric matrix, polysaccharides, proteins, and extracellular DNA which these bacteria generate and are imbedded within. Bacterial populations may harbour key gene loci implicated in biofilm formation, such as the ica gene encoding polysaccharide intracellular adhesion [27]. However, other researchers have shown that ica genes are not required [28], demonstrating the complexity and variability of bio-

N. Mannering (✉)
The University of Melbourne,
Parkville, VIC, Australia

R. Narulla
Prince of Wales Hospital, Randwick, NSW, Australia

B. Lenane
The University of New South Wales,
Sydney, NSW, Australia

© ISAKOS 2022
U. G. Longo et al. (eds.), *Infection in Knee Replacement,*
https://doi.org/10.1007/978-3-030-81553-0_4

"

film formation. Thomson et al. [3] described that *Pseudomonas aeruginosa* generated significantly increased biofilm compared to all *E. coli* strains tested, suggesting that this enhanced activity correlates with more aggressive in-vivo models of *P. aeruginosa* PJI. Investigators agree that biofilm is difficult to study in-vitro due to the protection against antibiotics that biofilm provides, along with bacterial species variation within biofilm and its propensity for prosthetic adherence.

4.1.3 Antimicrobial Efficacy

Adequate antimicrobial efficacy is crucial for controlling PJI, in terms of either definitive cure or long-term suppression. This is highlighted by the increasing incidence of difficult-to-treat infections, such as gram-negative PJI [29, 30] and methicillin resistant Staphylococcus Aureus (MRSA) [31]. Results of an in-vitro study utilizing a standardized medium, the Calgary Biofilm Device [32], demonstrated that Rifampicin and Tigecycline had low minimum biofilm eradication concentrations (MBEC), highlighting their antibiofilm activity against *S. aureus* and *S. epidermidis* which were isolated from patients diagnosed with PJI [33]. Similar results have been shown in other in-vitro studies [6], as well as in clinical evidence that supports the use of Rifampicin for PJI [31, 34].

In addition to systemic antibiotics, localized therapy using antibiotic-loaded cement spacers has demonstrated good efficacy in-vitro. Antibiotic elutions reach peak values within the first 2 or 3 days, inhibiting bacterial growth of *S. epidermidis* for 14–30 days [13]. Whilst there has been concern regarding the mechanical strength of antibiotic-loaded bone cement [35], a recent in-vitro study of a double layered spacer demonstrated beneficial biomechanical and drug-eluting properties [36]. Other constructs consisting of a vancomycin-loaded hydroxyapatite/poly amino acid scaffold [37] show consistent bactericidal effect on *S. aureus* and MRSA in-vitro, with good drug-eluting delivery over 38 days and also promote osteogenesis.

4.1.4 Modelling for Risk Factors

Some risk factors associated with PJI, including diabetes and obesity [38, 39], may also be studied in-vitro. It has been shown that elevated glucose levels aid the formation of biofilm [40] in an *E. faecalis* model. This may relate to findings that even perioperative hyperglycaemia in nondiabetic patients influences infection rates [41]. Whilst helpful, in-vitro studies have limited utility in this area, and these associations are potentially more relevant for in-vivo models.

4.1.5 Limitations

Whilst in-vitro models are effective for studying the cellular and biochemical responses to microorganisms and antibiotics, several elements are still lacking. Firstly, it is impossible to fully replicate in-vitro the complex bio-cellular environment that exists in an infected prosthetic joint. Secondly, bone metabolism and inflammatory responses occur in a dynamic weight bearing joint, which should be replicated experimentally. Thirdly, effectiveness of treatment needs to be examined in a living model which replicates as close as possible the biomechanical, immunological, and pharmacological dynamics in clinical PJI. Hence, in-vivo models in a controlled and ethical environment are required as the next step in the study of PJI pathogenesis and management.

4.2 In-Vivo Models of PJI

In-vivo models of prosthetic joint infection have developed significantly since Rodet's first experimental demonstrations in 1884 [42]. Rodet confirmed that osteomyelitis could be induced by inoculation of a "micrococcus" into rabbits, which formed localized infection at the femoral and tibial metaphysis. As a more recent guide, Carli et al. [43] described the ideal characteristics of a clinically representative model of PJI. In such a model: (1) biofilm can be formed on the prosthesis surface; (2) prosthesis materials should be similar to clinical materials and create a similar intra-articular environment; (3) animals chosen should have similar musculoskeletal and immunological systems compared with humans; and (4) bacteria, biofilm, and host immune responses can be measured quantitatively.

4.2.1 Animal Characteristics

The majority of in-vivo implant and prosthetic joint related infections have been modelled in rabbits [44], in particular the New Zealand rabbit. The use of rabbits presents several advantages, including their docility, relatively low costs, reasonable size, and ease of handling. In their review, Bottagisio et al. [44] identified that rabbit tibias were used in 60.9% of in-vivo surgical sites and rabbit femurs in 27% of surgical sites. However, due to their bone fragility, rabbits have been shown to have a high incidence of postoperative fracture [45]. Studies are further limited by the substantial biomechanical and kinematic differences between the rabbit knee and the human knee. Despite these limitations, rabbits are still the most widely used animals for PJI models.

The second most common model is the murine model [46], typically C57BL/6 wildtype mice [3, 47–51]. Some studies euthanized mice between 3 and 6 weeks for harvesting of bone/joint tissue and implants for sonication [3, 51]. Mice occupy less space than rabbits, are easy to monitor and maintain, and can be bioengineered to emit fluorescent signals from immune cells [50, 52].

4.2.2 Prosthetic Designs

Various prosthetic designs have been utilized to model PJI. One of the first animal models of PJI, performed in 1976, utilized stainless steel particles infected with *S. aureus* into the suprapatellar bursa of rabbits [53]. Since then, multiple iterations of implants have been described.

Determining the relevance of various animal prosthesis trials to the human total knee arthroplasty (TKA) can be difficult. For example,

Kirschner-wires (K-wires) have limitations in that the prosthesis is a non-weight bearing, non-articulating, stainless steel construct, as opposed to the titanium alloy (Ti-6Al-4V) and cobalt-chromium-molybdenum alloy in human TKA. Secondly, whilst tibial plateau replacement has been shown to develop biofilm [48], it is unable to replicate the biomechanical dynamics of a total anatomical prosthesis. Finally, there is minimal consensus on the type of animal prosthesis to best mimic TKA PJI [46], and authors appreciate the impracticality and difficulty of miniaturizing total joint prostheses in animals [17].

Nevertheless, PJI studies have been performed on knee joint arthroplasty designs in rabbits as early as 1996 [54]. Much later, having identified a deficiency in prosthetic designs, Carli et al. [48] were the first to apply a three-dimensional printed tibial prosthesis with Ti-6Al-4V in a PJI murine model. Using this prosthesis, Carli et al. [47] revised the tibial replacement with a mouse-sized vancomycin eluting cement spacer, mimicking the first stage of a standard two-stage revision procedure for PJI in humans. Mice treated with antibiotic spacers had significantly lower inflammatory markers, had more preserved tibial bone, and had no intra-articular purulence. Retrieved spacers demonstrated lower bacterial counts compared with Ti-6Al-4V implants, although they did not have the same effect in periprosthetic tissue, suggesting that local antimicrobial activity was limited to the joint.

4.2.3 Gram-Positive Models

Given the leading causative group of microorganisms for PJI is gram-positive [29, 55, 56], studies have strongly focused on developing animal models to replicate these pathogens in-vivo [48, 50, 51, 57–60].

In order to study intraoperative contamination, rabbit models of early onset PJI have involved the injection of a high inoculum of *S. aureus* derived from an infected joint replacement into the joint space of a rabbit [54]. It was found that <102 colony forming units (CFU) of

S. aureus are necessary to establish infection in a rabbit hip hemiarthroplasty model, compared with 104 CFU without a prosthetic implant. Infection remains within the joint space initially, then spreads to the adjacent metaphysis, with only the upper one-third of the metaphysis being involved at 3 weeks. Infection then progressed to involve the entire metaphysis of the periprosthetic bone. Other studies modelling haematogenous spread postulate that long bone osteomyelitis secondary to bacteraemia also begins in the metaphysis [42], then subsequently spreads to the implant. Furthermore, an in-vivo rabbit model of haematogenous spread demonstrated that lower levels of bacteraemia were needed to initiate PJI when inoculated in the immediate postoperative period compared to 3 weeks later [61].

In their mouse model of diabetes and implant related infection, Lovati et al. [62] demonstrated that diabetic mice showed severe infection resulting from *S. aureus* induced into the femur after an intramedullary pin implantation and an inability to respond to treatment with standard antibiotics alone. In their later work, Lovati et al. [63] showed that diabetic mice treated with a prostaglandin vasodilator in conjunction with antibiotics showed restrained signs of infection, pointing to a potential therapeutic combination in this at-risk group.

4.2.4 Gram-Negative Models

Gram-negative PJI was previously a rare complication, accounting for between 3 and 6% of all PJI [26, 64]. However, due to a rise in gram-negative PJI, between 15 and 36% [29, 30], a greater understanding of its pathogenesis will need to be developed. A model for the in-vivo experimentation of gram-negative PJI was established by Thompson et al. [3], which utilized an orthopaedic grade K-wire inserted into the femur of C57BL/6 mice with the implant protruding into the knee joint. Bacterial inoculation with either *P. aeruginosa* or *E. coli* was then injected into the joint before closure. It was found that 1 x 104 Colony Forming Units (CFU) of *P. aeruginosa* were needed to achieve ade-

quate bioluminescence imaging signals, compared to 1 x 105 CFU for *E. coli*. Furthermore, tissue and sonicated implants demonstrated greater bacterial growth of *P. aeruginosa* infected implants (67%), compared to *E. coli* infected implants (7%).

4.2.5 Biofilm Formation

Biofilm formation has been implicated as a major virulence mechanism of bacteria to adhere to tissue and protect the microorganism from antibiotics or the host immune system [65]. In a post-arthroplasty mouse model, Pribaz et al. [51] isolated four different strains of *S. aureus* and inoculated the knee joint of mice after implantation of stainless steel K-wire prostheses. All four strains demonstrated similar biofilm formation on scanning electron microscopy. In addition, these produced the same amount of infection induced inflammation as demonstrated by fluorescent neutrophil imaging. Thompson et al. [3] also utilized scanning electron microscopy for the detection of biofilm. They found implants infected with *P. aeruginosa* had more substantial biofilm formation on the intra-articular component of the implant, as well as adherent host immune cells, compared with *E. coli*. These results, together with the greater bacterial growth, suggest *P. aeruginosa* infection to be a more problematic disease.

4.2.6 Immune Reactions

Flow cytometry is commonly used to identify cell infiltrates into joint tissue. Whilst fewer pathogens are required to trigger infection in the presence of prosthetic implants, such implants induce substantial migration of cells including neutrophils and macrophages [3, 54]. Instead of activating phagocytosis, immune cells attempt to break down biofilm by releasing cytokines [66], reactive oxygen intermediates, and degradative enzymes. This process is complicated, however, by the depletion of local oxygen levels by bacterial communities, as well as restricted blood perfusion [67]. Whilst most of these processes may be similar, it is important to recognize that inflammatory reactions in rodent models differ from humans; for example, no homolog of the human genes IL-26, CXCL8, and CXCR1 exists in mice. Furthermore, neutrophils are the predominant circulating leukocyte in humans, whilst lymphocytes circulate in higher ratios in mice [68].

4.2.7 Limitations

In-vivo studies identify many important aetiological and potential treatment factors for PJI, but still carry significant limitations. Studies in animals cannot translate directly to the periprosthetic environment in humans, due to differences in anatomy and biomechanical characteristics of animal bone, poorly reproducible prostheses, and other physiological, immunological, and genetic differences. Furthermore, the International Consensus on Orthopaedic Infection acknowledges that there is no established ideal prosthetic design for use in modelling PJI [46]. However, as with in-vitro models, the relevance and importance of in-vivo models will only strengthen with time and rigorous scientific application.

4.3 Conclusion

Orthopaedic surgeons and researchers are constantly evaluating the diagnostic tools and treatments for prosthetic joint infections [69, 70]. Although not without important limitations, in-vitro and in-vivo models will continue to be a relevant and growing research field to aid the management of PJI. Emerging technologies and advances, such as three-dimensional printing, manufacturing techniques, drug delivery systems, and gene specific therapies, will create exciting modelling opportunities for further study. The increase in total joint arthroplasties performed worldwide will drive orthopaedic surgeons to seek new and innovative ways to combat PJI. In a truly interdisciplinary field, in-vitro and in-vivo models of PJI will help solve unanswered questions in the management of this complicated disease, which represents a significant clinical challenge and considerable burden for the entire orthopaedic community.

References

1. Holmberg A, et al. Biofilm formation by Propionibacterium acnes is a characteristic of invasive isolates. Clin Microbiol Infect. 2009;15(8):787–95.
2. McConda DB, et al. A novel co-culture model of murine K12 osteosarcoma cells and S. aureus on common orthopedic implant materials: 'the race to the surface' studied in vitro. Biofouling. 2016;32(6):627–34.
3. Thompson JM, et al. Mouse model of Gram-negative prosthetic joint infection reveals therapeutic targets. JCI Insight. 2018;3(17).
4. O'Toole G. Microtiter dish biofilm formation assay. J Vis Exp. 2011;47:2437.
5. Ashton NN, et al. In vitro testing of a first-in-class tri-alkylnorspermidine-biaryl antibiotic in an anti-biofilm silicone coating. Acta Biomater. 2019;93:25–35.
6. Coraça-Huber DC, et al. Staphylococcus aureus biofilm formation and antibiotic susceptibility tests on polystyrene and metal surfaces. J Appl Microbiol. 2012;112(6):1235–43.
7. Dunne N, et al. In vitro study of the efficacy of acrylic bone cement loaded with supplementary amounts of gentamicin: effect on mechanical properties, antibiotic release, and biofilm formation. Acta Orthop. 2007;78(6):774–85.
8. Ghimire N, et al. Direct microscopic observation of human neutrophil-*Staphylococcus aureus* interaction in vitro suggests a potential mechanism for initiation of biofilm infection on an implanted medical device. Infect Immun. 2019;87(12):e00745.
9. Stoodley P, et al. Molecular and imaging techniques for bacterial biofilms in joint arthroplasty infections. Clin Orthop Relat Res. 2005;437:31–40.
10. Hendriks JG, et al. The release of gentamicin from acrylic bone cements in a simulated prosthesis-related interfacial gap. J Biomed Mater Res B Appl Biomater. 2003;64(1):1–5.
11. Hsu YH, et al. Vancomycin and ceftazidime in bone cement as a potentially effective treatment for knee periprosthetic joint infection. J Bone Joint Surg Am. 2017;99(3):223–31.
12. Jones Z, et al. A resorbable antibiotic eluting bone void filler for periprosthetic joint infection prevention. J Biomed Mater Res B Appl Biomater. 2016;104(8):1632–42.
13. Kelm J, et al. In vivo and in vitro studies of antibiotic release from and bacterial growth inhibition by antibiotic-impregnated polymethylmethacrylate hip spacers. Antimicrob Agents Chemother. 2006;50(1):332–5.

14. Li D, et al. The immobilization of antibiotic-loaded polymeric coatings on osteoarticular Ti implants for the prevention of bone infections. Biomater Sci. 2017;5(11):2337–46.

15. Scott CP, Higham PA. Antibiotic bone cement for the treatment of Pseudomonas aeruginosa in joint arthroplasty: comparison of tobramycin and gentamicin-loaded cements. J Biomed Mater Res B Appl Biomater. 2003;64(2):94–8.

16. Ueng SW, et al. Efficacy of vancomycin-releasing biodegradable poly(lactide-co-glycolide) antibiotics beads for treatment of experimental bone infection due to Staphylococcus aureus. J Orthop Surg Res. 2016;11(1):52.

17. Moriarty TF, et al. Recommendations for design and conduct of preclinical in vivo studies of orthopedic device-related infection. J Orthop Res. 2019;37(2):271–87.

18. Arciola CR, et al. Hydroxyapatite-coated orthopaedic screws as infection resistant materials: in vitro study. Biomaterials. 1999;20(4):323–7.

19. Barth E, et al. In vitro and in vivo comparative colonization of Staphylococcus aureus and Staphylococcus epidermidis on orthopaedic implant materials. Biomaterials. 1989;10(5):325–8.

20. Gómez-Barrena E, et al. Bacterial adherence on UHMWPE with vitamin E: an in vitro study. J Mater Sci Mater Med. 2011;22(7):1701–6.

21. Bracco P, Oral E. Vitamin E-stabilized UHMWPE for total joint implants: a review. Clin Orthop Relat Res. 2011;469(8):2286–93.

22. Lambert B, et al. Effects of vitamin E incorporation in polyethylene on oxidative degradation, wear rates, immune response, and infections in total joint arthroplasty: a review of the current literature. Int Orthop. 2019;43(7):1549–57.

23. Turner A, et al. The antioxidant and non-antioxidant contributions of vitamin E in vitamin E blended ultra-high molecular weight polyethylene for total knee replacement. J Mech Behav Biomed Mater. 2014;31:21–30.

24. Affatato S, et al. In vitro wear performance of standard, crosslinked, and vitamin-E-blended UHMWPE. J Biomed Mater Res A. 2012;100A(3):554–60.

25. Costerton W, et al. The application of biofilm science to the study and control of chronic bacterial infections. J Clin Invest. 2003;112(10):1466–77.

26. Del Pozo JL, Patel R. Clinical practice. Infection associated with prosthetic joints. N Engl J Med. 2009;361(8):787–94.

27. Galdbart JO, et al. Screening for Staphylococcus epidermidis markers discriminating between skin-flora strains and those responsible for infections of joint prostheses. J Infect Dis. 2000;182(1):351–5.

28. Nilsdotter-Augustinsson A, et al. Characterization of coagulase-negative staphylococci isolated from patients with infected hip prostheses: use of phenotypic and genotypic analyses, including tests for the presence of the Ica operon. Eur J Clin Microbiol Infect Dis. 2007;26(4):255–65.

29. Benito N, et al. Time trends in the aetiology of prosthetic joint infections: a multicentre cohort study. Clin Microbiol Infect. 2016;22(8):732.e1–8.

30. Jamei O, et al. Which orthopaedic patients are infected with gram-negative non-fermenting rods? J Bone Joint Infect. 2017;2(2):73–6.

31. Soriano A, et al. Treatment of acute post-surgical infection of joint arthroplasty. Clin Microbiol Infect. 2006;12(9):930–3.

32. Ceri H, et al. The Calgary biofilm device: new technology for rapid determination of antibiotic susceptibilities of bacterial biofilms. J Clin Microbiol. 1999;37(6):1771–6.

33. Molina-Manso D, et al. In vitro susceptibility of Staphylococcus aureus and Staphylococcus epidermidis isolated from prosthetic joint infections. J Antibiot (Tokyo). 2012;65(10):505–8.

34. Spitzmüller R, et al. Duration of antibiotic treatment and risk of recurrence after surgical management of orthopaedic device infections: a multicenter case-control study. BMC Musculoskelet Disord. 2019;20(1):184.

35. Lee SH, et al. Elution and mechanical strength of vancomycin-loaded bone cement: in vitro study of the influence of brand combination. PLoS One. 2016;11(11):e0166545.

36. Ikeda S, et al. Double-layered antibiotic-loaded cement spacer as a novel alternative for managing periprosthetic joint infection: an in vitro study. J Orthop Surg Res. 2018;13(1):322.

37. Cao Z, et al. In vitro and in vivo drug release and antibacterial properties of the novel vancomycin-loaded bone-like hydroxyapatite/poly amino acid scaffold. Int J Nanomedicine. 2017;12:1841–51.

38. Malinzak RA, et al. Morbidly obese, diabetic, younger, and unilateral joint arthroplasty patients have elevated total joint arthroplasty infection rates. J Arthroplast. 2009;24(6 Suppl):84–8.

39. Namba RS, Inacio MC, Paxton EW. Risk factors associated with deep surgical site infections after primary total knee arthroplasty: an analysis of 56,216 knees. J Bone Joint Surg Am. 2013;95(9):775–82.

40. Seneviratne CJ, et al. Effect of culture media and nutrients on biofilm growth kinetics of laboratory and clinical strains of Enterococcus faecalis. Arch Oral Biol. 2013;58(10):1327–34.

41. Mraovic B, et al. Perioperative hyperglycemia and postoperative infection after lower limb arthroplasty. J Diabetes Sci Technol. 2011;5(2):412–8.

42. Cremieux AC, Carbon C. Experimental models of bone and prosthetic joint infections. Clin Infect Dis. 1997;25(6):1295–302.

43. Carli AV, et al. Developing a clinically representative model of periprosthetic joint infection. J Bone Joint Surg Am. 2016;98(19):1666–76.

44. Bottagisio M, Coman C, Lovati AB. Animal models of orthopaedic infections. A review of rabbit models used to induce long bone bacterial infections. J Med Microbiol. 2019;68(4):506–37.

45. Mapara M, Thomas BS, Bhat KM. Rabbit as an animal model for experimental research. Dent Res J (Isfahan). 2012;9(1):111–8.

46. Jie K, et al. Prosthesis design of animal models of periprosthetic joint infection following total knee arthroplasty: a systematic review. PLoS One. 2019;14(10):e0223402.

47. Carli AV, et al. Vancomycin-loaded polymethylmethacrylate spacers fail to eradicate periprosthetic joint infection in a clinically representative mouse model. J Bone Joint Surg Am. 2018;100(11):e76.

48. Carli AV, et al. Quantification of peri-implant bacterial load and in vivo biofilm formation in an innovative, clinically representative mouse model of periprosthetic joint infection. J Bone Joint Surg Am. 2017;99(6):e25.

49. Sheppard WL, et al. Novel in vivo mouse model of shoulder implant infection. J Shoulder Elb Surg. 2020;29:1412.

50. Bernthal NM, et al. A mouse model of post-arthroplasty Staphylococcus aureus joint infection to evaluate in vivo the efficacy of antimicrobial implant coatings. PLoS One. 2010;5(9):e12580.

51. Pribaz JR, et al. Mouse model of chronic post-arthroplasty infection: noninvasive in vivo bioluminescence imaging to monitor bacterial burden for long-term study. J Orthop Res. 2012;30(3):335–40.

52. Bernthal NM, et al. Combined in vivo optical and μCT imaging to monitor infection, inflammation, and bone anatomy in an orthopaedic implant infection in mice. J Vis Exp. 2014;92:e51612.

53. Schurman DJ, Johnson BL Jr, Amstutz HC. Knee joint infections with Staphylococcus aureus and Micrococcus species. J Bone Joint Surg Am. 1975;57(1):40–9.

54. Belmatoug N, et al. A new model of experimental prosthetic joint infection due to methicillin-resistant Staphylococcus aureus: a microbiologic, histopathologic, and magnetic resonance imaging characterization. J Infect Dis. 1996;174(2):414–7.

55. Benito N, et al. The different microbial etiology of prosthetic joint infections according to route of acquisition and time after prosthesis implantation, including the role of multidrug-resistant organisms. J Clin Med. 2019;8(5):673.

56. Tande AJ, Patel R. Prosthetic joint infection. Clin Microbiol Rev. 2014;27(2):302–45.

57. Achermann Y, et al. Factors associated with rifampin resistance in staphylococcal periprosthetic joint infections (PJI): a matched case-control study. Infection. 2013;41(2):431–7.

58. Bernthal NM, et al. Protective role of IL-1β against post-arthroplasty Staphylococcus aureus infection. J Orthop Res. 2011;29(10):1621–6.

59. Das SS, et al. (99m)Tc-ciprofloxacin scintigraphy in rabbit model of prosthetic joint infection. J Nucl Med. 2003;44(2):317–9; author reply 319–20.

60. Scherr TD, et al. Mouse model of post-arthroplasty Staphylococcus epidermidis joint infection. Methods Mol Biol. 2014;1106:173–81.

61. Southwood RT, et al. Infection in experimental hip arthroplasties. J Bone Joint Surg Br. 1985;67(2):229–31.

62. Lovati AB, et al. Diabetic mouse model of orthopaedic implant-related Staphylococcus aureus infection. PLoS One. 2013;8(6):e67628.

63. Lovati AB, et al. Does PGE_1 vasodilator prevent orthopaedic implant-related infection in diabetes? Preliminary results in a mouse model. PLoS One. 2014;9(4):e94758.

64. Zimmerli W, Trampuz A, Ochsner PE. Prosthetic-joint infections. N Engl J Med. 2004;351(16):1645–54.

65. Donlan RM, Costerton JW. Biofilms: survival mechanisms of clinically relevant microorganisms. Clin Microbiol Rev. 2002;15(2):167–93.

66. Heim CE, et al. IL-12 promotes myeloid-derived suppressor cell recruitment and bacterial persistence during Staphylococcus aureus orthopedic implant infection. J Immunol. 2015;194(8):3861–72.

67. Emslie KR, Fenner LM, Nade SM. Acute haematogenous osteomyelitis: II. The effect of a metaphyseal abscess on the surrounding blood supply. J Pathol. 1984;142(2):129–34.

68. Luthje FL, et al. The inflammatory response to bone infection - a review based on animal models and human patients. APMIS. 2020;128:275–86.

69. Parvizi J, et al. New definition for periprosthetic joint infection: from the Workgroup of the Musculoskeletal Infection Society. Clin Orthop Relat Res. 2011;469(11):2992–4.

70. Oussedik S, et al. Defining peri-prosthetic infection. J Bone Joint Surg Br. 2012;94-B(11):1455–6.

Part III

Clinical Manifestation

General and Local Symptoms of Infection in Knee Replacement

Giovanna Stelitano, Laura Risi Ambrogioni,
Calogero Di Naro, Vincenzo Candela,
Carlo Casciaro, Umile Giuseppe Longo,
and Vincenzo Denaro

5.1 Introduction

Infection of periprosthetic joints is among the leading complications following total knee arthroplasty (TKA). The length and complexity of the treatment represent a physical, psychological and economic challenge for both the patient and the doctor. Despite the low incidence rate of infection after TKA, efforts to prevent infection and reduce the overall impact of periprosthetic joint infections (PJIs) seem justified by the increasing prevalence of TKA. In general, the prevention of PJI is based on the improvement of the host's defences, on the optimization of the conditions of the surgical wound and the minimization of microbial contamination throughout the entire treatment period [1]. The outcome of the treatment seems to be influenced by multiple variables such as the type of microorganism involved, the patient's comorbidities and the extent of soft tissue and bone involvement and the physician's expertise. For these reasons, the management of PJIs has become more rigorous and standardized in recent decades, mainly as regards the approach to the routine use of local antibiotics with high dosage and the necessary

deferment of reimplantation. Several risk factors relating to patients predispose to deep postoperative infection. Host factors include rheumatoid arthritis; skin ulcers; diabetes mellitus; past cancers; obesity; smoking habits; liver transplantation; HIV immunodeficiency virus seropositivity; open sky on the knee or a periarticular fracture; previous septic arthritis or adjacent osteomyelitis. Definitive diagnosis requires constant and considerable attention to the slightest clinical suspicion in both early and late infections. A meticulous anamnesis, the clinical examination, the study of imaging, arthrocentesis and haematological tests are all an integral part of the diagnostic process in the suspected infection. The timing of the clinical presentation is a crucial factor in the choice of the appropriate management strategy.

5.2 General Consideration

The different modalities of clinical presentation of the patient have been well described to define the most suitable management approach to PJI [2]. Postoperative infections diagnosed through the positivity of intraoperative culture tests during prosthetic revision are usually triggered by virulence-lowering microorganisms such as coagulase-negative staphylococci and Propionibacterium. A timely and precise diagnosis is necessary to avoid delays that can lead to

G. Stelitano · L. Risi Ambrogioni · C. Di Naro
V. Candela · C. Casciaro · U. G. Longo (✉)
V. Denaro
Department of Orthopaedic and Trauma Surgery,
Campus Bio-Medico University, Rome, Italy
e-mail: g.longo@unicampus.it

© ISAKOS 2022
U. G. Longo et al. (eds.), *Infection in Knee Replacement*,
https://doi.org/10.1007/978-3-030-81553-0_5

diagnosing a prosthetic infection as chronic or late, which could instead be identified and treated in the acute phase. Pain is the main symptom of onset. Sustained wound secretion raises the highest suspicion of infection, which should be treated with arthrotomy, surgical toilet and flushing [3]. Culture tests for serous secretions are often challenging to portray and, therefore, they are not recommended. The empirical antibacterial therapy for persistent wound secretions should be prevented since it can merely relieve the clinical symptoms and can even delay the diagnosis, thus compromising the possibility of treating the infection without removing the prosthesis [4]. In the first few weeks after the surgical procedure, purposeful management of wound healing delays or marginal skin necrosis by the surgical toilet and closure by primary intention is desirable over empirical antibacterial treatment with long-term observation. This strategy may eventually result in the development of a profound infection [5]. An acute haematogenic infection typically occurs with unexpected onset of pain or tightness in a prosthesis that used to work well. An infectious outbreak elsewhere or a recent invasive procedure capable of triggering a battery should be evaluated as potential risk factors for the appearance of a haematogenic infection. The seriousness of symptoms such as pain, joint stiffness facilitates rapid diagnosis in these situations. Unfortunately, empirical antibiotic therapy is frequently prescribed for the appearance of painful symptoms without apparent cause in patients with prostheses, without attempting to make a precise diagnosis. This approach only serves to make subsequent attempts to detect a profound infection difficult. In the most infected TKA, the diagnosis is made in the subacute or chronic phase. The pain after surgery, prolonged secretion from the wound in the postoperative period, administration of antibiotic therapy for delayed healing and joint stiffness despite intense rehabilitation treatment are all elements that lay down for a deep infection. To date, PJI is defined as a variety of clinical symptoms and signs, tissue histological examination and culture examination. The certain diagnosis of infection is made if at least one of the following elements is found on knee examination: two or more cultures from arthrocentesis or from deep tissues taken surgically are positive for the same microorganism; histopathological evaluation of intraarticular tissues detects alterations attributable to acute inflammation; frankly purulent secretion during the surgical procedure; the potential occurrence of a secreting fistula [6]. The identification and treatment of the microorganism responsible for the infection can ensure optimal results, where possible, and by implementing the consequent therapeutic strategies. Joint inspection, evaluation of knee function and measurement of range of motion are features that must be evaluated. Examination of the spine and ipsilateral hip is essential to avoid radicular or referred pain, respectively. Both neurological and vascular examination of the leg complete the clinical evaluation of the patient.

5.3 Clinical Examination

The patient who complains of persistent pain after TKA should receive an appropriate objective examination to assess the limb properly. In addition to normal physiological parameters such as vital signs, height, weight, a detailed examination of the skin for lesions, erythema and signs of infection such as heat, effusion, vascular changes and sinus tract drainage should be performed (Fig. 5.1). The presence of signs of wound dehiscence may indicate an infectious aetiology (Figs. 5.2 and 5.3). The evaluation of the gait is useful to highlight the presence of an antalgic thrust varus and valgus. Measurement of active and passive range of motion and the capability to actively sustain full extension without extensor delay must be included in the physical examination. The stability of the knee can be assessed with varus and valgus forces at 0° and 30°. In comparison, stability in the sagittal plane can be determined with posterior flexion tests at 60° and 90° flexion. Both the manual strength test and the assessment of muscle atrophy need to be observed. The knee has to be probed and evaluated for sensitivity with the iliotibial band and pes anserine bursa to exclude bursitis or flexion

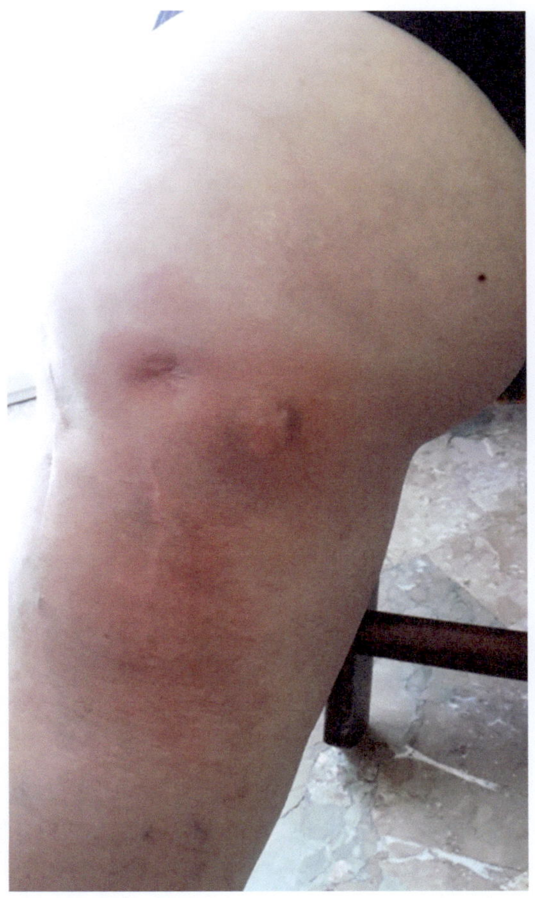

Fig. 5.1 Periprosthetic joint infection of total knee arthroplasty; local signs of infection

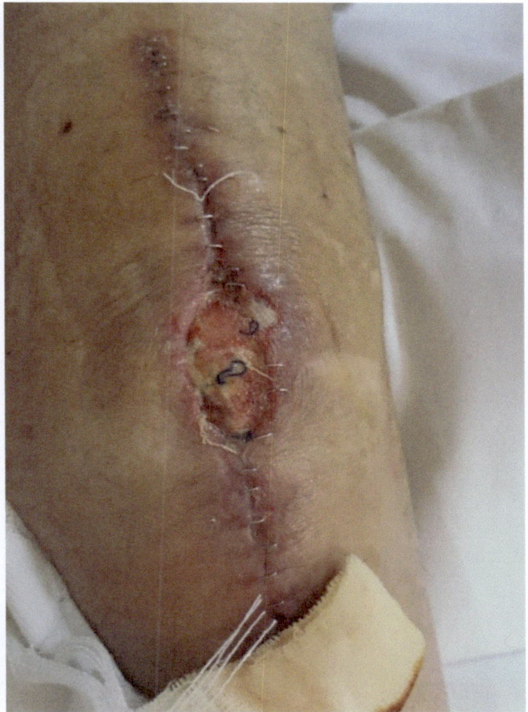

Fig. 5.2 Periprosthetic joint infection of total knee arthroplasty; wound dehiscence

instability. Because patellofemoral tracking is a common source of continuous pain after TKA, painful patellar crackling, patellar clunk syndrome, reduction in patellar size or patellar thickness, shortening of patellar tendon length, increased posterior femoral condylar offset, utilization of smaller femoral parts, thicker tibial polyethylene inserts and greater flexion of femoral constituents should be evaluated. These factors increase the contact of the quadriceps tendon with the upper aspect of the intercondylar box and, consequently, the risk of fibrosynovial proliferation increases. A neurovascular examination should be conducted to assess the quality and symmetry of peripheral pulses and the strength of both the quadriceps and the vastus medialis obliquus. The physical examination should con-

clude with an evaluation of the spine, and other joints to exclude other extra-articular causes of pain, such as lumbar radiculopathy, referred pain from coxarthrosis and vascular claudication. In some patients, the replacement can be clearly visible through a skin hole (Fig. 5.4).

5.4 Presenting Symptoms and Clinical Assessment

When a patient reports a painful TKA, the clinical suspicion of PJI should always be investigated even if there are no apparent signs of infection, such as redness or swelling. The clinical onset of PJIs after TKA is often blurred and insidious. History of wound drainage, invasive procedures or dental procedures and comorbidities such as diabetes mellitus or immunosuppressive conditions increase the risk of PJIs and, therefore, meticulous evaluated [7, 8]. Although the progress in laboratory and imaging techniques may

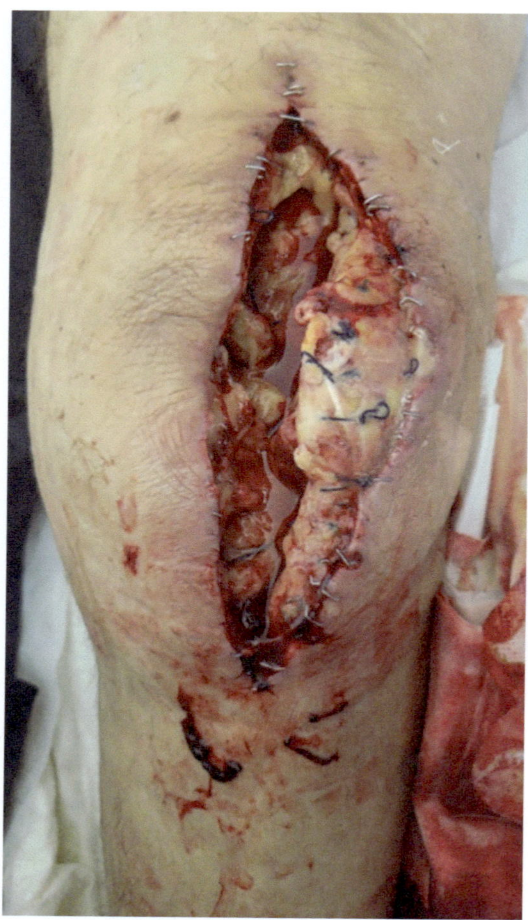

Fig. 5.3 Periprosthetic joint infection of total knee arthroplasty; wound dehiscence

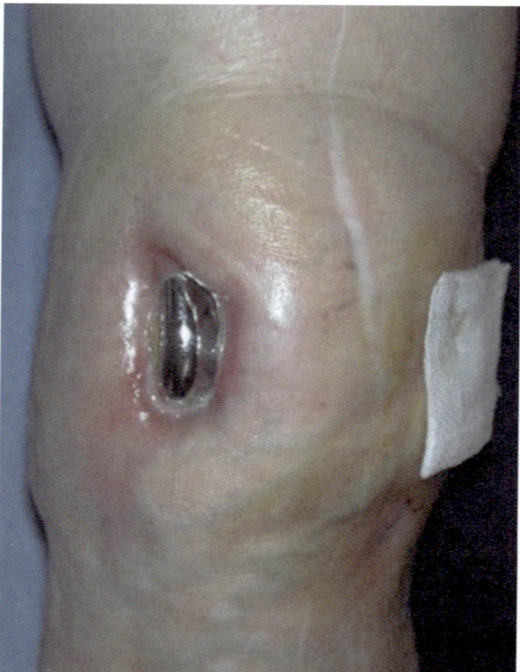

Fig. 5.4 The replacement visible through a skin hole

enhance the detection of PJI, the clinical presentation is still the basis for diagnosis. Stratification of the risk of the likelihood of infection is warranted in any patient presenting with a painful TKA [9]. The diagnosis of a PJI after TKA is critical because the treatment of infected patients is very different from the treatment of uncomplicated TKA. Faced with suspicion of PJI, a comprehensive and more thorough evaluation of the patient is necessary. Possible risk factors for infection are obesity, inflammatory arthritis, diabetes, malnutrition, early implant mobilization (<5 years) and early osteolysis (<5 years). The signs or symptoms most commonly complained of by patients with chronic PJI are fever, pain, joint effusion and periarticular erythema [10, 11]. Despite the clini-

cal presentation of the infection after TKA, to date, no study evaluates the role of physical examination for the diagnosis of PJI [12]. While aseptic prosthetic loosening pain increases with weight gain and decreases at rest, persistent and progressive pain at rest is one of the PJI's first symptoms. This pain occurs at the time of surgery and has been associated with superficial infection, leakage or healing problems of the wound. In contrast, an acute haematogenic infection can occur in a previously painless and well-functioning knee. The clinical picture of an infected prosthetic joint varies about the source of infection, the time required for the infection to develop and the viral load of the infecting organism. The classic presentation is that of a painful joint even at rest, hot and erythematous (Fig. 5.5). The most common symptom of prosthetic infections is pain, present in more than 90% of patients. As it is difficult to differentiate the pain caused by an aseptic mobilization from that of a prosthetic infection, this symptom alone has a low diagnostic prediction. Joint loosening pain occurs mainly with movement or load, while infection pain is less likely to be associated

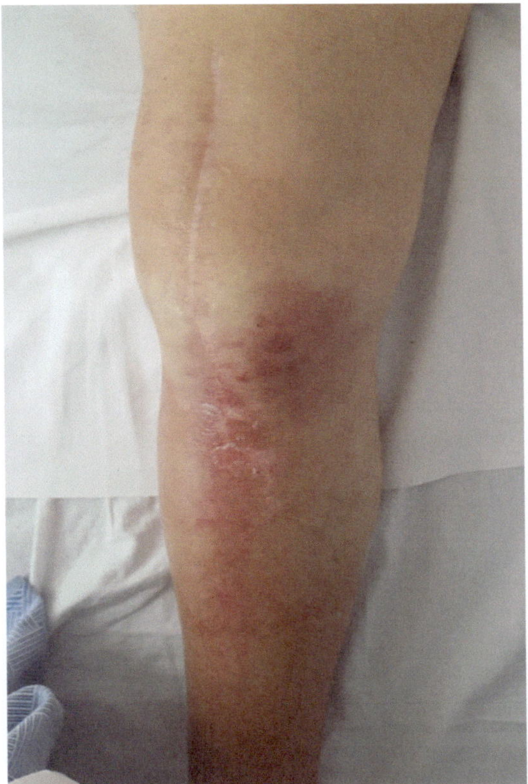

Fig. 5.5 Local signs of infection with hot and erythematous skin

with joint loading, has a more constant duration and a tendency to increase over time. Other symptoms, such as fever, swelling and suppuration, occur to a lesser extent, and their frequency and intensity are related to the patient's age. In very elderly subjects or therapy with corticosteroids or other anti-inflammatories, the febrile response may be modest or completely absent, especially in late infections or supported by low virulent strains. Rarely, the patient in good general condition and with age < 60 years comes to the observation with manifest septicemia, high fever, hypotension and multi-organ dysfunction. The triad of pain at rest, fever and localized oedema takes on high predictive value and constitutes, even in the absence of microbiological confirmation, sufficient reason to establish empirical therapy. In the presence of suspected infection, an arthrocentesis must always be performed and, if the conditions require it, an empirical therapy must be set up pending a crop assessment. Despite clinical presentation, treatment with empirical antibiotics for presumed cellulite or superficial infection is not recommended without a definite diagnosis. Antibiotic treatment can suppress clinical symptoms, decrease the ability to isolate the microorganism and delay diagnosis [13].

5.5 Wound Complications

Wound complications after TKA are dramatic and responsible for increased risk of PJI and other postoperative complications such as component resection, myofascial or fasciocutaneous flap reconstruction or amputation [14]. Wound healing may include three phases: inflammation, a fibroblastic proliferative phase and a wound maturation phase. The faster gains in wound strength occur during the first weeks of wound healing. In contrast, the maturation phase of the wound proceeds for several months as the collagen fibrils become increasingly structured and well-organized. There are several patient-specific, intraoperative and postoperative factors that can influence normal wound healing [14]. Intraoperative factors impacting the healing process include the site of the incision, soft tissue flap management and appropriate tissue handling.

Wound complications differ in prolonged postoperative drainage, superficial or full-thickness soft tissue necrosis. The increase in the severity of the infection occurs if the treatment of these complications is delayed. Although prolonged serous drainage is performed, this represents a difficult challenge after TKA. Initially, a chronically draining wound in the absence of erythema or purulence can be managed with local wound care, elevation and immobilization. Surgical debridement is required when drainage persists for more than 5–7 days. Persistent wound drainage is often due to the presence of a sizeable subcutaneous hematoma or intraarticular hemarthrosis. Hematomas increase the soft tissue tension and create an ideal medium for bacterial growth [15].

Small necrotic lesions with a diameter of less than 3 cm, usually located at the edges of the wound can be treated with local wound care and delayed secondary closure. Careful surveillance of these small necrotic lesions is imperative. Superficial soft tissue necrosis usually demands surgical debridement. Necrotic lesions with a diameter greater than 3 cm usually demand split-thickness skin grafts, fasciocutaenous flap or myocardial flap coverage. It has been shown that closing the wound with the aid of vacuum can reduce oedema from the extravascular space, improve blood supply and wound granulation, suppress bacterial proliferation and reduce wound size. Vacuum wound closure systems may be useful to reduce wound size before any soft tissue covering procedures or may facilitate wound healing without additional surgery. In cases of full-thickness necrosis, the prosthetic components are usually exposed, and immediate debridement is required. After irrigation and debridement, secondary closure is rarely successful. Vascularized tissue transfer with fasciocutaneous, myocutaneous and myotendinous flaps have been described [5]. Consultation plastic surgeon can aid in determining appropriate flap coverage.

5.6 Conclusions

The clinical presentation can be hugely useful to guide the diagnosis, but PJI must be confirmed by clinical tests. Differences in pre-test probability can also greatly influence the post-test probability of patients with similar laboratory results. For example, two patients with elevated ESR and PCR, but no other elevation of serum or synovial marker may have a different probability of PJI based on differences in their clinical presentation. While the importance of pre-test probability is recognized by the American Academy of Orthopaedic Surgeons (AAOS), no attention is given to the clinical presentation of the patient.

Although clinical presentation in PJI currently plays a marginal role in diagnostic guidelines, fever and erythema around the joint are suggestive findings of PJI. The existing diagnostic criteria are based on both cultures and laboratory results to define PJI [8, 16]. The analysis of the patient's signs and symptoms with PJI is non-

invasive, simple and can substantially guide the diagnosis. Pain may be the only symptom of chronic infection (especially in cases of low virulence) and is a sufficient symptom to warrant further evaluation to exclude PJI. Compared to aseptic revisions, the presence of joint effusion appears to be significantly higher in patients with PJI [17]. The difficulties encountered in treating infections following TKA can be considerable, and the treatment must be carefully planned after appropriate clinical and diagnostic work-up.

References

1. Hanssen AD, Osmon DR, Nelson CL. Prevention of deep periprosthetic joint infection. Instr Course Lect. 1997;46:555–67.
2. Segawa H, Tsukayama DT, Kyle RF, Becker DA, Gustilo RB. Infection after total knee arthroplasty. A retrospective study of the treatment of eighty-one infections. J Bone Joint Surg Am. 1999;81(10):1434–45.
3. Weiss AP, Krackow KA. Persistent wound drainage after primary total knee arthroplasty. J Arthroplast. 1993;8(3):285–9.
4. Brandt CM, Sistrunk WW, Duffy MC, Hanssen AD, Steckelberg JM, Ilstrup DM, et al. Staphylococcus aureus prosthetic joint infection treated with debridement and prosthesis retention. Clin Infect Dis. 1997;24(5):914–9.
5. Lian G, Cracchiolo A, Lesavoy M. Treatment of major wound necrosis following total knee arthroplasty. J Arthroplast. 1989;4(Suppl):S23–32.
6. Hanssen AD, Rand JA, Osmon DR. Treatment of the infected total knee arthroplasty with insertion of another prosthesis. The effect of antibiotic-impregnated bone cement. Clin Orthop Relat Res. 1994;309:44–55.
7. Parvizi J, Adeli B, Zmistowski B, Restrepo C, Greenwald AS. Management of periprosthetic joint infection: the current knowledge: AAOS exhibit selection. J Bone Joint Surg Am. 2012;94(14):e104.
8. Osmon DR, Berbari EF, Berendt AR, Lew D, Zimmerli W, Steckelberg JM, et al. Executive summary: diagnosis and management of prosthetic joint infection: clinical practice guidelines by the Infectious Diseases Society of America. Clin Infect Dis. 2013;56(1):1–10.
9. Ting NT, Della Valle CJ. Diagnosis of periprosthetic joint infection-an algorithm-based approach. J Arthroplast. 2017;32(7):2047–50.
10. Sendi P, Banderet F, Graber P, Zimmerli W. Clinical comparison between exogenous and haematogenous periprosthetic joint infections caused by Staphylococcus aureus. Clin Microbiol Infect. 2011;17(7):1098–100.

11. Tsaras G, Osmon DR, Mabry T, Lahr B, St Sauveur J, Yawn B, et al. Incidence, secular trends, and outcomes of prosthetic joint infection: a population-based study, olmsted county, Minnesota, 1969-2007. Infect Control Hosp Epidemiol. 2012;33(12):1207–12.

12. Shohat N, Goswami K, Tan TL, Henstenburg B, Makar G, Rondon AJ, et al. Fever and erythema are specific findings in detecting infection following total knee arthroplasty. J Bone Joint Infect. 2019;4(2):92–8.

13. Aresti N, Kassam J, Bartlett D, Kutty S. Primary care management of postoperative shoulder, hip, and knee arthroplasty. BMJ. 2017;359:j4431.

14. Galat DD, McGovern SC, Larson DR, Harrington JR, Hanssen AD, Clarke HD. Surgical treatment of early wound complications following primary total knee arthroplasty. J Bone Joint Surg Am. 2009;91(1):48–54.

15. Vince K, Chivas D, Droll KP. Wound complications after total knee arthroplasty. J Arthroplast. 2007;22(4 Suppl 1):39–44.

16. Parvizi J, Gehrke T, Chen AF. Proceedings of the international consensus on periprosthetic joint infection. Bone Joint J. 2013;95-B(11):1450–2.

17. Duff GP, Lachiewicz PF, Kelley SS. Aspiration of the knee joint before revision arthroplasty. Clin Orthop Relat Res. 1996;331:132–9.

Part IV

Diagnosis

Laboratory Diagnosis of Periprosthetic Joint Infections

Graham S. Goh and Javad Parvizi

6.1 Introduction

Total knee arthroplasty (TKA) is one of the most common elective surgical procedures in the world. The volume of primary and revision TKA has risen dramatically and is projected to grow over the next decade [1]. Periprosthetic joint infection (PJI) is a rare but devastating complication after TKA, with an estimated risk of 0.5–2% following primary procedures [2]. Despite the low incidence of this complication, PJI is the most common indication for revision in the Medicare population [3] and the main cause of failure in modern total joint arthroplasty (TJA) [4, 5]. With over a million joint replacement procedures performed each year in the USA [6], the overall burden of PJI will also invariably increase. Despite global efforts to reduce the incidence of PJI, several international arthroplasty registries have shown that the infection burden has in fact increased over time [7]. Furthermore, as the prevalence of risk factors such as obesity and diabetes increases around the world [8, 9], some authors have also projected an increase in PJI rates in the near future [10]. This rare but devastating complication is not only associated with a significantly increased risk of mortality and decreased quality of life [11, 12], but also poses a substantial economic burden to the healthcare system as costs can be up to four times higher than that of uninfected cases [13]. As the management of an infected knee arthroplasty is drastically different from aseptic cases, it is imperative that orthopedic surgeons definitively establish or rule out the diagnosis of PJI prior to revision surgery, helping patients avoid the increased morbidity and costs associated with this complication wherever possible.

The lack of a "gold standard" diagnostic test makes the diagnosis of PJI extremely challenging. Historically, there has been no standardized criteria or algorithm for the diagnosis of PJI, which led to the use of a wide variety of tests and procedures that were unnecessarily burdensome and costly for patients, often resulting in treatment delays or misdiagnosis. Recently, several evidence-based guidelines have been introduced to standardize the approach to a patient with a suspected PJI, including the American Academy of Orthopaedic Surgeons (AAOS) Clinical Practice Guidelines on Diagnosis of Periprosthetic Joint Infection [14] as well as the Proceedings of the 2018 International Consensus Meeting (ICM) on Periprosthetic Joint Infection (Fig. 6.1) [15]. These documents should be familiar to all orthopedic surgeons as well as other physicians who

G. S. Goh
Rothman Institute, Thomas Jefferson University, Philadelphia, PA, USA

J. Parvizi (✉)
Sidney Kimmel School of Medicine, Rothman Institute at Thomas Jefferson University, Philadelphia, PA, USA

© ISAKOS 2022
U. G. Longo et al. (eds.), *Infection in Knee Replacement*,
https://doi.org/10.1007/978-3-030-81553-0_6

Major criteria (at least one of the following)	Decision
Two positive cultures of the same organism	Infected
Sinus tract with evidence of communication to the joint or visualization of the prosthesis	

		Minor Criteria	Score	Decision
Preoperative Diagnosis	Serum	Elevated CRP _or_ D-Dimer	2	≥6 Infected
		Elevated ESR	1	
	Synovial	Elevated Synovial _WBC_ _or_ _LE_ (++)	3	2-5 Possibly Infected*
		Positive Alpha-defensin	3	
		Elevated Synovial PMN %	2	0-1 Not Infected
		Elevated Synovial CRP	1	

		*Inconclusive pre-op score _or_ dry tap	Score	Decision
Postoperative Diagnosis		Preoperative score	-	≥6 Infected
		Positive Histology	3	**4-5 Inconclusive****
		Positive Purulence	3	
		Positive Single Culture	2	≤3 Not Infected

Fig. 6.1 Evidence-based criteria for the diagnosis of periprosthetic joint infections as recommended by the 2018 International Consensus Meeting (ICM). *For patients with inconclusive minor criteria, operative criteria can also be used to fulfill definition for PJI for PJI. **Consider further molecular diagnostics such as Next-generation sequencing. (Reprinted with permission from "The 2018 Definition of Periprosthetic Hip and Knee Infection: An Evidence-Based and Validated Criteria." The Journal of Arthroplasty. Elsevier; 2018;)

frequently encounter patients with joint replacements in their practice.

The general approach to diagnosing a PJI is twofold. First, the presence or absence of a joint infection must be confirmed; second, the infecting microorganism(s) must be isolated and its antimicrobial susceptibility elucidated. In addition to clinical findings from history and physical examination, the diagnosis of PJI often relies on laboratory results from peripheral blood and synovial fluid, microbiological evaluation, histological examination of periprosthetic tissue, intraoperative findings, and in some cases, radiographic evaluation [16–18]. In particular, isolating the causative microorganism from cultures of fluid or tissue within the joint remains the cornerstone for diagnosis and targeted antibiotic therapy, which has been shown to increase the chances of treatment success [19] and influence the prognosis of patients with this condition [16]. This chapter reviews the laboratory tests available in an orthopedic surgeon's armamentarium to diagnose PJI following knee replacement surgery.

6.2 Peripheral Blood Tests

Serum biomarkers are useful adjuncts in the diagnosis of PJI [16, 17], especially in the absence of major diagnostic criteria such as a communicating sinus tract or two positive cultures [15]. Biomarkers are measurable biological substances that are part of a physiological or pathological pathway or the pharmacological response to therapeutic interventions [20]. Given their high accessibility, peripheral blood tests are often first-line investigations for any patient with a suspected PJI.

6.2.1 Erythrocyte Sedimentation Rate and C-Reactive Protein

Erythrocyte sedimentation rate (ESR) and C-reactive protein (CRP) are two of the most well-researched serological biomarkers in the diagnosis of PJI. CRP is an acute-phase reactant that is produced by the liver in response to systemic infections. ESR is the rate at which red blood cells form a sediment at the bottom of a standardized tube, which is increased by the presence of fibrinogen and other clotting factors that are produced during inflammation. While nonspecific for the diagnosis of localized infections due to their elevation in non-infectious inflammatory conditions, these tests are often used as first-line screening tools for PJI due to their high sensitivities exceeding 90%, making them particularly valuable in ruling out PJI [21–23]. When both ESR and CRP are below their diagnostic thresholds of 30 mm/h and 10 mg/L, respectively, the negative likelihood ratio of PJI ranges from 0 to 0.06 [21]. As such, the use of these markers in the first step of the evaluation of a patient with suspected PJI has been endorsed by the 2018 ICM (Fig. 6.2) [24].

Despite the accessibility and utility of these markers, ESR and CRP may be falsely low or normal in cases when the infecting organism is slow-growing and may not elicit an adequate

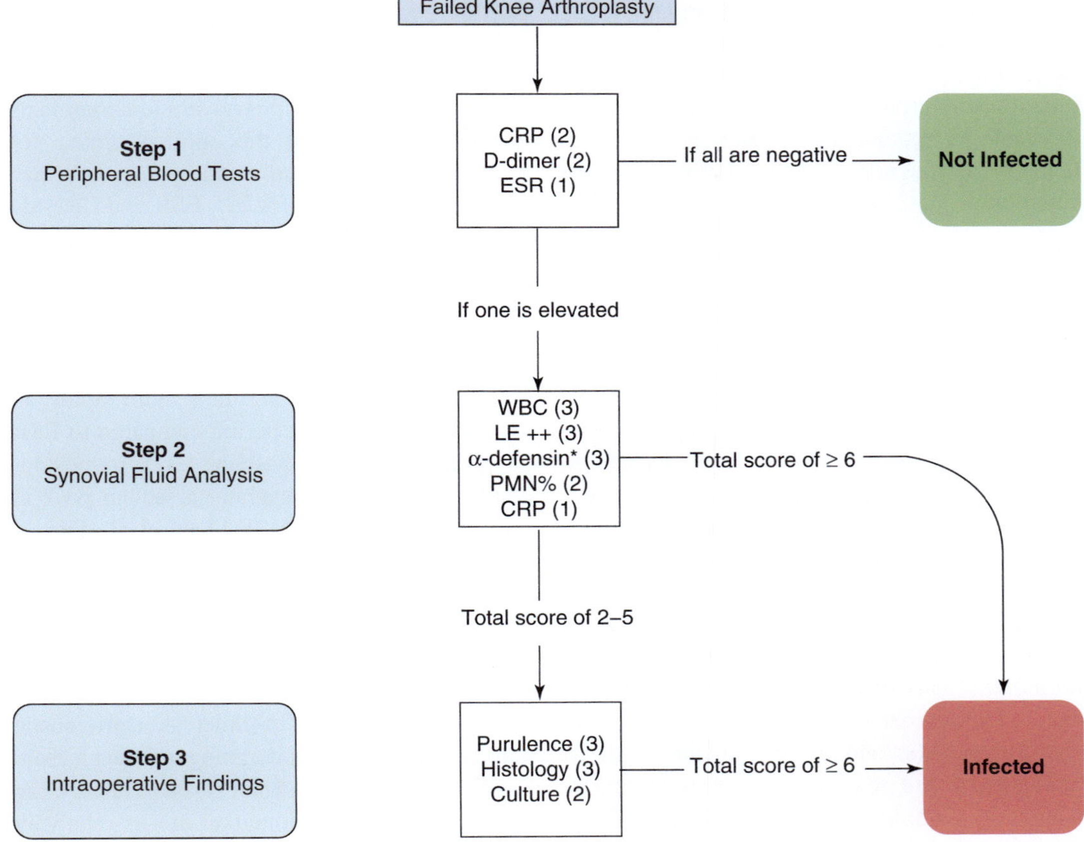

Fig. 6.2 Diagnostic algorithm to guide the selection of laboratory tests. *CRP* C-reactive protein, *ESR* erythrocyte sedimentation rate, *WBC* white blood cell count, *LE* leukocyte esterase, *PMN%* polymorphonuclear neutrophil percentage. Points are stated in parentheses. *Does not need to be performed routinely. (Reprinted with permission from "Development and Validation of an Evidence-Based Algorithm for Diagnosing Periprosthetic Joint Infection" The Journal of Arthroplasty. Elsevier; 2019;)

inflammatory response [25–28]. Perez et al. found that ESR and CRP were not as accurate in diagnosing PJI caused by low-virulence organisms such as coagulase-negative staphylococci, *Bacillus* spp, *Corynebacterium* spp, and *Cutibacterium acnes* (previously known as *Propionibacterium acnes*) [27]. Similarly, Akgün et al. demonstrated that CRP was not a reliable screening marker for PJI and led to high false-negative rates especially in cases with a low-virulence organism [28]. It is also worth noting that these markers are not specific for infection-induced inflammation and may be elevated in other inflammatory states including autoimmune diseases and tissue damage from trauma or surgery. Conversely, the anti-inflammatory effect of systemic corticosteroids may also decrease their concentrations [29]. Although Cipriano et al. demonstrated that ESR and CRP had a similar diagnostic accuracy in patients with and without inflammatory arthritis [30], their limited specificity cautions against the isolated use of these markers to diagnose PJI in complex clinical situations.

6.2.2 D-Dimer

Similar to traditional inflammatory markers such as CRP and ESR, the measurement of serum D-dimer has gained attention as a valuable prognostic tool in patients with systemic sepsis and bacteremia [31, 32]. Systemic and local infections are known to stimulate fibrinolytic activity and coagulation abnormalities as part of the host inflammatory response [33, 34]. This in turn leads to an elevation in breakdown products of fibrinolysis such as D-dimer [35]. The increased fibrinolytic activity and creation of byproducts are hypothesized to trap infecting microorganism(s) and/or inflammatory cells to limit the extent of systemic damage. Joint inflammation or infection in particular has been shown to elicit a rise in D-dimer levels due to the high concentration of fibrin released by inflamed synovium [31, 32, 34], which breaks down into degradation products and increases the concentration of D-dimer in serum and synovial fluid

[36]. In an *in vivo* study of foals with septic arthritis, Ribera et al. found that the concentration of D-dimer in synovial fluid was markedly elevated, reinforcing the notion that D-dimer is a mediator of joint inflammation or infection [34]. It is thus not surprising that recent studies in arthroplasty literature have extrapolated this concept and identified D-dimer as a promising biomarker for the diagnosis of PJI [37]. In the initial study on 245 primary and revision arthroplasty patients, Shahi et al. found that serum D-dimer was more accurate in diagnosing PJI than ESR and CRP combined, with a sensitivity and specificity of 89% and 93% compared to 84% and 47%, respectively [37]. Importantly, the authors also showed that D-dimer was only elevated in 12% of patients with an infection in sites other than the prosthetic joint, in contrast to ESR and CRP, which were elevated in 100% and 84% of these patients, respectively. Another advantage cited by proponents of this novel biomarker is its utility in ascertaining the optimal timing for reimplantation in patients undergoing two-stage exchange arthroplasty for PJI. ESR and CRP are not reliable in this aspect due to their elevated levels in the postoperative period [38, 39], which has led several authors to conclude that these markers are poorly predictive of treatment failure at the time of reimplantation [40, 41]. On the contrary, D-dimer rises and falls more rapidly in the early postoperative period compared to ESR and CRP, returning to baseline levels by postoperative day 2 before reaching a second peak at postoperative week 2 [42]. Shahi et al. demonstrated that two of five patients who were free of infection as defined by the Musculoskeletal Infection Society (MSIS) criteria but had elevated D-dimer levels at the time of the second stage subsequently failed treatment for PJI [37], thus supporting the role of D-dimer as a prognostic marker for patients undergoing reimplantation. Practical considerations that further enhance the appeal of this novel biomarker are its relatively low cost and high accessibility in routine clinical practice [37]. These factors have culminated in the endorsement of serum D-dimer as an inexpensive and reliable test for the diagnostic workup of PJI [24].

Despite its utility, recent studies have questioned the usefulness of D-dimer for the diagnosis of PJI. Li et al. identified 565 patients who underwent revision surgery (95 PJI cases, 470 aseptic cases) and found that the area under the curve (AUC) for plasma D-dimer was 0.657, with an optimal threshold of 1250 ng/mL, sensitivity of 64%, and specificity of 65% [43]. The authors postulated that the use of plasma D-dimer instead of serum D-dimer as well as the predominantly Asian cohort could have accounted for the inconsistent findings when compared to the study by Shahi et al. [37]. Serum samples, unlike plasma ones, are obtained following the consumption of coagulation factors, which may hence alter D-dimer levels. Despite this methodological difference in measurement, current evidence suggests that plasma and serum D-dimer concentrations are very highly correlated and show a strong linear relationship [44, 45]. In another study evaluating plasma D-dimer, Xu et al. found that a threshold of 1.02 mg/L fibrinogen equivalent units (FEU) to discriminate between infected and non-infected revisions demonstrated poor sensitivity (68%) and specificity (51%) [46]. Similarly, Pannu et al. found that the threshold of 850 ng/mL led to a good sensitivity (96%) but poor specificity (32%) with an AUC of 0.742 [47], whereas a different cutoff point of 2300 ng/mL had a moderate sensitivity of 71% and improved specificity of 74%, although these values were still much lower than the values reported in the original study by Shahi et al. [37]. It is possible that the lack of consensus regarding the diagnostic threshold for D-dimer in the literature could have arisen from the inconsistencies in laboratory techniques used to measure this biomarker. The lack of standardization among the various assays has been a topic of dispute, with several authors questioning the clinical utility of D-dimer in view of the high variability in its measurement and reporting [48]. An additional reason could be that the proposed threshold by Shahi et al. may not be the optimal one, as evidenced from the aforementioned studies. While D-dimer is an inexpensive and accessible assay in routine practice that has the potential to detect PJI with a higher sensitivity and specificity, additional studies with consistent laboratory measurement methods are needed to confirm its superior diagnostic performance over traditional tests and determine the optimal threshold value for this marker.

6.2.3 Fibrinogen

Similar to the rationale for the use of D-dimer in systemic and local infections [33, 34], other fibrinolytic markers such as fibrinogen and fibrinogen degradation product (FDP) have gained recognition for their accuracy in diagnosing PJI [43]. Fibrinogen is a glycoprotein found in human plasma that is converted into fibrin by thrombin for the formation of a fibrin-based blood clot in the final steps of the coagulation cascade [33]. It is also a positive acute-phase reactant that increases in concentration during inflammation. When evaluating the relationship between thrombosis and infection, Kirschenbaum et al. found that fibrinogen played an integral role in neutrophil adherence during systemic sepsis [49], while Horn et al. found that neutrophil alpha-defensins stimulated the production of fibrinogen and thrombospondin-1 amyloid-like structures to entrap infecting microorganisms [50]. Not surprisingly, the use of fibrinogen has also garnered attention from the arthroplasty community recently. In the study by Li et al., plasma fibrinogen was found to be a promising biomarker with the highest AUC compared to plasma D-dimer, ESR, or CRP [43]. When 4.01 g/L was used as the cutoff point, the sensitivity and specificity were 76% and 86%, respectively. In another study, Wu et al. noted that the AUC for fibrinogen was higher than that of FDP or D-dimer [51]. The authors determined the optimal threshold for fibrinogen to be 3.61 g/L, with 76% sensitivity and 86% specificity. Similar to this study, Xu et al. found that plasma fibrinogen was useful for diagnosing PJI as well as confirming the presence of persistent infection at the time of reimplantation [52]. These encouraging findings support the use of plasma fibrinogen in the evaluation of a patient with suspected PJI before revision surgery and at the time of reimplantation, although further studies are needed to validate these findings in more diverse populations.

6.2.4 Interleukin-6

Interleukin-6 (IL-6) is pleiotropic cytokine produced by macrophages in response to tissue injury. It stimulates the production of acute-phase reactants such as CRP, regulates pyrexia by pituitary hormones, modulates bone resorption, promotes hematopoiesis, and induces plasma cell development [53]. Serum IL-6 has been established as a valuable inflammatory marker in association with sepsis, trauma, and major surgery [54, 55]. Given that IL-6 lies upstream of other markers, such as CRP, in the inflammatory cascade [56], it is postulated to be a more rapid and sensitive marker for the detection of PJI [57]. IL-6 exhibits a more rapid increase and return to baseline levels following TJA compared to ESR or CRP, often peaking within the first 6–12 h after surgery and returning to baseline within the first two to three postoperative days, leading authors to conclude that IL-6 may be a superior indicator of an early-stage immune response [58, 59]. Importantly, studies have shown that IL-6 is more elevated in patients with PJI compared to patients with aseptic loosening [60]. Berbari et al. found that the pooled sensitivity and specificity for IL-6 in three studies were 97% and 87%, respectively [61], and the authors concluded that serum IL-6 had the highest accuracy in diagnosing PJI when compared to ESR and CRP. In a more recent meta-analysis of eleven studies, Xie et al. reported a pooled sensitivity and specificity of 72% and 89%, respectively, although the poorer sensitivity was likely due to the inclusion of two studies on shoulder PJIs that had a higher proportion of low-virulence organisms such as *Cutibacterium acnes* [57]. Overall, current literature suggests that serum IL-6 may be a promising marker for the diagnosis of PJI with a relatively high diagnostic accuracy. A growing interest in the use of IL-6 has led to its incorporation into the latest clinical practice guidelines by the AAOS [14]. Notwithstanding, serum IL-6 has only been evaluated in a small number of studies

and the optimal threshold for this marker has yet to be determined. Current barriers to its use include the relatively high cost and technical skills required to run the analysis. As serum IL-6 assays become more widely available for clinical use, this biomarker could be used in combination with other routine markers like serum CRP, further enhancing their diagnostic yield as shown in previous studies [62, 63].

6.2.5 Procalcitonin

Procalcitonin (PCT) is a protein produced by thyroid parafollicular C-cells and lung neuroendocrine cells. Serum PCT levels are undetectable in healthy individuals without evidence of infection and are greatly elevated in bacterial infections, giving the biomarker a high diagnostic accuracy for the identification of systemic infection [64]. The utility of serum PCT for diagnosing PJI has been investigated in several studies [62, 65, 66]. In a meta-analysis of six studies on PCT, the pooled sensitivity and specificity were 53% and 92%, respectively, making this test suitable as a rule-in rather than a rule-out diagnostic tool [66]. Similarly, Boettner et al. investigated the serum levels of PCT, IL-6, tumor necrosis factor (TNF)-α, ESR, and CRP in 78 patients undergoing revision arthroplasty for sepsis and found that serum PCT was very specific (98%) but had a very low sensitivity (33%) [62]. Based on current evidence, serum PCT has a limited diagnostic value as a biomarker for PJI due to its low sensitivity and should not be routinely used in the workup of an infected knee replacement.

6.2.6 Novel Serological Markers

In recent years, a myriad of serological markers have been evaluated for their diagnostic potential. Some examples of these novel biomarkers include TNF-α [62, 63], lipopolysaccharide-binding protein (LBP) [63, 67], toll-like receptor (TLRs) [68], intercellular adhesion molecule-1 (ICAM-1) [69, 70], soluble urokinase plasminogen activation receptor (su-PAR) [71], and CD64

[72]. While a few of these markers have shown a high diagnostic accuracy, practical considerations such as the high cost and technical competency required to run these tests remain important barriers to their adoption into clinical practice. Consequently, further research to discover accurate and clinically relevant serum biomarkers for the diagnosis of PJI is necessary.

6.3   Synovial Fluid Analysis

Joint aspiration is a crucial step in the diagnostic workup of any patient with a suspected joint infection [15]. Although listed as the second step in the ICM diagnostic algorithm [73], this procedure is commonly performed in the office alongside the abovementioned blood tests. Synovial fluid biomarkers play an integral role in the diagnosis of PJI and have been incorporated into recent guidelines as minor diagnostic criteria [15]. In a comprehensive meta-analysis by Carli et al., synovial fluid tests were found to have a superior diagnostic accuracy compared to serum or tissue-based diagnostic tests [74]. The authors identified five synovial fluid tests (alpha-defensin laboratory-based or lateral flow test, CRP, leukocyte esterase strips, polymorphonuclear neutrophil percentage, and white blood cell count) that had the best fitted hierarchical summary receiver operating characteristic (HSROC) curves and highest diagnostic performance of all 17 tests analyzed, concluding that any aspiration should utilize one of these five tests whenever PJI is suspected. This section will focus on these five synovial fluid biomarkers as well as new emerging tests for the diagnosis of PJI.

6.3.1   White Blood Cell Count and Polymorphonuclear Neutrophil Percentage

White blood cell (WBC) count and polymorphonuclear neutrophil percentage (PMN%) are two important synovial fluid tests that have been validated as minor criteria in the current evidence-based definition of PJI [15]. Multiple studies have evaluated the accuracy of these markers for the diagnosis of PJI [75–78]. Unlike other criteria, it is important to note that the diagnostic thresholds for these biomarkers vary based on the timing of infection. For acute PJI within 6 weeks postoperatively, a threshold of >10,000 cells/µL for synovial WBC count and >90% for synovial PMN% should be used to diagnose PJI, whereas for chronic PJI greater than 6 weeks postoperatively, a threshold of >3000 cells/µL and >80% should be used [15]. Using these cutoff points, Shahi et al. found a sensitivity and specificity of 86% and 83% for synovial WBC count, respectively, as well as a sensitivity and specificity of 86% and 81% for synovial PMN%, respectively [79].

When using these biomarkers, clinicians should be cognizant of certain clinical scenarios that may negatively influence the accuracy of results [80, 81]. As is the case with other tests, the type of microorganism and premature use of antimicrobials before joint aspiration have been shown to impact diagnostic thresholds [76, 82], although a concurrent diagnosis of inflammatory arthritis did not appear to do so [30]. In the setting of a traumatic aspiration, a validated formula that adjusts for the synovial red blood cell, serum red blood cell, and serum WBC counts should be used to calculate the corrected synovial WBC count [80]. Additionally, Kwon et al. noted that automated synovial fluid WBC count and PMN% could be unreliable in the context of a failed metal-on-metal implant or corrosion reaction [83]. As the presence of macrophages with phagocytosed metal or amorphous material, fragmented cells, or blood clots can lead to inaccuracies when performing an automated cell count [81], it has been recommended that such cases require a manual synovial WBC count to alert the surgeon of the possibility of a false-positive result [84]. Similarly, the inability to generate a WBC differential in this context should cast doubts on the reliability of the automated synovial fluid WBC count. In a previous study by Wyles et al., the authors found that of the 35 metal-on-metal THAs analyzed, 12 (34%) had a false-positive synovial fluid WBC count (>10,000 cells/IL) and the differential could not be generated in 16

(46%) samples [85]. While these caveats may be more relevant to hip corrosion, a recent study by Deirmengian et al. also found a high rate of false positivity using automated cell counters to analyze synovial fluid of hip and knee arthroplasties [86]. Although false-positive rates were higher in THAs (34%), the frequency (10%) and magnitude of false-positive automated synovial fluid WBC counts were also concerning for TKAs, with higher modified ICM scores and culture positivity confirming the accuracy of manual rather than automated WBC counts [86]. These findings highlight the need to verify the accuracy of positive automated synovial fluid WBC counts with manual counts, as well as the need to integrate other synovial fluid tests and minor diagnostic criteria to reconcile any inconsistencies.

6.3.2 Leukocyte Esterase

Leukocyte esterase is an enzyme secreted by activated neutrophils following their migration to the site of infection. It has traditionally been used in the diagnosis of urinary tract infections, although its diagnostic utility in the workup of PJI has also gained recognition recently [87]. Leukocyte esterase tests are readily available, point-of-care tests requiring the application of infected joint fluid onto colorimetric strips. Detection of the enzyme is then reflected as a color change on the test strip [87], providing almost immediate results and guiding intraoperative decision-making. Furthermore, leukocyte esterase testing is currently the simplest and cheapest test available with an estimated cost of 0.17 USD per test [88]. Despite its accessibility and ease of use, one major limitation is the potential for blood contamination within the fluid samples to interfere with the colorimetric changes of the test strip [89], although this may be overcome by centrifuging synovial fluid samples for 2–3 min prior to application [90]. Excellent diagnostic accuracy has been demonstrated in previous studies, with Wetters et al. reporting a sensitivity of 92.9–93.3% and specificity of 77.0–88.8% [89], and Tischler et al. reporting a sensitivity of 79% and specificity of 81% in 221 patients that fulfilled

MSIS criteria for PJI [91]. In a meta-analysis of five studies, Wyatt et al. also found a sensitivity and specificity of 81% (95% CI, 49–95%) and 97% (95% CI, 82–99%) using a (++) reading, respectively [88]. When considering (++) as the diagnostic threshold instead of (+), Carli et al. reported a higher specificity (97% vs. 84%) at the expense of a slightly lower sensitivity (93% vs. 96%) [74]. A third study compared its diagnostic accuracy with that of other laboratory tests and found the highest diagnostic odds ratio for the leukocyte esterase strip test (OR 30.06, 95% CI 17.8–50.7) [79].

6.3.3 Alpha-Defensin

Alpha-defensin is another synovial fluid biomarker that has a high accuracy when used in the diagnostic workup for PJI [92]. Defensins are naturally occurring antimicrobial peptides that are part of the innate immune response against most gram positive and negative bacteria, fungi, and enveloped viruses [93]. They are commonly secreted by neutrophils as well as certain macrophage cell lines, and their synthesis is induced by pro-inflammatory cytokines or microbiological products. While their precise antimicrobial mechanism has yet to be fully elucidated, alpha-defensins are generally believed to cause a disruption in pathogen membrane integrity, resulting in cell lysis [94, 95]. Current literature has demonstrated the utility of alpha-defensin as a diagnostic tool for PJI, with studies reporting a sensitivity and specificity of over 95% [96, 97]. Bingham et al. even suggested that the diagnostic accuracy of synovial fluid alpha-defensin assays exceeded that of all other available tests [98]. This was confirmed in a recent meta-analysis by Carli et al., which found that laboratory-based alpha-defensin tests and leukocyte esterase strips (++) had a near-perfect diagnostic performance with the best fitted HSROC curves compared to other tests [74]. However, it is important to distinguish between the two available methods to analyze alpha-defensin: (1) the laboratory-based alpha-defensin immunoassay, which is a quantitative test that takes up to 24 h to complete and

(2) the alpha-defensin lateral flow test, which is a standalone device that produces a qualitative binary result within approximately 10 min. In the aforementioned study by Carli et al., the lateral flow test kit had a lower pooled sensitivity of 82% compared to the laboratory-based test, although a high specificity was still maintained [74]. These findings were echoed by previous systematic reviews and meta-analyses on alpha-defensin [99–102]. Eriksson et al. found a lower overall diagnostic accuracy for the lateral flow test compared to the laboratory immunoassay (AUC 0.75 vs. 0.98), whereas no difference in specificity was found (90% vs. 96%; $p = 0.06$) [100]. Similarly, Suen et al. analyzed ten studies and reported a pooled sensitivity and specificity of 77% and 91% for the lateral flow test, which was lower than that of the immunoassay (sensitivity 95%, specificity 97%) [102]. Although a recent meta-analysis by Kuiper et al. questioned the difference in sensitivity [103], current evidence still suggests that the lateral flow test may be a more suitable test for ruling in rather than ruling out infection [100]. Notwithstanding, several advantages of the lateral flow device exist, such as the improved accessibility of a point-of-care test with a rapid response time, obviating the need to ship samples to a centralized laboratory for analysis as in the case of the laboratory-based immunoassay.

Specific clinical scenarios may influence the diagnostic performance of alpha-defensin. When comparing lateral flow test results of 109 cases with the 2013 ICM definition of PJI, Plate et al. found a higher false-positive rate in patients with a concurrent diagnosis of inflammatory arthritides including crystal deposition disease, concluding that an assessment for crystal deposition in synovial fluid aspirates should also be performed if this test is to be used for the diagnosis of PJI [104]. As is the case with synovial fluid WBC counts, corrosion reactions seen in failed metal-on-metal implants may lead to a false-positive rate of 31% when using the alpha-defensin test [105]. Nonetheless, alpha-defensin provides consistent accuracy irrespective of the infecting organism species or premature antibiotic administration [92, 106]. While the impressive performance of the laboratory-based alpha-defensin immunoassay has led to its incorporation into 2018 update of the ICM criteria for the diagnosis of PJI [15], it is important to acknowledge that relatively fewer studies have evaluated this novel biomarker compared to the wealth of literature on routine diagnostic tests [74], highlighting the need for additional investigations in more objective settings. Moreover, given the high costs of alpha-defensin (approximately USD 760) relative to leukocyte esterase (approximately 0.17 USD), future research should aim to evaluate the cost-effectiveness of this novel biomarker for the diagnosis of PJI.

6.3.4 Synovial CRP

As serum CRP is a marker of systemic inflammation, it has a limited specificity for localized infections and the potential for false-negatives in the presence of low-virulence biofilm infections [107]. Consequently, several authors have postulated that synovial fluid CRP could be a more specific and sensitive diagnostic test for PJI [108]. CRP functions by activating the complement system to eradicate foreign or dying cells. As a result, its concentration is often higher at the focus of inflammation, as shown in a previous study using synovial CRP to differentiate inflammatory from non-inflammatory monoarthritis [109]. In the initial study proposing its use for the diagnosis of PJI, Parvizi et al. found a sensitivity of 85% and specificity of 95% when using an automated turbidimetric method to analyze synovial CRP [110]. Similarly, Plate et al. studied 171 hip and knee PJIs and found an optimal synovial CRP threshold of 2.9 mg/L, with a sensitivity of 91% and specificity of 82% [111]. Although one study questioned the utility of this synovial fluid biomarker [112], the accuracy of synovial CRP was confirmed in a recent meta-analysis of seven studies, which yielded a pooled sensitivity and specificity of 92% (95% CI, 86–96%) and 90% (95% CI, 87–93%), respectively [113]. Furthermore, the combined measurement of CRP with other synovial fluid biomarkers such as synovial fluid WBC count [114], alpha-defensin

[115], and IL-6 [116] has been shown to greatly improve its diagnostic accuracy, with one study even demonstrating a sensitivity of 97% and specificity of 100% [97]. As with other biomarkers, synovial CRP levels are highly dependent on the causative microorganism, as higher false-negative rates may be observed in the context of less-virulent pathogens [117].

6.3.5 Novel Synovial Fluid Markers

The introduction of alpha-defensin into uniformly accepted diagnostic criteria for PJI has spurred the investigation and development of novel synovial fluid biomarkers in recent years [15, 118]. While some markers such as synovial fluid PCT have failed to demonstrate accuracy in the diagnosis of PJI [118], other markers including synovial fluid calprotectin [119], D-lactate [120], adenosine deaminase [114], and CD64 index (granulocyte:lymphocyte ratio of CD64 expression) [121] have shown promising results. Calprotectin is a protein component of the cytoplasmic membrane in neutrophils that is released following neutrophil activation [122]. While traditionally used in the diagnosis of inflammatory bowel disease, recent studies have shown that this marker can be analyzed in synovial fluid to monitor treatment in inflammatory arthritis [123]. A recent pilot study found that synovial calprotectin had a 89% sensitivity and 90% specificity for diagnosing PJI in a cohort of 61 patients (19 PJIs and 42 aseptic revisions) [119]. In the same vein, synovial D-lactate has been suggested to be an accurate biomarker for PJI diagnosis [124]. As human cells possess L-lactate dehydrogenase and can only produce the L-rotatory isomer of lactate [125], D-lactate has been identified as a bacteria-specific metabolite that can be quantified in synovial fluid and used as a specific marker for joint infections [126]. In a prospective study of 71 PJIs diagnosed based on MSIS criteria, Karbysheva et al. found that synovial D-lactate had a sensitivity and specificity of 94% and 78%, respectively [120]. Coupled with practical advantages such as a rapid turnaround duration and low costs of performing this test, the authors concluded that this biomarker could be a useful point-of-care screening tool for the diagnosis of PJI. Despite these encouraging results, current literature on these novel biomarkers are limited and require validation in future studies before their incorporation into diagnostic algorithms.

6.4 Frozen Section Histopathology

Periprosthetic tissue can be sent for histological evaluation to support the diagnosis of PJI. Specifically, pathologists can examine frozen tissue for neutrophilic infiltration that is suggestive of acute inflammation. One advantage of this diagnostic tool is the relatively short time needed to obtain the results from frozen section analysis, which can provide valuable information for the surgeon and guide intraoperative decision-making. Additionally, histological analysis is unlikely to be influenced by the administration of antibiotics preoperatively, which may be necessary in the rare cases that PJI is complicated by sepsis. On the contrary, technical expertise is needed to utilize this diagnostic tool reliably, as the result is highly operator-dependent and can vary based on the experience or technique of the pathologist reviewing the sample. Moreover, it has been suggested that less-virulent organisms including *C. acnes* and coagulase-negative staphylococci may not elicit a robust neutrophilic inflammatory response, thus increasing the risk of false-negative results in such cases [127]. In order to maximize the diagnostic yield of this test and reduce sampling error, it is important that surgeons sample the periprosthetic tissues that appear infected based on gross inspection intraoperatively. Traditional sites for periprosthetic tissue sampling include the joint pseudocapsule and periprosthetic interface membrane between the implant and adjacent bone. Based on the 2018 ICM definition of PJI, for frozen section histology to be positive, greater than five neutrophils per high-powered field must be identified in at least five separate microscopic fields under ×400 magnification [15].

The diagnostic accuracy of frozen section histopathology was reviewed in a previous meta-analysis of 26 studies involving 3269 patients (796 culture-positive PJIs) [128]. When considering a diagnostic threshold of 5 PMNs per high-powered field, the authors reported a positive likelihood ratio of 10.3 (95% CI 6.3–16.6) and negative likelihood ratio of 0.24 (95 CI, 0.14–0.39), suggesting that intraoperative frozen sections are more useful for confirming the diagnosis of PJI but moderately accurate excluding this diagnosis due to low sensitivity. This was confirmed in a subsequent study utilizing the MSIS criteria as a reference standard for PJI, which reported a sensitivity of 74% and specificity of 94% based on 200 samples sent for frozen section [129]. As frozen section histology appears to be more reliable for ruling in compared to ruling out a diagnosis of PJI, surgeons should consider limiting the use of frozen section histology to patients categorized into the "inconclusive" group preoperatively based on the 2018 ICM criteria. Given the high costs and increased procedural time associated with collecting samples, processing them in the laboratory and performing histological examinations, this more conservative approach could lead to substantial cost savings for the patient.

6.5 Microorganism Identification

The second goal in the diagnosis of PJI consists of identifying the causative organism(s) and determining its antimicrobial susceptibility. While multiple synovial fluid biomarkers have demonstrated superior sensitivity (alpha-defensin, leukocyte esterase, synovial CRP, WBC count, and PMN%) compared to that of culture-based tests [74], synovial fluid and/or periprosthetic tissue cultures still play a major role in any diagnostic algorithm as it allows clinicians to identify the infecting microorganism and administer targeted antibiotic therapy, thereby maximizing the chance of treatment success [19]. Microbial identification also provides valuable prognostic information for patients and guides perioperative counseling [16]. According to the 2018 ICM definition of PJI, the isolation of the same pathogen from two separate tissue or fluid samples is diagnostic of PJI [15]. However, while multiple clinical guidelines on the appropriate surgical and laboratory techniques to maximize culture yield have been published [130], an estimated 7–12% of patients still have negative cultures despite clear clinical evidence of infection such as a draining sinus or a high synovial fluid WBC count [131–134], thus creating a diagnostic conundrum known as culture-negative PJI.

6.5.1 Synovial Fluid Cultures

Synovial fluid culture is an invaluable diagnostic tool as it offers surgeons the opportunity to identify the infecting microorganism(s) and determine its susceptibility prior to surgery. This knowledge can help to guide treatment decisions, especially in regard to the type of antibiotics to administer perioperatively and mix into the antibiotic-loaded polymethylmethacrylate (PMMA) spacer. Following joint aspiration, synovial fluid should be transported to the microbiology laboratory and inoculated onto solid or liquid media as soon as possible, as long transportation times can lead to higher false-negative rates [135]. If this is not feasible, aspirated fluid can also be inoculated into blood culture bottles in the procedure suite to decrease the risk of contamination and improve pathogen recovery while awaiting sample processing [135]. Although cultures are part of major and minor criteria in the recent ICM definition of PJI [15], it must be acknowledged that preoperative aspiration culture only has a moderate-to-high sensitivity for diagnosing PJI. In a meta-analysis of 34 studies with a total of 3332 patients, Qu et al. reported a pooled sensitivity and specificity of 72% (95% CI, 65–78%) and 95% (95% CI, 93–97%), respectively, with subgroup analyses showing a trend toward poorer diagnostic accuracy for hip aspirations compared to knee aspirations (sensitivity 70% vs. 78%; specificity, 94% vs. 96%) [136]. Similarly, the meta-analysis by Carli et al. concluded that this test had a poorer fitted HSROC curve and lower pooled sensitivity compared with other synovial fluid biomarkers [74]. Notwithstanding, the potential to identify the causative pathogen preoperatively should not be discounted, and synovial fluid cultures should remain a part of the workup for any patient with a suspected prosthetic knee infection.

6.5.2 Intraoperative Tissue Cultures

Isolation of the same pathogen from two separate cultures is considered to be diagnostic for PJI based on the 2018 ICM definition, whereas a single positive culture may be considered a contaminant and should be reconciled with other minor criteria [15]. However, it is important to note that cultures not only help to support or confirm the diagnosis of PJI, but also provide guidance in antimicrobial selection. Although cultures have traditionally been used as the gold standard reference for assessing the accuracy of novel diagnostic tests, it is now recognized that up to 30% of PJI cases have negative cultures [24, 133, 137], owing to their lower sensitivity and inability to rule out PJI [138]. Conversely, as it is well established that a varying degree of clinically relevant PJI may be detected in some cases of presumed aseptic loosening based on positive intraoperative cultures [139], it is imperative that intraoperative cultures be taken regardless of the preoperative diagnosis [138]. To maximize culture yield, recommendations from the 2018 ICM state that at least three intraoperative samples should be sent for culture as this produced the highest negative predictive value to rule out infection without reducing the positive predictive value [138]. Samples should be taken from the areas of infection based on gross inspection, which should include synovial, femoral, and tibial tissue [138]. These should then be incubated for 5–14 days. For suspected culture-negative PJI cases or cases in which the organism is suspected to be less-virulent or fastidious (e.g. *Cutibacterium* species), a longer incubation time should be used [133]. Swab cultures should not be taken due to their low diagnostic yield [140].

6.5.3 Sonication Fluid Cultures

Current evidence suggests that low-intensity sonication of explanted prostheses is an effective means to disrupt biofilm on the prosthetic surface to increase the sensitivity of microbiological isolation compared to traditional sampling of synovial fluid or periprosthetic tissues [141–144]. Sonication may also improve culture yield by dislodging sessile organisms on explanted prostheses [145, 146]. Cultures of sonication fluid have demonstrated an improved sensitivity (78–97%) in microorganism identification without compromising specificity (81–99%) [142, 145, 147–149]. Trampuz et al. studied 331 patients and found a sensitivity of 79% for sonication fluid cultures, which was significantly greater than that of tissue cultures (61%) [142]. Interestingly, these findings persisted even in the presence of antimicrobial therapy within 14 days prior to surgery (75% vs. 45%). Similarly, Rothenberg et al. reported a higher sensitivity for sonication fluid cultures in MSIS-confirmed PJIs compared to tissue cultures (97% vs. 57%) with no difference in specificity [149], while Janz et al. showed that these parameters could be improved to 100% by separating components into multiple sonication fluid cultures [150]. In a meta-analysis of 12 studies evaluating sonication fluid cultures, Zhai et al. found a pooled sensitivity and specificity of 80% (95% CI, 0.74–0.84) and 95% (95% CI, 0.90–0.98), respectively [151]. Despite these promising results, some authors have suggested that the accuracy of sonication fluid cultures may vary based on the sonication technique used [152] as well as timing of PJI [153]. False-positive results have also been observed and attributed to contamination during the sonication process [150]. To overcome this limitation, most authors have recommended a diagnostic threshold of at least five five colony-forming units (CFUs) for sonication fluid cultures [142, 149, 151]. In view of the overwhelming evidence demonstrating improved pathogen isolation with the use of sonication fluid cultures relative to traditional synovial fluid or tissue cultures, current guidelines support the use of sonication in every patient suspected of having a PJI [138].

6.5.4 Culture-Negative Infections

The isolation of an organism from microbiological cultures is not always possible despite clinical evidence confirming the presence of PJI—a phenomenon commonly referred to as culture-negative periprosthetic joint infections (CN-PJI) [131]. False-negative results not only preclude the selection of targeted antimicrobial therapy and lead to lower rates of treatment success [154], but also result in unnecessary anxiety for patients who may challenge the diagnosis of PJI due to an inability to isolate a pathogen [133]. Furthermore, empirical treatment of CN-PJI usually entails administering broad-spectrum or multiple antibiotics to cover the most common microorganisms according to epidemiological surveys, which may be less effective and increases the risk of adverse reactions or systemic toxicity. The prevalence of CN-PJI has been noted to be as high as 30% [24, 133, 137]. Possible reasons for negative cultures have been proposed, such as infection by fastidious pathogens, biofilm encapsulation, uncommon organisms (e.g. fungi or mycobacteria) that do not replicate on routine culture media, inadequate sampling, or transportation, as well as insufficient resuscitation in the laboratory [16, 130, 135, 155]. Nonetheless, the most important cause of failure to isolate an organism is the administration of antibiotics before obtaining samples from the infected joint [131, 133, 155, 156].

6.5.5 Antibiotics and Culture Yield

Sub-therapeutic or mistargeted antimicrobial treatment has been shown to induce a viable but non-culturable (VBNC) physiological state in many pathogens [157–161], rendering the results of these cultures falsely negative [131, 133]. While most pathogens are generally unable to cause infection in a VBNC state, these bacteria still retain their virulence and can cause infection after being resuscitated [162], likely accounting for the phenomenon of CN-PJI. Current evidence cautions against the use of antibiotics in the period leading up to revision arthroplasty [82,

131, 142, 156]. Trampuz et al. demonstrated that any administration of antibiotics in the 2 weeks before obtaining intraarticular cultures adversely influenced the sensitivity of cultures and was associated with a higher false-negative rate (55% vs. 23%) [142]. In another case-control study of 60 patients, Berbari et al. found that 53% of patients who had CN-PJI received antimicrobial therapy within 3 months before the diagnosis and 23% received the antimicrobial agent up to the time samples were taken from the infected joint [131]. Similarly, Malekzadeh et al. found that patients with CN-PJI were 4 times more likely to have received antimicrobial therapy in the preceding 3 months before diagnosis [156], while Shahi et al. reported that patients with antibiotic use before aspiration had a higher rate of CN-PJI compared to those without any antibiotic history [82]. Given these considerations, clinical practice guidelines from the AAOS have recommended against preemptive treatment before a thorough evaluation for PJI, advising clinicians to withhold antibiotic therapy for at least 2 weeks before intraoperative specimen collection to improve culture yield [163]. However, whether these recommendations can be applied uniformly to all suspected cases of PJI remains unknown. In particular, several authors have proposed that an even longer period without antimicrobial exposure may be required to culture certain fastidious organisms [142, 164–166]. Future research is needed to refine the present guidelines with regard to the effect of different antimicrobial agents on the culture yield of differing organisms, as well as to define the optimal antibiotic-free period before obtaining samples in patients with suspected PJI.

It is important to distinguish between therapeutic antibiotics (which often requires a prolonged course of treatment) and prophylactic antibiotics (which often comprises a single dose administered perioperatively [167]). While the abovementioned studies have demonstrated that antibiotic administration prior to identifying the causative pathogen increases the risk of false-negative cultures [156], the need to withhold pre-incision prophylactic antibiotics remains a controversial issue in orthopedic surgery [168–174]. Prophylactic antibiotics were traditionally believed to interfere with culture yields from intraoperative samples, leading some investigators to advocate against their use in the context of revision arthroplasty for suspected PJI [164, 175, 176]. Although this practice appears logical, withholding prophylactic antibiotics may increase the risk of surgical site infection or systemic dissemination perioperatively. Moreover, recent evidence has largely refuted this belief [168–174]. In particular, two randomized controlled trials have demonstrated identical rates of positive intraoperative cultures [169] and concordant cultures [170] in patients who did or did not receive prophylactic antibiotics before incision. A large cohort study of 425 revision TKAs also reported no difference in the percentage of positive cultures (26% vs. 27%) as well as the species of bacteria cultured [174]. Given the large body of evidence suggesting that the practice of withholding prophylactic antibiotics to maximize culture yield may not be as critical as previously thought, the 2018 ICM recommended that perioperative antibiotic administration for revision TJA should not be routinely withheld, but should instead be guided by the degree of clinical suspicion for PJI and whether or not a causative organism has been isolated before surgery [130].

6.5.6 Molecular Tests

The overreliance on cultures as the gold standard for microorganism identification has led to the conundrum of CN-PJI. Molecular techniques to detect bacterial DNA present a unique opportunity to improve the accuracy of diagnosis for PJI, particularly in the setting of negative cultures [133]. Multiplex polymerase chain reaction (PCR)-based assays allow the detection of common microorganisms and their resistance genes, improving sensitivity and reducing the time to diagnosis compared with traditional cultures [177–179]. However, the requirement for specific primers often results in the failure to detect atypical or less common pathogens as well as resistance mechanisms [180, 181]. Another molecular technique currently available is 16S rRNA gene sequencing [178]. Unlike PCR-based assays, this method allows the detection of a wider variety of bacterial species, prompting some authors to suggest that 16S rRNA sequencing may have a higher sensitivity compared to bacterial cultures and PCR-based techniques [178, 182, 183]. Primers used in this technique are specific for highly conserved sequences that are found in almost all bacteria, as well as variable regions in between them, thereby allowing the identification of a broad range of bacteria. However, major limitations of this method include the inability to detect antimicrobial resistance genes and polymicrobial infections, which can only be determined using high-throughput sequencing methods rather than traditional capillary-based ones [184]. More recently, metagenomic next generation sequencing (mNGS) was introduced to overcome the shortcomings of previous molecular tests. This high-throughput sequencing technique enables the detection of complete bacterial genomes, including unculturable, unsuspected, and non-viable organisms in the sample [185–188]. Resistance genes can also be simultaneously detected using this technique [187]. Direct sequencing of specimens improves the diagnostic yield compared to traditional cultures [186], as recent studies have shown that mNGS was able to detect new organisms in 16–44% of CN-PJI cases and 4–67% of culture-positive cases [185–189].

In addition to improved diagnostic accuracy, other advantages of molecular testing have proposed. Current evidence suggests that molecular methods for pathogen identification are unaffected by prior antibiotic administration [181, 190], overcoming the limitations of traditional cultures. This advantage may be clinically useful in the management of patients undergoing two-stage exchange arthroplasty. As it is often is difficult to ascertain whether infection has been eradicated following a course of 4–6 weeks of systemic antibiotics in the interim stage, current practice often involves rechecking inflammatory markers such as ESR and CRP, although this has been shown to correlate poorly with the likelihood of residual infection at the time of reimplantation [40, 41, 191, 192]. Alternatively, synovial fluid cultures may be taken after an "antibiotic holiday" of 2 weeks prior to reimplantation to improve diagnostic yield. In such cases, molecular testing not only circumvents the need for an "antibiotic holiday," but also provides more sensitive diagnostic information that can guide clinical decisions such as the appropriateness and timing of reimplantation [193]. The utility of molecular methods may further extend to patients on chronic suppressive antibiotic therapy, providing a reliable method for monitoring bacterial load as well as the development of antimicrobial resistance. However, it is important to note that while the ability to detect bacterial DNA even after cell death from antimicrobial therapy may seem advantageous in these situations, this is in fact a double-edged sword, as these techniques cannot differentiate between active vs. eradicated infections [194, 195]. Previous studies have demonstrated that DNA can also be isolated from non-viable bacteria in sterile joints, especially in patients with inflammatory arthritis [196, 197]. Consequently, the importance of clinical correlation and adjunctive tests to support the diagnosis of PJI cannot be further emphasized [15]. Currently, high costs and complex laboratory workflows are the main obstacles hindering the adoption of molecular testing. As these methods become more cost-efficient over time, their speed of detection as well as improved sensitivity especially in the setting of prior antibiotic administration will allow clinicians to initiate targeted antimicrobial therapy at an earlier time, potentially improving the treatment outcomes for PJI in the future.

6.6 Conclusion

Infection following knee arthroplasty is a rare but devastating complication that not only increases the risk of mortality and diminishes the quality of life of orthopedic patients [11, 12], but also poses a substantial economic burden to the healthcare system [13]. Due to the vast differences in the management of aseptic failure and PJI, obtaining an early and accurate diagnosis remains paramount [132]. Despite the extraordinary efforts by the orthopedic community, the diagnosis of PJI still poses a formidable challenge to every surgeon. No single test can confirm or rule out the diagnosis, hence current diagnostic criteria are based on clinical findings as well as a combination of laboratory tests described in this chapter. Over the past decade, a plethora of novel serological and synovial fluid biomarkers have emerged as highly accurate tools for diagnosing PJI, some of which have been included in the latest 2018 definition of PJI [15]. Notwithstanding, surgeons should be cognizant of the challenging clinical scenarios and subpopulations that may alter the diagnostic performance of these laboratory tests, including patient comorbidities, timing of infection, pathogen virulence, and premature antibiotic use. Furthermore, one of the most difficult challenges in the diagnosis of PJI is the isolation of the causative microorganism. The limitations of traditional microbiological cultures have been highlighted repeatedly in orthopedic literature, culminating in a new diagnostic conundrum known as CN-PJI. To this end, molecular tests hold much promise in pathogen identification, maintaining their diagnostic accuracy in a variety of clinical situations. However, further research is necessary to translate this new technology into routine practice and validate its clinical utility in enhancing patient care, controlling healthcare costs and improving antimicrobial stewardship.

References

1. Sloan M, Premkumar A, Sheth NP. Projected volume of primary total joint arthroplasty in the U.S., 2014 to 2030. J Bone Joint Surg. 2018;100:1455–60. https://doi.org/10.2106/JBJS.17.01617.
2. Namba RS, Inacio MC, Paxton EW. Risk factors associated with deep surgical site infections after primary total knee arthroplasty: an analysis of 56,216 knees. J Bone Joint Surg Am. 2013;95:775–82.
3. Kurtz SM, Ong KL, Lau E, Bozic KJ, Berry D, Parvizi J. Prosthetic joint infection risk after TKA in the Medicare population. Clin Orthop Relat Res. 2010;468:52–6.
4. Koh CK, Zeng I, Ravi S, Zhu M, Vince KG, Young SW. Periprosthetic joint infection is the main cause of failure for modern knee arthroplasty: an analysis of 11,134 knees. Clin Orthop Relat

Res. 2017;475:2194–201. https://doi.org/10.1007/s11999-017-5396-4.

5. Dyrhovden GS, Lygre SHL, Badawy M, Gøthesen Ø, Furnes O. Have the causes of revision for total and unicompartmental knee arthroplasties changed during the past two decades? Clin Orthop Relat Res. 2017;475:1874–86. https://doi.org/10.1007/s11999-017-5316-7.

6. Steiner C, Andrews R, Barrett M, Weiss A. HCUP projections: mobility/orthopedic procedures 2003 to 2012. Washington, DC: US Agency for Healthcare Research and Quality; 2012.

7. Springer BD, Cahue S, Etkin CD, Lewallen DG, McGrory BJ. Infection burden in total hip and knee arthroplasties: an international registry-based perspective. Arthroplast Today. 2017;3:137–40. https://doi.org/10.1016/j.artd.2017.05.003.

8. Narayan KMV, Boyle JP, Geiss LS, Saaddine JB, Thompson TJ. Impact of recent increase in incidence on future diabetes burden: U.S., 2005-2050. Diabetes Care. 2006;29:2114–6. https://doi.org/10.2337/dc06-1136.

9. Flegal KM, Carroll MD, Ogden CL, Curtin LR. Prevalence and trends in obesity among US adults, 1999-2008. JAMA. 2010;303:235–41. https://doi.org/10.1001/jama.2009.2014.

10. O'Toole P, Maltenfort MG, Chen AF, Parvizi J. Projected increase in periprosthetic joint infections secondary to rise in diabetes and obesity. J Arthroplasty. 2016;31:7–10. https://doi.org/10.1016/j.arth.2015.07.034.

11. Zmistowski B, Karam JA, Durinka JB, Casper DS, Parvizi J. Periprosthetic joint infection increases the risk of one-year mortality. J Bone Joint Surg Am. 2013;95:2177–84. https://doi.org/10.2106/JBJS.L.00789.

12. Helwig P, Morlock J, Oberst M, Hauschild O, Hübner J, Borde J, et al. Periprosthetic joint infection—effect on quality of life. Int Orthop. 2014;38:1077–81. https://doi.org/10.1007/s00264-013-2265-y.

13. Kurtz SM, Lau E, Watson H, Schmier JK, Parvizi J. Economic burden of periprosthetic joint infection in the United States. J Arthroplasty. 2012;27:61–65. e1. https://doi.org/10.1016/j.arth.2012.02.022.

14. American Academy of Orthopaedic Surgeons. American Academy of Orthopaedic Surgeons clinical practice guideline on the diagnosis and prevention of periprosthetic joint infections. AAOS Quality & Practice Resources. n.d. https://www.aaos.org/contentassets/9a006edd608c468ba066624defca5502/pji-clinical-practice-guideline-final-9-18-19-.pdf. Accessed 30 Nov 2020.

15. Parvizi J, Tan TL, Goswami K, Higuera C, Della Valle C, Chen AF, et al. The 2018 definition of periprosthetic hip and knee infection: an evidence-based and validated criteria. J Arthroplasty. 2018;33:1309–1314.e2. https://doi.org/10.1016/j.arth.2018.02.078.

16. Patel R, Osmon DR, Hanssen AD. The diagnosis of prosthetic joint infection: current techniques and emerging technologies. Clin Orthop Relat Res. 2005;437:55–8.

17. Parvizi J, Ghanem E, Sharkey P, Aggarwal A, Burnett RSJ, Barrack RL. Diagnosis of infected total knee: findings of a multicenter database. Clin Orthop Relat Res. 2008;466:2628–33.

18. Parvizi J, Fassihi SC, Enayatollahi MA. Diagnosis of periprosthetic joint infection following hip and knee arthroplasty. Orthop Clin North Am. 2016;47:505–15. https://doi.org/10.1016/j.ocl.2016.03.001.

19. Yang J, Parvizi J, Hansen EN, Culvern CN, Segreti JC, Tan T, et al. 2020 Mark Coventry Award: Microorganism-directed oral antibiotics reduce the rate of failure due to further infection after two-stage revision hip or knee arthroplasty for chronic infection: a multicentre randomized controlled trial at a minimum of two years. Bone Joint J. 2020;102-B:3–9. https://doi.org/10.1302/0301-620X.102B6.BJJ-2019-1596.R1.

20. Nora D, Salluh J, Martin-Loeches I, Póvoa P. Biomarker-guided antibiotic therapy—strengths and limitations. Ann Transl Med. 2017;5:208. https://doi.org/10.21037/atm.2017.04.04.

21. Della Valle C, Parvizi J, Bauer TW, DiCesare PE, Evans RP, Segreti J, et al. Diagnosis of periprosthetic joint infections of the hip and knee. J Am Acad Orthop Surg. 2010;18:760–70.

22. Greidanus NV, Masri BA, Garbuz DS, Wilson SD, McAlinden MG, Xu M, et al. Use of erythrocyte sedimentation rate and C-reactive protein level to diagnose infection before revision total knee arthroplasty. J Bone Joint Surg. 2007;89:1409–16. https://doi.org/10.2106/jbjs.d.02602.

23. Schinsky MF, Valle CJD, Sporer SM, Paprosky WG. Perioperative testing for joint infection in patients undergoing revision total hip arthroplasty. J Bone Joint Surg Am. 2008;90:1869–75. https://doi.org/10.2106/jbjs.g.01255.

24. Abdel Karim M, Andrawis J, Bengoa F, Bracho C, Compagnoni R, Cross M, et al. Hip and knee section, diagnosis, algorithm: proceedings of international consensus on orthopedic infections. J Arthroplasty. 2019;34:S339–50. https://doi.org/10.1016/j.arth.2018.09.018.

25. Piper KE, Fernandez-Sampedro M, Steckelberg KE, Mandrekar JN, Karau MJ, Steckelberg JM, et al. C-reactive protein, erythrocyte sedimentation rate and orthopedic implant infection. PLoS One. 2010;5:e9358. https://doi.org/10.1371/journal.pone.0009358.

26. Nodzo SR, Westrich GH, Henry MW, Miller AO. Clinical analysis of Propionibacterium acnes infection after total knee arthroplasty. J Arthroplasty. 2016;31:1986–9. https://doi.org/10.1016/j.arth.2016.02.025.

27. Pérez-Prieto D, Portillo ME, Puig-Verdié L, Alier A, Martínez S, Sorlí L, et al. C-reactive protein may misdiagnose prosthetic joint infections, particularly chronic and low-grade infections. Int

Orthop. 2017;41:1315–9. https://doi.org/10.1007/s00264-017-3430-5.

28. Akgün D, Müller M, Perka C, Winkler T. The serum level of C-reactive protein alone cannot be used for the diagnosis of prosthetic joint infections, especially in those caused by organisms of low virulence. Bone Joint J. 2018;100-B:1482–6. https://doi.org/10.1302/0301-620X.100B11.BJJ-2018-0514.R1.

29. Greenberg SB. Infections in the immunocompromised rheumatologic patient. Crit Care Clin. 2002;18:931.

30. Cipriano CA, Brown NM, Michael AM, Moric M, Sporer SM, Della Valle CJ. Serum and synovial fluid analysis for diagnosing chronic periprosthetic infection in patients with inflammatory arthritis. J Bone Joint Surg Am. 2012;94:594–600. https://doi.org/10.2106/JBJS.J.01318.

31. Bouvier S, Cochery-Nouvellon E, Faillie J-L, Lissalde-Lavigne G, Lefrant J-Y, Gris J-C. Fibrin-related markers in patients with septic shock: individual comparison of D-dimers and fibrin monomers impacts on prognosis. Thromb Haemost. 2011;106:1228–30. https://doi.org/10.1160/th11-07-0489.

32. Schwameis M, Steiner MM, Schoergenhofer C, Lagler H, Buchtele N, Jilma-Stohlawetz P, et al. D-dimer and histamine in early stage bacteremia: a prospective controlled cohort study. Eur J Intern Med. 2015;26:782–6. https://doi.org/10.1016/j.ejim.2015.10.024.

33. Gando S. Role of fibrinolysis in sepsis. Semin Thromb Hemost. 2013;39:392–9. https://doi.org/10.1055/s-0033-1334140.

34. Ribera T, Monreal L, Armengou L, Ríos J, Prades M. Synovial fluid D-dimer concentration in foals with septic joint disease. J Vet Intern Med. 2011;25:1113–7. https://doi.org/10.1111/j.1939-1676.2011.0758.x.

35. Rodelo JR, De la Rosa G, Valencia ML, Ospina S, Arango CM, Gómez CI, et al. D-dimer is a significant prognostic factor in patients with suspected infection and sepsis. Am J Emerg Med. 2012;30:1991–9.

36. Busso N, Hamilton JA. Extravascular coagulation and the plasminogen activator/plasmin system in rheumatoid arthritis. Arthritis Rheum. 2002;46:2268–79.

37. Shahi A, Kheir MM, Tarabichi M, Hosseinzadeh HRS, Tan TL, Parvizi J. Serum D-dimer test is promising for the diagnosis of periprosthetic joint infection and timing of reimplantation. J Bone Joint Surg. 2017;99:1419–27. https://doi.org/10.2106/JBJS.16.01395.

38. Larsson S, Thelander U, Friberg S. C-reactive protein (CRP) levels after elective orthopedic surgery. Clin Orthop Relat Res. 1992:237–42. https://doi.org/10.1097/00003086-199202000-00035.

39. Bilgen Ö, Atici T, Durak K, Karaeminoğullari O, Bilgen MS. C-reactive protein values and erythrocyte sedimentation rates after total hip and total knee arthroplasty. J Int Med Res. 2001;29:7–12. https://doi.org/10.1177/147323000102900102.

40. Ghanem E, Azzam K, Seeley M, Joshi A, Parvizi J. Staged revision for knee arthroplasty infection: what is the role of serologic tests before reimplantation? Clin Orthop Relat Res. 2009;467:1699–705. https://doi.org/10.1007/s11999-009-0742-9.

41. Kusuma SK, Ward J, Jacofsky M, Sporer SM, Valle CJD. What is the role of serological testing between stages of two-stage reconstruction of the infected prosthetic knee? Clin Orthop Relat Res. 2010;469:1002–8. https://doi.org/10.1007/s11999-010-1619-7.

42. Lee YS, Lee Y-K, Han SB, Nam CH, Parvizi J, Koo K-H. Natural progress of D-dimer following total joint arthroplasty: a baseline for the diagnosis of the early postoperative infection. J Orthop Surg Res. 2018;13:36. https://doi.org/10.1186/s13018-018-0730-4.

43. Li R, Shao H-Y, Hao L-B, Yu B-Z, Qu P-F, Zhou Y-X, et al. Plasma fibrinogen exhibits better performance than plasma D-dimer in the diagnosis of periprosthetic joint infection: a multicenter retrospective study. J Bone Joint Surg. 2019;101:613–9. https://doi.org/10.2106/JBJS.18.00624.

44. Boisclair MD, Lane DA, Wilde JT, Ireland H, Preston FE, Ofosu FA. A comparative evaluation of assays for markers of activated coagulation and/or fibrinolysis: thrombin–antithrombin complex, D-dimer and fibrinogen/fibrin fragment E antigen. Br J Haematol. 1990;74:471–9. https://doi.org/10.1111/j.1365-2141.1990.tb06337.x.

45. Korte W, Riesen WF. Comparability of serum and plasma concentrations of haemostasis activation markers. Clin Chem Lab Med. 2001;39 https://doi.org/10.1515/cclm.2001.101.

46. Xu H, Xie J, Huang Q, Lei Y, Zhang S, Pei F. Plasma fibrin degradation product and D-dimer are of limited value for diagnosing periprosthetic joint infection. J Arthroplasty. 2019;34:2454–60. https://doi.org/10.1016/j.arth.2019.05.009.

47. Pannu TS, Villa JM, Patel PD, Riesgo AM, Barsoum WK, Higuera CA. The utility of serum d-dimer for the diagnosis of periprosthetic joint infection in revision total hip and knee arthroplasty. J Arthroplasty. 2020;35:1692–5. https://doi.org/10.1016/j.arth.2020.01.034.

48. Moser KA, Pearson LN, Pelt CE, Olson JD, Goodwin AJ, Isom JA, et al. Letter to the editor on "The 2018 Definition of Periprosthetic Hip and Knee Infection: An Evidence-Based and Validated Criteria". J Arthroplasty. 2020;35:2682–3. https://doi.org/10.1016/j.arth.2020.05.002.

49. Kirschenbaum LA, McKevitt D, Rullan M, Reisbeck B, Fujii T, Astiz ME. Importance of platelets and fibrinogen in neutrophil-endothelial cell interactions in septic shock. Crit Care Med. 2004;32:1904–9.

50. Horn M, Bertling A, Brodde MF, Müller A, Roth J, Van Aken H, et al. Human neutrophil alpha-

defensins induce formation of fibrinogen and thrombospondin-1 amyloid-like structures and activate platelets via glycoprotein IIb/IIIa. J Thromb Haemost. 2012;10:647–61.

51. Wu H, Meng Z, Pan L, Liu H, Yang X, Yongping C. Plasma fibrinogen performs better than plasma d-dimer and fibrin degradation product in the diagnosis of periprosthetic joint infection and determination of reimplantation timing. J Arthroplasty. 2020;35:2230–6. https://doi.org/10.1016/j.arth.2020.03.055.

52. Xu C, Qu P-F, Chai W, Li R, Chen J-Y. Plasma fibrinogen may predict persistent infection before reimplantation in two-stage exchange arthroplasty for periprosthetic hip infection. J Orthop Surg Res. 2019;14:133. https://doi.org/10.1186/s13018-019-1179-9.

53. Barton BE. IL-6: insights into novel biological activities. Clin Immunol Immunopathol. 1997;85:16–20. https://doi.org/10.1006/clin.1997.4420.

54. Damas P, Ledoux D, Nys M, Vrindts Y, De Groote D, Franchimont P, et al. Cytokine serum level during severe sepsis in human IL-6 as a marker of severity. Ann Surg. 1992;215:356–62. https://doi.org/10.1097/00000658-199204000-00009.

55. Pape HC, Schmidt RE, Rice J, van Griensven M, das Gupta R, Krettek C, et al. Biochemical changes after trauma and skeletal surgery of the lower extremity: quantification of the operative burden. Crit Care Med. 2000;28:3441–8. https://doi.org/10.1097/00003246-200010000-00012.

56. Selberg O, Hecker H, Martin M, Klos A, Bautsch W, Köhl J. Discrimination of sepsis and systemic inflammatory response syndrome by determination of circulating plasma concentrations of procalcitonin, protein complement 3a, and interleukin-6. Crit Care Med. 2000;28:2793–8.

57. Xie K, Dai K, Qu X, Yan M. Serum and synovial fluid interleukin-6 for the diagnosis of periprosthetic joint infection. Sci Rep. 2017;7:1496. https://doi.org/10.1038/s41598-017-01713-4.

58. Di Cesare PE, Chang E, Preston CF, Liu C. Serum interleukin-6 as a marker of periprosthetic infection following total hip and knee arthroplasty. J Bone Joint Surg Am. 2005;87:1921–7. https://doi.org/10.2106/JBJS.D.01803.

59. Wirtz DC, Heller K-D, Miltner O, Zilkens K-W, Wolff JM. Interleukin-6: a potential inflammatory marker after total joint replacement. Int Orthop. 2000;24:194–6.

60. Randau TM, Friedrich MJ, Wimmer MD, Reichert B, Kuberra D, Stoffel-Wagner B, et al. Interleukin-6 in serum and in synovial fluid enhances the differentiation between periprosthetic joint infection and aseptic loosening. PLoS One. 2014;9:e89045. https://doi.org/10.1371/journal.pone.0089045.

61. Berbari E, Mabry T, Tsaras G, Spangehl M, Erwin PJ, Murad MH, et al. Inflammatory blood laboratory levels as markers of prosthetic joint infection: a systematic review and meta-analysis. J Bone Joint Surg Am. 2010;92:2102–9. https://doi.org/10.2106/JBJS.I.01199.

62. Bottner F, Wegner A, Winkelmann W, Becker K, Erren M, Götze C. Interleukin-6, procalcitonin and TNF-α: markers of peri-prosthetic infection following total joint replacement. J Bone Joint Surg. 2007;89-B:94–9. https://doi.org/10.1302/0301-620X.89B1.17485.

63. Ettinger M, Calliess T, Kielstein JT, Sibai J, Brückner T, Lichtinghagen R, et al. Circulating biomarkers for discrimination between aseptic joint failure, low-grade infection, and high-grade septic failure. Clin Infect Dis. 2015;61:332–41. https://doi.org/10.1093/cid/civ286.

64. Simon L, Gauvin F, Amre DK, Saint-Louis P, Lacroix J. Serum procalcitonin and C-reactive protein levels as markers of bacterial infection: a systematic review and meta-analysis. Clin Infect Dis. 2004;39:206–17.

65. Xie K, Qu X, Yan M. Procalcitonin and α-Defensin for Diagnosis of Periprosthetic Joint Infections. J Arthroplasty. 2017;32:1387–94. https://doi.org/10.1016/j.arth.2016.10.001.

66. Yoon J-R, Yang S-H, Shin Y-S. Diagnostic accuracy of interleukin-6 and procalcitonin in patients with periprosthetic joint infection: a systematic review and meta-analysis. Int Orthop. 2018;42:1213–26. https://doi.org/10.1007/s00264-017-3744-3.

67. Friedrich MJ, Randau TM, Wimmer MD, Reichert B, Kuberra D, Stoffel-Wagner B, et al. Lipopolysaccharide-binding protein: a valuable biomarker in the differentiation between periprosthetic joint infection and aseptic loosening? Int Orthop. 2014;38:2201–7. https://doi.org/10.1007/s00264-014-2351-9.

68. Galliera E, Drago L, Vassena C, Romanò C, Marazzi MG, Salcito L, et al. Toll-like receptor 2 in serum: a potential diagnostic marker of prosthetic joint infection? J Clin Microbiol. 2014;52:620–3.

69. Drago L, Vassena C, Dozio E, Corsi MM, Vecchi ED, Mattina R, et al. Procalcitonin, C-reactive protein, interleukin-6, and soluble intercellular adhesion molecule-1 as markers of postoperative orthopaedic joint prosthesis infections. Int J Immunopathol Pharmacol. 2011;24:433–40. https://doi.org/10.1177/039463201102400216.

70. Worthington T, Dunlop D, Casey A, Lambert P, Luscombe J, Elliott T. Serum procalcitonin, interleukin-6, soluble intercellular adhesin molecule-1 and IgG to shortchain exocellular lipoteichoic acid as predictors of infection in total joint prosthesis revision. Br J Biomed Sci. 2010;67:71–6. https://doi.org/10.1080/09674845.2010.11730294.

71. Galliera E, Drago L, Marazzi MG, Romano C, Vassena C, Romanelli MMC. Soluble urokinase-type plasminogen activator receptor (suPAR) as new biomarker of the prosthetic joint infection: correlation with inflammatory cytokines. Clin Chim Acta. 2015;441:23–8.

72. Fjaertoft G, Douhan Håkansson L, Pauksens K, Sisask G, Venge P. Neutrophil CD64 (FcγRI) expres-

sion is a specific marker of bacterial infection: a study on the kinetics and the impact of major surgery. Scand J Infect Dis. 2007;39:525–35.

73. Shohat N, Tan TL, Della Valle CJ, Calkins TE, George J, Higuera C, et al. Development and validation of an evidence-based algorithm for diagnosing periprosthetic joint infection. J Arthroplasty. 2019:S0883540319305868. https://doi.org/10.1016/j.arth.2019.06.016.

74. Carli AV, Abdelbary H, Ahmadzai N, Cheng W, Shea B, Hutton B, et al. Diagnostic accuracy of serum, synovial, and tissue testing for chronic periprosthetic joint infection after hip and knee replacements: a systematic review. J Bone Joint Surg. 2019;101:635–49. https://doi.org/10.2106/JBJS.18.00632.

75. Mason JB, Fehring TK, Odum SM, Griffin WL, Nussman DS. The value of white blood cell counts before revision total knee arthroplasty. J Arthroplasty. 2003;18:1038–43. https://doi.org/10.1016/s0883-5403(03)00448-0.

76. Trampuz A, Hanssen AD, Osmon DR, Mandrekar J, Steckelberg JM, Patel R. Synovial fluid leukocyte count and differential for the diagnosis of prosthetic knee infection. Am J Med. 2004;117:556–62. https://doi.org/10.1016/j.amjmed.2004.06.022.

77. Bedair H, Ting N, Jacovides C, Saxena A, Moric M, Parvizi J, et al. The Mark Coventry award: diagnosis of early postoperative TKA infection using synovial fluid analysis. Clin Orthop Relat Res. 2010;469:34–40. https://doi.org/10.1007/s11999-010-1433-2.

78. Dinneen A, Guyot A, Clements J, Bradley N. Synovial fluid white cell and differential count in the diagnosis or exclusion of prosthetic joint infection. Bone Joint J. 2013;95-B:554–7. https://doi.org/10.1302/0301-620X.95B4.30388.

79. Shahi A, Tan TL, Kheir MM, Tan DD, Parvizi J. Diagnosing periprosthetic joint infection: and the winner is? J Arthroplasty. 2017;32:S232–5. https://doi.org/10.1016/j.arth.2017.06.005.

80. Ghanem E, Houssock C, Pulido L, Han S, Jaberi FM, Parvizi J. Determining "true" leukocytosis in bloody joint aspiration. J Arthroplasty. 2008;23:182–7. https://doi.org/10.1016/j.arth.2007.08.016.

81. Yi PH, Cross MB, Moric M, Levine BR, Sporer SM, Paprosky WG, et al. Do serologic and synovial tests help diagnose infection in revision hip arthroplasty with metal-on-metal bearings or corrosion? Clin Orthop Relat Res. 2015;473:498–505. https://doi.org/10.1007/s11999-014-3902-5.

82. Shahi A, Deirmengian C, Higuera C, Chen A, Restrepo C, Zmistowski B, et al. Premature therapeutic antimicrobial treatments can compromise the diagnosis of late periprosthetic joint infection. Clin Orthop Relat Res. 2015;473:2244–9. https://doi.org/10.1007/s11999-015-4142-z.

83. Kwon Y-M, Antoci V, Leone WA, Tsai T-Y, Dimitriou D, Liow MHL. Utility of serum inflammatory and synovial fluid counts in the diagnosis of infection in taper corrosion of dual taper modular stems. J Arthroplasty. 2016;31:1997–2003. https://doi.org/10.1016/j.arth.2016.02.020.

84. Lombardi AV Jr, Barrack RL, Berend KR, Cuckler JM, Jacobs JJ, Mont MA, et al. The Hip Society: algorithmic approach to diagnosis and management of metal-on-metal arthroplasty. J Bone Joint Surg. 2012;94-B:14–8. https://doi.org/10.1302/0301-620X.94B11.30680.

85. Wyles CC, Van Demark RE, Sierra RJ, Trousdale RT. High rate of infection after aseptic revision of failed metal-on-metal total hip arthroplasty. Clin Orthop Relat Res. 2014;472:509–16. https://doi.org/10.1007/s11999-013-3157-6.

86. Deirmengian CA, Kazarian GS, Feeley SP, Sizer SC. False-positive automated synovial fluid white blood cell counting is a concern for both hip and knee arthroplasty aspirates. J Arthroplasty. 2020;35:S304–7. https://doi.org/10.1016/j.arth.2020.01.060.

87. Parvizi J, Jacovides C, Antoci V, Ghanem E. Diagnosis of periprosthetic joint infection: the utility of a simple yet unappreciated enzyme. J Bone Joint Surg. 2011;93:2242–8.

88. Wyatt MC, Beswick AD, Kunutsor SK, Wilson MJ, Whitehouse MR, Blom AW. The alpha-defensin immunoassay and leukocyte esterase colorimetric strip test for the diagnosis of periprosthetic infection: a systematic review and meta-analysis. J Bone Joint Surg. 2016;98:992–1000. https://doi.org/10.2106/JBJS.15.01142.

89. Wetters NG, Berend KR, Lombardi AV, Morris MJ, Tucker TL, Della Valle CJ. Leukocyte esterase reagent strips for the rapid diagnosis of periprosthetic joint infection. J Arthroplasty. 2012;27:8–11. https://doi.org/10.1016/j.arth.2012.03.037.

90. Aggarwal VK, Tischler E, Ghanem E, Parvizi J. Leukocyte esterase from synovial fluid aspirate. J Arthroplasty. 2013;28:193–5. https://doi.org/10.1016/j.arth.2012.06.023.

91. Tischler EH, Cavanaugh PK, Parvizi J. Leukocyte esterase strip test: matched for musculoskeletal infection society criteria. J Bone Joint Surg Am. 2014;96:1917–20. https://doi.org/10.2106/JBJS.M.01591.

92. Deirmengian C, Kardos K, Kilmartin P, Gulati S, Citrano P, Booth RE. The alpha-defensin test for periprosthetic joint infection responds to a wide spectrum of organisms. Clin Orthop Relat Res. 2015;473:2229–35. https://doi.org/10.1007/s11999-015-4152-x.

93. White SH, Wimley WC, Selsted ME. Structure, function, and membrane integration of defensins. Curr Opin Struct Biol. 1995;5:521–7. https://doi.org/10.1016/0959-440x(95)80038-7.

94. Mathew B, Nagaraj R. Antimicrobial activity of human alpha-defensin 5 and its linear analogs: N-terminal fatty acylation results in enhanced antimicrobial activity of the linear analogs. Peptides. 2015;71:128–40. https://doi.org/10.1016/j.peptides.2015.07.009.

95. Xie Z, Feng J, Yang W, Xiang F, Yang F, Zhao Y, et al. Human alpha-defensins are immune-related Kv1.3 channel inhibitors: new support for their roles in adaptive immunity. FASEB J. 2015;29:4324–33. https://doi.org/10.1096/fj.15-274787.

96. Frangiamore SJ, Gajewski ND, Saleh A, Farias-Kovac M, Barsoum WK, Higuera CA. α-Defensin accuracy to diagnose periprosthetic joint infection—best available test? J Arthroplasty. 2016;31:456–60. https://doi.org/10.1016/j.arth.2015.09.035.

97. Deirmengian C, Kardos K, Kilmartin P, Cameron A, Schiller K, Parvizi J. Combined measurement of synovial fluid α-defensin and C-reactive protein levels: highly accurate for diagnosing periprosthetic joint infection. J Bone Joint Surg. 2014;96:1439–45. https://doi.org/10.2106/JBJS.M.01316.

98. Bingham J, Clarke H, Spangehl M, Schwartz A, Beauchamp C, Goldberg B. The alpha defensin-1 biomarker assay can be used to evaluate the potentially infected total joint arthroplasty. Clin Orthop Relat Res. 2014;472:4006–9. https://doi.org/10.1007/s11999-014-3900-7.

99. Ahmad SS, Hirschmann MT, Becker R, Shaker A, Ateschrang A, Keel MJB, et al. A meta-analysis of synovial biomarkers in periprosthetic joint infection: Synovasure™ is less effective than the ELISA-based alpha-defensin test. Knee Surg Sports Traumatol Arthrosc. 2018;26:3039–47. https://doi.org/10.1007/s00167-018-4904-8.

100. Eriksson HK, Nordström J, Gabrysch K, Hailer NP, Lazarinis S. Does the alpha-defensin immunoassay or the lateral flow test have better diagnostic value for periprosthetic joint infection? A systematic review. Clin Orthop Relat Res. 2018;476:1065–72. https://doi.org/10.1007/s11999.0000000000000244.

101. Marson BA, Deshmukh SR, Grindlay DJC, Scammell BE. Alpha-defensin and the Synovasure lateral flow device for the diagnosis of prosthetic joint infection: a systematic review and meta-analysis. Bone Joint J. 2018;100-B:703–11. https://doi.org/10.1302/0301-620X.100B6.BJJ-2017-1563.R1.

102. Suen K, Keeka M, Ailabouni R, Tran P. Synovasure 'quick test' is not as accurate as the laboratory-based α-defensin immunoassay: a systematic review and meta-analysis. Bone Joint. 2018;100-B:66–72. https://doi.org/10.1302/0301-620X.100B1.BJJ-2017-0630.R1.

103. Kuiper JWP, Verberne SJ, Vos SJ, van Egmond PW. Does the alpha defensin ELISA test perform better than the alpha defensin lateral flow test for PJI diagnosis? A systematic review and meta-analysis of prospective studies. Clin Orthop Relat Res. 2020;478:1333–44. https://doi.org/10.1097/CORR.0000000000001225.

104. Plate A, Stadler L, Sutter R, Anagnostopoulos A, Frustaci D, Zbinden R, et al. Inflammatory disorders mimicking periprosthetic joint infections may result in false-positive α-defensin. Clin Microbiol Infect. 2018;24:1212.e1–6. https://doi.org/10.1016/j.cmi.2018.02.019.

105. Okroj KT, Calkins TE, Kayupov E, Kheir MM, Bingham JS, Beauchamp CP, et al. The alpha-defensin test for diagnosing periprosthetic joint infection in the setting of an adverse local tissue reaction secondary to a failed metal-on-metal bearing or corrosion at the head-neck junction. J Arthroplasty. 2018;33:1896–8. https://doi.org/10.1016/j.arth.2018.01.007.

106. Shahi A, Parvizi J, Kazarian GS, Higuera C, Frangiamore S, Bingham J, et al. The alpha-defensin test for periprosthetic joint infections is not affected by prior antibiotic administration. Clin Orthop Relat Res. 2016;474:1610–5. https://doi.org/10.1007/s11999-016-4726-2.

107. Johnson AJ, Zywiel MG, Stroh A, Marker DR, Mont MA. Serological markers can lead to false negative diagnoses of periprosthetic infections following total knee arthroplasty. Int Orthop. 2011;35:1621–6.

108. Parvizi J, Jacovides C, Adeli B, Jung KA, Hozack WJ, Mark B. Coventry Award: synovial C-reactive protein: a prospective evaluation of a molecular marker for periprosthetic knee joint infection. Clin Orthop Relat Res. 2012;470:54–60. https://doi.org/10.1007/s11999-011-1991-y.

109. Zamani B, Jamali R, Ehteram H. Synovial fluid adenosine deaminase and high-sensitivity C-reactive protein activity in differentiating monoarthritis. Rheumatol Int. 2012;32:183–8.

110. Parvizi J, McKenzie JC, Cashman JP. Diagnosis of periprosthetic joint infection using synovial C-reactive protein. J Arthroplasty. 2012;27:12–6. https://doi.org/10.1016/j.arth.2012.03.018.

111. Plate A, Anagnostopoulos A, Glanzmann J, Stadler L, Weigelt L, Sutter R, et al. Synovial C-reactive protein features high negative predictive value but is not useful as a single diagnostic parameter in suspected periprosthetic joint infection (PJI). J Infect. 2019;78:439–44. https://doi.org/10.1016/j.jinf.2019.04.003.

112. Tetreault MW, Wetters NG, Moric M, Gross CE, Della Valle CJ. Is synovial c-reactive protein a useful marker for periprosthetic joint infection? Clin Orthop Relat Res. 2014;472:3997–4003. https://doi.org/10.1007/s11999-014-3828-y.

113. Wang C, Wang Q, Li R, Duan J-Y, Wang C-B. Synovial fluid C-reactive protein as a diagnostic marker for periprosthetic joint infection: a systematic review and meta-analysis. Chin Med J (Engl). 2016;129:1987–93. https://doi.org/10.4103/0366-6999.187857.

114. Sousa R, Serrano P, Gomes Dias J, Oliveira JC, Oliveira A. Improving the accuracy of synovial fluid analysis in the diagnosis of prosthetic joint infection with simple and inexpensive biomarkers: C-reactive protein and adenosine deaminase. Bone Joint J. 2017;99-B:351–7. https://doi.org/10.1302/0301-620X.99B3.BJJ-2016-0684.R1.

115. Stone WZ, Gray CF, Parvataneni HK, Al-Rashid M, Vlasak RG, Horodyski M, et al. Clinical evaluation of synovial alpha defensin and synovial C-reactive

protein in the diagnosis of periprosthetic joint infection. J Bone Joint Surg. 2018;100:1184–90. https://doi.org/10.2106/JBJS.17.00556.

116. Gallo J, Svoboda M, Zapletalova J, Proskova J, Juranova J. Serum IL-6 in combination with synovial IL-6/CRP shows excellent diagnostic power to detect hip and knee prosthetic joint infection. PLoS One. 2018;13:e0199226. https://doi.org/10.1371/journal.pone.0199226.

117. Deirmengian CA, Citrano PA, Gulati S, Kazarian ER, Stave JW, Kardos KW. The C-reactive protein may not detect infections caused by less-virulent organisms. J Arthroplasty. 2016;31:152–5. https://doi.org/10.1016/j.arth.2016.01.060.

118. Deirmengian C, Kardos K, Kilmartin P, Cameron A, Schiller K, Parvizi J. Diagnosing periprosthetic joint infection: has the era of the biomarker arrived? Clin Orthop Relat Res. 2014;472:3254–62. https://doi.org/10.1007/s11999-014-3543-8.

119. Wouthuyzen-Bakker M, Ploegmakers JJW, Kampinga GA, Wagenmakers-Huizenga L, Jutte PC, Muller Kobold AC. Synovial calprotectin: a potential biomarker to exclude a prosthetic joint infection. Bone Joint J. 2017;99-B:660–5. https://doi.org/10.1302/0301-620X.99B5.BJJ-2016-0913.R2.

120. Karbysheva S, Yermak K, Grigoricheva L, Renz N, Perka C, Trampuz A. Synovial fluid d-lactate—a novel pathogen-specific biomarker for the diagnosis of periprosthetic joint infection. J Arthroplasty. 2020;35:2223–2229.e2. https://doi.org/10.1016/j.arth.2020.03.016.

121. Qin L, Hu N, Li X, Chen Y, Wang J, Huang W. Evaluation of synovial fluid neutrophil CD64 index as a screening biomarker of prosthetic joint infection. Bone Joint J. 2020;102-B:463–9. https://doi.org/10.1302/0301-620X.102B4.BJJ-2019-1271.R1.

122. Nakashige TG, Zhang B, Krebs C, Nolan EM. Human calprotectin is an iron-sequestering host-defense protein. Nat Chem Biol. 2015;11:765–71.

123. Abildtrup M, Kingsley GH, Scott DL. Calprotectin as a biomarker for rheumatoid arthritis: a systematic review. J Rheumatol. 2015;42:760–70.

124. Yermak K, Karbysheva S, Perka C, Trampuz A, Renz N. Performance of synovial fluid D-lactate for the diagnosis of periprosthetic joint infection: a prospective observational study. J Infect. 2019;79:123–9. https://doi.org/10.1016/j.jinf.2019.05.015.

125. Ewaschuk JB, Naylor JM, Zello GA. D-lactate in human and ruminant metabolism. J Nutr. 2005;135:1619–25.

126. Gratacos J, Vila J, Moya F, Marcos MA, Collado A, Sanmartí R, et al. D-lactic acid in synovial fluid. A rapid diagnostic test for bacterial synovitis. J Rheumatol. 1995;22:1504–8.

127. Bori G, Soriano A, García S, Gallart X, Mallofre C, Mensa J. Neutrophils in frozen section and type of microorganism isolated at the time of resection arthroplasty for the treatment of infection. Arch Orthop Trauma Surg. 2009;129:591.

128. Tsaras G, Maduka-Ezeh A, Inwards CY, Mabry T, Erwin PJ, Murad MH, et al. Utility of intraoperative frozen section histopathology in the diagnosis of periprosthetic joint infection: a systematic review and meta-analysis. J Bone Joint Surg Am. 2012;94:1700–11. https://doi.org/10.2106/JBJS.J.00756.

129. Kwiecien G, George J, Klika AK, Zhang Y, Bauer TW, Rueda CAH. Intraoperative frozen section histology: matched for musculoskeletal infection society criteria. J Arthroplasty. 2017;32:223–7. https://doi.org/10.1016/j.arth.2016.06.019.

130. Ascione T, Barrack R, Benito N, Blevins K, Brause B, Cornu O, et al. General assembly, diagnosis, pathogen isolation - culture matters: proceedings of International Consensus on Orthopedic Infections. J Arthroplasty. 2019;34:S197–206. https://doi.org/10.1016/j.arth.2018.09.071.

131. Berbari EF, Marculescu C, Sia I, Lahr BD, Hanssen AD, Steckelberg JM, et al. Culture-negative prosthetic joint infection. Clin Infect Dis. 2007;45:1113–9. https://doi.org/10.1086/522184.

132. Parvizi J, Ghanem E, Menashe S, Barrack RL, Bauer TW. Periprosthetic infection: what are the diagnostic challenges? J Bone Joint Surg. 2006;88:138–47.

133. Parvizi J, Erkocak OF, Della Valle CJ. Culture-negative periprosthetic joint infection. J Bone Joint Surg Am. 2014;96:430–6. https://doi.org/10.2106/JBJS.L.01793.

134. Kalbian I, Park JW, Goswami K, Lee Y-K, Parvizi J, Koo K-H. Culture-negative periprosthetic joint infection: prevalence, aetiology, evaluation, recommendations, and treatment. Int Orthop. 2020;44:1255–61. https://doi.org/10.1007/s00264-020-04627-5.

135. Hughes JG, Vetter EA, Patel R, Schleck CD, Harmsen S, Turgeant LT, et al. Culture with BACTEC Peds Plus/F bottle compared with conventional methods for detection of bacteria in synovial fluid. J Clin Microbiol. 2001;39:4468–71.

136. Qu X, Zhai Z, Wu C, Jin F, Li H, Wang L, et al. Preoperative aspiration culture for preoperative diagnosis of infection in total hip or knee arthroplasty. J Clin Microbiol. 2013;51:3830–4. https://doi.org/10.1128/JCM.01467-13.

137. Tande AJ, Patel R. Prosthetic joint infection. Clin Microbiol Rev. 2014;27:302–45. https://doi.org/10.1128/CMR.00111-13.

138. Abdel MP, Akgün D, Akin G, Akinola B, Alencar P, Amanatullah DF, et al. Hip and knee section, diagnosis, pathogen isolation, culture: proceedings of International Consensus on Orthopedic Infections. J Arthroplasty. 2019;34:S361–7. https://doi.org/10.1016/j.arth.2018.09.020.

139. Jacobs AME, Bénard M, Meis JF, van Hellemondt G, Goosen JHM. The unsuspected prosthetic joint infection: incidence and consequences of positive intra-operative cultures in presumed aseptic knee and hip revisions. Bone Joint J. 2017;99-B:1482–9. https://doi.org/10.1302/0301-620X.99B11.BJJ--2016-0655.R2.

140. Aggarwal VK, Higuera C, Deirmengian G, Parvizi J, Austin MS. Swab cultures are not as effective as tissue cultures for diagnosis of periprosthetic joint infection. Clin Orthop Relat Res. 2013;471:3196–203. https://doi.org/10.1007/s11999-013-2974-y.

141. Nguyen LL, Nelson CL, Saccente M, Smeltzer MS, Wassell DL, McLaren SG. Detecting bacterial colonization of implanted orthopaedic devices by ultrasonication. Clin Orthop Relat Res. 2002;403:29–37. https://doi.org/10.1097/00003086-200210000-00006.

142. Trampuz A, Piper KE, Jacobson MJ, Hanssen AD, Unni KK, Osmon DR, et al. Sonication of removed hip and knee prostheses for diagnosis of infection. N Engl J Med. 2007;357:654–63. https://doi.org/10.1056/NEJMoa061588.

143. Shen H, Tang J, Wang Q, Jiang Y, Zhang X. Sonication of explanted prosthesis combined with incubation in BD Bactec bottles for pathogen-based diagnosis of prosthetic joint infection. J Clin Microbiol. 2014;53:777–81. https://doi.org/10.1128/jcm.02863-14.

144. Hischebeth GTR, Randau TM, Molitor E, Wimmer MD, Hoerauf A, Bekeredjian-Ding I, et al. Comparison of bacterial growth in sonication fluid cultures with periprosthetic membranes and with cultures of biopsies for diagnosing periprosthetic joint infection. Diagn Microbiol Infect Dis. 2016;84:112–5. https://doi.org/10.1016/j.diagmicrobio.2015.09.007.

145. Holinka J, Bauer L, Hirschl AM, Graninger W, Windhager R, Presterl E. Sonication cultures of explanted components as an add-on test to routinely conducted microbiological diagnostics improve pathogen detection. J Orthop Res. 2010;29:617–22. https://doi.org/10.1002/jor.21286.

146. Scorzolini L, Lichtner M, Iannetta M, Mengoni F, Russo G, Panni AS, et al. Sonication technique improves microbiological diagnosis in patients treated with antibiotics before surgery for prosthetic joint infections. New Microbiol. 2014;37:321–8.

147. Puig-Verdié L, Alentorn-Geli E, González-Cuevas A, Sorlí L, Salvadó M, Alier A, et al. Implant sonication increases the diagnostic accuracy of infection in patients with delayed, but not early, orthopaedic implant failure. Bone Joint J. 2013;95-B:244–9. https://doi.org/10.1302/0301-620x.95b2.30486.

148. Janz V, Wassilew GI, Hasart O, Matziolis G, Tohtz S, Perka C. Evaluation of sonicate fluid cultures in comparison to histological analysis of the periprosthetic membrane for the detection of periprosthetic joint infection. Int Orthop. 2013;37:931–6. https://doi.org/10.1007/s00264-013-1853-1.

149. Rothenberg AC, Wilson AE, Hayes JP, O'Malley MJ, Klatt BA. Sonication of arthroplasty implants improves accuracy of periprosthetic joint infection cultures. Clin Orthop Relat Res. 2017;475:1827–36. https://doi.org/10.1007/s11999-017-5315-8.

150. Janz V, Wassilew GI, Hasart O, Tohtz S, Perka C. Improvement in the detection rate of PJI in total hip arthroplasty through multiple sonicate fluid cultures: multiple sonicate cultures for PJI. J Orthop Res. 2013;31:2021–4. https://doi.org/10.1002/jor.22451.

151. Zhai Z, Li H, Qin A, Liu G, Liu X, Wu C, et al. Meta-analysis of sonication fluid samples from prosthetic components for diagnosis of infection after total joint arthroplasty. J Clin Microbiol. 2014;52:1730–6. https://doi.org/10.1128/JCM.03138-13.

152. Van Diek FM, Albers CGM, Van Hooff ML, Meis JF, Goosen JHM. Low sensitivity of implant sonication when screening for infection in revision surgery. Acta Orthop. 2017;88:294–9. https://doi.org/10.1080/17453674.2017.1300021.

153. Prieto-Borja L, Auñón Á, Blanco A, Fernández-Roblas R, Gadea I, García-Cañete J, et al. Evaluation of the use of sonication of retrieved implants for the diagnosis of prosthetic joint infection in a routine setting. Eur J Clin Microbiol Infect Dis. 2018;37:715–22. https://doi.org/10.1007/s10096-017-3164-8.

154. Tan TL, Kheir MM, Shohat N, Tan DD, Kheir M, Chen C, et al. Culture-negative periprosthetic joint infection: an update on what to expect. J Bone Joint Surg Open Access. 2018;3:e0060. https://doi.org/10.2106/JBJS.OA.17.00060.

155. Trampuz A, Piper KE, Hanssen AD, Osmon DR, Cockerill FR, Steckelberg JM, et al. Sonication of explanted prosthetic components in bags for diagnosis of prosthetic joint infection is associated with risk of contamination. J Clin Microbiol. 2006;44:628–31. https://doi.org/10.1128/JCM.44.2.628-631.2006.

156. Malekzadeh D, Osmon DR, Lahr BD, Hanssen AD, Berbari EF. Prior use of antimicrobial therapy is a risk factor for culture-negative prosthetic joint infection. Clin Orthop Relat Res. 2010;468:2039–45. https://doi.org/10.1007/s11999-010-1338-0.

157. Pasquaroli S, Zandri G, Vignaroli C, Vuotto C, Donelli G, Biavasco F. Antibiotic pressure can induce the viable but non-culturable state in Staphylococcus aureus growing in biofilms. J Antimicrob Chemother. 2013;68:1812–7. https://doi.org/10.1093/jac/dkt086.

158. Pasquaroli S, Citterio B, Cesare A, Amiri M, Manti A, Vuotto C, et al. Role of daptomycin in the induction and persistence of the viable but non-culturable state of Staphylococcus aureus biofilms. Pathogens. 2014;3:759–68. https://doi.org/10.3390/pathogens3030759.

159. Zhao X, Zhong J, Wei C, Lin C-W, Ding T. Current perspectives on viable but non-culturable state in foodborne pathogens. Front Microbiol. 2017;8 https://doi.org/10.3389/fmicb.2017.00580.

160. Li L, Mendis N, Trigui H, Oliver JD, Faucher SP. The importance of the viable but non-culturable state in human bacterial pathogens. Front Microbiol. 2014;5 https://doi.org/10.3389/fmicb.2014.00258.

161. Oliver JD. Recent findings on the viable but non-culturable state in pathogenic bacteria. FEMS Microbiol Rev. 2010;34:415–25. https://doi.org/10.1111/j.1574-6976.2009.00200.x.

162. Sun F, Chen J, Zhong L, Zhang X, Wang R, Guo Q, et al. Characterization and virulence retention of viable but nonculturable Vibrio harveyi. FEMS Microbiol Ecol. 2008;64:37–44.

163. Della Valle C, Parvizi J, Bauer TW, DiCesare PE, Evans RP, Segreti J, et al. American Academy of Orthopaedic Surgeons clinical practice guideline on: the diagnosis of periprosthetic joint infections of the hip and knee. J Bone Joint Surg. 2011;93:1355–7.

164. Barrack RL, Jennings RW, Wolfe MW, Bertot AJ. The value of preoperative aspiration before total knee revision. Clin Orthop Relat Res. 1997;345:8–16. https://doi.org/10.1097/00003086-199712000-00003.

165. Mont MA, Waldman BJ, Hungerford DS. Evaluation of preoperative cultures before second-stage reimplantation of a total knee prosthesis complicated by infection. J Bone Joint Surg Am. 2000;82:1552–7. https://doi.org/10.2106/00004623-200011000-00006.

166. Burnett RSJ, Kelly MA, Hanssen AD, Barrack RL. Technique and timing of two-stage exchange for infection in TKA. Clin Orthop Relat Res. 2007;464:164–78. https://doi.org/10.1097/blo.0b013e318157eb1e.

167. Tan TL, Shohat N, Rondon AJ, Foltz C, Goswami K, Ryan SP, et al. Perioperative antibiotic prophylaxis in total joint arthroplasty: a single dose is as effective as multiple doses. J Bone Joint Surg. 2019;101:429–37. https://doi.org/10.2106/JBJS.18.00336.

168. Ghanem E, Parvizi J, Clohisy J, Burnett S, Sharkey PF, Barrack R. Perioperative antibiotics should not be withheld in proven cases of periprosthetic infection. Clin Orthop Relat Res. 2007;461:44–7. https://doi.org/10.1097/BLO.0b013e318065b780.

169. Pérez-Prieto D, Portillo ME, Puig-Verdié L, Alier A, Gamba C, Guirro P, et al. Preoperative antibiotic prophylaxis in prosthetic joint infections: not a concern for intraoperative cultures. Diagn Microbiol Infect Dis. 2016;86:442–5. https://doi.org/10.1016/j.diagmicrobio.2016.09.014.

170. Tetreault MW, Wetters NG, Aggarwal V, Mont M, Parvizi J, Della Valle CJ. The Chitranjan Ranawat Award: should prophylactic antibiotics be withheld before revision surgery to obtain appropriate cultures? Clin Orthop Relat Res. 2014;472:52–6. https://doi.org/10.1007/s11999-013-3016-5.

171. Bedenčič K, Kavčič M, Faganeli N, Mihalič R, Mavčič B, Dolenc J, et al. Does preoperative antimicrobial prophylaxis influence the diagnostic potential of periprosthetic tissues in hip or knee infections? Clin Orthop Relat Res. 2016;474:258–64. https://doi.org/10.1007/s11999-015-4486-4.

172. Burnett RSJ, Aggarwal A, Givens SA, McClure JT, Morgan PM, Barrack RL. Prophylactic antibiotics do not affect cultures in the treatment of an infected TKA: a prospective trial. Clin Orthop Relat Res. 2010;468:127–34. https://doi.org/10.1007/s11999-009-1014-4.

173. Wouthuyzen-Bakker M, Benito N, Soriano A. The effect of preoperative antimicrobial prophylaxis on intraoperative culture results in patients with a suspected or confirmed prosthetic joint infection: a systematic review. J Clin Microbiol. 2017;55:2765–74. https://doi.org/10.1128/JCM.00640-17.

174. Wouthuyzen-Bakker M, Tornero E, Claret G, Bosch J, Martinez-Pastor JC, Combalia A, et al. Withholding preoperative antibiotic prophylaxis in knee prosthesis revision: a retrospective analysis on culture results and risk of infection. J Arthroplasty. 2017;32:2829–33. https://doi.org/10.1016/j.arth.2017.03.064.

175. Spangehl MJ, Masri BA, O'Connell JX, Duncan CP. Prospective analysis of preoperative and intraoperative investigations for the diagnosis of infection at the sites of two hundred and two revision total hip arthroplasties\ast. J Bone Joint Surg. 1999;81:672–83. https://doi.org/10.2106/00004623-199905000-00008.

176. Toms AD, Davidson D, Masri BA, Duncan CP. The management of peri-prosthetic infection in total joint arthroplasty. J Bone Joint Surg. 2006;88-B:149–55. https://doi.org/10.1302/0301-620x.88b2.17058.

177. Achermann Y, Vogt M, Leunig M, Wust J, Trampuz A. Improved diagnosis of periprosthetic joint infection by multiplex PCR of sonication fluid from removed implants. J Clin Microbiol. 2010;48:1208–14. https://doi.org/10.1128/jcm.00006-10.

178. Janz V, Schoon J, Morgenstern C, Preininger B, Reinke S, Duda G, et al. Rapid detection of periprosthetic joint infection using a combination of 16s rDNA polymerase chain reaction and lateral flow immunoassay. Bone Joint Res. 2018;7:12–9. https://doi.org/10.1302/2046-3758.71.bjr-2017-0103.r2.

179. Sigmund IK, Holinka J, Sevelda F, Staats K, Heisinger S, Kubista B, et al. Performance of automated multiplex polymerase chain reaction (mPCR) using synovial fluid in the diagnosis of native joint septic arthritis in adults. Bone Joint J. 2019;101-B:288–96. https://doi.org/10.1302/0301--620x.101b3.bjj-2018-0868.r1.

180. Fenollar F, Roux V, Stein A, Drancourt M, Raoult D. Analysis of 525 samples to determine the usefulness of PCR amplification and sequencing of the 16S rRNA gene for diagnosis of bone and joint infections. J Clin Microbiol. 2006;44:1018–28. https://doi.org/10.1128/jcm.44.3.1018-1028.2006.

181. Cazanave C, Greenwood-Quaintance KE, Hanssen AD, Karau MJ, Schmidt SM, Gomez Urena EO, et al. Rapid molecular microbiologic diagnosis of prosthetic joint infection. J Clin Microbiol. 2013;51:2280–7. https://doi.org/10.1128/JCM.00335-13.

182. Tsang STJ, McHugh MP, Guerendiain D, Gwynne PJ, Boyd J, Simpson AHRW, et al. Underestimation of Staphylococcus aureus (MRSA and MSSA) carriage associated with standard culturing techniques. Bone Joint Res. 2018;7:79–84. https://doi.org/10.1302/2046-3758.71.bjr-2017-0175.r1.

183. Chen M-F, Chang C-H, Chiang-Ni C, Hsieh P-H, Shih H-N, Ueng SWN, et al. Rapid analysis of bacterial composition in prosthetic joint infection by

16S rRNA metagenomic sequencing. Bone Joint Res. 2019;8:367–77. https://doi.org/10.1302/2046-3758.88.bjr-2019-0003.r2.

184. Janda JM, Abbott SL. 16S rRNA gene sequencing for bacterial identification in the diagnostic laboratory: pluses, perils, and pitfalls. J Clin Microbiol. 2007;45:2761–4. https://doi.org/10.1128/JCM.01228-07.

185. Tarabichi M, Alvand A, Shohat N, Goswami K, Parvizi J. Diagnosis of Streptococcus canis periprosthetic joint infection: the utility of next-generation sequencing. Arthroplast Today. 2018;4:20–3. https://doi.org/10.1016/j.artd.2017.08.005.

186. Street TL, Sanderson ND, Atkins BL, Brent AJ, Cole K, Foster D, et al. Molecular diagnosis of orthopaedic device infection direct from sonication fluid by metagenomic sequencing. J Clin Microbiol. 2017; https://doi.org/10.1101/118026.

187. Ruppé E, Lazarevic V, Girard M, Mouton W, Ferry T, Laurent F, et al. Clinical metagenomics of bone and joint infections: a proof of concept study. Sci Rep. 2017;7 https://doi.org/10.1038/s41598-017-07546-5.

188. Thoendel MJ, Jeraldo PR, Greenwood-Quaintance KE, Yao JZ, Chia N, Hanssen AD, et al. Identification of prosthetic joint infection pathogens using a shotgun metagenomics approach. Clin Infect Dis. 2018;67:1333–8. https://doi.org/10.1093/cid/ciy303.

189. Huang Z, Zhang C, Li W, Fang X, Wang Q, Xing L, et al. Metagenomic next-generation sequencing contribution in identifying prosthetic joint infection due to Parvimonas micra: a case report. J Bone Joint Infect. 2019;4:50–5. https://doi.org/10.7150/jbji.30615.

190. Fang X, Li W, Zhang C, Huang Z, Zeng H, Dong Z, et al. Detecting the presence of bacterial DNA and RNA by polymerase chain reaction to diagnose suspected periprosthetic joint infection after antibiotic therapy: diagnose of PJI by DNA and RNA-based PCR. Orthop Surg. 2018;10:40–6. https://doi.org/10.1111/os.12359.

191. Shukla SK, Ward JP, Jacofsky MC, Sporer SM, Paprosky WG, Valle CJD. Perioperative testing for persistent sepsis following resection arthroplasty of the hip for periprosthetic infection. J Arthroplasty. 2010;25:87–91. https://doi.org/10.1016/j.arth.2010.05.006.

192. Melendez DP, Greenwood-Quaintance KE, Berbari EF, Osmon DR, Mandrekar JN, Hanssen AD, et al. Evaluation of a genus- and group-specific rapid PCR assay panel on synovial fluid for diagnosis of prosthetic knee infection. J Clin Microbiol. 2016;54:120–6. https://doi.org/10.1128/JCM.02302-15.

193. Tan TL, Gomez MM, Manrique J, Parvizi J, Chen AF. Positive culture during reimplantation increases the risk of subsequent failure in two-stage exchange arthroplasty. J Bone Joint Surg. 2016;98:1313–9. https://doi.org/10.2106/jbjs.15.01469.

194. Canvin JM, Goutcher SC, Hagig M, Gemmell CG, Sturrock RD. Persistence of Staphylococcus aureus as detected by polymerase chain reaction in the synovial fluid of a patient with septic arthritis. Rheumatology. 1997;36:203–6. https://doi.org/10.1093/rheumatology/36.2.203.

195. Van Der Heijden IM, Wilbrink B, Vije AE, Schouls LM, Breedveld FC, Tak PP. Detection of bacterial DNA in serial synovial samples obtained during antibiotic treatment from patients with septic arthritis. Arthritis Rheumat. 1999;42:2198–203.

196. Chen T, Rimpiläinen M, Luukkainen R, Möttönen T, Yli-Jama T, Jalava J, et al. Bacterial components in the synovial tissue of patients with advanced rheumatoid arthritis or osteoarthritis: analysis with gas chromatography-mass spectrometry and pan-bacterial polymerase chain reaction. Arthritis Care Res. 2003;49:328–34. https://doi.org/10.1002/art.11119.

197. Wilbrink B, Hazes JMW, Breedveld FC, Tak PP. Detection of bacterial DNA in joint samples from patients with undifferentiated arthritis and reactive arthritis, using polymerase chain reaction with universal 16S ribosomal RNA primers. Arthritis Rheum. 1998;41:535–43.

Microbiological Diagnosis of Knee Prosthesis Infections

Camille Kolenda, Céline Dupieux,
Sébastien Lustig, Tristan Ferry,
and Frédéric Laurent

7.1 Introduction

Microbiological analyses are one of the cornerstones of the management of knee prosthesis infections (KPIs) as the culture and isolation of the pathogen is a major criterion for their diagnosis [1, 2]. Then, bacterial identification and antimicrobial susceptibility testing are required to adapt and/or optimize antimicrobial treatment.

As bacteria responsible for acute and chronic infections can be different, microbiological analysis must be carried out in order to identify a wide panel of pathogens combining culture protocols adapted to slow growing bacteria, but also mycobacteria and fungi, and molecular approaches. Indeed, while bacteria causing acute infections are usually virulent and easy to grow pathogens (*Staphylococcus aureus* and beta-hemolytic streptococci, *Enterobacteriaceae*), the bacteriological diagnosis of chronic infections can be much more challenging. Bacteria involved in chronic infections are more diverse including low-grade pathogens corresponding to bacteria belonging to commensal skin flora (e.g., coagulase negative staphylococci, corynebacteria, *P. acnes*) [3]. Identification of such bacteria can trigger difficulties of distinction between contamination and true infection. The formation of biofilm, the presence of metabolic variants, named *small colony variants* (SCVs), and the

C. Kolenda (✉) · C. Dupieux · F. Laurent
Institut des Agents Infectieux, Laboratoire de bactériologie, Centre National de référence des staphylocoques, Hôpital de la Croix-Rousse, Lyon, France

Centre de référence des infections ostéo-articulaires complexes - Lyon (CRIOAc Lyon), Hôpital de la Croix-Rousse, Lyon, France

CIRI – Centre International de Recherche en Infectiologie, Inserm, U1111, Université Claude Bernard Lyon 1, CNRS, UMR5308, Ecole Normale Supérieure de Lyon, Lyon, France
e-mail: camille.kolenda@chu-lyon.fr; celine.dupieux@chu-lyon.fr; frederic.laurent@univ-lyon1.fr

S. Lustig
Centre de référence des infections ostéo-articulaires complexes - Lyon (CRIOAc Lyon), Hôpital de la Croix-Rousse, Lyon, France

Service de chirurgie orthopédique, Hôpital de la Croix-Rousse, Lyon, France

T. Ferry
Centre de référence des infections ostéo-articulaires complexes - Lyon (CRIOAc Lyon), Hôpital de la Croix-Rousse, Lyon, France

CIRI – Centre International de Recherche en Infectiologie, Inserm, U1111, Université Claude Bernard Lyon 1, CNRS, UMR5308, Ecole Normale Supérieure de Lyon, Lyon, France

Service des maladies infectieuses et tropicales, Hospices Civils de Lyon, Hôpital de la Croix-Rousse, Lyon, France
e-mail: tristan.ferry@univ-lyon1.fr

© ISAKOS 2022
U. G. Longo et al. (eds.), *Infection in Knee Replacement*,
https://doi.org/10.1007/978-3-030-81553-0_7

low microbial inoculum in chronic infections can also affect the sensitivity of microbiological diagnosis [4, 5]. Finally, some bacteria can be very difficult to grow or can only be identified with molecular biology techniques (*Mycoplasma* spp., *Tropheryma whipplei*).

7.2 Types of Samples

General rules have to be applied to improve the yield of microbiological diagnosis of KPIs:

- To prevent false negative samples, it is recommended to respect a minimum of 15 days without any antibiotherapy (except in case of sepsis) before the samples, 1 month if rifampicin, fluoroquinolones, or cyclins.
- To prevent false positive samples, it is recommended to respect a strict surgical asepsis.

7.2.1 Preoperative Samples

When abscesses or fluid collections in the joint or in the soft tissue are present, aspiration can be performed, with ultrasound guidance if needed. Vials for aerobic and anaerobic blood cultures should be inoculated with aspirated fluid immediately to increase the sensitivity but an aliquot must always be kept for microscopic examinations, conventional cultures, and molecular analyses [6]. Preoperative aspiration culture has a moderate sensitivity but a very high specificity [7]. Ultrasound guided percutaneous biopsies can also be taken when aspiration is not feasible. Superficial samples from wounds or fistulae using a swab must be avoided since they are most often contaminated by cutaneous flora and their results correlate poorly with those obtained with deep samples, with the only exception of *S. aureus* [8].

7.2.2 Peri-operative Samples

Multiple samples must be collected, from different anatomical sites and, if possible, from sites which are macroscopically pathological, due to the heterogeneous distribution of pathogenic bacteria inside the infected site and the possible presence of commensal bacteria. These samples can be fluid (e.g., pus, articular fluid), solid samples (e.g., granulomatous tissue, bone tissue, interposition tissue, and any suspicious tissue), or osteosynthesis material (e.g., screws, cement, rods). International guidelines recommend that ideally five or six periprosthetic samples be obtained, but recent studies suggest that this number could be reduced to four samples [2, 9, 10]. Culture positivity rates can vary depending on the sample type including joint fluid and tissue samples being more frequently positive than bone samples [10]. A low number (<3) of samples may lead to a lack of sensitivity of culture or a misinterpretation of a single positive culture and a higher number to an increased probability of contamination without evidence of improved sensitivity of the examination. It is recommended to use new sterile instruments for each tissue specimen to avoid cross-contamination. Sampling with a swab must be avoided as the culture sensitivity is low, compared with tissue samples [11].

In case of implant-associated infections, prostheses and other devices can also be sent to the laboratory combined with culture of periprosthetic tissue samples to increase the sensitivity in cases with strong suspicion of KPI without microbiological documentation or prior antibiotic administration, but must be processed specifically, using mechanical methods such as sonication to dislodge bacteria from the biofilm formed on the material [1, 12, 13]. Particular attention must be paid during the collection of prosthetic/biomaterial components to avoid contamination which should be transferred into a non-perforable, sterile, leak-proof container of suitable size. Results from sonicate fluid must be interpreted with caution and remains a subject on debate.

In addition, the taking of paired blood cultures routinely in case of fever or sepsis associated with KPI, of arthritis, and presence of a secondary infected site must be encouraged and never forgotten. If positive, these blood cultures can be useful to guide the diagnosis if culture of periprosthetic samples remains negative or confirm the pathogenic nature of bacteria isolated in such samples.

7.3 Bacteriological Analysis

Transport is an important pre-analysis step for these types of samples and should be organized involving the surgical, laboratory, and logistics departments. The different samples must be transferred at room temperature as quickly as possible, ideally within 2 h. If this deadline cannot be met, transport medium to keep fragile bacteria and anaerobes alive must be used. It is essential to mention for the clinical lab the date and time of sampling, the anatomical site, and clinical information (e.g., antibiotherapy, use of a prosthesis).

It is essential to particularly pay attention to the risk of contamination of these samples in the lab as commensal bacteria can be involved in KPIs. They must be handled in BSC-2 by a technician wearing a disposable overall and gloves (changed regularly) and using sterile equipment.

Solid samples (bone fragments or tissue) must be crushed for example using sterile glass beads before examination, in order to homogenate the specimens and to release bacteria [14]. Molecular grade water should be preferred to culture broth as a diluent so that further molecular analyses (particularly broad range PCR) are not compromised. Sonication of prosthetic devices has been proposed especially to release bacteria from biofilm [12, 13]. The use of a solution of dithiotheritol has been proposed as an alternative to bead mill processing of the samples [15].

The part of the sample which is not inoculated must be preserved by freezing (− 20 °C) until definitive diagnosis is reached in case additional tests are needed (e.g., testing for mycobacterium, fungi, molecular biology).

7.3.1 Microscopic Examination

Microscopic examination includes:

– Direct microscopic examination for synovial fluids (e.g., on Malassez cell) to search for micro-crystals (for differential diagnosis of chondrocalcinosis and acute articular gout) and quantify leukocytes, followed by May-Grunwald-Giemsa staining for quantification of polymorphonuclear neutrophils (PMNs). A percentage of PMNS >65% or a leukocyte count of >1.7 × 10³/μL is indicative of KPI [16].
– Gram's staining to test for bacteria. It has a high specificity but a very low sensitivity [17]. It is useful mainly in acute infections.

7.3.2 Culture

Culture methods include the use of solid agar plates as well as broth media for enrichment incubated at approximately 35 ± 2 °C in various atmospheres.

Given the bacterial epidemiology of the KPI, samples are classically inoculated at least onto:

– A blood agar incubated aerobically with early reading on D1–D2 and late on D5,
– A supplemented chocolate agar incubated in a 5% CO_2 atmosphere with early reading on D1–D2 and late reading on D5,
– A blood agar or Schaedler agar incubated in anaerobic conditions with early reading at D3–D5 and late reading D14,
– An enriched anaerobic liquid medium such as Schaedler or Rosenow's broth with regular reading up to D14 if necessary, in order to increase the culture sensitivity, notably for the culture of slow growing anaerobic bacteria such as *Cutibacterium acnes* [18].

Inoculation of periprosthetic tissue samples after being crushed directly into blood culture bottles has been reported to increase sensitivity of culture, reduce time to culture positivity, and allows to reduce costs associated with the use of multiple plates and broths used for multiple samples [9, 10].

Reading of plates must be attentive to the examination for different appearances of colonies, notably micro-colonies which could signal the presence of metabolic variants (SCV). An early positive culture in a solid medium does not exclude continued readings and complete incubation to look for additional bacteria of slower growth, polymicrobial infections representing 10–15% of infections. In order to limit the risks of false positives linked to contamination of boxes during their iterative openings at early readings, some authors recommend doubling the inoculation of the anaerobic agar plates and chocolate agar plates. In this case, one plate is used for early reading and the second plate is only opened for late reading. All reading procedures, re-inoculation, and handling of medium should be systematically performed in a BSC-2.

Identification and antibiotic susceptibility testing (according to EUCAST/CLSI recommendations) must be performed on all isolates and different colony morphotypes (such as SCV) of the same bacterial species because they may show different antimicrobial susceptibility profiles.

Additional cultures for fungi and mycobacteria should be performed depending on the clinical context on specific request.

7.4 Molecular Biology

If culture remains the current gold-standard for diagnosis of KPIs, the pathogen is not identified in up to 40% of cases [19]. To face this situation and overcome these difficulties, molecular assays have been developed during the last decades. Compared to culture, PCR is theoretically more sensitive, faster, and not as affected by antibiotic treatment. Broad range 16S rRNA PCR or specific PCR targeting frequent KPI pathogens can be used. The former has the advantage to detect all bacteria but requires sequencing of the PCR product for bacterial identification, may be non-specific (due to background bacterial DNA in samples/reagents), and polymicrobial infection may be missed by sequencing. Reports of sensitivities and specificities of these PCR vary depending on the study and the samples types (synovial fluid, tissue samples, sonication fluids) [20–24]. Published studies mainly report the evaluation of broad range PCR assays but more recently, multiplex specific PCR have been developed but some of them do not include primers for the common PJI targets such as coagulase nega-

tive staphylococci and *C. acnes* [21, 22]. On the whole, reported data do not support superiority of these molecular assays compared with traditional culture methods except in case of treatment with antibiotics at the time of surgery or infection by fastidious bacteria [20–24]. Molecular biology methods complement conventional cultures without replacing them and should be used in case of strong suspicion of infection with negative cultures but not routinely because of their high cost.

More recently, the use of next generation sequencing in the diagnosis of KPIs has been evaluated as an alternative to PCR assays, not suited to detect polymicrobial infections in the case of broad range PCR or uncommon pathogens not included in panels of specific PCR assays [25–28]. Metagenomic sequencing offers the possibility of directly detecting all nucleic acids from a clinical sample, giving access in theory to more information than just bacterial identification by sequencing of the whole bacterial genome necessary for antimicrobial resistance prediction. However, samples obtained in the context of KPIs are challenging sample types as they couple low bacterial load with high levels of contaminating human cells affecting the sensitivity [25]. More studies exploring protocols allowing bacterial DNA enrichment are required to assess the performance of these techniques for bacterial identification and antimicrobial resistance prediction to justify their expensive cost compared to conventional culture or PCR assays [29, 30].

7.5 Interpretation

According to different international guidelines, a prosthesis infection is defined by the presence of one major diagnosis criteria including two positive periprosthetic cultures with phenotypically identical organisms or by a combination of three minor criteria including a single positive culture [1, 2, 31]. However, clinically, PKI may be present without meeting these criteria. Interpretation of the bacteriological results in the context of KPI is thus often complex. It must take into account the clinical context, as the bacterial inoculum is lower in chronic than acute infections and in case of previous antimicrobial therapy, affecting performances of microbial diagnosis. Bacterial species identified should also be interpreted regarding the number of positive samples and the number of positive culture media. Growth of a virulent microorganism (e.g., *S. aureus*, haemolytic streptococci, *Enterobacteriaceae,* etc.) in a single specimen may also represent PKI while one culture that yielding a bacteria part of the normal skin flora may be indicative of a contamination (e.g., coagulase negative staphylococci, *C. acnes*) and should be evaluated in the context of other available evidence [2].

References

1. Gehrke T, Parvizi J. Proceedings on the international consensus meeting on periprosthetic joint infection; 2018.
2. Osmon DR, Berbari EF, Berendt AR, Lew D, Zimmerli W, Steckelberg JM, et al. Diagnosis and management of prosthetic joint infection: clinical practice guidelines by the Infectious Diseases Society of America. Clin Infect Dis. 2013;56(1):e1–25.
3. Triffault-Fillit C, Ferry T, Laurent F, Pradat P, Dupieux C, Conrad A, et al. Microbiologic epidemiology depending on time to occurrence of prosthetic joint infection: a prospective cohort study. Clin Microbiol Infect. 2018;25(5):353–8.
4. McConoughey SJ, Howlin R, Granger JF, Manring MM, Calhoun JH, Shirtliff M, et al. Biofilms in periprosthetic orthopedic infections. Future Microbiol. 2014;9(8):987–1007.
5. von Eiff C, Peters G, Becker K. The small colony variant (SCV) concept - the role of staphylococcal SCVs in persistent infections. Injury. 2006;37(Suppl 2):S26–33.
6. Hughes JG, Vetter EA, Patel R, Schleck CD, Harmsen S, Turgeant LT, et al. Culture with BACTEC Peds plus/F bottle compared with conventional methods for detection of bacteria in synovial fluid. J Clin Microbiol. 2001;39(12):4468–71.
7. Qu X, Zhai Z, Wu C, Jin F, Li H, Wang L, et al. Preoperative aspiration culture for preoperative diagnosis of infection in total hip or knee arthroplasty. J Clin Microbiol. 2013;51(11):3830–4.
8. Cuñé J, Soriano A, Martínez JC, García S, Mensa J. A superficial swab culture is useful for microbiologic diagnosis in acute prosthetic joint infections. Clin Orthop Relat Res. 2009;467(2):531–5.
9. Peel TN, Spelman T, Dylla BL, Hughes JG, Greenwood-Quaintance KE, Cheng AC, et al. Optimal periprosthetic tissue specimen number for diagnosis of prosthetic joint infection. J Clin Microbiol. 2017;55(1):234–43.
10. Bémer P, Léger J, Tandé D, Plouzeau C, Valentin AS, Jolivet-Gougeon A, et al. How many samples and how many culture media to diagnose a prosthetic joint infection: a clinical and microbiological prospective multicenter study. J Clin Microbiol. 2016;54(2):385–91.
11. Aggarwal VK, Higuera C, Deirmengian G, Parvizi J, Austin MS. Swab cultures are not as effective as tissue cultures for diagnosis of periprosthetic joint infection. Clin Orthop Relat Res. 2013;471(10):3196–203.
12. Dudareva M, Barrett L, Figtree M, Scarborough M, Watanabe M, Newnham R, et al. Sonication versus tissue sampling for diagnosis of prosthetic joint and other orthopedic device-related infections. J Clin Microbiol. 2018;56(12):e00688–18.
13. Trampuz A, Piper KE, Jacobson MJ, Hanssen AD, Unni KK, Osmon DR, et al. Sonication of removed hip and knee prostheses for diagnosis of infection. N Engl J Med. 2007;357(7):654–63.
14. Roux A-L, Sivadon-Tardy V, Bauer T, Lortat-Jacob A, Herrmann J-L, Gaillard J-L, et al. Diagnosis of prosthetic joint infection by beadmill processing of a periprosthetic specimen. Clin Microbiol Infect. 2011;17(3):447–50.
15. Drago L, Signori V, De Vecchi E, Vassena C, Palazzi E, Cappelletti L, et al. Use of dithiothreitol to improve the diagnosis of prosthetic joint infections. J Orthop Res. 2013;31(11):1694–9.
16. Trampuz A, Hanssen AD, Osmon DR, Mandrekar J, Steckelberg JM, Patel R. Synovial fluid leukocyte count and differential for the diagnosis of prosthetic knee infection. Am J Med. 2004;117(8):556–62.
17. Zimmerli W, Trampuz A, Ochsner PE. Prosthetic-joint infections. N Engl J Med. 2004;351(16):1645–54.
18. Butler-Wu SM, Burns EM, Pottinger PS, Magaret AS, Rakeman JL, Matsen FA, et al. Optimization of periprosthetic culture for diagnosis of *Propionibacterium acnes* prosthetic joint infection. J Clin Microbiol. 2011;49(7):2490–5.
19. Yoon H-K, Cho S-H, Lee D-Y, Kang B-H, Lee S-H, Moon D-G, et al. A review of the literature on culture-negative periprosthetic joint infection: epidemiology, diagnosis and treatment. Knee Surg Relat Res. 2017;29(3):155–64.
20. Ryu SY, Greenwood-Quaintance KE, Hanssen AD, Mandrekar JN, Patel R. Low sensitivity of periprosthetic tissue PCR for prosthetic knee infection diagnosis. Diagn Microbiol Infect Dis. 2014;79(4):448–53.
21. Malandain D, Bémer P, Leroy AG, Léger J, Plouzeau C, Valentin AS, et al. Assessment of the automated multiplex-PCR Unyvero i60 ITI® cartridge system to diagnose prosthetic joint infection: a multicentre study. Clin Microbiol Infect. 2018;24(1):83.e1–6.
22. Achermann Y, Vogt M, Leunig M, Wust J, Trampuz A. Improved diagnosis of periprosthetic joint infection by multiplex PCR of sonication fluid from removed implants. J Clin Microbiol. 2010;48(4):1208–14.

23. Bemer P, Plouzeau C, Tande D, Leger J, Giraudeau B, Valentin AS, et al. Evaluation of 16S rRNA gene PCR sensitivity and specificity for diagnosis of prosthetic joint infection: a prospective multicenter cross-sectional study. J Clin Microbiol. 2014;52(10):3583–9.
24. Melendez DP, Greenwood-Quaintance KE, Berbari EF, Osmon DR, Mandrekar JN, Hanssen AD, et al. Evaluation of a genus- and group-specific rapid PCR assay panel on synovial fluid for diagnosis of prosthetic knee infection. Carroll KC, editor. J Clin Microbiol. 2016;54(1):120–6.
25. Street TL, Sanderson ND, Atkins BL, Brent AJ, Cole K, Foster D, et al. Molecular diagnosis of orthopedic-device-related infection directly from sonication fluid by metagenomic sequencing. J Clin Microbiol. 2017;55(8):2334–47.
26. Sanderson ND, Street TL, Foster D, Swann J, Atkins BL, Brent AJ, et al. Real-time analysis of nanopore-based metagenomic sequencing from infected orthopaedic devices. BMC Genomics. 2018;19(1):714.
27. Thoendel MJ, Jeraldo PR, Greenwood-Quaintance KE, Yao JZ, Chia N, Hanssen AD, et al. Identification of prosthetic joint infection pathogens using a shotgun metagenomics approach. Clin Inf Dis. 2018;67(9):1333–8.
28. Ivy MI, Thoendel MJ, Jeraldo PR, Greenwood-Quaintance KE, Hanssen AD, Abdel MP, et al. Direct detection and identification of prosthetic joint infection pathogens in synovial fluid by metagenomic shotgun sequencing. J Clin Microbiol. 2018;56(9):e00402–18.
29. Wang C, Huang Z, Fang W, Zhang Z, Fang X, Li W, et al. Preliminary assessment of nanopore-based metagenomic sequencing for the diagnosis of prosthetic joint infection. Int J Infect Dis. 2020;97:54–9.
30. Thoendel M, Jeraldo PR, Greenwood-Quaintance KE, Yao JZ, Chia N, Hanssen AD, et al. Comparison of microbial DNA enrichment tools for metagenomic whole genome sequencing. J Microbiol Methods. 2016;127:141–5.
31. Parvizi J, Tan TL, Goswami K, Higuera C, Della Valle C, Chen AF, et al. The 2018 Definition of periprosthetic hip and knee infection: an evidence-based and validated criteria. J Arthroplasty. 2018;33(5):1309–1314.e2.

Molecular Analysis and Histological Evaluation

Vishal Hegde, Douglas A. Dennis, and Charlie C. Yang

8.1   Introduction

Periprosthetic joint infection (PJI) is one of the most serious and debilitating complications suffered by patients after total joint arthroplasty. The reported incidence of PJI for total knee arthroplasty has ranged from 0.8 to 1.9% and for total hip arthroplasty from 0.3 to 1.7% [1]. When faced with a periprosthetic joint infection, early and accurate diagnosis continues to be critical to deliver successful targeted treatment to the patient. Currently, under clinical suspicion, a combination of radiological, serological, synovial, microbiological, and histological investigation is performed to assist in diagnosis and isolate the offending organism(s) [2]. Although considerable advances have been made in the diagnostic armamentarium available to the clinician, microbiological culture continues to be the gold standard to identify pathogens and their antimicrobial sensitivities.

Although valuable in a considerable subset of cases, problems remain with the use of culture in the isolation of pathogenic organisms in PJI. In spite of strategies to optimize yield, such as an increasing number of samples, longer culture incubation period, and implant sonication, the sensitivity of culture is only 39–70% [3–6]. In addition, cultures yield a negative result in 7–50% of PJI cases [3, 7, 8]. These culture-negative PJI cases prevent the selection of targeted antimicrobial therapy for the patient and result in poorer outcomes. Studies suggest that patients with a culture-negative PJI have a 4.5 times greater rate of re-operation than those with positive cultures [9].

Several factors have been implicated in the decreased yield of culture for certain PJI patients. Historically, it has been proven difficult to isolate sessile organisms that reside within a biofilm in comparison to their traditional planktonic state. Prior antibiotic therapy can also decrease the yield of culture, with 53% of culture-negative PJI having had preceding antibiotic therapy in some studies [10]. Both bacteria in biofilm and those exposed to antibiotics have been shown to enter a viable but non-culturable state (VBNC), characterized by a loss of culturability on routine agar medium [11]. Certain fastidious organisms, including *Cutibacterium acnes*, *Brucella*, and *C. burnetii* can be difficult to isolate with standard culture methods even when not in a VBNC state and require specialized microbiological techniques to detect [12]. Finally, polymicrobial infections pose a unique challenge when

V. Hegde · C. C. Yang (✉)
Colorado Joint Replacement, Denver, CO, USA
e-mail: vhegde2@jh.edu

D. A. Dennis
Colorado Joint Replacement, Denver, CO, USA

Department of Mechanical and Materials Engineering, University of Denver, Denver, CO, USA
e-mail: douglasdennis@centura.org

© ISAKOS 2022
U. G. Longo et al. (eds.), *Infection in Knee Replacement*,
https://doi.org/10.1007/978-3-030-81553-0_8

using traditional culture methods, with a detection rate as low as 13–17% [13]. When culturing these infections, secondary bacteria can be hidden due to overgrowth by a rapidly growing primary species.

With these limitations of traditional microbiological culture in mind, there has been an increasing interest in alternative molecular diagnostic techniques to isolate pathological organisms in PJI, such as polymerase chain reaction (PCR), next-generation sequencing (NGS), and metagenomic sequencing. As these techniques gradually occupy an increased role in the diagnosis of PJI, it is important to understand the advantages and limitations of each technique and consider what their role should be within the diagnostic framework for PJI in the future.

8.2 Molecular Analysis

8.2.1 PCR

Techniques for molecular analysis have expanded rapidly in recent years and have increasing roles in the diagnosis of genetic disease, cancer, and infection. The simplest of these techniques is pathogen specific polymerase chain reaction (PCR), which uses a primer to detect a specific organism (e.g. *S. aureus*) or a group of closely related species (e.g. all staphylococcal species) (Fig. 8.1). This primer targets a known DNA sequence and amplifies this fragment, which can be from a particular gene or non-coding region of bacterial DNA. Originally, techniques such as gel electrophoresis were used for "end-point" detec-

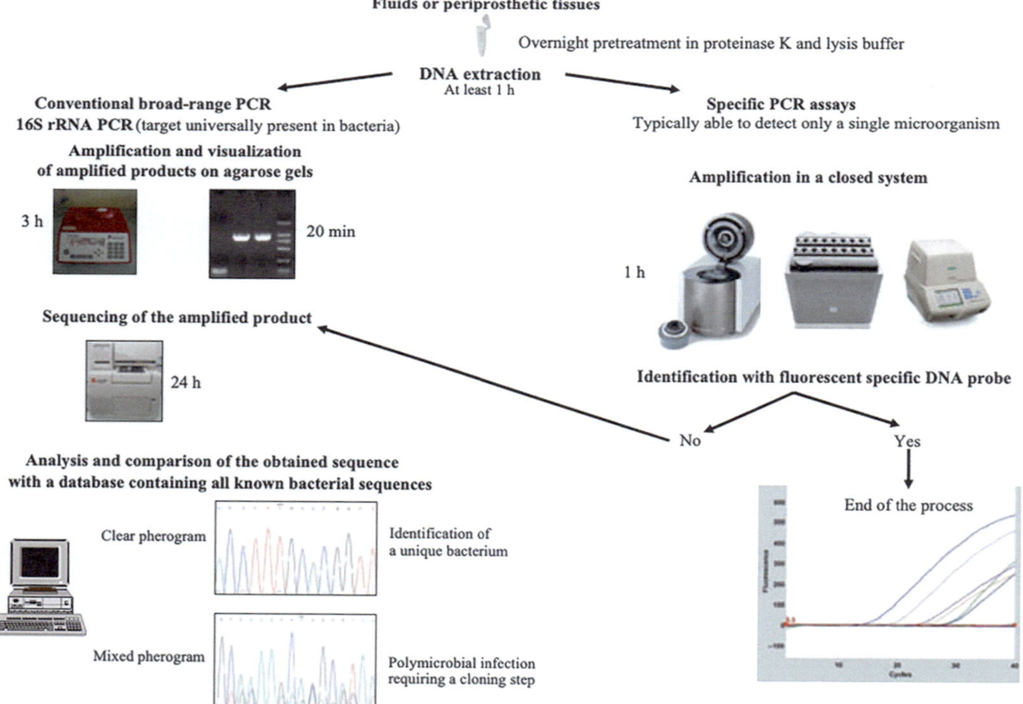

Fig. 8.1 Methodology of conventional broad-range PCR and specific PCR assays. (Reprinted from Lévy PY, Fenollar F. The role of molecular diagnostics in implant-associated bone and joint infection. Clin Microbiol Infect. 2012 Sept;18:1168–1175, with permission from Elsevier)

tion (positive or negative) of this PCR product or "amplicon." More recently, real-time PCR, where the PCR machine detects the amplicon in real time using fluorescent dyes, has been developed. This technique is both more sensitive than gel-based PCR and gives the user a quantitative result [14]. A primer can be designed that is unique for any organism and has the advantage of being extremely sensitive, potentially detecting even a single copy of the target DNA. Unfortunately, pathogen specific PCR has limited applicability in the diagnosis of PJI, due to its detection of only a single organism. Attempts to address this have been made with multiplex PCR assays, which use a group of specific primers to detect bacteria and fungi that are common in PJI. Unfortunately, these tests are labor intensive and may still overlook rare organisms. Studies have demonstrated that multiplex PCR does not outperform culture, with a sensitivity of 81% and a false positive rate of 88%, limiting its utility [15, 16].

Broad-range PCR provides the ability to find DNA from any bacteria. Most broad-range PCR techniques are based on the gene coding for the small subunit of the bacterial ribosome (16S rDNA) [14]. This gene contains highly conserved regions that are pan-bacterial, as well as more variable regions that are different among bacterial species. These highly conserved regions enable broad-range PCR assays to amplify DNA from any bacterial species, after which the specific identity of the bacterial species is subsequently determined by analyzing at least one variable region contained within the amplicon. Using traditional Sanger sequencing technology, direct analysis of the amplicon is only interpretable if a single sequence makes up greater than 70% of the total amplicon [14]. This makes interpretation difficult in the setting of a polymicrobial infection, which will result in mixed sequence data.

In addition to its inability to detect a polymicrobial infection, the main limitations of broad-range PCR relate to issues with contamination and sensitivity. As PCR can be an extremely sensitive assay, contamination from bacterial DNA introduced during the collection and handling of the sample, as well as DNA present in PCR reagents can lead to false positive results. Development of techniques to remove extraneous DNA, such as UV irradiation or DNase treatment, have been partially successful in addressing this problem, but can actually reduce the activity of the *Taq* polymerase, thus considerably reducing the sensitivity of the PCR assay [17–19]. Reducing the number of PCR cycles can also avoid the effects of low-level reagent contamination, but results in a 100–1000 times lower sensitivity than pathogen specific PCR assays [14]. Newer methods, such as a PCR-based system with mass spectroscopic identification of pathogens (Ibis Biosciences T5000 biosensor system) have also been developed in an attempt to increase sensitivity. This technique appears to be less affected by prior antimicrobial therapy than traditional culture, with a sensitivity of 85.7% among subjects receiving antimicrobial therapy within 14–28 days of surgery [20]. A recent meta-analysis of all PCR studies found a pooled specificity of 94% and a pooled sensitivity of 76% [21].

8.2.2 NGS

In contrast to traditional Sanger sequencing, next-generation sequencing (NGS) parallelizes the sequencing process, so thousands of sequencing processes are able to occur in one reaction system concurrently [22]. This decreases both the time required and cost; NGS requires only 12 h to complete a workflow of whole genome sequencing, and multi-gene sequencing with NGS costs about the same as single-gene Sanger sequencing [23, 24]. In addition, fewer DNA or RNA samples are required [23]. In a recent meta-analysis, NGS sequencing by synthesis was demonstrated to have a similar specificity to Sanger sequencing at 96.3% vs. 96.7%, respectively [25].

Studies examining the efficacy of NGS for PJI demonstrate considerable promise. In a prospective study by Parvizi et al. examining 65 revision arthroplasties and 17 primary arthroplasties, NGS had a sensitivity of 90%, compared to culture with 60.7% [26]. NGS had a

88.2% concordance with culture and was able to detect a potential pathogen in 81.8% of culture-negative PJI. In 9 of the 11 culture-negative PJI cases, NGS detected a polymicrobial infection. Interestingly, NGS was positive in 35% of primary and 25% of aseptic revision cases, indicating a high false positive rate. In many of these cases, *C. acnes* was the predominant organism detected. Other organisms isolated were mostly microbiota, the significance of which is unclear in the context of our limited understanding of the joint microbiome. Further emerging data using NGS also indicates that a greater number of PJI cases may be polymicrobial at the DNA level than previously thought based on traditional culture. Data presented at the 2019 American Academy of Orthopedic Surgeons meeting suggests that 88.7% of PJI patients who subsequently failed during longitudinal follow-up with a new organism detected by culture had that infective organism isolated using NGS during the initial treatment resection arthroplasty [27].

A further evolution of NGS technology involves metagenomic shotgun sequencing. Instead of targeting a specific highly conserved region of interest, such as the 16S rDNA for bacteria or the internal transcribed spacer for fungi, shotgun metagenomics extracts and sequences of all nucleic acid in a sample both from the host and any microorganisms are present [28]. This data is then compared against comprehensive curated library databases containing all known pathogens [29, 30]. Using this "open read" technology, shotgun metagenomics is only limited by missing or incomplete taxonomic representation in databases, which may produce a false negative result. This technique can even detect organisms that are transcriptionally active (metatranscriptome), shedding light on potential antimicrobial resistance [31]. A study using shotgun metagenomic sequencing by Thoendel et al. was able to identify known pathogens in 94.8% of culture-positive PJI and new pathogens in 43.9% of culture-negative PJI. The rate of false positive detection of microorganisms from uninfected aseptic failure cases was in this study was 3.6%, and the authors noted that the presence of human

and contaminant microbial DNA continues to be a challenge when using this technique [28].

While it seems likely that NGS holds promise and will see an increasing role in the diagnosis of PJI in the future, there are important issues that remain to be determined regarding its clinical utility. Currently, NGS is a costly technology that requires highly specialized equipment, trained technicians, and bioinformatics expertise that is currently only available in a few institutions [27]. A recent cost analysis comparing traditional culture with NGS found NGS to be cost-effective when the pre-test probability of PJI is greater than 45.5% [32]. This reinforces the concept that NGS does not provide a definitive answer as to whether a patient has a PJI, but adds data that must be interpreted along with the clinical picture and other laboratory investigations that help determine the pre-test probability of a PJI. Further study is also required to determine the significance of the DNA signal that is identified by NGS. Due to its high sensitivity, it is currently unclear whether the polymicrobial signals detected by NGS represent pathologic entities, contaminants, or organisms natively present as a part of the natural microbiome of the joint. Moving forward, it will be critical to understand the clinical relevance of these polymicrobial metagenomic signals, in particular due to the antimicrobial stewardship implications of the broad-spectrum treatment that would be required if these signals are deemed to be pathologic.

8.2.3 Histological Evaluation

In cases where preoperative testing is equivocal, the histological study of periprosthetic tissue has long been an important tool used to confirm or rule out a PJI. The presence of a polymorphonuclear neutrophil (PMN) infiltrate has traditionally been considered indicative of septic implant failure. This is reflected in the inclusion of positive histology as an intraoperative finding in the 2018 Musculoskeletal Infection Society's (MSIS) evidence-based definition for diagnosing PJI [33]. Within, the MSIS considers positive histology "greater than 5 neutrophils per high-power field in 5 high-power fields observed from histologic analysis of periprosthetic tissue at ×400 magnification." In a meta-analysis of intraoperative frozen section histopathology in the diagnosis of PJI, this criterion was shown to be an accurate predictor of culture-positive PJI, with a likelihood ratio of 10.25 [34].

The MSIS criteria built on the work of Feldman et al., who, recognizing the difficulty of identifying a PMN infiltrate using standard hematoxylin-eosin staining, established five criteria to ensure the adequate analysis of specimens [35]. First, the tissue has to be pink-tan, and not simply white scar, to avoid analysis of dense fibrous tissue or fibrin. Second, at least two specific tissue samples are used in order to minimize the risk of sampling error. Third, the five most cellular areas in the tissue sample are chosen for evaluation. Fourth, all PMNs have to have defined cytoplasmic borders to be included. Debris that appears to be the result of nuclear fragmentation is excluded, as it cannot be categorized definitively as a PMN. Fifth, five separate fields are evaluated under high power magnification (HPF).

When obtaining samples, good surgical technique is important to ensure accurate results. To limit false positive results, tissue should be obtained using sharp dissection rather than cautery [36, 37]. Furthermore, the best sample to obtain for histological study is the periprosthetic membrane. A study by Bori et al. demonstrated that the proportion of patients with PJI that had a positive interface membrane was significantly higher than those with a positive pseudocapsule (83% vs. 42%, $p = 0.04$) [38]. This may be due either to the fact that fibrosis in the pseudocapsule hinders neutrophil infiltration, or that the largest bacterial biofilm is found at the implant–bone interface.

There are special circumstances in which the traditionally accepted histological cutoff of five PMNs per HPF in five HPFs may lead to inaccurate conclusions, either increasing the rate of false negative or false positive results. One such patient population are those who have been previously implanted with a cement spacer and have returned for reimplantation with a definitive prosthesis. Studies examining these patients have concluded that histology has a low sensitivity, with one study showing histology was positive in only two of the seven patients who had positive cultures at the time of reimplantation and another showing a sensitivity of 25% (one of the four patients) [39, 40]. There are also two subsets of patients in which histology will produce a high false positive result: patients with underlying inflammatory disease and those receiving a prosthetic replacement in the setting of a periprosthetic fracture. A study by Kataoka et al. examined synovial tissue from 60 rheumatoid arthritis patients at the time of their total joint arthroplasty and found 16.6% (10 out of 60) had greater than five PMNs per HPF [41]. The authors postulated that there is a persistent neutrophil infiltration in the rheumatoid synovium due to the underlying active disease, and this common microscopic finding is not necessarily consistent with an infection. Another study by Muñoz-Mahamud et al., examining 11 patients undergoing arthroplasty due to periprosthetic fracture, found a 66.6% (four out of six cases) false positive rate using histology [42]. In these patients, it may be the case that a neutrophil infiltration can occur in the periprosthetic membrane secondary to inflammation caused by the fracture and injured surrounding vasculature and not solely due to an infectious process.

Although much of this work has been done with frozen section, as intraoperative histology is most useful to guide surgical decision making, it is important to note that the morphological identification of PMNs and their differentiation from other inflammatory components within periprosthetic tissue may be more difficult in frozen sections than in permanent paraffin sections [43]. Some authors, such as Stroh et al., report few differences between the results of frozen and paraffin sections, with a concordance of 97.7% (297 of 304 sections) and the difference not affecting the final outcome of any patient [44]. This is in contrast to a study by Tohtz et al., which found a 21.8% (14 of 64 cases) discrepancy between frozen and paraffin sections [37, 43, 44]. In 18.8% (12 patients) of cases, the frozen section diagnosis was unclear and permanent sections confirmed the diagnosis (8 patients had aseptic loosening and 4 had septic loosening). In 3.2% (2 patients) of cases, the frozen section diagnosis was aseptic loosening and the permanent section diagnosis was septic loosening.

Even when examining paraffin sections, prosthetic wear particles and bone fragments, which are common in periprosthetic membranes, make the processing of tissue difficult and lead to artifacts or thick sections that complicate the identification of PMNs [45]. As a result, there is interest in developing more precise methods for the detection of PMNs, using molecular markers. In one study, by Morawietz et al., CD15 immunohistochemistry was used to identify PMNs, resulting in a sensitivity of 73% and a specificity of 95% in culture-positive PJI [46]. The authors

concluded that with their methods, only 23 PMNs in 10 HPFs are indicative of a PJI. Another study by Kashima et al. used chloroacetate esterase (CAE) enzyme histochemistry, which resulted in a sensitivity of 83% and a specificity of 96% in culture-positive PJI (Fig. 8.2) [43, 45, 46]. The authors noted that if the criterion for histological diagnosis of PJI was lowered to two PMNs per HPF, the sensitivity and specificity increased to 94% and 96%, respectively. In 17% (five out of 29) of the culture-positive PJI cases, the histology had between two and five PMNs per HPF, while in all culture-negative cases, there were fewer than two PMNs per HPF. The exception to this was two cases which were culture negative, but still met the MSIS criteria for PJI, both of

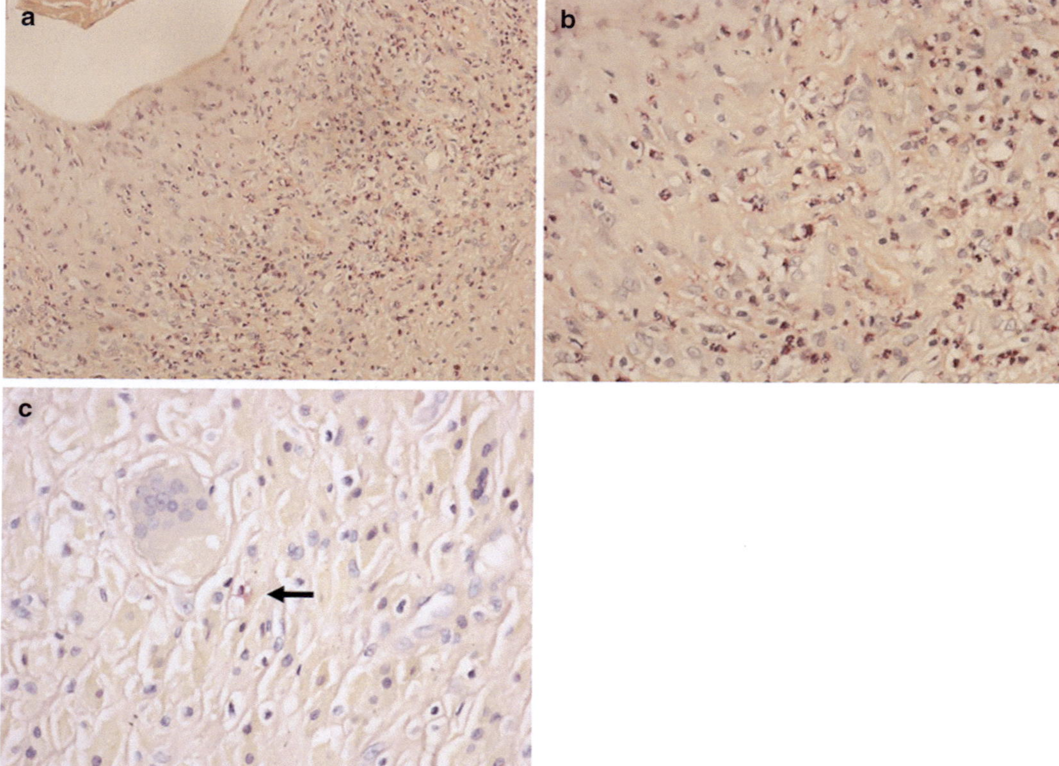

Fig. 8.2 CAE staining of paraffin sections of peri-implant tissues showing (**a**) low-power and (**b**) high-power views of a case of septic implant failure. There are numerous neutrophil polymorphs which show bright red cytoplasmic staining, whereas background foreign body macrophages are unstained. (**c**) Absence of CAE staining in a case of aseptic implant failure. Macrophages and a macrophage polykaryon are unstained. The inflammatory infiltrate including a CAE-positive mast cell (arrow). (Reprinted from Kashima TG, Inagaki Y, Grammatopoulos G, Athanasou NA. Use of chloroacetate esterase staining for the histological diagnosis of prosthetic joint infection. Virchows Arch. 6 ed. 2015 Feb 17;466 (5):595–601, with permission from Springer)

which had between two and five PMNs per HPF. Both studies concluded that the MSIS criteria of 5 PMNs per HPF in 5 HPFs are too high and may miss some infections, in particular those caused by lower virulence organisms such as *C. acnes* [47].

Considerable work is now being done to help identify molecular biomarkers that are uniquely present in infected periprosthetic tissues. In the future, tissue biomarkers such as CD15 and certain toll-like receptors (TLR) may help us achieve a more reliable histological diagnosis of PJI [43].

8.3 Conclusions

Despite the progress in the study of PJI over the last 40 years, its diagnosis continues to be an elusive issue after total hip and knee arthroplasty. The current MSIS histological criteria for PJI remains the same as the one proposed by Mirra et al. in 1976 [43]. Increasing accuracy in the identification of bacteria and PMNs may assist clinicians in increasing the precision of their diagnosis by lowering currently established thresholds for PJI. The next step in this process may be examination not just on the cellular but also the molecular level.

References

1. Del Pozo JL, Patel R. Clinical practice. Infection associated with prosthetic joints. N Engl J Med. 2009;361(8):787–94.
2. Karim MA, Andrawis J, Bengoa F, Bracho C, Compagnoni R, Cross M, et al. Hip and knee section, diagnosis, algorithm: proceedings of International Consensus on Orthopedic Infections. J Arthroplasty. 2019;34(Suppl):S339–50.
3. Parvizi J, Erkocak OF, Valle Della CJ. Culture-negative periprosthetic joint infection. J Bone Joint Surg. 2014;96(5):430–6.
4. Tan TL, Kheir MM, Shohat N, Tan DD, Kheir M, Chen C, et al. Culture-negative periprosthetic joint infection: an update on what to expect. JBJS Open Access. 2018;3(3):e0060.
5. Larsen LH, Lange J, Xu Y, Schønheyder HC. Optimizing culture methods for diagnosis of prosthetic joint infections: a summary of modifications and improvements reported since 1995. J Med Microbiol. 2012;61(3):309–16.
6. Peel TN, Spelman T, Dylla BL, Hughes JG, Greenwood-Quaintance KE, Cheng AC, et al. Optimal periprosthetic tissue specimen number for diagnosis of prosthetic joint infection. J Clin Microbiol. 2017;55(1):234–43.
7. Tarabichi M, Shohat N, Goswami K, Alvand A, Silibovsky R, Belden K, et al. Diagnosis of Periprosthetic joint infection. J Bone Joint Surg. 2018;100(2):147–54.
8. Font-Vizcarra L, García S, Martínez-Pastor JC, Sierra JM, Soriano A. Blood culture flasks for culturing synovial fluid in prosthetic joint infections. Clin Orthop Relat Res. 2010;468(8):2238–43.
9. Mortazavi SMJ, Vegari D, Ho A, Zmistowski B, Parvizi J. Two-stage exchange arthroplasty for infected Total knee arthroplasty: predictors of failure. Clin Orthop Relat Res. 2011;469(11):3049–54.
10. Berbari EF, Marculescu C, Sia I, Lahr BD, Hanssen AD, Steckelberg JM, Gullerud R, Osmon DR. Culture-negative prosthetic joint infection. Clin Infect Dis. 2007;45(9):1113–9.
11. Li L, Mendis N, Trigui H, Oliver JD, Faucher SP. The importance of the viable but non-culturable state in human bacterial pathogens. Front Microbiol. 2014;5(70):130.
12. Parikh MS, Antony S. A comprehensive review of the diagnosis and management of prosthetic joint infections in the absence of positive cultures. J Infect Public Health. 2016;9(5):545–56.
13. Lévy PY, Fenollar F. The role of molecular diagnostics in implant-associated bone and joint infection. Clin Microbiol Infect. 2012;18(12):1168–75.
14. Hartley JC, Harris KA. Molecular techniques for diagnosing prosthetic joint infections. J Antimicrob Chemother. 2014;69(Suppl 1):i21–4.
15. Jacovides CL, Kreft R, Adeli B, Hozack B, Ehrlich GD, Parvizi J. Successful identification of pathogens by polymerase chain reaction (PCR)-based Electron spray ionization time-of-flight mass spectrometry (ESI-TOF-MS) in culture-negative Periprosthetic joint infection. J Bone Joint Surg. 2012;94(24):2247–54.
16. Melendez DP, Uhl JR, Greenwood-Quaintance KE, Hanssen AD, Sampath R, Patel R. Detection of prosthetic joint infection by use of PCR-electrospray ionization mass spectrometry applied to synovial fluid. J Clin Microbiol. 2014;52(6):2202–5.
17. Harris KA, Hartley JC. Development of broad-range 16S rDNA PCR for use in the routine diagnostic clinical microbiology service. J Med Microbiol Society. 2003;52(Pt 8):685–91.
18. Levine MJ, Mariani BA. Molecular genetic diagnosis of infected total joint arthroplasty. 1995. europepmc.org.
19. Mariani BD, Martin DS, Levine MJ, Booth RE, Tuan RS. The Coventry Award. Polymerase chain reaction detection of bacterial infection in total knee arthroplasty. Clin Orthop Relat Res. 1996;331(331):11–22.
20. Greenwood-Quaintance KE, Uhl JR, Hanssen AD, Sampath R, Mandrekar JN, Patel R. Diagnosis of

prosthetic joint infection by use of PCR-electrospray ionization mass spectrometry. J Clin Microbiol. 2014;52(2):642–9.

21. Jun Y, Jianghua L. Diagnosis of periprosthetic joint infection using polymerase chain reaction: an updated systematic review and Meta-analysis. Surg Infect. 2018;19(6):555–65.

22. Grada A, Weinbrecht K. Next-generation sequencing: methodology and application. J Invest Dermatol. 2013;133(8):e11–4.

23. Verma M, Kulshrestha S, Puri A. Genome sequencing. Methods Mol Biol. 2017;1525(2):3–33.

24. Lohmann K, Klein C. Next generation sequencing and the future of genetic diagnosis. Neurotherapeutics. 2014;11(4):699–707.

25. Li M, Zeng Y, Wu Y, Si H, Bao X, Bin Shen B. Performance of sequencing assays in diagnosis of prosthetic joint infection: a systematic review and meta-analysis. J Arthroplasty. 2019;34(7):1514.

26. Tarabichi M, Shohat N, Goswami K, Alvand A, Silibovsky R, Belden K, et al. Diagnosis of Periprosthetic joint infection: the potential of next-generation sequencing. J Bone Joint Surg. 2018;100(2):147–54.

27. Goswami K, Parvizi J. Culture-negative periprosthetic joint infection: is there a diagnostic role for next-generation sequencing? Exp Rev Mol Diagn. 2020;20(3):269–72.

28. Thoendel MJ, Jeraldo PR, Greenwood-Quaintance KE, Yao JZ, Chia N, Hanssen AD, et al. Identification of prosthetic joint infection pathogens using a shotgun metagenomics approach. Clin Infect Dis. 2018;67(9):1333–8.

29. Fulkerson E, Valle CJD, Wise B, Walsh M, Preston C, Di Cesare PE. Antibiotic susceptibility of bacteria infecting total joint arthroplasty sites. J Bone Joint Surg. 2006;88(6):1231–7.

30. Dunne WM, Westblade LF, Ford B. Next-generation and whole-genome sequencing in the diagnostic clinical microbiology laboratory. Eur J Clin Microbiol Infect Dis. 2012;31(8):1719–26.

31. Aguiar-Pulido V, Huang W, Suarez-Ulloa V, Cickovski T, Mathee K, Narasimhan G. Metagenomics, metatranscriptomics, and metabolomics approaches for microbiome analysis. Evol Bioinformatics Online. 2016;12(Suppl 1):5–16.

32. Torchia MT, Austin DC, Kunkel ST, Dwyer KW, Moschetti WE. Next-generation sequencing vs culture-based methods for diagnosing periprosthetic joint infection after total knee arthroplasty: a cost-effectiveness analysis. J Arthroplasty. 2019;34(7):1333–41.

33. Parvizi J, Tan TL, Goswami K, Higuera C, Valle Della C, Chen AF, et al. The 2018 definition of periprosthetic hip and knee infection: an evidence-based and validated criteria. J Arthroplasty. 2018;33(5):1309–1314.e2.

34. Tsaras G, Maduka-Ezeh A, Inwards CY, Mabry T, Erwin PJ, Murad MH, et al. Utility of intraoperative frozen section histopathology in the diagnosis of periprosthetic joint infection. J Bone Joint Surg. 2012;94(18):1700–11.

35. Feldman DS, Lonner JH, Desai P, Zuckerman JD. The role of intraoperative frozen sections in revision total joint arthroplasty. J Bone Joint Surg. 1995;77(12):1807–13.

36. Zmistowski B, Valle Della C, Bauer TW, Malizos KN, Alavi A, Bedair H, et al. Diagnosis of periprosthetic joint infection. 2014. p. 77–83.

37. Enayatollahi MA, Parvizi J. Diagnosis of infected total hip arthroplasty. Hip Int. 2015;25(4):294–300.

38. Bori G, Muñoz-Mahamud E, Garcia S, Mallofre C, Gallart X, Bosch J, Garcia E, Riba J, Mensa J, Soriano A. Interface membrane is the best sample for histological study to diagnose prosthetic joint infection. Mod Pathol. 2011;24(4):579–84.

39. Valle Della CJ, Bogner E, Desai P, Lonner JH, Adler E, Zuckerman JD, et al. Analysis of frozen sections of intraoperative specimens obtained at the time of reoperation after hip or knee resection arthroplasty for the treatment of infection. J Bone Joint Surg. 1999;81(5):684–9.

40. Bori G, Soriano A, García S, Mallofre C, Riba J, Mensa J. Usefulness of histological analysis for predicting the presence of microorganisms at the time of reimplantation after hip resection arthroplasty for the treatment of infection. J Bone Joint Surg. 2007;89(6):1232–7.

41. Kataoka M, Torisu T, Tsumura H, Yoshida S, Takashita M. An assessment of histopathological criteria for infection in joint arthroplasty in rheumatoid synovium. Clin Rheumatol. 2014;21(2):159–63.

42. Muñoz-Mahamud E, Bori G, García S, Ramírez J, Riba J, Soriano A. Usefulness of histology for predicting infection at the time of hip revision for the treatment of Vancouver B2 periprosthetic fractures. J Arthroplasty. 2013;28(8):1247–50.

43. Bori G, McNally MA, Athanasou N. Histopathology in periprosthetic joint infection: when will the Morphomolecular diagnosis be a reality? Biomed Res Int. 2018;2018(304):1–10.

44. Stroh DA, Johnson AJ, Naziri Q, Mont MA. Discrepancies between frozen and paraffin tissue sections have little effect on outcome of staged total knee arthroplasty revision for infection. J Bone Joint Surg. 2012;94(18):1662–7.

45. Morawietz L, Tiddens O, Mueller M, Tohtz S, Gansukh T, Schroeder JH, et al. Twenty-three neutrophil granulocytes in 10 high-power fields is the best histopathological threshold to differentiate between aseptic and septic endoprosthesis loosening. Histopathology. 2009;54(7):847–53.

46. Kashima TG, Inagaki Y, Grammatopoulos G, Athanasou NA. Use of chloroacetate esterase staining for the histological diagnosis of prosthetic joint infection. Virchows Arch. 2015;466(5):595–601.

47. Mirra JM, Amstutz HC, Matos M, Gold R. The pathology of the joint tissues and its clinical relevance in prosthesis failure. Clin Orthop Relat Res. 1976;(117):221. europepmcorg.

Imaging

Vincenzo Candela, Sergio De Salvatore,
Calogero Di Naro, Giovanna Stelitano,
Carlo Casciaro, Laura Risi Ambrogioni,
Umile Giuseppe Longo, and Vincenzo Denaro

9.1 Introduction

Infection is one of the most debilitating complications following knee arthroplasty. A timely diagnosis of periprosthetic joint infection (PJI) is crucial for maintaining the joint function, avoid systemic sepsis, and limit the use of hospital and physician resources. Distinguishing PJI from aseptic mobilization is challenging but useful for the correct management of patients. Imaging can help in this purpose.

Imaging includes radiographs, resonance imaging (MR), computerized tomography (CT), ultrasound (US), and nuclear studies.

In addition to imaging, the AAOS study group recommended the erythrocyte sedimentation rate (ESR) and C-reactive protein (CRP) testing.

An X-ray could show periprosthetic radiolucency and the presence of intraarticular gas. MR imaging using metal artefact reduction techniques may detect osteolysis around the knee arthroplasty. CT scan may assist in distinguishing between septic and aseptic loosening. Nuclear techniques are used in patients with an uncertain diagnosis. They include labelled leukocyte imaging with bone or bone marrow scan, fluorodeoxyglucose-positron emission tomography (FDG-PET), gallium, or labelled leukocyte imaging. Nowadays, nuclear medicine is valuable for joint arthroplasty assessment.

9.2 Ultrasound (US)

US is a useful imaging method to diagnose joint effusion and synovial hypertrophy, Baker's cysts, and synovitis. It is commonly used for guided arthrocentesis, aspiration of fluid around the joints, synovial and soft tissue biopsy, or abscess drainage [1, 2]. It can also be used for dynamic examination of the knee joint. Infected joint fluid often displays heterogeneous echoes with irregular hyperechoic synovial thickening and hypoechoic or non-echoic synovial fluid. Active synovial inflammation and the infection show strength or hyperaemia with colour-Doppler ultrasound. Advantages of US tests include accessibility, lack of ionizing radiation, no imaging contraindications, low cost, and a generally high tolerance for patients. However, US is operator dependent and has a constrained utility in the evaluation of osseous structures and surgical hardware.

9.3 Radiography

Radiography is usually the first imaging modality performed to assess a painful knee arthroplasty. It is used in the evaluation of total knee arthroplas-

V. Candela · S. De Salvatore · C. Di Naro
G. Stelitano · C. Casciaro · L. Risi Ambrogioni
U. G. Longo (✉) · V. Denaro
Department of Orthopaedic and Trauma Surgery,
Campus Bio-Medico University, Rome, Italy
e-mail: g.longo@unicampus.it

© ISAKOS 2022
U. G. Longo et al. (eds.), *Infection in Knee Replacement*,
https://doi.org/10.1007/978-3-030-81553-0_9

ties (TKAs) in both the immediate postoperative period and during the follow-up. The correct alignment of TKA, the type of implant used, the fixation interfaces, ligamentous laxity, and polyethylene wear are usually analysed through a weight-bearing X-ray. However, radiography lacks sensitivity and specificity in the assessment of PJI.

Radiographic signs of infected TKA, with low specificity, are swelling of soft tissue, periprosthetic lucency (Fig. 9.1), reflecting erosions (usually at the edges of the prosthesis) (Fig. 9.2), presence of intraarticular gas, and loosening of the elements.

Abnormalities like radiolucent lines are evaluated on AP views of the tibial component, on lateral views of the femoral component and skyline views of the patella. Changes in component position very reliably predict loosening. It is difficult to distinguish septic loosening from aseptic loosening. Septic loosening usually produces extensive radiolucent zones and a periosteal reaction.

However, X-ray could show no abnormalities or nonspecific findings. These are periostitis, broad radiolucent lines, and focal osteolysis [3]. Li et al. showed that postoperative soft tissue gas on radiography is predictive of early PJI and is associated with a broader spectrum of microorganisms [1].

9.4 Resonance Imaging

MR imaging of the postoperative knee could be challenging. Knee arthroplasty produces significant susceptibility artefacts, which distort the appearance of the adjacent bony and soft tissue structures.

Cobalt, chrome, and molybdenum are usually associated with more extensive metal artefact compared with titanium or zirconium [2]. MR

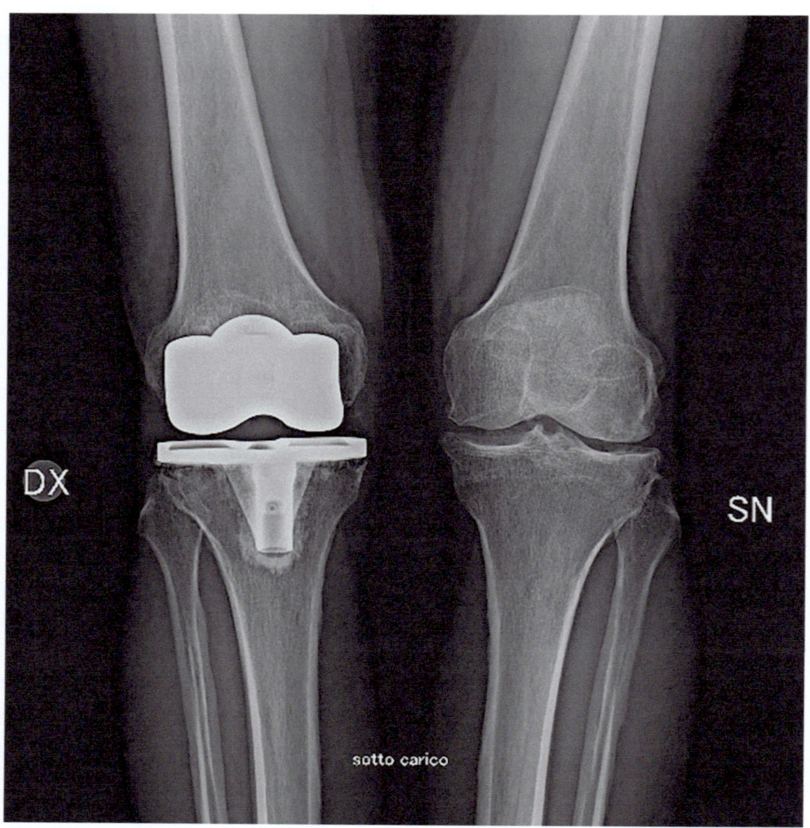

Fig. 9.1 Periprosthetic lucency

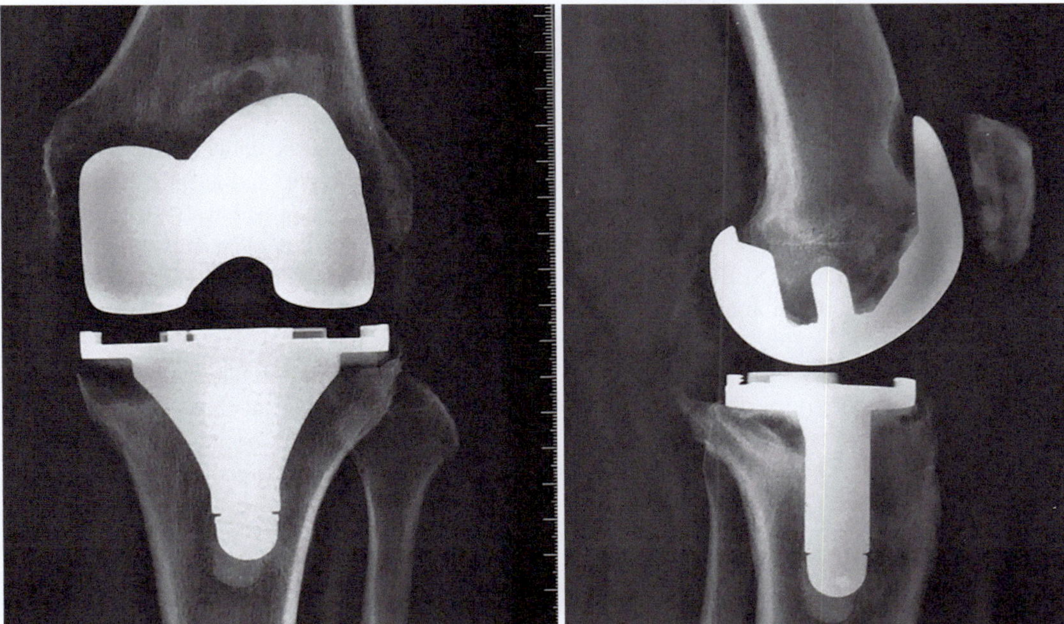

Fig. 9.2 Periprosthetic lucency

imaging using metal artefact reduction techniques, such as "section encoding for metal artefact correction (SEMAC)" and "multiacquisition variable-resonance image combination (MAVRIC)", may detect osteolysis around the knee arthroplasty [4].

Several authors report lamellar and hyperintensive synovitis during MR examination in patients with infected knee arthroplasty [5]. MR imaging can provide helpful information in patients with suspected periprosthetic joint infection. In acute infections, MR imaging can demonstrate the presence of a wound complication like a hematoma or abscess. The MR imaging demonstration of a sinus tract is diagnostic for joint infection.

9.5 Computerized Tomography Imaging

Computerized tomography (CT) scan may assist in distinguishing between septic and aseptic loosening [6]. Beam sclerosis artefacts limit the evaluation of adjacent bone and soft tissue structures, so dual-energy CT can achieve metal suppression artefacts and is often used to detect radiographically hidden periosteal osteolysis. CT is better than MR imaging in isolating foreign bodies and gaseous lesions in the bone. CT imaging with enhanced contrast helps to outline soft tissue abscesses around the joints, synovitis, anatomical location, and the extent of soft tissue and bone infections [7]. MR and CT with intravenous contrast could detect soft tissue and intraosseous abscesses or active enhancing synovitis.

9.6 Single-Photon Emission Computed Tomography with Computerized Tomography (SPECT/CT)

Single-photon emission computed tomography (SPECT) is a nuclear medicine tomographic imaging technique using gamma rays. It may integrate and improves CT defects. Single-photon emission computed tomography with CT (SPECT/CT) provides information on the site of infection [8]. Several radiopharmaceuticals have been used for SPECT/CT imaging. They include 99mTc-labelled diphosphonates, radiolabelled white blood cells with 111In, 99mTc-hexamethylpropylene amine oxime, 67Ga citrate, and other new tracers. Kim et al. [8] report that the sensitivity and specificity of SPECT/CT with 99mTc-hexamethylpropylene labelled leukocyte are both 93.3%. Graute et al. [9] underline that the SPECT/CT in addition to planar scintigraphy with 99mTc-labelled antigranulocyte antibodies for diagnosing and localizing low-grade joint infections has a sensitivity and specificity of 89% and 73%, respectively. Moreover, SPECT/CT provides an accurate anatomic localization of all positive areas, allowing a correct diagnosis of prosthesis versus soft tissue involvement.

9.7 Bone Scintigraphy/Three-Phase Bone Scan

Bone scintigraphy is a nuclear medicine procedure that uses small amounts of radioactive material to diagnose and assess the severity of a variety of bone diseases and conditions, including bone fractures, heterotopic ossifications, cancer, arthritis, aseptic loosening, and infection. It is the first method in nuclear medicine usually performed in cases of suspected PJI, and it is typically performed using 99mTc-methylene diphosphonate (99mTc-MDP), which accumulates on the surface of the mineral bone matrix.

Increased uptake on all three phases of the bone scan is indicative of infected TKA.

Bone scintigraphy can be positive as a standard postoperative appearance up to 2 years after TKA placement [10]. Moreover, osteolysis or synovitis from PE wear debris generally may simulate a PJI.

Bone scintigraphy is characterized by high sensitivity (95%) but low specificity for the diagnosis of PJI. Nevertheless, a negative three-phase Tc bone scan typically excludes infection [11–13].

9.8 Gallium-67 Citrate Scintigraphy

Gallium-67 (67Ga) is a radionuclide. It was initially used to diagnose cancer [14]. 67Ga accumulates in both septic and aseptic inflammation sites. The exact reason why 67Ga accumulates in infection sites is still unclear. It is probably associated with the migration of lactoferrin, leukocytes, and siderophores produced by bacteria in inflammatory areas [12]. 67Ga binds to lactoferrin and leukocytes in the plasma, and it migrates in inflammatory foci at high concentrations. However, Gallium-67 citrate scintigraphy has low specificity in the diagnosis of PJI, so it has been almost entirely replaced by other radiopharmaceuticals [10].

9.9 Indium-111 Leukocyte Scan

Indium-111 leukocyte scan is the most widely used for suspected PJI. Leukocyte labelling is usually performed with indium-111 (111In) or 99mTc-hexamethylpropylene amine oxime (99mTc-HMPAO). Patient white blood cells are radiolabelled in vitro and then reinjected into the patients [10, 12]. Indium labelled leukocytes accumulate in areas of inflammation or infection or postoperative healing wounds. The evaluation of a negative indium scan is a strong predictor of the absence of infected TKA, but a positive indium scan has, unfortunately, a very limited value [12].

9.10 Dual-Isotope Imaging with In-111-Labelled Leukocytes and Tc-99m Sulphur Colloid Bone Marrow Scan

Dual-isotope imaging with In-111-labelled leukocytes and Tc-99m sulphur colloid bone marrow scan test is considered the most vigorous technique for detecting PJIs. However, it has some limitations. Patients leukocytes are labelled with In-111 and reinjected.

Simultaneously, Tc-99m sulphur colloid bone marrow scan (Tc-99m hexamethylpropyleneamineoxime [HMPAO]) is performed and delayed imaging after 24 h are acquired. The in vitro labelling process is challenging and requires the direct processing of blood products, which risks the contamination of the final product [15]. Sulphur colloid accumulates throughout the reticuloendothelial system, in the bone marrow, and in the liver and the spleen. In acute PJIs, chemotactic factors are secreted, so leukocytes migrate from the peripheral blood to the periprosthetic sites [12]. In chronic, long-standing infections, however, neutrophil recruitment is less evident. In PJIs an increased radiotracer uptake on both the three-phase bone scan and labelled leukocyte scan, in the same anatomical location, is found [11, 12]. A positive labelled leukocyte test has high sensitivity but low specificity. The conjunction of dual-isotope imaging with In-111-labelled leukocytes and Tc-99m sulphur colloid bone marrow scan test improves specificity and accuracy. Palestro et al. found that dual-isotope imaging with an In-111 and Tc-99m sulphur colloid bone marrow scan has 95% accuracy for the diagnosis of PJIs.

9.11 Labelled Leukocyte Scintigraphy with Antigranulocyte Antibody

99m Tc-antigranulocyte scintigraphy (AGS) is an alternative to autologous WBC scintigraphy in the detection of PJI. Leukocytes are labelled using monoclonal antibodies and antibody fragments against specific surface receptors on granulocytes [11]. Besilesomab and sulesomab are the monoclonal antibodies most commonly used. The sensitivity and specificity of besilesomab for PJI range from 67–91% to 57–75%, respectively [16]. AGS is a promising diagnostic tool, but, since the antibodies used are murine-derived, they could trigger a human anti-murine antibody (HAMA) response.

9.12 Positron Emission Tomography with 18F-Fluorodeoxyglucose (18F-FDG/PET)

Positron emission tomography (PET) is an imaging technique performed using a radioactive substance to visualize and measure metabolic processes in the body. PET with 18F-fluorodeoxyglucose (18F-FDG/PET) detects inflammatory cells with increased glucose uptake in infection sites [17]. This technique gives high-quality imaging with high spatial resolution, adequate capacity to determine anatomical location, and no need to manipulate blood products in vitro [18]. Fluorodeoxyglucose arrives in the cells via glucose transporters, where it is phosphorylated by hexokinase to 18F-2-18F FDG-6 phosphate. The uptake of fluorodeoxyglucose depends on the cellular metabolic rate, on the affinity, and on the number of glucose transporters, both of which are prevalent in the inflammatory cells. Scanning is performed 30–60 min after radiotracer injection.

Positron emission tomography with 18F-FDG can also be used to examine the potentially infected painful knee arthroplasty. High uptake at the prosthesis–bone interface indicates an infection. On the other side, an intermediate uptake suggests aseptic loosening. FDG uptake is usually estimated using SUV score [19].

Zhuang et al. [19] reported that 18F-FDG/PET has a sensitivity of 91%, a specificity of 72%, and an accuracy of 78% to assess total infected knee replacement.

Love et al. reported that 18F-FDG/PET has low specificity, so it can be used to exclude infection if the test is negative [11]. 18F-FDG/PET can quantify disease activity. It can be used to assess patients with infections during various phases of the disease [20].

Many authors have concluded from their results that 18F-FDG/PET is a promising tool to distinguish septic loosening from aseptic, with a sensitivity of approximately 80–100% and specificity of almost 90–100% [19]. More studies compare the value of FDG-PET with combined 111In-labelled leukocyte/99mTc-sulphur colloid bone marrow imaging for diagnosing infection in knee prostheses. Compared to 111In-labelled leukocyte/99mTc-sulphur colloid bone marrow imaging, positron emission tomography with 18F-fluorodeoxyglucose has many advantages, including the availability, the presence of only one radiotracer injection, and the short execution time (less than 2 h) [15]. Moreover, positron emission tomography with 18F-fluorodeoxyglucose provides superior spatial resolution compared to 111In-labelled leukocyte/99mTc-sulphur colloid bone imaging [21].

9.13 Conclusion

In conjunction with the clinical examination and laboratory testing, radiologic imaging represents an important adjunct in the diagnosis of PJI. Radiologic imaging includes radiographs, MR, CT, US, and nuclear studies. MR and CT imaging are frequently used to evaluate the extent of disease and exclude other or additional pathologic and traumatic findings. With the presence of surgical hardware, both MR and CT imaging may be degraded by metal artefact that may be decreased with the utilization of metal suppression techniques. Various nuclear imaging studies are helpful in the diagnosis of PJI including SPECT/CT, Bone Scintigraphy, Gallium-67 Citrate Scintigraphy, Indium-111 Leukocyte Scan, Dual-Isotope Imaging with In-111-Labelled Leukocytes and Tc-99m Sulphur Colloid Bone Marrow Scan, Labelled Leukocyte Scintigraphy with Antigranulocyte Antibody and 18F-FDG/PET.

References

1. Li N, Kagan R, Hanrahan CJ, Hansford BG. Radiographic evidence of soft-tissue gas 14 days after total knee arthroplasty is predictive of early prosthetic joint infection. AJR Am J Roentgenol. 2020;214(1):171–6. PubMed PMID: 31573855. Epub 2019/10/01.
2. Heyse TJ, Chong Le R, Davis J, Boettner F, Haas SB, Potter HG. MRI analysis for rotation of total knee components. Knee. 2012;19(5):571–5. PubMed PMID: 22364925.
3. Duff GP, Lachiewicz PF, Kelley SS. Aspiration of the knee joint before revision arthroplasty. Clin Orthop Relat Res. 1996;(331):132–9. PubMed PMID: 8895629.
4. Fritz J, Lurie B, Potter HG. MR imaging of knee arthroplasty implants. Radiographics. 2015;35(5):1483–501. PubMed PMID: 26295591. Pubmed Central PMCID: PMC4613886. Epub 2015/08/21.
5. Plodkowski AJ, Hayter CL, Miller TT, Nguyen JT, Potter HG. Lamellated hyperintense synovitis: potential MR imaging sign of an infected knee arthroplasty. Radiology. 2013;266(1):256–60. PubMed PMID: 23091176.
6. Cyteval C, Hamm V, Sarrabère MP, Lopez FM, Maury P, Taourel P. Painful infection at the site of hip prosthesis: CT imaging. Radiology. 2002;224(2):477–83. PubMed PMID: 12147845.
7. Fayad LM, Patra A, Fishman EK. Value of 3D CT in defining skeletal complications of orthopedic hardware in the postoperative patient. AJR Am J Roentgenol. 2009;193(4):1155–63. PubMed PMID: 19770342.
8. Kim HO, Na SJ, Oh SJ, Jung BS, Lee SH, Chang JS, et al. Usefulness of adding SPECT/CT to 99mTc-hexamethylpropylene amine oxime (HMPAO)-labeled leukocyte imaging for diagnosing prosthetic joint infections. J Comput Assist Tomogr. 2014;38(2):313–9. PubMed PMID: 24625603.
9. Graute V, Feist M, Lehner S, Haug A, Müller PE, Bartenstein P, et al. Detection of low-grade prosthetic joint infections using 99mTc-antigranulocyte SPECT/CT: initial clinical results. Eur J Nucl Med Mol Imaging. 2010;37(9):1751–9. PubMed PMID: 20309680. Epub 2010/03/23.
10. Glaudemans AW, Galli F, Pacilio M, Signore A. Leukocyte and bacteria imaging in prosthetic joint infection. Eur Cell Mater. 2013;25:61–77. PubMed PMID: 23325539. Epub 2013/01/16.
11. Love C, Marwin SE, Palestro CJ. Nuclear medicine and the infected joint replacement. Semin Nucl Med. 2009;39(1):66–78. PubMed PMID: 19038601.
12. Palestro CJ, Love C. Role of nuclear medicine for diagnosing infection of recently implanted lower extremity arthroplasties. Semin Nucl Med. 2017;47(6):630–8. PubMed PMID: 28969761.
13. Palestro CJ. Nuclear medicine and the failed joint replacement: past, present, and future. World J Radiol. 2014;6(7):446–58. PubMed PMID: 25071885. Pubmed Central PMCID: 4109096.
14. Cyteval C, Bourdon A. Imaging orthopedic implant infections. Diagn Interv Imaging. 2012;93(6):547–57. PubMed PMID: 22521777. Epub 2012/04/20.
15. Basu S, Kwee TC, Saboury B, Garino JP, Nelson CL, Zhuang H, et al. FDG PET for diagnosing infection in hip and knee prostheses: prospective study in 221 prostheses and subgroup comparison with combined (111)In-labeled leukocyte/(99m)Tc-sulfur colloid

bone marrow imaging in 88 prostheses. Clin Nucl Med. 2014;39(7):609–15. PubMed PMID: 24873788. Pubmed Central PMCID: PMC4113396.

16. Boubaker A, Delaloye AB, Blanc CH, Dutoit M, Leyvraz PF, Delaloye B. Immunoscintigraphy with antigranulocyte monoclonal antibodies for the diagnosis of septic loosening of hip prostheses. Eur J Nucl Med. 1995;22(2):139–47. PubMed PMID: 7758501.

17. Parvizi J, Ghanem E, Menashe S, Barrack RL, Bauer TW. Periprosthetic infection: what are the diagnostic challenges? J Bone Joint Surg Am. 2006;88(Suppl 4):138–47. PubMed PMID: 17142443.

18. Gemmel F, Van den Wyngaert H, Love C, Welling MM, Gemmel P, Palestro CJ. Prosthetic joint infections: radionuclide state-of-the-art imaging. Eur J Nucl Med Mol Imaging. 2012;39(5):892–909. PubMed PMID: 22361912. Epub 2012/02/24.

19. Zhuang H, Duarte PS, Pourdehnad M, Maes A, Van Acker F, Shnier D, et al. The promising role of 18F-FDG PET in detecting infected lower limb prosthesis implants. J Nucl Med. 2001;42(1):44–8. PubMed PMID: 11197979.

20. Houshmand S, Salavati A, Hess S, Werner TJ, Alavi A, Zaidi H. An update on novel quantitative techniques in the context of evolving whole-body PET imaging. PET Clin. 2015;10(1):45–58. PubMed PMID: 25455879. Epub 2014/11/22.

21. Basu S, Zhuang H, Torigian DA, Rosenbaum J, Chen W, Alavi A. Functional imaging of inflammatory diseases using nuclear medicine techniques. Semin Nucl Med. 2009;39(2):124–45. PubMed PMID: 19187805.

Elie Kozaily, Noam Shohat, and Javad Parvizi

Since periprosthetic joint infection (PJI) has emerged as a devastating complication after knee replacement, scientific societies have been mobilized to find valid criteria to define a PJI.

The first definition was proposed in 2011 by a group of experts convened by Musculoskeletal Infection Society (MSIS). Since then, many working groups outlined definition criteria for PJI. In fact, the Infection Disease Society of North America (IDSA) published a definition in 2013 then international experts met in Philadelphia for the International Consensus Meeting (ICM) in 2013 and later in 2018.

Accordingly, we walk you through the evolution of the PJI definition from its earliest version by MSIS 2011 to its latest 2018 version by ICM.

The MSIS 2011 criteria have been consistently used by clinicians and researchers. The working group describes two groups of patients who can be safely diagnosed with PJI by fulfilling one of the two major criteria (or both): The patients who present with a sinus tract communicating with the prosthesis and the patients in whom two separate

E. Kozaily · J. Parvizi (✉)
Rothman Orthopaedics Institute at Thomas Jefferson University, Philadelphia, PA, USA
e-mail: admin@parvizisurgical.com

N. Shohat
Rothman Orthopaedics Institute at Thomas Jefferson University, Philadelphia, PA, USA

Assaf Harofeh Medical Center, Tel Aviv University, Tel Aviv, Israel

tissue or fluid samples—obtained from the affected prosthetic joint—put to evidence the same pathogen by culture. Otherwise, MSIS group recommends that four out of six minor criteria be present to diagnose a PJI. The minor criteria include: elevated serum erythrocyte sedimentation rate (ESR) and serum C-reactive protein (CRP), elevated synovial leukocyte count, elevated synovial neutrophil percentage, purulence in the affected joint, isolation of a microorganism in one culture of periprosthetic tissue or fluid, greater than five neutrophils per high-power field in five high-power fields on from histologic analysis of periprosthetic tissue [1].

Of note, the group acknowledged that PJI may be present even if fewer than four of these minor criteria are met. For instance, some of these criteria may be negative in low-grade infections.

The following points need to be considered when interpreting the MSIS criteria:

- Serum biomarkers thresholds for ESR and CRP were 30 mm/h and 10 mg/dL respectively.
- However, ESR and CRP interpretation can be challenging as their serum level depends on a myriad of patient-related factors (inflammatory arthritis, obesity) and the time from index joint replacement among others.
- Synovial fluid markers, white blood cells WBC and PMNs percentage, for knee chronic PJI were reported to range from 1100 to

© ISAKOS 2022
U. G. Longo et al. (eds.), *Infection in Knee Replacement*,
https://doi.org/10.1007/978-3-030-81553-0_10

4000 cells/µL and 64 to 69% respectively. In acute knee PJI, occurring 3 months or prior from index surgery, numbers were higher 20,000 cells/µL and 89% for WBC and PMNs percentage respectively.

- Tissue samples sent for microbiology should be obtained from representative periprosthetic tissue or (synovial) fluid. At least three and no more than five samples should be sent for culture; gram stain and other tests may not be perfectly accurate for diagnosing a PJI. The isolated pathogen in the two samples should be confirmed identical based on its phenotype and anti-microbial susceptibility in vitro [*since genetic testing like polymerase chain reaction (PCR) or next-generation sequencing (NGS) are not routinely ordered*].
- Histology studies should take the clinical picture into consideration as the pathologist looks for at least five polymorphonuclears (PMNs) per high-power field (HPF) on surgical tissue examination.
- For instance, elevated neutrophil count may be present in a periprosthetic fracture or inflammatory arthritis. Other challenges include presence of foreign body macrophages that mimic neutrophils and neutrophils entrapped in superficial fibrin or adherent to endothelium or small veins as those should be disregarded.

In August 2013, hundreds of international experts gathered for the first consensus meeting in Philadelphia, USA. This International Consensus Meeting (ICM) endorsed the MSIS definition. The ICM added leukocyte esterase test as a minor criterion equivalent to elevated WBC count in synovial fluid and excluded the purulence surrounding the prosthesis from the minor criteria. Thus, out of the five minor criteria left, three should be present in order to diagnose PJI [2].

Furthermore, the ICM determined acceptable thresholds for minor criteria based on time from index arthroplasty, acute (within 90 days) vs. chronic infections. The thresholds in acute infections tend to be higher compared to chronic infections, respectively, serum CRP (100 vs. 10 mg/L), synovial fluid WBC (10,000 vs. 3000 cells/µL), and PMN counts (90% vs. 80%). The criteria were similar for leukocyte esterase

and histological analysis in acute and chronic settings. Yet, no threshold was determined for ESR in acute infection compared to well-defined 30 mm/h in chronic infection [2].

In the same year 2013, the IDSA panelists followed the classical process for establishing guidelines, thereby commanding a strength for each of the criteria based on quality of evidence, changing the concept of major and minor criteria. The panel's definition included the presence of a single culture with virulent organism as a criterion for PJI diagnosis [3].

With new biomarkers surfacing along with traditional biomarkers' interpretation changing, the international experts met for the second edition of the ICM, in Philadelphia, USA in 2018 to refine and update PJI definition criteria in order to improve outcomes [4] (Table 10.1).

The ICM acknowledged that minor differences may exist between PJI after hip and knee replacement yet the proposed definition applies to both joints.

Although the definition did not reach a strong consensus with 68% of the experts agreeing, 28% disagreeing, and 4% abstaining, these recent ICM criteria have shown consistent validity. For instance, a higher sensitivity and a similar specificity compared to MSIS and previous ICM, 97.7% and 99.5% respectively. Similarly, thresholds for biomarkers have been chosen to optimize sensitivity in early stage PJI and specificity in advanced stage PJI.

Of note, chronicity of infection as well as invasiveness of the diagnostic tests is considered in this definition in order to set the ground for an algorithm-based approach. Relative weights for each of the findings and biomarkers have been put in place hence a scoring system, based on American Academy of Orthopedic Surgery (AAOS) guidelines.

The major benefit from these new criteria is the potential to establish a pre-operative diagnosis. In fact, in many cases, the diagnosis of PJI could not be definitive until the surgeon goes for a revision surgery and relies on peri-operative findings like intraoperative purulence or frozen section results. The role of joint aspiration preoperatively has become pivotal, allowing more than 80% of cases to be diagnosed before going to revision diagnostic and therapeutic surgery.

Table 10.1 PJI definition criteria. Reprinted from Shohat N, Tan TL, Della Valle CJ, Calkins TE, George J, Higuera C, et al. Development and Validation of an Evidence-Based Algorithm for Diagnosing Periprosthetic Joint Infection. J Arthroplasty 2019 Nov;34 (11):2730–2736.e1, Copyright (2019), with permission from Elsevier

Major criteria (at least one of the following)	Decision
Two positive cultures of the same organism	Infected
Sinus tract with evidence of communication to the joint or visualization of the prosthesis	Infected

		Minor Criteria	Score	Decision
Preoperative Diagnosis	Serum	Elevated CRP *or* D-Dimer	2	≥6 Infected
		Elevated ESR	1	
	Synovial	Elevated Synovial *WBC or LE* (++)	3	2-5 Possibly Infected[a]
		Positive Alpha-defensin	3	
		Elevated Synovial PMN %	2	0-1 Not Infected
		Elevated Synovial CRP	1	

	*Inconclusive pre-op score *or* dry tap	Score	Decision
Preoperative Diagnosis	Preoperative score	-	≥6 Infected
	Positive Histology	3	**4-5 Inconclusive[b]**
	Positive Purulence	3	
	Positive Single Culture	2	≤3 Not Infected

[a]For patients with inconclusive minor criteria, operative criteria can also be used to fulfill definition for PJI
[b]Consider further molecule diagnostics such as Next-generation sequencing

New biomarkers like serum D-dimer and synovial fluid alpha-defensin have been introduced.

In fact, a high serum D-dimer can be as relevant as a high CRP in chronic PJI; however, more studies are needed to validate serum D-dimer role in diagnosing acute PJI and PJI in general.

Even though synovial fluid alpha-defensin has been criticized as it is an expensive and not routinely ordered test, the experts still assert that the introduction of alpha-defensin aims to help specialists diagnose challenging cases and/or interpret and integrate this test's results, if available.

Of note, optimal thresholds for synovial fluid biomarkers in diagnosing chronic knee PJI were defined as higher than 3000 cells/μL for WBC and higher than 80% for PMNs [5].

Next-generation sequencing (NGS) can be valuable when the diagnosis is difficult to make, for example, when PJI is strongly suspected but serum and/or synovial markers are within normal or the pathogen is not isolated by traditional culture.

Nonetheless, the working force behind the new criteria has reported several limitations and controversies. For instance, these criteria are mainly validated on chronic PJIs (at least 6 weeks from index joint replacement), Plus, in many instances like adverse local tissue reactions, inflammatory arthritis these criteria may not be applicable.

Like in previous recommendations, the experts reaffirm that patients can have a PJI but not meet the criteria and vice versa. Clinical judgment by the specialist should prevail to guide the management.

10.1 Algorithm for Diagnosis

The American Academy of Orthopaedic Surgeons (AAOS) provides guidelines in 2010 for the diagnosis of knee and hip PJI using serum and synovial markers. Based on expert opinion and systematic review of the literature, this algorithm simplified a very confusing and challenging process. These guidelines were indorsed by the ICM on PJI in 2013 with slight modifications, and both algorithms have served physicians around the globe in daily clinical practice [6]. Developments in PJI diagnosis including new synovial and serum markers [7–12] has increased confusion among many surgeons who were unsure how to incorporate these tests into their practice and into the previously established guidelines.

In light of these developments, and the 2018 scoring system, Shohat et al. proposed an algorithm that would incorporate recent developments in the field [13]. The study relied on previous AAOS and ICM guidelines to develop an evidence-based, validated diagnostic algorithm. Using data from three centers and machine learning analysis, a stepwise approach to diagnosing PJI was proposed. Step 1 included serum testing and clinical findings which are evident at the first patient encounter. Step 2 included synovial markers, and the final step, step 3 included intraoperative findings. The proposed algorithm relies on the 2108 PJI definition and was formally validated on an external cohort and demonstrated a high overall sensitivity (96.9%) and specificity (99.5%). Given the significant advantages of this algorithm, it has been introduced in the 2018 ICM on PJI and received a 73% agreement (super majority, strong consensus) (Fig. 10.1).

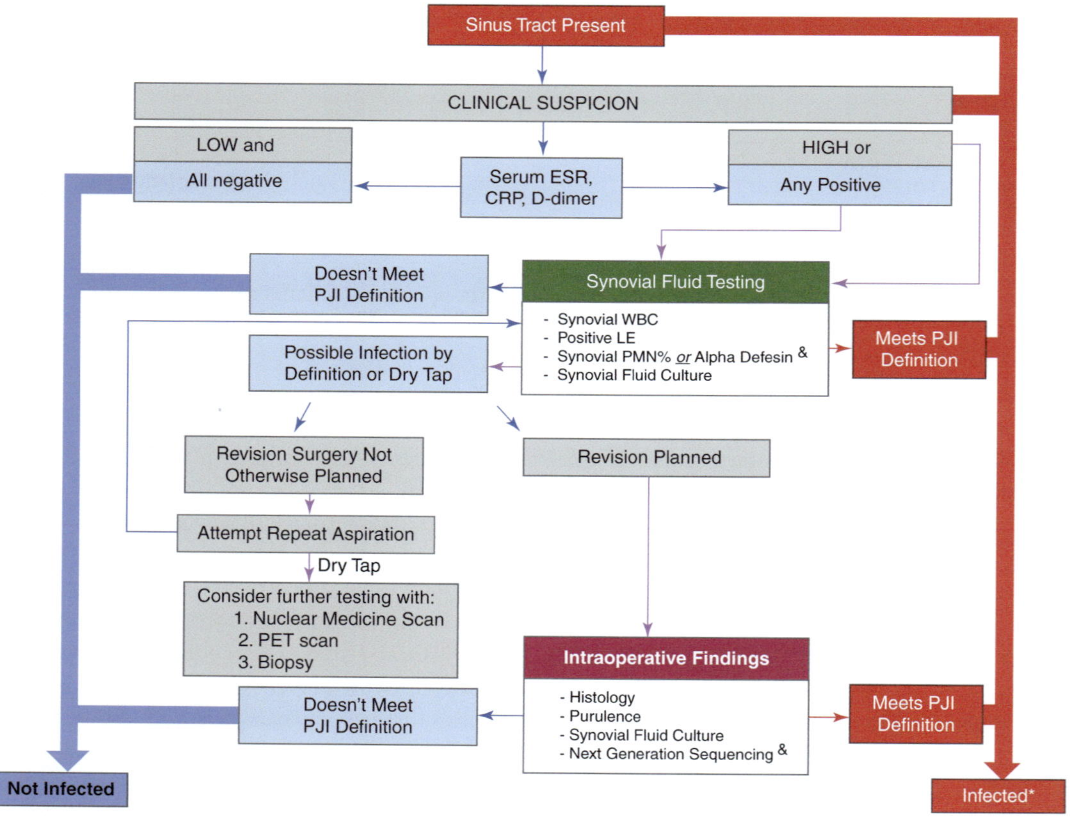

Fig. 10.1 Algorithm for the diagnosis of PJI. (Reprinted from Shohat N, Tan TL, Della Valle CJ, Calkins TE, George J, Higuera C, et al. Development and Validation of an Evidence-Based Algorithm for Diagnosing Periprosthetic Joint Infection. J Arthroplasty 2019 Nov;34(11):2730-2736.e1, Copyright (2019), with permission from Elsevier)

The first step in evaluating PJI should include serum testing for C-reactive protein, D-dimer, and erythrocyte sedimentation rate. If one of the three is elevated, physicians should proceed with a joint aspiration. However, the authors also noted that in 2.8% of PJI cases all three markers will be negative—and that emphasizes the importance of clinical findings and high clinical suspicion. Patients undergoing revision surgery less than 2 years from index surgery, those with more than 1 surgery on the same joint in the past, signs of erythema, tachycardia, reduced ROM, and serum PMN% above 70 should raise suspicion of PJI and in those cases the joint should be aspirated even if serum markers are negative.

The synovial fluid should be routinely investigated for white blood-cell count with differential and leukocyte esterase testing. Alpha-defensin received special attention as it is an expensive test and not routinely ordered. The authors found that alpha defensing does not add to the performance of the algorithm which implies it should not be ordered routinely. This step would rule in or out PJI in most patients and in those that a diagnosis cannot be reached, intraoperative findings will need to be taken into consideration. Intraoperative findings including purulence, histology, and next-generation sequencing (NGS) or a single positive culture can aid in these cases where the diagnosis has not been conclusive.

It is important to note that it is possible that the diagnosis of PJI may not be made even after reaching the third stage or may be inconclusive after obtaining synovial tests. These patients are often encountered in clinical practice and represent a real diagnostic challenge. Furthermore, it is important to note that the proposed algorithm and the definition of PJI may be inaccurate and require a modification in the tests utilized for the following conditions: adverse local tissue reactions, crystalline deposition arthropathy, inflammatory arthroplasty flares, and infection with slow growing organisms, such as *P acnes*.

Overall the proposed algorithm has several advantages compared to previous published guidelines. The algorithm allows us to account for the interplay between the individual or combined diagnostic test results and their influence on the probability for infection at different stages/times throughout the workup for infection. This interplay has a significant effect on the overall diagnostic performance [14–16]. It also allows clinicians to reach an educated conclusion before continuing forward to more invasive and costly tests. Furthermore, it minimizes the number of tests performed in each step and has the potential to reduce costs of unnecessary expensive tests, which are currently oftentimes performed.

Bibliography

1. Parvizi J, Zmistowski B, Berbari EF, Bauer TW, Springer BD, Della Valle CJ, et al. New definition for periprosthetic joint infection: from the Workgroup of the Musculoskeletal Infection Society. Clin Orthop. 2011;469(11):2992–4.
2. Parvizi J, Gehrke T. Definition of periprosthetic joint infection. J Arthroplast. 2014;29(7):1331.
3. Osmon DR, Berbari EF, Berendt AR, Lew D, Zimmerli W, Steckelberg JM, et al. Diagnosis and management of prosthetic joint infection: clinical practice guidelines by the Infectious Diseases Society of America. Clin Infect Dis. 2013;56(1):e1–25.
4. Parvizi J, Tan TL, Goswami K, Higuera C, Della Valle C, Chen AF, et al. The 2018 definition of periprosthetic hip and knee infection: an evidence-based and validated criteria. J Arthroplasty. 2018;33(5):1309–1314.e2.
5. Balato G, Franceschini V, Ascione T, Lamberti A, Balboni F, Baldini A. Diagnostic accuracy of synovial fluid, blood markers, and microbiological testing in chronic knee prosthetic infections. Arch Orthop Trauma Surg. 2018;138(2):165–71.
6. Zmistowski B, Della Valle C, Bauer TW, Malizos KN, Alavi A, Bedair H, et al. Diagnosis of periprosthetic joint infection. J Arthroplast. 2014;29(2 Suppl):77–83.
7. Tarabichi M, Shohat N, Goswami K, Alvand A, Silibovsky R, Belden K, et al. Diagnosis of periprosthetic joint infection: the potential of next-generation sequencing. J Bone Joint Surg Am. 2018;100(2):147–54.
8. Saleh A, George J, Faour M, Klika AK, Higuera CA. Serum biomarkers in periprosthetic joint infections. Bone Joint Res. 2018;7(1):85–93.
9. Shahi A, Kheir MM, Tarabichi M, Hosseinzadeh HRS, Tan TL, Parvizi J. Serum D-dimer test is promising for the diagnosis of periprosthetic joint infection and timing of reimplantation. J Bone Joint Surg Am. 2017;99(17):1419–27.
10. Ahmad SS, Hirschmann MT, Becker R, Shaker A, Ateschrang A, Keel MJB, et al. A meta-analysis of synovial biomarkers in periprosthetic joint infection: Synovasure™ is less effective than the ELISA-based

alpha-defensin test. Knee Surg Sports Traumatol Arthrosc. 2018;26:3039–47.

11. Wyatt MC, Beswick AD, Kunutsor SK, Wilson MJ, Whitehouse MR, Blom AW. The alpha-defensin immunoassay and leukocyte esterase colorimetric strip test for the diagnosis of periprosthetic infection: a systematic review and Meta-analysis. J Bone Joint Surg Am. 2016;98(12):992–1000.

12. Lee YS, Koo K-H, Kim HJ, Tian S, Kim T-Y, Maltenfort MG, et al. Synovial fluid biomarkers for the diagnosis of periprosthetic joint infection: a systematic review and Meta-analysis. J Bone Joint Surg Am. 2017;99(24):2077–84.

13. Development and validation of an evidence-based algorithm for diagnosing periprosthetic joint infection [cited 2020 Feb 2]. https://www.ncbi.nlm.nih.gov/pubmed/31279603.

14. Sousa R, Serrano P, Gomes Dias J, Oliveira JC, Oliveira A. Improving the accuracy of synovial fluid analysis in the diagnosis of prosthetic joint infection with simple and inexpensive biomarkers: C-reactive protein and adenosine deaminase. Bone Joint J. 2017;99-B(3):351–7.

15. Tarabichi M, Fleischman AN, Shahi A, Tian S, Parvizi J. Interpretation of leukocyte esterase for the detection of periprosthetic joint infection based on serologic markers. J Arthroplasty. 2017;32(9S):S97–S100.e1.

16. Deirmengian C, Kardos K, Kilmartin P, Cameron A, Schiller K, Parvizi J. Combined measurement of synovial fluid α-defensin and C-reactive protein levels: highly accurate for diagnosing periprosthetic joint infection. J Bone Joint Surg Am. 2014;96(17):1439–45.

Ilan Small, Nicolaas C. Budhiparama,
and Noam Shohat

11.1 Introduction

Pain is the most common symptom in PJI and is present in the majority of cases [1, 2]. In a recent study evaluating patients undergoing revision surgery for failed TKA due to PJI and aseptic causes [3], over 90% of patients in both groups complained of pain, making pain alone a very non-specific complaint. As so, any potential cause for pain following TKA should be included in the differential diagnosis of PJI. Causes for pain following TKA can be divided into those present immediately after surgery and those emerging after a period of time that surgery was considered successful (Table 11.1).

Common causes for persistent pain or new onset pain immediately after surgery should be first classified as extrinsic or intrinsic. Extrinsic causes of pain may be a result of poor indication or dual pathology from sources outside the artificial joint, including the hip joint, spinal radiculopathy, vascular claudication, local bursitis or tendinopathy, and systemic conditions such as autoimmune diseases. Intrinsic causes of pain following surgery result from the artificial joint itself and include instability, malalignment, component mal-positioning and impingement, recurrent hemarthrosis, arthrofibrosis, and extensor mechanism problems.

When pain presents in an artificial joint that was previously pain free, wear, osteolysis, and aseptic loosening should be considered [4, 5]. Aseptic loosening is a frequent cause of pain and revision surgery [6]. It can be caused by various reasons with the end result being failure of the bond between an implant and bone in the absence of infection [7]. While usually occurring 10–20 years from index TKA, it can occur earlier due to patient characteristics and component material and positioning [8, 9]. Symptoms of aseptic causes of failure include pain, joint effusion, erythema, and restricted range of motion among others. These symptoms may present similarly to PJI, thus making it a difficult task to differentiate between these two different pathologies [10–13]. While at times, some of these aseptic causes for failure are overt, making it tempting to make a diagnosis of aseptic failure, PJI must always be ruled out before any revision surgery takes place as 12% of the so-called aseptic cases have an underlying PJI [14, 15].

I. Small
Department of Orthopaedic Surgery, Sackler Faculty of Medicine, Tel Aviv University, Ramat Aviv, Israel

N. C. Budhiparama (✉)
Nicolaas Institute of Constructive Orthopaedic Research and Education Foundation for Arthroplasty and Sports Medicine, Jakarta, Indonesia

N. Shohat
Rothman Institute, Thomas Jefferson University, Philadelphia, PA, USA

Sackler Faculty of Medicine, Tel Aviv University, Ramat Aviv, Israel

© ISAKOS 2022
U. G. Longo et al. (eds.), *Infection in Knee Replacement*,
https://doi.org/10.1007/978-3-030-81553-0_11

Table 11.1 Causes for pain following TKA

Extra-articular	Intra-articular
Radiating: • Hip • Spine	Early onset: • Maltracking • Malalignment • Instability • Impingement • Clunk
Local: • Bursitis • Tendinitis	Late onset: • Wear • Osteolysis • Loosening
Vascular: • Claudication • DVT • Bleeding	
Systemic: • Inflammatory • Neuropathic	

11.2 Serum Negative Infections

Serum screening tests (C-reactive protein [CRP] and erythrocyte sedimentation rate [ESR]) are usually the first step in the workup of a painful TKA as they are readily available and minimally invasive. While extremely useful, numerous studies have showed low sensitivity and specificity [16, 17]. Berbari et al. in a meta-analysis of 23 papers reported a pooled sensitivity of 75% (95% CI, 72–77%) for ESR and 88% (95% CI, 86–90%) for the CRP level. Pooled specificity for the same markers was 70% (95% CI, 68–72%) and 74% (95% CI) [18]. Kheir et al. calculated a false negative rate of 14.5% for ESR and 8.6% for CRP [17]. Parvizi et al. using machine learning found that 2.5% of patients with PJI will have negative serum screening workup, emphasizing the problem of relying solely on serum testing for screening [19]. This is especially true in infections caused by low-virulence organisms [20–22].

It is therefore fundamental to include clinical acumen in every investigation to ensure that diagnosis of PJI is not missed. In a recent paper investigating the efficacy of clinical findings in the workup of PJI, fever and erythema were found to be the most specific signs for diagnosing PJI with a positive likelihood ratio (LR) of 10.78 and 8.08, respectively. The authors concluded that clinical presentation can and should be used to guide which future diagnostic tests should be ordered and in the interpretation of their results [12]. Parvizi et al. using random forest analysis found that the presence of fever, erythema, reduced range of motion, tachycardia, failure occurring less than 2 years from index arthroplasty, and a history of more than one surgery in the index joint are all important parameters that should raise suspicion for PJI and prompt aspiration of the joint even if serum markers are negative for infection [19].

11.3 Culture Negative and Slow Growing Organism Infections

Bacterial infections may be culture negative organisms or slow growing, which elicits a relatively subtle immune response, which makes establishing a diagnosis more challenging [17]. Culture negative PJI accounts for up to 40% of cases in some reports [23]. Kheir et al. performed a retrospective study on over 1000 revision arthroplasty cases (549 for PJI, 653 for aseptic causes) and compared commonly used serum and synovial marker cutoffs stratified based on the underlying organism causing infection [17]. Interestingly, they reported that culture negative and slow growing organisms such as coagulase-negative Staphylococcus had lower levels of ESR, CRP as well as synovial WBC and PMN%, thus are prone to being misdiagnosed as aseptic failure if not receiving special attention.

Taking these findings into consideration, all efforts should be taken to maximize the utility of culture growth. If a PJI is suspected, the use of empirical antimicrobials prior to fluid aspiration should be avoided to prevent sterilization prior to culture to prevent a false negative result [7, 24]. The American Academy of Orthopaedic Surgeons recommends against prescribing antimicrobials for 2 weeks for patients with suspected PJI until the infection is verified [25]. Fluid aspiration should be repeated and the aspirate incubated for 2–3 weeks on aerobic, anaerobic, fungal, and acid-fast bacilli cultures. One to 2 weeks is rec-

Table 11.2 Red flag patients

Red flag patients	Presentation	Useful markers	Comments
Slow growing organisms	Pain, effusion, erythema, reduced ROM	Serum and synovial markers using 2018 PJI definition molecular testing	In cases where a diagnosis is suspected and cannot me made using conventional methods, molecular testing should be ordered
Inflammatory arthritis	Pain, effusion, erythema, reduced ROM, fever	CRP, ESR, synovial WBC, synovial PMN, alpha defensin	Conventional thresholds should be adhered to, except in cases where a flare up is suspected
Crystalline deposit disease	Pain, effusion, erythema, reduced ROM, fever	Uric acid, calcium pyrophosphate, CRP, ESR, synovial fluid	Crystalline deposit may be present in small amounts which may be misclassified or missed
Hemarthrosis	Pain, effusion, erythema, reduced ROM	Serum PT, PTT, INR Joint aspiration	Joint aspiration will show sanguineous fluid containing red blood cells
Metal allergy	Pain, allergic dermatitis, prosthetic loosening	Eosinophils	Skin patch test, leukocyte migration inhibition test, lymphocyte transformation test may all be useful

ommended for the growth of *P. acnes* and some coagulase-negative staphylococci [8, 15]. During surgery, three to five samples should be taken from the interphase and the pseudocapsule, and tissue should be sent for histopathological analysis.

Previous diagnostic criteria were specific but lacked sensitivity to diagnose less obvious infections. Recently, new diagnostic criteria have been developed to better diagnose these culture negative and low-grade infections [8, 26]. Parvizi et al. in their evidence-based definition for PJI have increased sensitivity for diagnosis to 97.7% (95% CI 94.7%–99.3%) compared to previous criteria showing sensitivity of 79.3–86.9%. Although they were able to capture a substantial amount of PJI patients, in 2.3% of the cohort a diagnosis was inconclusive which they define "gray area" patients, i.e. not clear if infected or not. These patients are often encountered in clinical practice and represent a real diagnostic challenge. Interestingly, all patients with an inconclusive diagnosis had negative cultures, and the authors propose they may benefit from molecular diagnostic testing.

In cases where a PJI diagnosis is still not confirmed, increasing evidence supports the use of genome sequencing [9–11, 26]. Using metagenomics shotgun sequencing, Thoendel et al. detected a wide range of PJI pathogens and suggested this method may aid in identifying the

infecting organism in culture negative PJI [27]. They were able to identify new potential pathogens in 43.9% (43/98) of culture negative PJIs. While the translation of sequencing data into a clinically useful instrument in the setting of PJI remains critically limited, it seems likely that genome sequencing may occupy an increased role for the diagnosis of infection in the future.

Red flag patients are reported in Table 11.2.

In certain populations, conventional workup and diagnostic criteria may be inaccurate. Due to the relative rarity of these patients and possible outliers, many studies exclude them from the analysis. Furthermore guidelines are established and rely on investigations of PJI in primarily patients without these underlying diseases [28].

11.3.1 Inflammatory Arthritis

Autoimmune and chronic diseases have similar clinical symptoms as PJI and obtaining a thorough patient history, including past medical history, is vital in determining the cause of joint failure. Rheumatoid arthritis (RA) has received the most focus as its complications are a common cause for joint arthroplasty [29]. Elevated serum CRP and ESR levels are diagnostic criteria for PJI and are also commonly used to aid in the diagnosis of RA. Thus, applying the same thresholds in RA patients as in the general population raises concern over identification and false positive results. Yeganeh et al. and Shohat et al. examined whether different thresholds for commonly used serum and synovial markers should be used in patients with inflammatory arthritis, the majority with rheumatoid arthritis [29, 30]. Both studies concluded that conventional PJI thresholds for serum and synovial diagnostic markers are sufficient for differential diagnosis with respect to RA. Special attention should be given to patients presenting with an acute flare as these studies were performed on patients presenting in various stages of the disease activity.

11.3.2 Crystalline Deposit Diseases

Patients with a suspected PJI and a history of crystalline deposit diseases, such as gout and pseudogout, should have synovial fluid analysis performed before administration of antibiotics to avoid falsely negative cultures as infections may precipitate crystalline deposit disease as crystalline deposits may act as a nidus for infection [31, 32]. George et al. reported on 22 patients with crystalline deposition within the affected joint that fueled inflammation and presented with edema, erythema, fever, and pain within the joint; symptoms similar to that of a PJI [31]. As these two pathologies require different treatment, it is important for the physician to be aware of the proper diagnostic workup to proceed accordingly. Diagnostic studies of the aspirated fluid should include microscopic studies looking for uric acid crystals to detect gout and calcium pyrophosphate in suspected pseudogout. Overlapping manifestations of crystalline deposit disease and PJIs include elevated white blood cell count, ESR, and CRP. Synovial fluid aspiration should be examined for crystals, cultures should be taken, and uric acid levels measured. These crystalline deposit diseases are difficult to diagnose because of the small amount of crystals, which may be misclassified or missed entirely by physicians with limited clinical experience.

11.3.3 Hemarthrosis

Hemarthrosis occurs due to bleeding into the joint and may present similarly to PJI, including decreased range of motion, edema, erythema, and pain [33]. Hemarthrosis should be suspected based on previous history of the patient and may occur from traumatic or atraumatic causes, such as coagulopathies and anticoagulant medication. Hemarthrosis can be diagnosed via imaging or aspiration of the joint. Joint aspiration will show sanguineous fluid containing red blood cells. Additional diagnostic studies should include cell differentials, gram stain, and culture to confirm the diagnosis.

11.3.4 Metal Allergy

While rare, metal hypersensitivity is also a potential cause of pain following TKA that may mimic PJI [34, 35]. The most common allergy-inducing metals are nickel (19.7–24.4%), cobalt (2–8.8%), and chromium (2.4–5.9%). Clinical symptoms of metal hypersensitivity include local or systemic allergic dermatitis, pain, and prosthetic loosening due to chronic aseptic inflammation [36]. With respect to standard laboratory examinations, the skin patch test, leukocyte migration inhibition test (LMIT), and lymphocyte transformation test (LTT) are the most popular diagnostic tests for metal hypersensitivity. However, none of the tests has been universally accepted and applied.

11.4 Conclusion

As the number of knee arthroplasties continues to increase each year, physicians will increasingly encounter unsatisfied patients and those with chronic pain and will need to recognize the cause of the pain and treat the patient accordingly. PJI is a severe complication following knee arthroplasty with several differential diagnoses that surgeons should be aware of. A working diagnosis of suspected PJI will be able to improve quality of care for patients through proper treatment. Future research should focus on cases where differences between PJI and aseptic cases are subtle in an effort to improve diagnosis and subsequent treatment.

References

1. Aggarwal VK, Rasouli MR, Parvizi J. Periprosthetic joint infection: current concept. Indian J Orthop. 2013;47(1):10.
2. Kurtz SM, Lau E, Watson H, Schmier JK, Parvizi J. Economic burden of periprosthetic joint infection in the United States. J Arthroplast. 2012;27(8):61–5.
3. Suarez J, Griffin W, Springer B, Fehring T, Mason JB, Odum S. Why do revision knee arthroplasties fail? J Arthroplast. 2008;23(6):99–103.
4. Beam E, Osmon D. Prosthetic joint infection update. Infect Dis Clin. 2018;32(4):843–59.
5. Runner RP, Mener A, Roberson JR, Bradbury TL, Guild GN, Boden SD, Erens GA. Prosthetic joint infection trends at a dedicated orthopaedics specialty hospital. Adv Orthop. 2019;2019:4629503.
6. Sundfeldt M, Carlsson LV, Johansson CB, Thomsen P, Gretzer C. Aseptic loosening, not only a question of wear: a review of different theories. Acta Orthop. 2006;77(2):177–97.
7. Kutzner I, Hallan G, Høl PJ, Furnes O, Gøthesen Ø, Figved W, Ellison P. Early aseptic loosening of a mobile-bearing total knee replacement: a case-control study with retrieval analyses. Acta Orthop. 2018;89(1):77–83.
8. Lee BS, Cho HI, Bin SI, Kim JM, Jo BK. Femoral component varus malposition is associated with tibial aseptic loosening after TKA. Clin Orthop Relat Res. 2018;476(2):400.
9. Peel TN, Cheng AC, Buising KL, Choong PF. Microbiological aetiology, epidemiology, and clinical profile of prosthetic joint infections: are current antibiotic prophylaxis guidelines effective? Antimicrob Agents Chemother. 2012;56(5):2386–91.
10. Duff GP, Lachiewicz PF, Kelley SS. Aspiration of the knee joint before revision arthroplasty. Clin Orthop Relat Res. 1996;331:132–9.
11. Sendi P, Banderet F, Graber P, Zimmerli W. Clinical comparison between exogenous and haematogenous periprosthetic joint infections caused by Staphylococcus aureus. Clin Microbiol Infect. 2011;17(7):1098–100.
12. Shohat N, Goswami K, Tan TL, Henstenburg B, Makar G, Rondon AJ, Parvizi J. Fever and erythema are specific findings in detecting infection following total knee arthroplasty. J Bone Joint Infect. 2019;4(2):92.
13. Parvizi J, Gehrke T, Chen AF. Proceedings of the international consensus on periprosthetic joint infection. Bone Joint J. 2013;95(11):1450–2.
14. Sloan M, Premkumar A, Sheth NP. Projected volume of primary total joint arthroplasty in the US, 2014 to 2030. J Bone Joint Surg. 2018;100(17):1455–60.
15. Parvizi J, Zmistowski B, Berbari EF, Bauer TW, Springer BD, Della Valle CJ, et al. New definition for periprosthetic joint infection: from the Workgroup of the Musculoskeletal Infection Society. Clin Orthop Relat Res. 2011;469(11):2992.
16. Saleh A, George J, Faour M, Klika AK, Higuera CA. Serum biomarkers in periprosthetic joint infections. Bone Joint Res. 2018;7(1):85–93.
17. Kheir MM, Tan TL, Shohat N, Foltz C, Parvizi J. Routine diagnostic tests for periprosthetic joint infection demonstrate a high false-negative rate and are influenced by the infecting organism. J Bone Joint Surg. 2018;100(23):2057–65.
18. Berbari E, Mabry T, Tsaras G, Spangehl M, Erwin PJ, Murad MH, et al. Inflammatory blood laboratory levels as markers of prosthetic joint infection: a systematic review and meta-analysis. J Bone Joint Surg. 2010;92(11):2102–9.
19. Shohat N, Tan TL, Della Valle CJ, Calkins TE, George J, Higuera C, Parvizi J. Development and validation of an evidence-based algorithm for diagnosing periprosthetic joint infection. J Arthroplast. 2019;34(11):2730–6.
20. Parvizi J, McKenzie JC, Cashman JP. Diagnosis of periprosthetic joint infection using synovial C-reactive protein. J Arthroplast. 2012;27(8):12–6.
21. Ecker NU, Suero EM, Gehrke T, Haasper C, Zahar A, Lausmann C, et al. Serum C-reactive protein relationship in high-versus low-virulence pathogens in the diagnosis of periprosthetic joint infection. J Med Microbiol. 2019;68(6):910–7.
22. Palan J, Nolan C, Sarantos K, Westerman R, King R, Foguet P. Culture-negative periprosthetic joint infections. EFORT Open Rev. 2019;4(10):585–94.
23. Yoon JR, Han SB, Jee MK, Shin YS. Comparison of kinematic and mechanical alignment techniques in primary total knee arthroplasty: a meta-analysis. Medicine. 2017;96(39):e8157.
24. Tan TL, Kheir MM, Shohat N, Tan DD, Kheir M, Chen C, Parvizi J. Culture-negative periprosthetic joint infection: an update on what to expect. J Bone Joint Surg. 2018;3(3):e0060.
25. Parvizi J, Tan TL, Goswami K, Higuera C, Della Valle C, Chen AF, Shohat N. The 2018 definition of periprosthetic hip and knee infection: an evidence-based and validated criteria. J Arthroplast. 2018;33(5):1309–14.
26. Patel R, Alijanipour P, Parvizi J. Suppl-2, M8: advancements in diagnosing periprosthetic joint infections after total hip and knee arthroplasty. Open Orthop J. 2016;10:654.
27. Thoendel MJ, Jeraldo PR, Greenwood-Quaintance KE, Yao JZ, Chia N, Hanssen AD, et al. Identification of prosthetic joint infection pathogens using a shotgun metagenomics approach. Clin Infect Dis. 2018;67(9):1333–8.
28. Premkumar A, Morse K, Levack AE, Bostrom MP, Carli AV. Periprosthetic joint infection in patients with inflammatory joint disease: prevention and diagnosis. Curr Rheumatol Rep. 2018;20(11):68.
29. Shohat N, Goswami K, Fillingham Y, Tan TL, Calkins T, Della Valle CJ, et al. Diagnosing periprosthetic joint infection in inflammatory arthritis: assumption is the enemy of true understanding. J Arthroplast. 2018;33(11):3561–6.

30. Yeganeh MH, Kheir MM, Shahi A, Parvizi J. Rheumatoid arthritis, disease modifying agents, and periprosthetic joint infection: what does a joint surgeon need to know? J Arthroplast. 2018;33(4):1258–64.
31. George MP, Ernste FC, Tande A, Osmon D, Mabry T, Berbari EF. Clinical presentation, management, and prognosis of pseudogout in joint arthroplasty: a retrospective cohort study. J Bone Joint Infect. 2019;4(1):20.
32. Plate A, Stadler L, Sutter R, Anagnostopoulos A, Frustaci D, Zbinden R, et al. Inflammatory disorders mimicking periprosthetic joint infections may result in false-positive α-defensin. Clin Microbiol Infect. 2018;24(11):1212–1.
33. Tande AJ, Patel R. Prosthetic joint infection. Clin Microbiol Rev. 2014;27(2):302–45.
34. Bao W, He Y, Fan Y, Liao Y. Metal allergy in total-joint arthroplasty: case report and literature review. Medicine. 2018;97(38):e12475.
35. Hallab N, Merritt K, Jacobs JJ. Metal sensitivity in patients with orthopaedic implants. J Bone Joint Surg. 2001;83(3):428.
36. Basko-Plluska JL, Thyssen JP, Schalock PC. Cutaneous and systemic hypersensitivity reactions to metallic implants. Dermatitis. 2011;22(2):65–79.

Part V

Treatment of Knee Replacement Infections

Systemic Antibiotic Therapy

Philip P. Roessler, Gunnar T. R. Hischebeth, and Sascha Gravius

12.1 Introduction

Both systemic antibiotic therapy and surgery are crucial for the management of periprosthetic joint infections (PJI) of the knee [1]. Sometimes, antibiotic therapy is used as a standalone suppression therapy in patients where surgical intervention is impossible.

Delivery of systemic antibiotic agents can either be achieved orally or intravenously. While the intake of oral antibiotics generally is much more convenient and may even be managed in an outpatient setting, intravenous antibiotics usually exhibit a better bioavailability but, as a downside, may require inpatient therapy and a thorough monitoring [2, 3].

Common goal of all systemic antibiotic treatments is to eradicate the cause of infection that should be identified prior to therapy induction (see Sect. 12.3) [4]. In case a bacterium is unknown, treatment with broad spectrum antibiotics should be considered at the beginning [5]. However, joint aspiration and biopsies are required first to ensure later optimization of any antibiotic treatment. The secondary goals of systemic antibiotic therapy are to deal with the biofilm, formed through bacterial colonization, e.g. with *Staphylococcus* spp. or *Streptococcus* spp. (see Sect. 12.1) or to prevent biofilm formation on newly implanted hardware in the first place [6].

Although being crucial to an effective antimicrobial therapy in cases of PJI, most systemic antibiotics do not reach an effective local concentration alone and thus require a synergistic use of a local antibiotics [7]. The importance of these locally delivered antibiotics (e.g. from cement spacers) will be discussed later (see Chap. 13). Quorum quenching, meaning the disruption of bacterial communication—the so-called quorum sensing—of certain species [8] as well as chemotherapeutic approaches [9] are technically not considered systemic antibiotic treatments in a narrower sense and will therefore be detailed later (see Chap. 13).

P. P. Roessler (✉)
Gelenkzentrum Mittelrhein, Koblenz, Germany

Medical Faculty, University of Bonn, Bonn, Germany
e-mail: philip.roessler@uni-bonn.de

G. T. R. Hischebeth
Institute of Medical Microbiology, Immunology and Parasitology, University Hospital Bonn, Bonn, Germany
e-mail: gunnar.hischebeth@ukbonn.de

S. Gravius
Center for Orthopaedics and Trauma Surgery, University Hospital Mannheim, Mannheim, Germany
e-mail: sascha.gravius@umm.de

© ISAKOS 2022
U. G. Longo et al. (eds.), *Infection in Knee Replacement*,
https://doi.org/10.1007/978-3-030-81553-0_12

12.2 Principles and Timing

As a basic principle, any antibiotic therapy should be delayed until culture specimens have been taken (see Sect. 12.3). Only this assures an increased probability to eventually start a focused therapy at a certain time point [10]. In contrast, some recent publications advocate to start with antibiotic treatment as soon as possible since culture yields may eventually be the same, but later recurrence rates of PJI are considerably lower [11]. However, systemic antibiotic treatment should always be planned in advance, taking into consideration all available diagnostic and clinical information of the given case. In an ideal scenario, antibiotic treatment is usually initiated in an interdisciplinary consensus between orthopedic surgeons, clinical microbiologists, and all other involved specialists [12].

In each case of TKA revision the need for an initial empirical therapy has to be waged against its clinical implications. Especially in PJI cases accompanied by acute sepsis or positive systemic inflammatory response syndrome (SIRS) criteria, early systemic antibiotic treatment should not be delayed in order to improve clinical outcomes [13]. It may also be helpful to identify the most common infective agents in your hospital or department to enable an individualized empiric response, even differentiating between acute and chronic infections. Wherever possible, empirical antibiotic therapy should be converted into a focused therapy depending on culture results in the course of the treatment. While delayed systemic therapy applies for those cases with septic implant removal without previous cultures, systemic therapy in one-stage revision or mobile parts exchange procedures should usually be initiated 15–60 min before tourniquet inflation or skin incision [14, 15]. Dosage and duration of recommended antibiotic therapies are shown in Table 12.1.

In cases of retained hardware, biofilm-activity is a major requirement for an ideal systemic antibiotic treatment. Cases without hardware on the other hand mainly require an antibiotic therapy with preferable tissue penetration (e.g. to treat osteitis).

12.3 Debridement, Antibiotics, and Implant Retention (Dair)

This treatment strategy may either involve an empiric therapy with an antibiotic agent of a much broader spectrum, in case the pathogen is still unknown, or a focused therapy, in case the pathogen has already been identified. Duration and dosages are documented in Table 12.1. In cases of DAIR, it is of crucial importance to also add biofilm-active substances (e.g. Rifampicin) to the antibiotic therapy regimen if they are needed (e.g. against *Staphylococcus* spp. or *Cutibacterium* spp.). Pathogens that belong to the difficult-to-treat (DTT) group, meaning those causative agents for which no biofilm-active antibiotics are available, can only be suppressed by prolongation of systemic antibiotic treatment [16]. In these cases, later suppressive therapy may be a valid option. Gram-negative bacteria should be treated with fluoroquinolones like Ciprofloxacin intravenously and even during a later sequential phase. Administration of Rifampicin should be avoided in cases of gram-negative infections [17].

Generally, an interdisciplinary approach together with a clinical microbiologist is advised to select the best possible biofilm-active agent in cases of multi-resistant bacteria strains [18]. All other causative agents are treated as described in paragraph 12.2 and in Table 12.1. In summary, the key to success of DAIR is a proven susceptibility of the identified pathogen to biofilm-active substances paired with a thorough surgical debridement.

12.4 One-Stage Exchange

The same principles as for DAIR also apply for the concept of one-stage exchanges. Even here, the main goal is a biofilm-active therapy. Duration and dosages of various substances are also documented in Table 12.1. However, no clear evidence exists for the ideal duration of intravenous and sequential therapy [16].

Table 12.1 Systemic antibiotic treatment: proposed substances, sequence, duration, and dosage

Microorganism	Antibiotic substance	Dosage (route)
Staphylococcus spp.		
Methicillin/oxacillin-susceptible (with remaining hardware, DAIR)	Flucloxacillin *OR*	3 × 4 g or 4 × 3 g (i.v.)
	Cefazolin *OR*	3 × 2 g (i.v.)
	Daptomycin	1 × 8–10 mg/kg (i.v.)
	+ Rifampicin[a] (each)	2 × 0.45 g (p.o.)
	Followed by (depending on susceptibility testing)	
	Levofloxacin *OR*	2 × 0.5 g (p.o.)
	Doxycycline *OR*	2 × 0.1 g (p.o.)
	Cotrimoxazole	3 × 0.96 mg (p.o.)
	+ Rifampicin[a] (each)	2 × 0.45 mg (p.o.)
Methicillin/oxacillin-resistant (with remaining hardware, DAIR)	Daptomycin *OR*	1 × 12 mg/kg (i.v.)
	Vancomycin[b]	2 × 15 mg/kg (i.v.)
	+ Rifampicin[a] (each)	2 × 0.45 g (p.o.)
	Followed by (depending on susceptibility testing)	
	Levofloxacin *OR*	2 × 0.5 g (p.o.)
	Doxycycline *OR*	2 × 0.1 g (p.o.)
	Cotrimoxazole	3 × 0.96 mg (p.o.)
	+ Rifampicin[a] (each)	2 × 0.45 mg (p.o.)
Rifampicin-resistant	Daptomycin *OR*	1 × 10 mg/kg (i.v.)
	Vancomycin[b]	2 × 15 mg/kg (i.v.)
	i.v. for 2–4 weeks, followed by life-long suppression therapy (Cotrimoxazole, Doxycycline) under certain circumstances	
Streptococcus spp.		
Penicillin-susceptible	Penicillin G *OR*	4 × 5-10 M U (i.v.)
	Ceftriaxone	2 × 1–2 g (i.v.)
	i.v. for 2 weeks, followed by	
	Amoxicillin *OR*	3 × 1 g (p.o.)
	Levofloxacin	2 × 0.5 g (p.o.)
Penicillin-resistant	Vancomycin[b] *OR*	2 × 15 mg/kg (i.v.)
	Daptomycin	1 × 10 mg/kg (i.v.)
	i.v. for 2 weeks, followed by	
	Levofloxacin *OR*	2 × 0.5 g (p.o.)
	Clindamycin	3 × 0.6–0.9 g (p.o.)
Enterococcus spp.		
Penicillin/Ampicillin-susceptible	Ampicillin	3 × 5 g (i.v.)
	+ Gentamicin	1 × 6–7 mg/kg (i.v.)
	i.v. for 2–3 weeks, followed by	
	Amoxicillin *OR*	3 × 1 g (p.o.)
	Linezolid (in cases of known allergies, max. 4 weeks)	2 × 0.6 g (p.o.)
Penicillin/Ampicillin-resistant	Daptomycin *OR*	1 × 10–12 mg/kg (i.v.)
	Vancomycin[b]	2 × 15 mg/kg (i.v.)
	+ Gentamicin	1 × 6–7 mg/kg (i.v.)
	i.v. for 2–4 weeks, followed by	
	Linezolid (max. 4 weeks)	2 × 0.6 g (p.o.)

(continued)

Table 12.1 (continued)

Microorganism	Antibiotic substance	Dosage (route)
Vancomycin-resistant (VRE)	Daptomycin *OR*	1 × 10–12 mg/kg (i.v.)
	Linezolid (max. 4 weeks)	2 × 600 mg (i.v.)
	Followed by life-long suppression therapy under certain circumstances	
Enterobacterales		
	Ciprofloxacin	2 × 750 mg (p.o.)
Quinolone-susceptible	+ Ampicillin/Sulbactam OR	4 × 3 g (i.v.)
	Piperacillin/Tazobactam	4 × 4.5 g (i.v.)
	i.v. for 2 weeks	
Quinolone-resistant	Meropenem *OR*	3 × 2 g (i.v.)
	Piperacillin/Tazobactam *OR*	4 × 4.5 g (i.v.)
	Colistin	Loading dose 1 × 9 M U, then 3 × 3 M U (i.v.) OR 2 × 4.5 M U (i.v.)
	+ Fosfomycin	3 × 4–5 g (i.v.)
	i.v. for 2 weeks, followed by sequential therapy in consensus with microbiologist	
Non-fermenters		
(e.g. *Pseudomonas aeruginosa, A. baumannii*)	Meropenem OR	3 × 2 g (i.v.)
	Piperacillin/Tazobactam OR	4 × 4.5 g (i.v.)
	Ceftazidime	3 × 2 g (i.v.)
	+ Tobramycin	1 × 6–7 mg/kg (i.v.)
	i.v. for 2 weeks, followed by (depending on susceptibility testing)	
	Ciprofloxacin	2 × 0.75 g (p.o.)
(e.g. *Pseudomonas aeruginosa, A. baumannii*) multi-resistant	*Adapted therapy in consensus with microbiologist*	
Anaerobes		
Cutibacterium acnes	Penicillin G *OR*	4 × 5–10 M U (i.v.)
	Clindamycin (in cases of known allergies)	3 × 600 mg (i.v.)
	+ Rifampicin[a]	2 × 0.45 g (p.o.)
	i.v. for 2 weeks, followed by	
	Amoxicillin *OR*	3 × 1 g (p.o.)
	Levofloxacin	2 × 0.5 g (p.o.)
	+ Rifampicin[a]	2 × 0.45 g (p.o.)
Gram-positive anaerobes		
Non *Cutibacterium acnes*	Ampicillin/Sulbactam *OR*	4 × 3 g (i.v.)
	Piperacillin/Tazobactam *OR*	4 × 4.5 g (i.v.)
	Moxifloxacin	1 × 400 mg (p.o.)
	i.v. for 2 weeks	
Gram-negative anaerobes		
	Ampicillin/Sulbactam *OR*	4 × 3 g (i.v.)
	Piperacillin/Tazobactam *OR*	4 × 4.5 g (i.v.)
	i.v. for 2 weeks, followed by	
	Metronidazole	3 × 400 mg (p.o.)
Candida spp.		

Table 12.1 (continued)

Microorganism	Antibiotic substance	Dosage (route)
Fluconazole-susceptible	Caspofungin[c] *OR*	Loading dose 1 × 70 mg, then 1 × 50 mg (i.v.)
	Anidulafungin *OR*	Loading dose 1 × 200 mg, then 1 × 100 mg (i.v.)
	Fluconazole	1 × 400 mg (p.o.)
	Followed by life-long suppression therapy under certain circumstances	
Fluconazole-resistant	Caspofungin[c] *OR*	Loading dose 1 × 70 mg, then 1 × 50 mg (i.v.)
	Anidulafungin *OR*	Loading dose 1 × 200 mg, Then 1 × 100 mg (i.v.)
	Voriconazole	2 × 200 mg (p.o.)
Culture-negative PJI		
	Ampicillin/Sulbactam	4 × 3 g (i.v.)
	+/− Rifampicin[a]	2 × 0.45 g (p.o.)

DAIR debridement, antibiotics, and implant retention, *i.v.* intravenously, *p.o.* per os, *VRE* vancomycin-resistant Enterococcus; *PJI* periprosthetic joint infection. Comments: Generally, dose-adjustment according to regularly monitored renal and liver function as well as body weight is advised

[a]Biofilm-active antibiotics (e.g. Rifampicin) should not be given over the course of a temporal cement spacer treatment or while surgical drains are still in situ. Patients aged 75 years and older should receive a reduced dosage of Rifampin with 2 × 0.30 g (p.o.)

[b]Vancomycin levels of concentration should be monitored closely every 2–3 days before administration of the next dose (low plasma-levels, ideal range 15–20 mg/L)

[c]Caspofungin should be administered with a maintenance dose of 1 × 70 mg, if body weight exceeds 80 kg

12.5 Two-Stage Exchange

Any two-stage exchange procedure can be divided into two distinctive steps: (1) prosthesis removal and (2) prosthesis re-implantation. The first step is followed by a phase where the joint remains without an implant or with a spacer (e.g. bone cement). The main goal during this phase is an antibiotic therapy with a good tissue penetration to treat osteitis or osteomyelitis as well as soft tissue infections. Biofilm-active substances are unnecessary, even when the cement spacer remains in situ [19]. The surgical approach and subsequent strategies are explained in detail in Sect. 12.4. The duration between the first and second step is usually between 2 and 6 weeks, depending on the concept that was chosen. Drug holidays—a phase without systemic antibiotic treatment in between—is no longer recommended, as their effect is not supported by the literature [16]. Following the second step there is a new prosthesis in situ yet again and thus the main goal then is to protect it against colonization with biofilm-active antibiotics. In cases of DTT a prolonged duration of systemic antibiotics or life-long suppressive therapy may be required.

12.6 Empiric Therapy

Main paradigm of an empiric systemic antibiotic therapy, especially in bacterial sepsis, is "hit early, hit hard." This requires substances covering a broad spectrum of bacteria including *Staphylococcus* spp. (including methicillin-resistant strains) and certain gram-negative bacteria (*Enterobacterales*, formerly *Enterobacteriaceae*). There should also be sufficient information about the pathogen-specific spectrum of germs of the department or region [16, 20].

In cases of acute sepsis or SIRS, joint aspiration and culture (in special small-volume sample media, e.g. pediatric blood culture flasks), native synovial fluid cell count (total leucocytes, total granulocytes, and leucocyte/granulocyte ratio) as well as two pairs of blood cultures are desirable before therapy initiation to eventually obtain a culture of the suspected causative agent [21]. Possible empiric treatment options include Vancomycin and a third or fourth generation cephalosporin or Piperacillin/Tazobactam (Table 12.1). Since therapeutic concentrations of cephalosporin in the knee joint can already be reached in standard dosage, no special adaption is required for an initial therapy [22]. One of the main causes of PJI with negative cultures is an early beginning of empiric treatment [23]. For this reason, individual patient risk must be calculated and weighed against a possibly unidentified causative agent during the course of further treatment. Empiric therapy should generally be administered intravenously [16, 24].

12.7 Focused Therapy

After gathering all available diagnostic information (see Sect. 12.3), initiation of a focused treatment can be discussed and planned. Ideally, histopathologic and microbiologic data, foremost culture results are the basis for an adequate antibiotic treatment using a single or in combined substances. The appropriate dosage but also the duration of therapy should be defined. Some antibiotics may require hematological testing on a regular basis in order to detect side effects. During this stage any already initiated empiric therapy should be revisited and adjusted. Antibiotic susceptibility profiles, which usually accompany extended microbiologic cultures, can help to identify the best possible treatment depending on the individual specifications of the causative agent [25, 26]. This tool becomes even more important in cases of mixed infections with

various bacteria in addition to further diagnostics like PCR (see Sect. 12.3).

An ideal systemic antibiotic agent will fulfill the following criteria [27]:

- Status and activity of the bacteria.
- Good tissue penetration of bone and other musculoskeletal tissues.
- High ratio of attainable local tissue concentration and minimal inhibitory concentration (MIC).
- Low rates of spontaneous resistance formation.
- Activity even against planktonic and biofilm-embedded bacteria (especially in cases of remaining hardware).
- Good tolerance and long-term tolerance for the patient.
- Suitability for sequential therapy (high oral bioavailability).

Moreover, the choice of any systemic antibiotic treatment also depends on the surgical approach [16, 28]. The principle of DAIR may require other substances and treatment durations than one-stage or two-stage revision of TKA [29, 30]. Focused or targeted therapy is usually started as a continuation of previous empiric therapy and should be administered intravenously for at least 2 weeks post-operatively (counting in the period of empiric therapy), before a conversion to oral administration is considered. Generally, a treatment period of 12 weeks is recommended for systemic antibiotic therapy starting from the time point of the index surgery and the first empiric antibiotic therapy. Intravenous antibiotics are given first during the perioperative period followed by oral therapy usually for 5–10 weeks [16]. The time frame between intravenous and oral antibiotic treatment will depend on the type of bacterium and the adequate antibiotic available for oral administration [31].

12.7.1 *Staphylococcus* spp.

Systemic antibiotics effective against methicillin-susceptible *S. aureus* (MSSA) are beta-lactam antibiotics like Oxacillin, Cefazolin and Ceftriaxone (Table 12.1). In case of a known hypersensitivity (e.g. history of previous anaphylaxis) against beta-lactams, Vancomycin or Daptomycin may be chosen [18]. However, care has to be taken with regard to correct dosage monitoring due to their side effects and a possible risk of later re-infection [32, 33]. Infections caused by methicillin-resistant *S. aureus* (MRSA) may be treated with Vancomycin, Daptomycin or even Teicoplanin [16, 31]. This includes almost all coagulase-negative strains with the exception of *S. lugdunensis* which usually is methicillin-susceptible and can therefore be treated with a beta-lactam (Table 12.1).

Since most species of *Staphylococcus* are considered to be biofilm-forming, systemic antibiotic treatment should be supplemented by an adjunctive, biofilm-active antibiotic like Rifampicin [20]. Through inhibition of bacterial transcription in mural synthesis, Rifampicin breaks up biofilms and thus increases the anti-infective effect of the combination therapy agent in certain cases—especially in patients whose implants are retained during DAIR procedures or who undergo one-stage revisions [9]. Meropenem, an alternative to Rifampicin, instead inhibits transpeptidases to achieve a comparable effect of biofilm breakage [34]. Rifampicin monotherapy should be avoided, because it is associated with a high risk of early resistance induction due to point mutation [35]. In combination therapies, it is discussed that potentially Rifampicin should be administered with a certain delay to surgical debridement providing a non-oozing, dry wound, and initiation of systemic antibiotic therapy with another antibacterial substance [35]. Moreover, Rifampicin may induce Cytochrome P450 (CYP3A) and thus alter serum blood levels of other medications. In general, adjunctive, biofilm-active antibiotics should not be given over the course of a temporal cement spacer treatment or while surgical drains are still in situ [16].

Staphylococcus spp. unsusceptible to biofilm-active substances like Rifampicin belong to the DTT group of causative agents.

12.7.2 *Streptococcus* spp.

Streptococcus spp. should be treated with intravenous beta-lactam antibiotics like Penicillin or Ampicillin (Table 12.1). In the outpatient setting, an intravenous treatment with Ceftriaxone appears favorable due to the ease of dosing [36]. Again, in case of a known hypersensitivity against beta-lactams, Vancomycin is the alternative of choice given the previously named precautions [33].

12.7.3 *Enterococcus* spp.

Enterococcus spp. show a broad variety in their susceptibility patterns and therefore susceptibility testing appears to be mandatory in order to choose the right combination of substances. Intravenous monotherapy with a beta-lactam antibiotic like Ampicillin can be sufficient, if local delivery of a second antibiotic like gentamicin via the coating of an implant or cement spacer is ensured [37]. However, one should be aware about the limited time of antibiotics release. Ampicillin-resistant *Enterococcus* spp. should be treated with Vancomycin or Daptomycin (Table 12.1).

12.7.4 Gram-Negative Bacteria

Systemic substances with an activity against gram-negative bacteria like *Enterobacterales* (*Escherichia coli, Klebsiella* spec., *Enterobacter* spec.) include beta-lactam antibiotics, carbapenems, and fluoroquinolones (Table 12.1). In cases of a suspected gram-negative infection, susceptibility testing is strongly advised to confirm the efficacy of the desired therapy agent [9, 16]. Since fluoroquinolones show a very high tissue penetration especially for bone, they should be considered primarily for oral treatment [16, 38].

Non-fermenters like *Pseudomonas aeruginosa* or *Acinetobacter* spp. represent difficult causative agents, since even radical surgical treatment sometimes is not able to eradicate infection. Proposed substances for systemic antibiotic treatment include Ciprofloxacin, Levofloxacin, Ceftazidime, Piperacillin/ Tazobactam, and Meropenem (Table 12.1). Ciprofloxacin-resistant gram-negative bacteria belong to the DTT group of causative agents [16].

12.7.5 Anaerobic Bacteria

Gram-positive anaerobic bacteria like *Cutibacterium acnes* (formerly *Propionibacterium acnes*) or *Peptostreptococcus* are more common in shoulder infections due to a proximity to the axilla but have also been reported to cause TKA infections [21, 39]. Suggested systemic substances are Penicillin or Ceftriaxone (Table 12.1). Gram-negative anaerobic bacteria like *Bacteroides* or *Fusobacterium* are usually treated by Ampicillin followed by Metronidazole [16].

12.7.6 Fungi

Fungi generally belong to the DTT group of causative agents [16] with *Candida* spp. making up for more than 80% of this group [40]. Infection with various fungi species are relatively rare but show a rising prevalence due to an increased rate of arthroplasty revision surgery [41]. They are often related to immunosuppression due to concomitant diseases or chronic treatment of medical conditions [40].

Systemic therapy options include Caspofungin, Anidulafungin, and Fluconazole (Table 12.1). Suppressive treatment with Fluconazole is recommended for more than 1 year in total, often even requiring more radical surgical approaches like total implant removal or even amputation due to recurrent infection.

12.8 Suppressive Therapy

In cases of PJI where surgical intervention is impossible (e.g. due to multimorbidity) or in DTT and recurrent infection despite numerous surgical interventions, chronic suppressive oral antibiotic therapy may be warranted [26, 42]. Such an approach is generally not to be considered therapeutic, but rather symptomatic in order to suppress the infection. More than 80% of cases show a re-infection once the suppressive therapy is discontinued [43].

There is no clear guideline regarding dosage and duration of such a therapy regimen, so all decisions have to be made based on clinical rationale considering the underlying causative agent as well as the patient's individual situation. Besides the persistent suppression of infection, one major concern of a suppressive therapy is the side effects of chronic antibiotic intake (e.g. liver damage, kidney damage, general immunosuppression, resistance formation) as well as further soft tissue damage or bone loss [16]. Appropriate substances for suppressive therapy include Doxycycline and Trimethoprim/ Sulfamethoxazole (Cotrimoxazole)—depending on susceptibility testing.

12.9 Conclusion

Multimodal management of PJI usually includes systemic antibiotic therapy as a major component. While an empiric intravenous therapy is usually started around the first surgical intervention, it has to be adapted to culture results throughout the course of treatment. A focused therapy with regard to the individual case should be continued for at least 2 weeks after the last surgical intervention before a conversion to an oral therapy is considered. In general, systemic antibiotic therapy has to be closely tailored to the chosen surgical approach. For this reason, there are no clear guidelines regarding timing and duration of such therapy since it has to be adapted to all concomitant interventions. Dosages of systemic antibiotics may vary with respect to culture results and susceptibility testing. In cases of DTT causative agents like multi-resistant bacteria strains or fungi, treatment can be complicated further, necessitating the use of additional interventions like more radical surgical approaches. Especially in cases of DAIR, one-stage revisions or re-implantations, the use of biofilm-active antibiotics should be considered to prevent biofilm formation and protect the implant surface. For elderly or multimorbid patients, chronic suppressive oral antibiotic therapy may be an option.

References

1. Karczewski D, et al. A standardized interdisciplinary algorithm for the treatment of prosthetic joint infections. Bone Joint J. 2019;101-B(2):132–9.
2. Li HK, et al. Oral versus intravenous antibiotics for bone and joint infection. N Engl J Med. 2019;380(5):425–36.
3. Li HK, et al. Oral versus intravenous antibiotic treatment for bone and joint infections (OVIVA): study protocol for a randomised controlled trial. Trials. 2015;16(1):583.
4. Li C, Renz N, Trampuz A. Management of periprosthetic joint infection. Hip Pelvis. 2018;30(3):138–46.
5. Trampuz A, Zimmerli W. New strategies for the treatment of infections associated with prosthetic joints. Curr Opin Investig Drugs. 2005;6(2):185–90.
6. Kunutsor SK, et al. Debridement, antibiotics and implant retention for periprosthetic joint infections: a systematic review and meta-analysis of treatment outcomes. J Infect. 2018;77(6):479–88.
7. Moreno MG, Trampuz A, Di Luca M. *Synergistic antibiotic activity against planktonic and biofilm-embedded Streptococcus agalactiae, Streptococcus pyogenes and Streptococcus oralis.* J Antimicrob Chemother. 2017;72:3085–92.
8. Paluch E, et al. Prevention of biofilm formation by quorum quenching. Appl Microbiol Biotechnol. 2020;104(5):1871–81.
9. McConoughey SJ, et al. Biofilms in periprosthetic orthopedic infections. Future Microbiol. 2014;9(8):987–1007.
10. Parvizi J, Ghazavi M, M.O.P.-O.A. Committee of the Consensus Meeting. Optimal timing and antibiotic prophylaxis in periprosthetic joint infection (PJI): literature review and world consensus (part three). Shafa Ortho J. 2014;2(3).
11. Wouthuyzen-Bakker M, et al. Withholding preoperative antibiotic prophylaxis in knee prosthesis revision: a retrospective analysis on culture results and risk of infection. J Arthroplasty. 2017;32(9):2829–33.
12. Wimmer MD, et al. Evaluation of an interdisciplinary therapy algorithm in patients with prosthetic joint infections. Int Orthop. 2013;37(11):2271–8.
13. Liang SY, Kumar A. Empiric antimicrobial therapy in severe sepsis and septic shock: optimizing pathogen clearance. Curr Infect Dis Rep. 2015;17(7):493.
14. W-Dahl A, et al. Timing of preoperative antibiotics for knee arthroplasties: improving the routines in Sweden. Patient Saf Surg. 2011;5:22.
15. Dellinger EP. Prophylactic antibiotics: administration and timing before operation are more important than administration after operation. Clin Infect Dis. 2007;44(7):928–30.
16. Izakovicova P, Borens O, Trampuz A. Periprosthetic joint infection: current concepts and outlook. EFORT Open Rev. 2019;4(7):482–94.
17. Widmer AF, et al. Killing of nongrowing and adherent Escherichia Coli determines drug efficacy in device-related infections. Antimicrob Agents Chemother. 1991;35(4):741–6.
18. Osmon DR, Berbari EF, Berendt AR. Diagnosis and management of prosthetic joint infection: clinical practice guidelines by the Infectious Diseases Society of America. Clin Infect Dis. 2013;56(1):e1–e25.
19. Tande AJ, et al. Prosthetic joint infection. Clin Microbiol Rev. 2014;27(2):302–45.
20. Anemuller R, et al. Hip and knee section, treatment, antimicrobials: proceedings of international consensus on orthopedic infections. J Arthroplasty. 2019;34(2S):S463–75.
21. Rakow A, et al. Origin and characteristics of haematogenous periprosthetic joint infection. Clin Microbiol Infect. 2019;25(7):845–50.
22. Ueng SW, et al. Antibacterial activity of joint fluid in cemented total-knee arthroplasty: an in vivo comparative study of polymethylmethacrylate with and without antibiotic loading. Antimicrob Agents Chemother. 2012;56(11):5541–6.
23. Parikh MS, Antony S. A comprehensive review of the diagnosis and management of prosthetic joint infections in the absence of positive cultures. J Infect Public Health. 2016;9(5):545–56.
24. Sousa R, et al. Empirical antibiotic therapy in prosthetic joint infections. Acta Orthop Belg. 2010;76(2):254–9.
25. Molina-Manso D, et al. In vitro susceptibility to antibiotics of staphylococci in biofilms isolated from orthopaedic infections. Int J Antimicrob Agents. 2013;41(6):521–3.
26. Gehrke T, Alijanipour P, Parvizi J. The management of an infected total knee arthroplasty. Bone Joint J. 2015;97-B(10 Suppl A):20–9.
27. Geipel U, Herrmann M. Das infizierte Implantat. Orthopade. 2004;33(12):1411–28.
28. Tande AJ, et al. Management of prosthetic joint infection. Infect Dis Clin North Am. 2017;31(2):237–52.
29. Byren I, et al. One hundred and twelve infected arthroplasties treated with 'DAIR' (debridement, antibiotics and implant retention): antibiotic duration and outcome. J Antimicrob Chemother. 2009;63(6):1264–71.
30. Thakrar RR, et al. Indications for a single-stage exchange arthroplasty for chronic prosthetic joint infection: a systematic review. Bone Joint J. 2019;101-B(1_Supple_A):19–24.
31. Voigt J, Mosier M, Darouiche R. Antibiotics and antiseptics for preventing infection in people receiving revision total hip and knee prostheses: a systematic review of randomized controlled trials. BMC Infect Dis. 2016;16(1):749.

32. Tan TL, et al. Is vancomycin-only prophylaxis for patients with penicillin allergy associated with increased risk of infection after arthroplasty? Clin Orthop Relat Res. 2016;474(7):1601–6.
33. Kheir MM, et al. Vancomycin prophylaxis for total joint arthroplasty: incorrectly dosed and has a higher rate of periprosthetic infection than Cefazolin. Clin Orthop Relat Res. 2017;475(7):1767–74.
34. Haagensen J, et al. Spatiotemporal pharmacodynamics of Meropenem- and tobramycin-treated Pseudomonas Aeruginosa biofilms. J Antimicrob Chemother. 2017;72(12):3357–65.
35. Achermann Y, et al. Factors associated with rifampin resistance in staphylococcal periprosthetic joint infections (PJI): a matched case-control study. Infection. 2013;41(2):431–7.
36. Tice AD, Hoaglund PA, Shoultz DA. Outcomes of osteomyelitis among patients treated with outpatient parenteral antimicrobial therapy. Am J Med. 2003;114(9):723–8.
37. Roy R, et al. Strategies for combating bacterial biofilms: a focus on anti-biofilm agents and their mechanisms of action. Virulence. 2018;9(1):522–54.
38. Yan CH, et al. Team approach: the management of infection after total knee replacement. JBJS Rev. 2018;6(4):e9.
39. Dodson CC, et al. Propionibacterium acnes infection after shoulder arthroplasty: a diagnostic challenge. J Shoulder Elbow Surg. 2010;19(2):303–7.
40. Jakobs O, et al. Fungal periprosthetic joint infection in total knee arthroplasty: a systematic review. Orthop Rev (Pavia). 2015;7(1):5623.
41. Keuning MC, Al Moujahid A, Zijlstra WP. Prosthetic joint infection of a revision knee arthroplasty with *Candida parapsilosis*. Case Rep Orthop. 2019;2019:3634519.
42. Prendki V, et al. Prolonged suppressive antibiotic therapy for prosthetic joint infection in the elderly: a national multicentre cohort study. Eur J Clin Microbiol Infect Dis. 2017;36(9):1577–85.
43. Della Valle C, et al. American Academy of Orthopaedic surgeons clinical practice guideline on: the diagnosis of periprosthetic joint infections of the hip and knee. J Bone Joint Surg Am. 2011;93(14):1355–7.

Local Delivery of Antibiotic and Antiseptic

13

Ivan De Martino, Fabio Mancino, Giorgio Cacciola, Vincenzo Di Matteo, and Giulio Maccauro

13.1 Introduction

Total knee arthroplasty (TKA) is considered one of the most cost-effective orthopedic surgical procedures with more than one million procedures performed every year [1]. Periprosthetic joint infection (PJI) is a rare but devastating complication associated with extensive economic, physical, and psychological costs. The number of THA and TKA performed every year has constantly grown during the last decades due to an active aging population [1]; however, PJI rates average between 0.5% and 2% in total joint arthroplasty (TJA) [2], and it is estimated that, in the USA alone, \$1.6 billion will be spent in 2020 on revision TJA for PJI [3]. PJI is considered the most frequent cause of reoperations within 2 years from the index surgery and the second overall cause of reoperations after TKA [4, 5]. Early PJI has been associated with preoperative bacterial infection of the patient, or intraopera-

tive bacterial contamination from surgical team, operative tools, and instruments [6]. Currently, the use of perioperative systemic antibiotics in total joint arthroplasty (TJA) is the only consensus recommendation by international authorities [4, 5]. In oreder to reduce the incidence of PJI, multiple prevention strategies have been progressively introduced in the preoperative, intraoperative and postoperative phases [7, 8], including operating room ventilation and temperature, body exhaust suits, preoperative patient optimization, perioperative skin preparation and wound management. However, their efficacy has to be proven yet [4, 5].

Despite the growing attention in preventing postoperative infection, the projected increased volume of TJAs ensures that this complication will be encountered with greater frequency in the future [1]. In this chapter, we discuss the use of antiseptic intraoperative irrigation before wound closure, local delivery of antibiotic through powder or beads, and implant coatings, developed in order to prevent and treat infections in primary and revision TKA.

I. De Martino (✉) · F. Mancino · V. Di Matteo
G. Maccauro
Division of Orthopaedics and Traumatology, Department of Aging, Neurological, Orthopaedic and Head-Neck Studies, Fondazione Policlinico Universitario Agostino Gemelli IRCCS, Università Cattolica del Sacro Cuore, Rome, Italy
e-mail: ivan.demartino@policlinicogemelli.it; giulio.maccauro@policlinicogemelli.it

G. Cacciola
GIOMI Istituto Ortopedico del Mezzogiorno d'Italia Franco Scalabrino, Ganzirri, Messina, Italy

13.2 Antiseptic Intraoperative Lavage

Wound irrigation during TJA is a routine practice among orthopedic surgeons for preventing PJI. Multiple potential options have been

© ISAKOS 2022
U. G. Longo et al. (eds.), *Infection in Knee Replacement*,
https://doi.org/10.1007/978-3-030-81553-0_13

described including the use of 0.9% saline, castile soap, antibiotic solutions, and antiseptics like povidone-iodine, chlorhexidine gluconate, or hydrogen peroxide. However, no consensus has been reached yet due to a lack of evidence and a paucity of studies in the current literature. Intraoperative irrigation with antiseptic solutions could be considered a potential tool in reducing the risk of early PJI after TKA by preventing the formation of bacterial biofilm [9]. A 2014 focus group discussed evidence for standardization of surgical wound irrigation protocols and determined that, given a lack evidence-based science regarding this topic, they were unable to conclude on which solution, delivery method, or amount should be recommended [10]. However, the United States Center for Disease Control and Prevention guidelines for the prevention of surgical site infection (SSI) [4] and the World Health Organization (WHO) suggest the use of intraoperative irrigation with antiseptic solution considering its effectiveness in reducing the risk of SSI and deep infection [5]. Most of the available data in the current literature comes from in vitro studies, and only few clinical reports have been already published [11].

To date, there is no shared consensus regarding the usage of the best antiseptic solution in order to prevent and/or eradicate biofilm formation [11]. In this section we will review the clinical evidence available on intraoperative lavage with povidone-iodine and chlorhexidine gluconate solutions in TKA.

13.2.1 Povidone-Iodine Intraoperative Lavage

Intraoperative irrigation before wound closure with dilute povidone-iodine solution at different concentration has been associated with a decreased rate of postoperative infection in orthopedic (up to 1% dilution), urologic (1% dilution), cardiovascular (0.5% dilution), and general surgery (1% dilution) [12, 13]. Povidone-iodine is a stable chemical complex of polyvinylpyrrolidone (PVP) and elemental iodine (I) that progressively releases free iodine, a toxic element for microor-

ganisms [14, 15]. Hoekstra et al. [16], in an in vitro study, reported that diluted PVP-I was shown to be equivalent to, and in many cases better than, its competitors in the eradication of bacterial biofilm over 24 h and that was highly effective against *Pseudomonas aeruginosa*, *Candida albicans,* and *Methicillin-Resistant Staphylococcus aureus* (MRSA) at both 4 and 24 h. This highlighted its potential to be used as treatment of choice of highly exuding chronic biofilm-infected wounds. Similarly, Kanno et al. [17] reported that irrigation with 1% diluted PVP-I solution reduced bacterial count on contaminated wound's surface, especially when highly contaminated with *P. aeruginosa*. Despite its effectiveness toward a broad-spectrum of potentially infectious microorganisms, it is important to clarify that PVP-I solution may cause adverse reactions in human tissues. In an in vitro study it was reported that diluted PVP-I irrigation was found to be cytotoxic to bovine articular cartilage cells; however, Von Keudell et al. [18] found this effect to be much less evident in the 0.35% diluted solution in 1- to 3-min incubation periods. In addition, Kaysinger et al. [19] reported that diluted PVP-I solution at a concentration of 5% or greater was cytotoxic to embryo chick tibia and osteoblast cells.

However, only a few studies reported the outcomes of intraoperative irrigation with diluted PVP-I before wound closure in TKA [20–22]. Brown et al. [20] retrospectively analyzed 2250 primary TJA and compared the outcomes of 414 TKA and 274 total hip arthroplasty (THA) where 3 min irrigation with 0.35% dilute povidone-iodine solution was performed, followed by skin disinfection with 10% povidone-iodine solution prior to the final wound closure, with the outcomes of 1862 TJA where dilute povidone-iodine solution was not used (1232 TKA, 630 THA). The authors reported 18 early postoperative infections among the cases where irrigation with dilute PVP-I was not performed and 1 in the PVP-I irrigation group (0.97% and 0.15%, respectively; $p = 0.04$). The authors stated that a 3-min dilute PVP-I lavage combined with disinfection of the skin with 10% Betadine before surgical closure was associated

Table 13.1 Summary of orthopedic literature on the use of irrigation solutions containing povidone-iodine and/or chlorhexidine gluconate to prevent SSI

Author	Joint	N	Comparison	Solution	Outcome/%		p-value
Brown et al. (2012)	Hip and knee	274 THAs and 414 TKAs	630 THAs and 1232 TKAs	0.35% diluted PVP-I	Acute deep infection	0.15% vs. 0.97	0.04
Frish et al. (2017)	Knee and hip	386 TJAs	664 TJAs	0.05% CHG solution	Surgical site infection/deep infection	0.8% and 0.7%/1.2% vs. 0.8%	0.913/0.534
Hernandez et al. (2019)	Knee	2410 TKAs	3794 TKAs	0.25% diluted PVP-I	Reoperation for infection	0.8% vs. 0.5%	0.525
Calkins et al. (2019)	Knee and hip	81 THAs and 153 TKAs	79 THAs and 144 TKAs	0.35% diluted PVP-I	Acute deep infection	0.4% and 3.4%	0.038

THA total hip arthroplasty, *TKA* total knee arthroplasty, *PVP-I* polyvinylpyrrolidone-iodine, *SSI* surgical site infection

with a significant reduction in the infection rate after primary TKA and THA. Hernandez et al. [21], in a register-based study, retrospectively analyzed 6204 primary TKA and reported the outcomes of 2410 TKA where a 0.25% diluted PVP-I irrigation was performed before wound closure, compared with 3794 TKA where the irrigation was performed with normal saline solution. The authors reported that no significant differences between the two groups were observed regarding reoperation rate at 3-months follow-up (0.8% vs. 0.3%; $p = 0.06$), and a higher reoperation rate was observed in the PVP-I group at 1-year follow-up (1.2% vs. 0.6%; $p = 0.03$). However, no differences were reported regarding reoperations due to infection after the application of propensity score. Calkins et al. [22] analyzed the outcomes of 478 patients who underwent aseptic revision TKA and THA and that were randomized to receive a 3-min dilute PVP-I lavage (0.35%) or normal saline lavage before surgical wound closure. Among them, 234 patients (153 knees, 81 hips) received normal saline lavage and 223 (144 knees, 79 hips) received dilute PVP-I lavage. Within 90 days postoperatively, the authors reported eight infections in the saline group and one in the PVP-I group (3.4% vs. 0.4%, $p = 0.038$) and no difference in wound complications between groups (1.3% vs. 0%, $p = 0.248$).

In addition, PVP-I is safe, inexpensive, simple to use, and it has a broad-spectrum bactericidal activity that includes MRSA [15, 23].

Finally, based on the current literature, dilute PVP-I irrigation before surgical wound closure in primary and revision TJA appears to be a simple, safe, and effective option to reduce the risk of acute postoperative PJI (Table 13.1).

13.2.2 Chlorhexidine Intraoperative Lavage

Chlorhexidine gluconate (CHG) is a widely used antiseptic agent and is present in a variety of preparations to prevent infection, including pre-operative skin cleaning, surgical site preparation, intraoperative irrigation, CHG impregnated postoperative dressings, and hand antisepsis [24]. CHG has a broad-spectrum biocide bacteriostatic and bactericidal effect against Gram-Positive and Gram-Negative bacteria, and it has a faster onset of action than PVP-I [25]. It is a bactericidal agent, acting primarily disrupting the cell membrane [26, 27]. In addition, CHG has a particularly strong affinity for binding to skin and mucous membranes, theoretically enhancing the efficacy in prevention of SSI [28]. It has been previously stated in several animal studies that CHG could be safety used on wounds, and its potential use for wound lavage has been demonstrated by the studies on prevention of infection in humans [29]. In addition, it is considered effective in biofilm eradication when used to scrub an MRSA-coated titanium disc [30]. However, in an in vitro study, it has been reported that the clinically used concentration of CHX (2%) permanently halts cell migration and significantly reduces survival of fibroblasts, myoblasts, and osteoblasts, regardless of the exposure duration [31]. Nevertheless, to date there is a paucity of literature regarding the safety of CHG as an intrawound irrigation agent and peri-incisional topical antiseptic.

Despite many studies have reported the efficacy of CHG in skin preparation before total knee arthroplasty [24, 32], there is currently only one study that reported the outcomes of intraoperative CHG lavage in TJAs. Frisch et al. [24] evaluated the effect of CHG intraoperative irrigation on infection rates following THA and TKA. Intraoperative irrigation was performed with 0.9% saline and periodic 0.05% CHG solution followed by a final 1-min soak in CHG with immediate closure afterward. The authors reported no significant differences in terms of SSI ($p = 0.913$) and deep infections at 1-year follow-up ($p = 0.534$) when compared 411 TKAs where intraoperative irrigation was performed with normal saline solution before wound closure, with 248 TKAs where intraoperative irrigation was performed with CHG solution. The authors suggested that intraoperative CHG during TJA had a comparable infection rate to different protocols using PVP-I in THA and 0.9% saline in TKA.

Intraoperative irrigation with diluted antiseptic solutions like PVP-I or CHG before wound closure may contribute to the prevention of the biofilm formation and reduce the incidence of early PJI in TKA. However, despite promising in vitro evidence, further in vivo studies are required to examine and optimize safety and efficacy when intraoperatively applied before wound closure (Table 13.1).

13.3 Antibiotic Local Delivery

The application of antimicrobial agents at the site of musculoskeletal infections has been widely documented, ranging from the direct intra-articular infusion of antibiotic after TKA [33] to the intrawound placement of antibiotic powder to prevent infection in spinal surgery [34–40]. Due to a lack of clarification regarding the long-term efficacy of locally administrated antibiotics, the combination of antibiotics with implantable materials has been progressively investigated in order to provide a predictable release profile [41].

13.3.1 Antibiotic Powder

Intrawound vancomycin powder (VP) was recently considered in orthopedics to decrease SSIs and subsequent deep infections for its capacity to provide a high local concentration of the antibiotic, maximizing local bactericidal effect while minimizing adverse systemic reactions. Previous reports showed that intrawound VP did not increase the rate of side effects [34–38] and that after local administration, serum vancomycin concentrations remained below toxic levels [35–37].

The use of VP in spinal surgery has been widely documented by several reports indicating a reduced rate of SSIs [34–37, 39, 40]; however, Ghobrial et al. [34] reported that wound complications, including seroma formation, were associated with intrawound VP after spinal surgery. Despite the promising results of VP in spinal surgery, information regarding its use in TJA are still not clear. In front of a lack of clinical data, preclinical results have been supported by Cavanaugh et al. [42] and Edelstein et al. [43], suggesting the effectiveness of intrawound VP on clearing *S. aureus* from contaminated femoral implants in in vivo rats investigations. However, numerous questions are still unanswered regarding this procedure in TJA, including clear information about seroma formation, bearing wear, nephrotoxicity, and ototoxicity. Third body wear remains a real concern in the setting of TJA. Although vancomycin is a soluble molecule, there is a paucity of information about its use outside of plasma and about its solubility and possibility to precipitate in other body fluids. In a closed space such as knee or hip joint, with a prosthetic implant, undissolved particulate of antibiotic could reach portions of the prosthetic implant and cause abnormal wear and potentially early failure.

Quadir et al. [44], in a biomechanical study, demonstrated that crystalline antibiotics do not alter wear rates in Cobalt-Chrome (Co-Cr) on ultra-high molecular weight polyethylene (UHMWPE) secondary to third body wear in simulated ten million cycles. However, the long-term effect on polyethylene wear is still unknown.

Otte et al. [45] retrospectively compared over a 2-year period the rate of early PJI in patients who underwent primary or revision THA and TKA with and without the use of intrawound VP. The authors reported a significant decrease in the early PJI rate in the revision settings (THA and TKA) when VP was used (0 of 134, 0%) compared to when VP was not used (7 of 180, 3.89%; $p = 0.0217$). Similarly, Patel et al. [46] retrospectively reviewed 460 primary THAs and TKAs and compared the early PJI rate in the VP group ($n = 348$) with the control group ($n = 112$). The authors reported a decreased overall infection rate (0.57% vs. 2.7%; $p = 0.031$) and PJI rate (0.29% vs. 2.7%; $p = 0.009$) in the VP group compared to the control group with a lower readmission rate due to infection (0.57% vs. 2.7%; $p = 0.031$). In addition, the authors determined a number needed to treat (NNT) of 47.5, suggesting that the cost to prevent 1 infection with the addition of intrawound vancomycin was $816 (based on their institution costs) compared to the estimated average hospital cost per case in the USA of infected THA ($30,329) and TKA ($25,155) [47]. Matziolis et al. [48] retrospectively evaluated 8945 primary TJA and reported two infections among the TKA treated with intraoperative intrawound VP group (out of 650 TKAs, 0.4%) compared to 44 infections (out of 3471 TKAs, 1.3%; $p = 0.033$) in a control group. The differences noted among the two groups of patients who underwent THA did not achieve statistical significance; however, the infection rate in the control group was twofold greater compared to the VP group, and no wound complications were observed as a result of application of local vancomycin. Conversely, Dial et al. [38] retrospectively reviewed 265 consecutive THAs and despite a reduced deep infection rate when intrawound VP was used (0.7%) compared to the control group (5.5%, $p = 0.031$), the authors

reported an increased rate of sterile wound complications in the VP group (4.4% vs. 0%; $p = 0.030$). Similarly, Hanada et al. [6] prospectively evaluated 166 consecutive patients who underwent primary TKA or unicompartmental knee arthroplasty (UKA) and evaluated the efficacy and side effects of local intrawound VP. Despite a considerably high PJI rate in both groups (7.6% control group; 4.5% VP group), no significant difference was found among them (ns). However, operative wound complications were significantly more frequent in the VP group (11.8%) compared to the control group (4.3%) so that the authors did not recommend its use in the setting of primary TKA and UKA.

In conclusion, despite a paucity of available data in the current literature and contrasting opinion by authors, intrawound VP shows promising results in reducing early PJI, particularly if an increased rate of PJI is present due to the surgical procedure or the high-risk population involved. In addition, VP is a low-cost tool with an effective NNT (Table 13.2).

13.3.2 Nonabsorbable Polymethylmethacrylate (PMMA) Beads

Antibiotics have been used in combination with poly-methyl-methacrylate (PMMA) for decades [49], and it has been widely used as a fundamental tool in primary TKA in case of patients at high risk of infection or in revision TKA for PJI for cementing the implant components, as antibiotic-loaded articulated spacers or beads [50, 51]. The use of antibiotic-loaded cement has reported a significant reduction in infection rates in the settings of primary or revision THA [52] and TKA [53]. However, other studies reported limited clinical benefit of antibiotic-loaded cement in the treatment of PJI compared with systemic antibiotics and clinical data are not sufficient to support recommendations on dosages [54, 55]. In this paragraph we will discuss the role of antibiotic beads in TJA.

Gentamicin, vancomycin, and tobramycin-loaded PMMA beads are considered an effective

Table 13.2 Summary of orthopedic literature on the use of intrawound vancomycin powder and/or calcium sulfate beads to prevent SSI

Author	Joint	N	Comparison	Local antibiotic	Outcome/%		p-value
Otte et al. (2017)	Knee and hip	816 TJAs	824 TJAs	Intrawound VP	Early PJI	0% vs. 3.89%	0.0217
Flierl et al. (2017)	Hip and knee	32 TJAs	No control group	Calcium sulfate beads	PJI	48%	/
Dial et al. (2018)	Hip	137 THAs	128 THAs	Intrawound VP	PJI	0.7% vs. 5.5%	0.031
Patel et al. (2018)	Knee and hip	348 TJAs	1122 TJAs	Intrawound VP	Overall infection rate/ PJI rate	0.57% vs. 2.7%/0.29% vs. 2.7%	0.031/0.009
Lum et al. (2018)	Knee and hip	56 TJAs	No control group	Calcium sulfate beads	PJI	0%	/
Calanna et al. (2019)	Knee	10 TKAs	No control group	Calcium sulfate beads	PJI	20%	/
Gramlich et al. (2019)	Knee	42 TKAs	No control group	Calcium sulfate beads	PJI	26.2%	/
Hanada et al. (2019)	Knee	92 TKAs	90 TKAs	Intrawound VP	PJI	4.5% vs. 7.6%	NS
Matziolis et al. (2020)	Knee	650 TKAs	3471 TKAs	Intrawound VP	PJI	0.4% vs. 1.3%	0.033

TKA total knee arthroplasty, *THA* total hip arthroplasty, *TJA* total joint arthroplasty, *VP* vancomycin powder, *PJI* periprosthetic joint infection, *SSI* surgical site infection, *NS* not significant

drug delivery system for local antibiotic therapy in bone and soft-tissue infections with subsequent antibiotic concentrations above the minimum inhibitory concentration (MIC) for the infecting organisms [56]. The release of the antibiotics from the PMMA beads is a diffusion process, as in all antibiotic-loaded bone cements [57]. However, due to the increased surface area of the many, relatively small beads, much more antibiotic is released compared to solid bone cement plugs. Usually, gentamicin-loaded beads are held in situ approximately 14 days, after which 20–70% of the total amount of gentamicin has been released into the body, so that the main antibiotic efficacy is immediately after implantation [58]. Despite the multiple advantages, once the antibiotics have eluted from the nonabsorbable cement, the surface becomes a foreign body that is potentially subjected to bacterial colonization and biofilm formation [59, 60]. Neut et al. [61] analyzed in an extensive laboratory procedure the gentamicin-loaded beads from 20 patients treated for PJI and reported the presence of bacteria on the beads in 18 of the 20 patients involved, and that 19 of 28 bacterial strains isolated were gentamicin-resistant or highly resistant sub-populations. The authors suggested that despite their antibiotic release, the PMMA beads act as a biomaterial surface to which bacteria preferentially adhere, grow, and potentially develop antibiotic resistance. In a retrieval analysis of gentamicin-loaded beads left in situ for 5 years, it was reported that the gentamicin-release test revealed residual antibiotic release, and extensive microbiological sampling resulted in recovery of a gentamicin-resistant staphylococcal strain from the bead surface [62]. This case showed that even after 5 years, PMMA beads remained able to release subinhibitory concentration of antibiotics, approximately 0.4 mg of gentamicin per bead, stimulating the introduction of gentamicin-resistant strains. Finally, considering that every biomaterial left in the human body must be considered as a potential focus for infection [60], biodegradable beads are preferred as carriers for antibiotics as they do not show long-term release of subinhibitory antibiotic concentrations, do not require removal, and do not leave any biomaterial in situ to act as a potential focus for infection. In addition, in vitro results have shown that tobramycin impregnated beads made of polycaprolactone, a bioresorbable polymer, have even superior antibiotic elution characteristics compared with PMMA beads, suggesting more effective antibiotic delivery vehicle [63].

13.3.3 Absorbable Calcium Sulfate Beads

Calcium sulfate (CS), (CaSO$_4$ • 1/2 H$_2$O), also known as plaster of Paris, was introduced in orthopedic surgery in 1892 by Dreesman et al. as a filler for bone void [64]. Currently, antibiotic bone substitution materials/bone void fillers are based on biodegradable or resorbable materials such as polylactic acid, chitosan, or new combinations based on calcium sulfate [65]. Absorbable mineral-based bone cements, despite inferior mechanical characteristics compared to acrylic cements, provide multiple advantages regarding antibiotic delivery and infection control. Unlike PMMA beads, these materials do not have to be removed, they have the capacity to accommodate a wider range of antibiotics since there is little temperature increase during setting, and the antibiotics are slowly released meanwhile the material dissolves [59]. CS beads are suitable for application in the presence of infection, nonunion, or bone loss, and as the beads are absorbed, CS releases 100% of the antibiotic load, resulting in superior elution characteristics and higher sustained antibiotic concentrations over several weeks [41].

CS is a well-studied, non-immunogenic, biocompatible bone void filler used in orthopedic applications since the nineteenth century and currently used as substitute for bone cement in multiple settings of orthopedic surgery [66–72]. To date, multiple studies reported the outcome of antibiotic-loaded CS beads in the treatment of chronic osteomyelitis of long bone [73, 74]. McKee et al. [75] reported that tobramycin-loaded CS beads were as effective as PMMA beads in the treatment of chronic osteomyelitis and infected non-unions. Despite promising results, occasionally, non-infectious inflammatory reactions have been observed after the

implantation of resorbable beads, suspected to be caused by calcium-rich fluid generated in the process of rapid graft resorption [76, 77]. Currently there are only a few studies that evaluated the outcomes of CS beads in TKA. Three studies reported outcomes after debridement, antibiotics, and implant retention (DAIR) procedure with antibiotic-loaded CS beads, and two studies where the beads were used in the setting of two-stage revisions for PJI [78–80]. A DAIR procedure is usually performed for acute infections without complicating factors such as significant comorbidity or implant loosening. Antibiotic-loaded CS beads are available in three commercial products, Stimulan® (Biocomposite Ltd., Staffordshire, England), OSTEOSET®-T (Wright Medical Technology Inc., Arlington, TN, USA), and Herafill® beads G (Heraeus Medical GmbH, Wehrheim, Germany).

Calanna et al. [81] described a modified surgical technique called debridement, antibiotic pearls, and retention of the implant (DAPRI). In order to reduce the risk of persistent infection, they performed a methylene-blue guided debridement, defined as "tumor like," synovectomy, followed by Argon beam electrical stimulation of metallic surface, and by 4% dilute CHG irrigation. They added the CS beads loaded with vancomycin, tobramycin, and a third antibiotic based on preoperative antibiogram in the suprapatellar pouch, around the proximal tibia and the distal femur. The authors finally reported, at a mean follow-up of 24 months, that the procedure was considered a failure in 2 of 10 (20%) patients. Similarly, Flierl et al. [78] retrospectively evaluated at a mean follow-up of 13 months 32 patients (27 TKAs, 6 THAs) with acute hematogenous or acute postoperative PJI who underwent irrigation and debridement with implant retention and addition of antibiotic-impregnated CS beads. The authors reported an overall failure rate of 48%, in addition, acute hematogenous and acute postoperative PJI had similar failure rates of 47% and 50%, respectively ($p = 0.88$), suggesting that the addition of antibiotic-impregnated CS beads did not improve outcomes of DAIR in the setting of acute hematogenous or acute postoperative PJI. Kallala et al. [79] prospectively evaluated at a mean follow-up of 35 months, the outcomes of 755 patients who underwent 456 revision TKAs and 299 revision THAs. The procedures included one-stage revisions, the first or second stage of two-stage revisions, and DAIR with the implantation of Stimulan beads. The first of stage of the two-stage revision included washout, debridement, components removal, and implantation of PMMA spacer and antibiotic-impregnated CS beads. The second stage included spacer removal and implantation of revision components followed by antibiotic-impregnated CS beads. The authors found no significant difference in beads volume between patient drainage groups ($p > 0.05$). In addition, they found an overall difference in the volume of the beads involved in variable types of complication, with a larger volume in the group with hypercalcemia compared to patients without complications ($p = 0.0014$). It is reported in the literature that wound drainage tends to occur more frequently in patients in whom a higher volume of beads had been used, with more subcutaneous placement and in those with a poor host grade, such as McPherson grade C [82]. Gramlich et al. [80] evaluated at a mean of 23-months follow-up the outcomes of 42 patients treated using a single-stage algorithm consisting of DAIR, followed by implantation of antibiotic-loaded beads chosen in accordance with an antibiogram (OSTEOSET-T® and Herafill-Gentamycin®). The authors reported that permanent remission was achieved in 73.8% of the cases, while 11.9% showed chronic PJI under implant retention, suggesting good outcomes of DAIR and antibiotic-loaded CS beads in patients with recurrent PJI where DAIR is typically considered inappropriate. Marczak et al. [83] evaluated the outcomes at mean 52-months follow-up of two groups formed by 28 consecutive patients who underwent two-stage revision TKA for PJI, one group received Herafill beads, while the control group did not. The authors reported no cases of reinfections in the study group, while five were seen in the control group. No other differences were observed between the two groups, and no side effects related to the use of Herafill were noted. Lum et al. [84] evaluated postoperative complications following the use of antibiotic-loaded CS beads in 56 patients who underwent complex primary or revision hip or knee arthroplasty (26 knees and 30 hips). The authors reported one case (1.7%) of persistent wound drainage in a revision TKA that required subsequent surgical irrigation and a poly-exchange, and no postoperative infections were seen suggesting that CS beads may help to reduce postoperative wound complications and may be a safe adjunct tool in local antibiotic delivery.

The use of antibiotic-loaded beads for the treatment of PJI in TKA is reported in a limited number of studies in the current literature. Given the lack of evidence, the second International Consensus Meeting on PJI did not recommend the use of calcium sulfate/phosphate or PMMA beads, as local antibiotic carrier to prevent surgical site infection and PJI [85]. In addition, despite the encouraging clinical results in reducing the incidence of PJI, CS beads have been associated with multiple complications including hypercalcemia, persistent wound discharge, and heterotopic ossification [79, 86]. However, degradable, local antibiotics based on calcium sulfate could offer advantages and can be a reasonable addition to already established systems in the treatment of PJI (Table 13.2).

13.4 Coated Implant

Different implant-coating alternatives have been developed to reduce the risk of early PJI. The goal is to create a local environment favorable to the host and hostile to the microorganisms in order to reduce the bacterial adhesion to the implant and the subsequent biofilm formation. According to Romanò et al. [87], antibacterial coatings have been classified by their mechanism of action in passive surface, active surface finishing/modification, and perioperative antibacterial local carriers or coatings. The first one is based on preventing or reducing bacterial adhesion to implants through surface chemistry and/or structure modifications, without the use of any pharmacologically active substance. Examples of this approach include modified titanium dioxide surface or polymer coatings. The second one is based on pharmacologically active pre-incorporated bactericidal agents, such as antibiotics, antiseptics, metal ions, or other organic and inorganic substances that are actively released from the implant in order to reduce bacterial adhesion. Examples of this approach are "contact killing" active surface with silver- or iodine-coated joint implants. The third one is based on local antibacterial carriers, or coatings, that are not built into the device, but rather are applied during surgery, prior to the insertion of the implant. Those carriers or coatings may have direct or synergistic antibacterial/anti-adhesive activity or may deliver high local concentrations of loaded antibiotics or antibacterial.

13.4.1 Silver-Coated Implant

Silver is considered a promising coating as it has a broad-spectrum of antibacterial activity against planktonic and sessile Gram-positive and Gram-negative bacteria, including multiresistant bacteria [88, 89]. The bactericidal ability of silver depends on the capacity of dissolved cations to interfere with bacterial cell membrane and bacterial metabolism. In addition, silver cations in an aqueous medium contribute to the formation of reactive oxygen species that potentially harm prokaryotic cells [87].

Calcium phosphates like hydroxyapatite containing silver have shown to reduce the bacterial adhesion against *S. epidermidis, P. aeruginosa,* and *S. aureus* when compared to surfaces without silver [90, 91]. In addition, silver deposited on surfaces such as titanium and stainless steel has shown a toxic effect toward bacterial pathogens within specified doses of silver [92–95]. Currently there are only few studies that reported the outcomes of patients that underwent surgeries with silver-coated implants [95–97]. Hardes et al. [95] prospectively evaluated over a 5-year period the infection rate in 51 patients with sarcoma of proximal femur or proximal tibia who received a silver-coated megaprosthesis compared with 74 patients who received an uncoated titanium megaprosthesis was implanted. The authors reported a substantial reduction of the infection

rate from 17.6% in the titanium group to 5.9% in the silver-coated group ($p = 0.062$). In a subsequent study, the same authors [96] assessed the infection rate in 98 patients with sarcoma or giant-cell tumor of the proximal tibia who underwent placement of a titanium uncoated ($n = 42$) or silver-coated ($n = 56$) megaprosthesis. The authors reported an infection rate of 16.7% in the titanium group compared to 8.9% in the silver-coated group ($p = 0.247$), resulting in 5-year survivorship of the implants of 90% and 84% in the silver and uncoated titanium group, respectively. Zajonz et al. [97] retrospectively evaluated the reinfection rate of 34 patients treated with modular mega-endoprosthesis after a cured bone infection of the lower limb (femur or tibia). The authors reported, over a median follow-up of 72 months, a reinfection rate of 40% in the silver-coated group (8 of 20) and of 57% in the non-silver-coated group (8 of 14). However, these results were not statistically significant due to the low number of cases. Wafa et al. [98] retrospectively evaluated the outcomes of silver-coated tumor prostheses in 85 patients compared with 85 matched control patients treated for primary reconstruction (30%), one-stage revision (47%), and two-stage revision for infection (23%). At a minimum follow-up of 12 months there was a significant reduction in the overall postoperative infection rate from 22.4% to 11.8% ($p = 0.03$) in favor of the silver-coated implant group.

Despite this broad clinical use, little is known about the stability of silver-coated alloys, their efficacy on biofilm formation, and the kinetics of release. The main concerns about the use of silver-coated implants are directed toward the toxicity of silver ions. The same effects on prokaryotic cells could apply to eukaryotic cells leading to toxicity on bone cells, and the silver ions released could produce adverse reactions by accumulating in further districts within the body [99]. In addition, silver has a wide range of bacterial targets [100, 101], including the respiratory chain, and has been shown to induce resistance in Gram-negative bacteria and toxicity in eukaryotic cells [102, 103]. Moreover, concern is expressed toward the incomplete protection of the implant, since some modular components of the implants cannot be coated [87], and only a few implant designs are offered with silver-coating given a persistent relatively high cost of the technology when used outside oncology [104].

13.4.2 Iodine-Coated Implant

The use of PVP-I as an electrolyte was reported by Shirai et al. [105], in an in vitro study, and resulted in the formation of an adhesive porous anodic oxide with the antiseptic properties of iodine, suggesting the antibacterial attachment effect and cytocompatibility of iodine-supported implants. Similarly, Inoue et al. [106] showed that iodine-supported implants have a good antibacterial attachment effect in vivo and inhibit biofilm formation and growth by preventing initial bacterial attachment on the metal surface. Tsuchiya et al. [107] prospectively evaluated at a mean follow-up of 18 months 222 patients with postoperative infection or compromised status that were treated using a variety of iodine-supported titanium implants (spinal instrumentation, plates for osteosynthesis, pins, and wires). In 158 patients the iodine-supported implants were used to prevent infections while in 64 patients to treat active infections. The authors reported that acute infection developed in three tumor cases among the 158 patients on preventive therapy, and that infection was eradicated in all 64 infected patients suggesting that iodine-supported titanium implants can be very effective in preventing and treating infections after orthopedic surgery. Similarly, Shirai et al. [108] evaluated at a mean follow-up of 30 months 47 patients with malignant bone tumor or pyogenic arthritis treated with iodine-supported titanium megaprosthesis. The authors reported that only one patient (out of the 21) got infected and that in the 26 patients treated with one- or two-stage revision surgery, infection was eradicated without any additional surgery. In addition, Kabata et al. [109] retrospectively evaluated at a mean follow-up of 33 months the outcomes of a consecutive series of 30 hips including 13 primary THAs in compromised

immune system conditions or pyogenic arthritis, 14 revision THAs after PJI, and 3 conversions from hemiarthroplasty to THA in immunosuppressive conditions. The authors reported no signs of infection in any patient at the latest follow-up.

Finally, based on these findings, iodine-supported implants can be considered highly effective in preventing and treating postoperative infection while no adverse event has been reported to date. However, longer-term effects of local application of iodine coating and the effects on materials other than titanium have not been clarified yet and clinical trials are currently ongoing in order to confirm these preliminary results.

13.4.3 DAC® Hydrogel Coated Implant

Defensive Antibacterial Coating (DAC®) is a fast-resorbable hydrogel coating composed of covalently linked hyaluronan and poly-D,L-lactide (PLLA) (Novagenit Srl, Mezzolombardo, Italy) specifically designed to protect implanted biomaterials [110]. The rationale of this device is the capacity of hyaluronic acid to reduce biofilm formation on material surfaces exposed to bacterial contamination and affect different microbial species and, sometimes, different strains belonging to the same species [108, 109]. DAC® has been found to have a synergistic antibiofilm activity with various antibacterials and to be effectively manually spread onto the surface of various biomaterials commonly used in orthopedics, trauma, and dental surgery [111]. The adhesion density of *S. aureus* on titanium discs pre-treated with DAC® was significantly lower than adhesion on untreated controls at each time point. In particular, reductions of adhered bacteria equal to 86.8%, 80.4%, 74.6%, and 66.7% vs. untreated discs were observed after 15, 30, 60, and 120 min of incubation, respectively, while an increase of adhesion density during time was observed for both control and pre-treated discs [112]. In addition, DAC® hydrogel showed similar or superior in vitro activity, compared to gentamycin and vancomycin, and a synergistic activity when used in combination with antibiotics providing a larger reduction of biofilm formation (approximately 75 to 80% in comparison with untreated controls) [113]. It has been reported the capacity of DAC® to entrap different antibacterial agents at concentrations ranging from 2% to 10% and then to slowly release them locally for up to 72 h at levels considerably higher than the minimum inhibitory concentration (MIC) [114]. Romanò et al. [115] evaluated 380 patients who underwent cementless or hybrid fixation primary ($n = 270$) or revision ($n = 110$) THA ($n = 298$) and TKA ($n = 82$) with and without the antibiotic-loaded DAC® coating, in a multicenter randomized prospective study, at a mean follow-up of 15 months. The authors reported 11 early surgical site infections in the non-coated group (6%) and only one in the coated group (0.6%, $p = 0.003$). No local or systemic side effects related to the DAC® hydrogel coating were observed, and no detectable interference with implant fixation was noted. Similarly, Malizos et al. [116], in a multicenter randomized controlled prospective study, evaluated at a mean follow-up of 18 months 256 patients who underwent osteosynthesis for a closed fracture and were randomly assigned to receive implants with antibiotic-loaded DAC® coating or without coating. The authors reported six surgical site infections in the coated group (4.6%), compared to none in the non-coated group ($p < 0.03$). No local or systemic side effects related to the DAC® hydrogel coating were observed, and no detectable interference with bone healing was noted. Recently, Capuano et al. [117] retrospectively evaluated at a mean follow-up of 29 months 22 patients treated with a one-stage revision for PJI using implants coated with an antibiotic-loaded DAC® hydrogel, and compared them with 22 matched controls treated with a two-stage revision procedure using non-coated implants. The authors reported, although in a relatively limited series of patients, a similar infection recurrence rate after one-stage exchange with DAC®-coated implants (9%) compared to two-stage revision

without coating (14%), with reduced overall hospitalization time and antibiotic treatment duration. Zagra et al. [118] retrospectively evaluated at a mean follow-up of 2.8 years 27 patients who underwent a two-stage revision THA for PJI, using cementless implants coated with the antibiotic-loaded DAC® hydrogel, and compared them with 27 matched controls, who underwent a two-stage cementless revision THA with non-coated implants. The authors reported no evidence of infection, implant loosening, or adverse events in the DAC®-coated group, compared to four cases of infection recurrence in the non-coated group ($p = 0.11$).

In conclusion, despite these encouraging results, longer-term data are required in order to evaluate the incidence of delayed or late PJIs. In fact, the fast resorption of the hydrogel protects from long-term side effect but may limit the protection of the implant from late, hematogenous infections.

13.5 Conclusions

In conclusion, implant-related infections have a pronounced social and economic impact with increased rates of morbidity and mortality after THA and TKA [119, 120]. According to the current literature these complications will become a growing burden to healthcare systems over the coming decades unless novel and effective measures are not taken to reduce the incidence of PJIs [1]. Despite the promising results of the newer technologies, only a few of them are currently available in orthopedic surgery. Some potentially effective solutions may be excluded from the daily practice due to cytotoxicity, immunoreactivity, or interference with bone healing and osseointegration. Conversely, other technologies safely tested in vitro and in vivo may not be able to be used on a large scale, due to biotechnological, economic, and regulatory issues. Finally, effort should be made in order to increase the awareness of healthcare providers and their patients regarding the newer technologies and their possible contribution to mitigate septic complication.

References

1. Kurtz S, Ong K, Lau E, Mowat F, Halpern M. Projections of primary and revision hip and knee arthroplasty in the United States from 2005 to 2030. J Bone Joint Surg Am. 2007;89(4):780–5.
2. Kurtz SM, Lau E, Schmier J, Ong KL, Zhao K, Parvizi J. Infection burden for hip and knee arthroplasty in the United States. J Arthoplasty. 2008;23(7):984–91.
3. Haddad FS, Ngu A, Negus JJ. Prosthetic joint infections and cost analysis? Adv Exp Med Biol. 2017;971:93–100.
4. Berríos-Torres SI, Umscheid CA, Bratzler DW, et al. Centers for Disease Control and Prevention guideline for the prevention of surgical site infection. JAMA Surg. 2017;152(8):784–91.
5. Allegranzi B, Zayed B, Bischoff P, et al. New WHO recommendations on intraoperative and postoperative measures for surgical site infection prevention: an evidence-based global perspective. Lancet Infect Dis. 2016;16(12):e288–303.
6. Hanada M, Nishikino S, Hotta K, Furuhashi H, Hoshino H, Matsuyama Y. Intrawound vancomycin powder increases post-operative wound complications and does not decrease periprosthetic joint infection in primary total and unicompartmental knee arthroplasty. Knee Surg Sports Traumatol Arthrosc. 2019;27:2322–7.
7. Bosco JA, Bookman J, Slover J, Edusei E, Levine B. Principles of antibiotic prophylaxis in total joint arthroplasty: current concepts. J Am Acad Orthop Surg. 2015;23(8):e27–35.
8. Cacciola G, Mancino F, Malahias MA, Sculco PK, Maccauro G, De Martino I. Diluted povidone-iodine irrigation prior to wound closure in primary and revision total joint arthroplasty of hip and knee: a review of the evidence. J Biol Regul Homeost Agents. 2020;34(3 Suppl 2):57–62.
9. Kokavec M, Fristáková M. Efficacy of antiseptics in the prevention of post-operative infections of the proximal femur, hip and pelvis regions in orthopedic pediatric patients. Analysis of the first results. Acta Chir Orthop Traumatol Cech. 2008;75(2):106–9.
10. Barnes S, Spencer M, Graham D, Johnson HB. Surgical wound irrigation: a call for evidence-based standardization of practice. Am J Infect Control. 2014;42:525–9.
11. Blom A, Cho J, Fleischman A, et al. General assembly, prevention, antiseptic irrigation solution: proceedings of international consensus on orthopedic. J Arthroplasty. 2019;34(2S):S131–8.
12. Chundamala J, Wright JG. The efficacy and risks of using povidone-iodine irrigation to prevent surgical site infection: an evidence-based review. Can J Surg. 2007;50:473–81.
13. Cheng MT, Chang MC, Wang ST, et al. Efficacy of dilute Betadine solution irrigation in the prevention of postoperative infection of spinal surgery. Spine (Phila Pa 1976). 2005;30:1689–93.
14. Oduwole KO, Glynn AA, Molony DC, et al. Antibiofilm activity of sub-inhibitory povidone-iodine concentrations against Staphylococcus epidermidis and Staphylococcus aureus. J Orthop Res. 2010;28:1252–6.
15. Goldenheim PD. In vitro efficacy of povidone-iodine solution and cream against methicillin-resistant Staphylococcus aureus. Postgrad Med J. 1993;69(Suppl 3):S62.
16. Hoekstra MJ, Westgate SJ, Mueller S. Povidone-iodine ointment demonstrates in vitro efficacy against biofilm formation. Int Wound J. 2017;14(1):172–9.
17. Kanno E, Tanno H, Suzuki A, Kamimatsuno R, Tachi M. Reconsideration of iodine in wound irrigation: the effects on Pseudomonas aeruginosa biofilm formation. J Wound Care. 2016;25(6):335–9.
18. Von Keudell A, Canseco JA, Gomoll AH. Deleterious effects of diluted povidoneeiodine on articular cartilage. J Arthroplasty. 2013;28:918–21.
19. Kaysinger KK, Nicholson NC, Ramp WK, Kellam JF. Toxic effects of wound irrigation solutions on cultured tibiae and osteoblasts. J Orthop Trauma. 1995;9:303–11.
20. Brown NM, Cipriano CA, Moric M, Sporer SM, Della Valle CJ. Dilute betadine lavage before closure for the prevention of acute postoperative deep periprosthetic joint infection. J Arthroplasty. 2012;27(1):27–30.
21. Hernandez NM, Hart A, Taunton MJ, et al. Use of povidone-iodine irrigation prior to wound closure in primary Total hip and knee arthroplasty: an analysis of 11,738 cases. J Bone Joint Surg Am. 2019;101(13):1144–50.
22. Calkins TE, Culvern C, Nam D, et al. Dilute betadine lavage reduces the risk of acute postoperative periprosthetic joint infection in aseptic revision total knee and hip arthroplasty: a randomized controlled trial. J Arthroplasty. 2020;35(2):538–543.e1.
23. Haley CE, Marling-Cason M, Smith JW, et al. Bactericidal activity of antiseptics against methicillin-resistant Staphylococcus aureus. J Clin Microbiol. 1985;21:991–2.
24. George J, Klika AK, Higuera CA. Use of chlorhexidine preparations in total joint arthroplasty. J Bone Jt Infect. 2017;2(1):15–22.
25. Lim KS, Kam PC. Chlorhexidine-pharmacology and clinical applications. Anesth Intensive Care. 2008;36(4):502–12.
26. Sobel AD, Hohman D, Jones J, Bisson LJ. Chlorhexidine gluconate cleansing has no effect on the structural properties of human patellar tendon allografts. Arthroscopy. 2012;28(12):1862–6.
27. Kuyyakanond T, Quesnel LB. The mechanism of action of chlorhexidine. FEMS Microbiol Lett. 1992;100(1–3):211–5.
28. Mathur S, Mathur T, Shrivastava R, Khatri R. Chlorhexidine: the gold standard in chemical

plaque control. Natl J Physiol Pharm Pharmacol. 2011;1(2):45.

29. Frisch NB, Kadri OM, Tenbrunsel T, Abdul-Hak A, Qatu M, Davis JJ. Intraoperative chlorhexidine irrigation to prevent infection in total hip and knee arthroplasty. Arthroplast Today. 2017;3(4):294–7.

30. Smith DC, Maiman R, Schwechter EM, Kim SJ, Hirsh DM. Optimal irrigation and debridement of infected total joint implants with chlorhexidine gluconate. J Arthroplasty. 2015;30:1820–2.

31. Liu JX, Werner J, Kirsch T, Zuckerman JD, Virk MS. Cytotoxicity evaluation of chlorhexidine gluconate on human fibroblasts, myoblasts, and osteoblasts. J Bone Jt Infect. 2018;3(4):165–72.

32. Wang Z, Zheng J, Zhao Y, et al. Preoperative bathing with chlorhexidine reduces the incidence of surgical site infections after total knee arthroplasty: a meta-analysis. Medicine (Baltimore). 2017;96(47):e8321.

33. Whiteside LA, Peppers M, Nayfeh TA, Roy ME. Methicillin-resistant *Staphylococcus aureus* in TKA treated with revision and direct intra-articular antibiotic infusion. Clin Orthop Relat Res. 2011;469(1):26–33.

34. Ghobrial GM, Cadotte DW, Williams K Jr, Fehlings MG, Harrop JS. Complications from the use of intrawound vancomycin in lumbar spinal surgery: a systematic review. Neurosurg Focus. 2015;39:E11.

35. O'Neill KR, Smith JG, Abtahi AM, Archer KR, Spengler DM, McGirt MJ, Devin CJ. Reduced surgical site infections in patients undergoing posterior spinal stabilization of traumatic injuries using vancomycin powder. Spine J. 2011;11:641–6.

36. Strom RG, Pacione D, Kalhorn SP, Frempong-Boadu AK. Decreased risk of wound infection after posterior cervical fusion with routine local application of vancomycin powder. Spine (Phila Pa 1976). 2013;38:991–4.

37. Sweet FA, Roh M, Sliva C. Intrawound application of vancomycin for prophylaxis in instrumented thoracolumbar fusions: efficacy, drug levels, and patient outcomes. Spine (Phila Pa 1976). 2011;36:2084–8.

38. Dial BL, Lampley AJ, Green CL, Hallows R. Intrawound vancomycin powder in primary total hip arthroplasty increases rate of sterile wound complications. Hip Pelvis. 2018;30:37–44.

39. Bakhsheshian J, Dahdaleh NS, Lam SK, Savage JW, Smith ZA. The use of vancomycin powder in modern spine surgery: systematic review and meta-analysis of the clinical evidence. World Neurosurg. 2015;83:816–23.

40. Kang DG, Holekamp TF, Wagner SC, Lehman RA Jr. Intrasite vancomycin powder for the prevention of surgical site infection in spine surgery: a systematic literature review. Spine J. 2015;15:762–70.

41. Cooper JJ, Florance H, McKinnon JL, Laycock PA, Aiken SS. Elution profiles of tobramycin and vancomycin from high-purity calcium sulphate beads incubated in a range of simulated body fluids. J Biomater Appl. 2016;31(3):357–65.

42. Cavanaugh DL, Berry J, Yarboro SR, Dahners LE. Better prophylaxis against surgical site infection with local as well as systemic antibiotics. An in vivo study. J Bone Joint Surg Am. 2009;91(8):1907.

43. Edelstein AI, Weiner JA, Cook RW. Intra-articular vancomycin powder eliminates methicillin-resistant *S. aureus* in a rat model of a contaminated intraarticular implant. J Bone Joint Surg Am. 2017;99(3):232–8.

44. Qadir R, Ochsner JL, Chimento GF, Meyer MS, Waddell B, Zavatsky JM. Establishing a role for vancomycin powder application for prosthetic joint infection prevention-results of a wear simulation study. J Arthroplasty. 2014;29:1449–56.

45. Otte JE, Politi JR, Chambers B, Smith CA. Intrawound vancomycin powder reduces early prosthetic joint infections in revision hip and knee arthroplasty. Surg Technol Int. 2017;30:284–9.

46. Patel NN, Guild GN, Kumar AR. Intrawound vancomycin in primary hip and knee arthroplasty: a safe and cost-effective means to decrease early periprosthetic joint infection. Arthroplast Today. 2018;4:479–83.

47. Kurtz SM, Lau E, Watson H, Schmier JK, Parvizi J. Economic burden of periprosthetic joint infection in the United States. J Arthroplasty. 2012;27(8 Suppl):61.

48. Matziolis G, Brodt S, Böhle S, Kirschberg J, Jacob B, Röhner E. Intraarticular vancomycin powder is effective in preventing infections following total hip and knee arthroplasty. Sci Rep. 2020;10:13053.

49. Buchholz HW, Engelbrecht H. Depot effects of various antibiotics mixed with Palacos resins. Chirurg. 1970;41(11):511–5.

50. Anagnostakos K, Fürst O, Kelm J. Antibiotic-impregnated PMMA hip spacers: current status. Acta Orthop. 2006;77(4):628–37.

51. Cui Q, Mihalko WM, Shields JS, Ries M, Saleh KJ. Antibiotic-impregnated cement spacers for the treatment of infection associated with total hip or knee arthroplasty. J Bone Joint Surg Am. 2007;89(4):871–82.

52. Parvizi J, Saleh KJ, Ragland PS, Pour AE, Mont MA. Efficacy of antibiotic-impregnated cement in total hip replacement. Acta Orthop. 2008;79(3):335–41.

53. Jämsen E, Huhtala H, Puolakka T, Moilanen T. Risk factors for infection after knee arthroplasty. A register-based analysis of 43,149 cases. J Bone Joint Surg Am. 2009;91(1):38–47.

54. Iarikov D, Demian H, Rubin D, Alexander J, Nambiar S. Choice and doses of antibacterial agents for cement spacers in treatment of prosthetic joint infections: review of published studies. Clin Infect Dis. 2012;55(11):1474–80.

55. Hinarejos P, Guirro P, Leal J, et al. The use of erythromycin and colistin-loaded cement in total knee arthroplasty does not reduce the incidence of infection: a prospective randomized study in 3000 knees. J Bone Joint Surg Am. 2013;95(9):769–74.

56. Wahlig H, Dingeldein E, Bergmann R, Reuss K. The release of gentamicin from polymethylmethacrylate beads. An experimental and pharmacokinetic study. J Bone Joint Surg Br. 1978;60-B(2):270–5.

57. Wahlig H, Dingeldein E, Bergmann R, Reuss K. Experimentelle und pharmakokinetische Untersuchungen mit gentamycin-PMMA-Kugeln [experimental and pharmacokinetic studies with gentamicin PMMA beads (author's transl)]. Zentralbl Chir. 1979;104(14):923–33.

58. Walenkamp GH, Vree TB, van Rens TJ. Gentamicin-PMMA beads. Pharmacokinetic and nephrotoxicological study. Clin Orthop Relat Res. 1986;(205):171–83.

59. Howlin RP, Brayford MJ, Webb JS, Cooper JJ, Aiken SS, Stoodley P. Antibiotic-loaded synthetic calcium sulfate beads for prevention of bacterial colonization and biofilm formation in periprosthetic infections. Antimicrob Agents Chemother. 2015;59(1):111–20.

60. Gristina AG. Biomaterial-centered infection: microbial adhesion versus tissue integration. Science. 1987;237(4822):1588–95.

61. Neut D, van de Belt H, Stokroos I, van Horn JR, van der Mei HC, Busscher HJ. Biomaterial-associated infection of gentamicin-loaded PMMA beads in orthopaedic revision surgery. J Antimicrob Chemother. 2001;47(6):885–91.

62. Neut D, van de Belt H, van Horn JR, van der Mei HC, Busscher HJ. Residual gentamicin-release from antibiotic-loaded polymethylmethacrylate beads after 5 years of implantation. Biomaterials. 2003;24(10):1829–31.

63. Burd TA, Anglen JO, Lowry KJ, Hendricks KJ, Day D. In vitro elution of tobramycin from bioabsorbable polycaprolactone beads. J Orthop Trauma. 2001;15(6):424–8.

64. Peters CL, Hines JL, Bachus KN, Craig MA, Bloebaum RD. Biological effects of calcium sulfate as a bone graft substitute in ovine metaphyseal defects. J Biomed Mater Res A. 2006;76A(3):456–62.

65. Thomas MV, Puleo DA. Calcium sulfate: properties and clinical applications. J Biomed Mater Res B Appl Biomater. 2009;88(2):597–610.

66. Turner TM, Urban RM, et al. Radiographic and histologic assessment of calcium sulfate in experimental animal models and clinical use as a resorbable bone-graft substitute, a bone-graft expander, and a method for local antibiotic delivery. One institution's experience. J Bone Joint Surg Am. 2001;83-A Suppl 2(Pt 1):8–18.

67. Kelly CM, et al. The use of surgical grade calcium sulphate as a bone graft substitute. Clin Ortho Relat Res. 2001;382:42–50.

68. Gitelis S, et al. Use of calcium sulphate based bone graft substitute for benign bone lesions. Orthopaedics. 2001;4:162–6.

69. Mirzayan R, et al. The use of calcium sulphate in the treatment of benign bone lesions: a preliminary report. J Bone Joint Surg Am. 2001;83:355–8.

70. Peltier L. The use of plaster of Paris to fill large defects in bone. Am J Surg. 1959;97:311–5.

71. Borreli J, et al. Treatment of nonunions and osseous defects with bone graft and calcium sulphate. Clin Orthop Relat Res. 2003;411:245–54.

72. Evaniew N, Tan V, Parasu N, Jurriaans E, Finlay K, Deheshi B, Ghert M. Use of a calcium sulfate-calcium phosphate synthetic bone graft composite in the surgical management of primary bone tumours. Orthopedics. 2013;36(2):e216–22.

73. Lulu GA, Karunanidhi A, Mohamad Yusof L, et al. In vivo efficacy of tobramycin-loaded synthetic calcium phosphate beads in a rabbit model of staphylococcal osteomyelitis. Ann Clin Microbiol Antimicrob. 2018;17:46. https://doi.org/10.1186/s12941-018-0296-3.

74. Ferrando A, Part J, Baeza J. Treatment of Cavitary bone defects in chronic osteomyelitis: bioactive glass S53P4 vs. calcium Sulphate antibiotic beads. J Bone Jt Infect. 2017;2(4):194–201.

75. McKee MD, Li-Bland EA, Wild LM, Schemitsch EH. A prospective, randomized clinical trial comparing an antibiotic-impregnated bioabsorbable bone substitute with standard antibiotic-impregnated cement beads in the treatment of chronic osteomyelitis and infected nonunion. J Orthop Trauma. 2010;24(8):483–90.

76. Lee GH, Khoury JG, Bell JE, Buckwalter JA. Adverse reactions to OsteoSet bone graft substitute, the incidence in a consecutive series. Iowa Orthop J. 2002;22:35–8.

77. Robinson D, Alk D, Sandbank J, Farber R, Halperin N. Inflammatory reactions associated with a calcium sulfate bone substitute. Ann Transplant. 1999;4(3–4):91–7.

78. Flierl MA, Culp BM, Okroj KT, Springer BD, Levine BR, Della Valle CJ. Poor outcomes of irrigation and debridement in acute Periprosthetic joint infection with antibiotic-impregnated calcium sulfate beads. J Arthroplasty. 2017;32(8):2505–7.

79. Kallala R, Harris WE, Ibrahim M, Dipane M, McPherson E. Use of Stimulan absorbable calcium sulphate beads in revision lower limb arthroplasty: safety profile and complication rates. Bone Joint Res. 2018;7(10):570–9.

80. Gramlich Y, Walter G, Klug A, Harbering J, Kemmerer M, Hoffmann R. Procedure for single-stage implant retention for chronic periprosthetic infection using topical degradable calcium-based antibiotics. Int Orthop. 2019;43(7):1559–66.

81. Calanna F, Chen F, Risitano S, et al. Debridement, antibiotic pearls, and retention of the implant (DAPRI): a modified technique for implant retention in total knee arthroplasty PJI treatment. J Orthop Surg (Hong Kong). 2019;27(3):2309499019874413.

82. McPherson E, Dipane M, Sherif S. Dissolvable antibiotic beads in treatment of Periprosthetic joint infection and revision arthroplasty—the use of synthetic pure calcium sulfate (Stimulan®) impregnated

with Vancomycin & Tobramycin. Reconstr Rev. 2013;3:32–43.

83. Marczak D, Synder M, Sibiński M, Okoń T, Kowalczewski J. The use of calcium carbonate beads containing gentamicin in the second stage septic revision of total knee arthroplasty reduces reinfection rate. Knee. 2016;23(2):322–6.

84. Lum ZC, Pereira GC. Local bio-absorbable antibiotic delivery in calcium sulfate beads in hip and knee arthroplasty. J Orthop. 2018;15(2):676–8.

85. Baeza J, Cury MB, Fleischman A, et al. General assembly, prevention, local antimicrobials: proceedings of international consensus on orthopedic infections. J Arthroplasty. 2019;34(2S):S75–84.

86. Kallala R, Haddad FS. Hypercalcaemia following the use of antibiotic-eluting absorbable calcium sulphate beads in revision arthroplasty for infection. Bone Joint J. 2015;97-B(9):1237–41.

87. Romanò Morelli I, Battaglia AG, Drago L. Antibacterial coating of implants: are we missing something? Bone Joint Res. 2019;8(5):199–206.

88. Fromm KM. Silver coordination compounds with antimicrobial properties. Appl Organomet Chem. 2013;27:683–7.

89. Chernousova S, Epple M. Silver as antibacterial agent: ion, nanoparticle, and metal. Angem Chem Int Ed Engl. 2013;52:1636–53.

90. Roy M, Fielding GA, Beyenal H, Bandyopadhyay A, Bose S. Mechanical, in vitro antimicrobial, and biological properties of plasma-sprayed silver-doped hydroxyapatite coating. ACS Appl Mater Interfaces. 2012;4(3):1341–9.

91. Fielding GA, Roy M, Bandyopadhyay A, Bose S. Antibacterial and biological characteristics of silver containing and strontium doped plasma sprayed hydroxyapatite coatings. Acta Biomater. 2012;8(8):3144–52.

92. Bosetti M, Masse A, Tobin E, Cannas M. Silver coated materials for external fixation devices: in vitro biocompatibility and genotoxicity. Biomaterials. 2002;23(3):887–92.

93. Zhao L, Chu PK, Zhang Y, Wu Z. Antibacterial coatings on titanium implants. J Biomed Mater Res B Appl Biomater. 2009;91(1):470–80.

94. DeVasConCellos P, Bose S, Beyenal H, Bandyopadhyay A, Zirkle LG. Antimicrobial particulate silver coatings on stainless steel implants for fracture management. Mater Sci Eng C. 2012;32(5):1112–20.

95. Hardes J, Von Eiff C, Streitbuerger A, et al. Reduction of periprosthetic infection with silver-coated megaprostheses in patients with bone sarcoma. J Surg Oncol. 2010;101(5):389–95.

96. Hardes J, Henrichs MP, Hauschild G, Nottrott M, Guder W, Streitbuerger A. Silver-coated megaprosthesis of the proximal tibia in patients with sarcoma. J Arthroplasty. 2017;32(7):2208–13.

97. Zajonz D, Birke U, Ghanem M, et al. Silver-coated modular megaendoprostheses in salvage revision arthroplasty after periimplant infection with exten-sive bone loss—a pilot study of 34 patients. BMC Musculoskelet Disord. 2017;18(1):383.

98. Wafa H, Grimer RJ, Reddy K, et al. Retrospective evaluation of the incidence of early periprosthetic infection with silver-treated endoprostheses in high-risk patients: case-control study. Bone Joint J. 2015;97-B(2):252–7.

99. Mijnendonckx K, Leys N, Mahillon J, Silver S, Van Houdt R. Antimicrobial silver: uses, toxicity and potential for resistance. Biometals. 2013;26(4):609–21.

100. Feng QL, Wu J, Chen GQ, Cui FZ, Kim TN, Kim JO. A mechanistic study of the antibacterial effect of silver ions on *Escherichia coli* and *Staphylococcus aureus*. J Biomed Mater Res. 2002;52:662–8.

101. Gordon O, Vig Slenters T, Brunetto PS, Villarus AE, Sturdevant DE, Otto M, et al. Silver coordination polymers for prevention of implant infection: thiol interaction, impact on respiratory chain enzymes, and hydroxyl radical induction. Antimicrob Agents Chemother. 2010;54:4208–18.

102. Maillard JY, Hartemann P. Silver as an antimicrobial: facts and gaps in knowledge. Crit Rev Microbiol. 2013;39:373–83.

103. Randall CP, Gupta A, Jackson N, Busse D, O'Neil AJ. Silver resistance in gram-negative bacteria: a dissection of endogenous and exogenous mechanisms. J Antimicrob Chemother. 2015;70:1037–46.

104. Trentinaglia MT, Van Der Straeten C, Morelli I, Logoluso N, Drago L, Romanò CL. Economic evaluation of antibacterial coatings on healthcare costs in first year following total joint arthroplasty. J Arthroplasty. 2018;33(6):1656–62.

105. Shirai T, Shimizu T, Ohtani K, Zen Y, Takaya M, Tsuchiya H. Antibacterial iodine-supported titanium implants. Acta Biomater. 2011;7(4):1928–33.

106. Inoue D, Kabata T, Ohtani K, Kajino Y, Shirai T, Tsuchiya H. Inhibition of biofilm formation on iodine-supported titanium implants. Int Orthop. 2017;41(6):1093–9.

107. Tsuchiya H, Shirai T, Nishida H, et al. Innovative antimicrobial coating of titanium implants with iodine. J Orthop Sci. 2012;17(5):595–604.

108. Shirai T, Tsuchiya H, Nishida H, et al. Antimicrobial megaprostheses supported with iodine. J Biomater Appl. 2014;29(4):617–23.

109. Kabata T, Maeda T, Kajino Y, et al. Iodine-supported hip implants: short term clinical results. Biomed Res Int. 2015;2015:368124.

110. Pitarresi G, Palumbo FS, Calascibetta F, Fiorica C, Di Stefano M, Giammona G. Medicated hydrogels of hyaluronic acid derivatives for use in orthopedic field. Int J Pharm. 2013;449(1–2):84–94.

111. Junter GA, Thébault P, Lebrun L. Polysaccharide-based antibiofilm surfaces. Acta Biomater. 2016;30:13–25.

112. Ardizzoni A, Neglia RG, Baschieri MC, et al. Influence of hyaluronic acid on bacterial and

fungal species, including clinically relevant opportunistic pathogens. J Mater Sci Mater Med. 2011;22(10):2329–38.

113. Drago L, Boot W, Dimas K, et al. Does implant coating with antibacterial-loaded hydrogel reduce bacterial colonization and biofilm formation in vitro? Clin Orthop Relat Res. 2014;472(11):3311–23.

114. Romanò CL, De Vecchi E, Bortolin M, Morelli I, Drago L. Hyaluronic acid and its composites as a local antimicrobial/antiadhesive barrier. J Bone Jt Infect. 2017;2(1):63–72.

115. Romanò CL, Malizos K, Capuano N, et al. Does an antibiotic-loaded hydrogel coating reduce early post-surgical infection after joint arthroplasty? J Bone Jt Infect. 2016;1:34–41.

116. Malizos K, Blauth M, Danita A, et al. Fast-resorbable antibiotic-loaded hydrogel coating to reduce post-surgical infection after internal osteosynthesis: a multicenter randomized controlled trial. J Orthop Traumatol. 2017;18(2):159–69.

117. Capuano N, Logoluso N, Gallazzi E, Drago L, Romanò CL. One-stage exchange with antibacterial hydrogel coated implants provides similar results to two-stage revision, without the coating, for the treatment of peri-prosthetic infection. Knee Surg Sports Traumatol Arthrosc. 2018;26(11):3362–7.

118. Zagra L, Gallazzi E, Romanò D, Scarponi S, Romanò C. Two-stage cementless hip revision for peri-prosthetic infection with an antibacterial hydrogel coating: results of a comparative series. Int Orthop. 2019;43(1):111–5.

119. Parvizi J, Pawasarat IM, Azzam KA, Joshi A, Hansen EN, Bozic KJ. Periprosthetic joint infection: the economic impact of methicillin-resistant infections. J Arthroplasty. 2010;25(6 Suppl):103–7.

120. Berend KR, Lombardi AV Jr, Morris MJ, Bergeson AG, Adams JB, Sneller MA. Two-stage treatment of hip periprosthetic joint infection is associated with a high rate of infection control but high mortality. Clin Orthop Relat Res. 2013;471(2):510–8.

Surgical Approaches

14

Georgi P. Georgiev

14.1 Introduction

Nowadays, total knee arthroplasty (TKA) is performed after failure of non-operative treatment in cases of chronic pain in knee osteoarthritis and cases with significant knee deformities; usually, this procedure has significant success in pain relief and patient satisfaction [1]. However, following TKA, numerous complications have been reported in the literature; they include aseptic implant loosening with significant osteolysis, polyethylene wear, ligamentous laxity, periprosthetic fracture, arthrofibrosis, patellofemoral complications, and infections. Thus, revision surgery becomes necessary [2].

In revision TKA (rTKA), wound closure might be difficult. Precise anatomical knowledge of the knee and the appropriate surgical exposure could reduce the risk of complications and could dispose in good functional outcomes. The ideal approach ensures easy and straightforward joint exposure and facilitates the revision with minimum complication rates. Therefore, detailed knowledge of surgical approaches to the knee is essential. The surgeon should have various options in mind, even in cases when simple excision of previous scars ensures excellent visualization of the knee [3].

The preoperative planning of the surgical approach is crucial for rTKA. The correct approach depends on the selection of implants and allows for their optimal position and precise ligament balancing. After previous TKA, especially in an infected knee, subsequent approaches are impeded by scar formation in the deep tissue layers and the poor elasticity of the infected tissues. Existing debris and trauma of surrounding tissues due to instability additionally degrade tissue properties [4].

During rTKA, two essential rules should be borne in mind by the surgeon: safe approach and precise surgical technique during managing soft tissue flaps. At revision surgery, a medial parapatellar approach (MPA) with synovectomy, a quadriceps snip, a tibial tubercle osteotomy (TTO), a V-Y quadricepsplasty, a femoral peel (FP), and a medial epicondylar osteotomy (MEO) have been proposed [5]. Till now, no prospective randomized studies have presented and compared the results after different approaches for knee revision arthroplasty [4].

Detailed knowledge of the different surgical approaches described and discussed in this chapter, in the author's opinion, will be of help to knee surgeons in their works, as well as to the other colleagues who will perform this surgery in their future practice. The aim is to briefly summarize the characteristic anatomy of the area, discuss the

G. P. Georgiev (✉)
Department of Orthopedics and Traumatology,
University Hospital Queen Giovanna—ISUL,
Medical University of Sofia, Sofia, Bulgaria

© ISAKOS 2022
U. G. Longo et al. (eds.), *Infection in Knee Replacement*,
https://doi.org/10.1007/978-3-030-81553-0_14

possible complications and how to avoid them, and present the surgical approaches in detail. This information could be important in preventing damage to anatomical structures, especially in infected tissues, impeding surgical dissection.

14.2 Skin Incisions

The skin incision and approach should be considered to fully visualize the operated joint without excessive tension to the skin edges. However, before performing the incision, precise knowledge of the skin arterial blood supply, as well as the surrounding anatomical structures around the joint is mandatory. Detailed knowledge of anatomy will reduce the risk of possible iatrogenic damage during surgery and help avoid possible future complications.

The blood supply to the skin and the surrounding tissues around the knee is from the peripatellar arterial ring. This ring is formed by the supreme genicular, medial/lateral superior genicular, medial/lateral inferior genicular, and anterior tibial recurrent arteries [6]. The skin vascular supply is mainly ensured by subfascial arterioles that start from the medial side of the joint. Therefore, during the surgical approach, their protection without additional dissection is crucial. It should be pointed out that cutaneous blood supply may be disturbed after previous surgery, in rheumatoid or diabetic patients, after prolonged steroid/NSAIDs therapy, in cases of extra obesity, and older smokers [7].

A midline longitudinal incision is preferred because it better preserves the arterial supply of the skin. A large lateral flap should be avoided to minimize the complications in wound healing. This corresponds to the report of Johnson et al. [8], in which they established lower skin oxygenation of the lateral flap. Aso et al. [9], in midline skin incisions below 12 cm, did not establish any differences in oxygenation of the skin and pointed out that hypoxia was significant in the distal edges and might be due to excessive retraction during operation.

A straight longitudinal incision starts 6–12 cm proximally to the proximal border of the patella, passes over its midpoint, and reaches the medial border of the tibial tuberosity [7]. As an alternative, the incision could make a gentle medial curve over the patella [10]. Of course, the extent of the incision reflects the surgery requirements. As mentioned above, the skin is supplied by perforating arteries running through the fascia; therefore, a soft-tissue flap should be developed deep into the fascia to avoid skin necrosis [7]. The incision is extended through the underlying tissues to ensure enough skin flaps superficial to the extensor mechanism. With a proper skin incision, the surgeon reduces skin retraction and the risk of postoperative necrosis [11].

In the case of a previous anterior scar in a proper position, it should be incorporated in the new approach. In cases of multiple previous incisions, the most lateral should be preferred with full-thickness flaps [12]. Khan et al. [13] recommend the most recent, longitudinal, and lateral skin incision to be used after a prior TKA [13]. Daines [14] advocates a midline approach if multiple scars existed from surgeries a long time ago. In extensive fibrosis, the extension of the incision into normal tissue helps in deep dissection. Previous transverse approaches need to be crossed perpendicularly, and a new incision with an angle of below 60° to a previous scar is not recommended [15]. Windsor et al. [15] considered that skin bridges need to be over 7 cm wide to reduce the risk of flap necrosis. If the surgeon needs another new approach, a safe distance between the incisions should be ensured. Thienpont [4] points out that a skin bridge of at least 2.5 cm to 8 cm is needed.

In summary, a previous skin incision should be used if possible, except in cases of direct medial, lateral, or transverse incisions [7]. In infected rTKA, the skin incision should be safe and anatomically considered. After limb draping, previous scars should be well visible [5, 16]. Firstly, the debridement starts with the excision of the previous cicatrix, and in the case of a fistula, it should also be included in the excised tissue. If any sinus tracts are present, they should be excised to the joint capsule together with radical synovectomy [17].

14.3 Medial Parapatellar Approach

The MPA has been accepted as the workhorse of rTKA [18]. In 1878, von Langenbeck [19] described this approach for the first time. In over 90% of revision knee arthroplasties, a medial parapatellar arthrotomy has been preferred [4]. Della Valle et al. [16] present that in 92% of patients, the MPA in rTKA gave an adequate view of the knee joint.

Usually, a longitudinal midline skin incision is used. The incision of the parapatellar retinaculum is extended proximally, just lateral to the medial border of the quadriceps tendon, with a 3- to 4-mm intact part of the tendon on the vastus medialis for better closure of the approach; distally, the incision is extended along the medial border of the patella and the patellar tendon, leaving enough soft tissues on the patella for later closure [7] (Fig. 14.1). As an alternative, the so-called *wandering resident's approach* could be used. In this technique, detachment of the distal part of the quadriceps tendon in an oblique proximal-lateral direction from its insertion to the patella could be performed [3] (Fig. 14.2). A medial parapatellar arthrotomy ensures lateral eversion of the patella and maximally preserves the lymphatic and nerve branches [12].

The advantages of MPA include an excellent view and an easy and safe performance. The reported disadvantages are disruption of the quadriceps mechanism and destabilized patella [19], injury of the superior lateral genicular artery, and injury of the infrapatellar branch of the saphenous nerve with a painful neuroma [20].

In rTKA, the MPA with an extensive synovectomy is usually performed. Excision of all adhesions from the suprapatellar pouch and the deep surface of the quadriceps tendon ensures better visualization of the joint; thereafter, with the knee extended, the medial and lateral gutters should be released. Elevation of a subperiosteal flap of the medial retinaculum and the deep medial collateral ligament down to the semimembranosus insertion allows for external rotation of the tibia and thus facilitates access to the knee [5]. The extensor apparatus should be mobilized

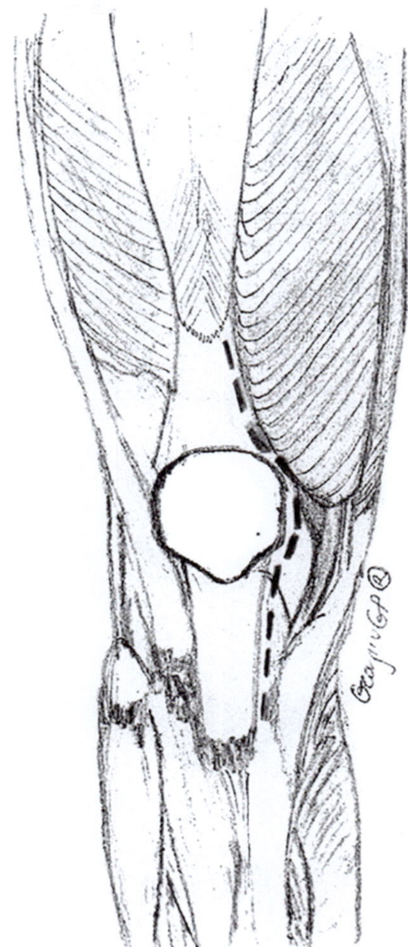

Fig. 14.1 Medial parapatellar approach

safely after releasing and excising the scar tissue between the patellar tendon and the anterolateral tibia, as well as adhesions on the lateral side of the patella to allow for patellar subluxation. This reduces the risk of patellar tendon injury [5]. Eversion of the patella is ensured by external rotation of the tibia together with knee flexion until anterior subluxation of the tibia occurs [13]. With severe adhesions and limited visualization, a lateral release should be performed for patellar mobilization. In cases of risk for avulsion of the tendon, a pin on the tendon insertion should be used [13]. Then, removal of the polyethylene inlay could be done [4]. Removing the polyethylene liner allows for better visualization and is

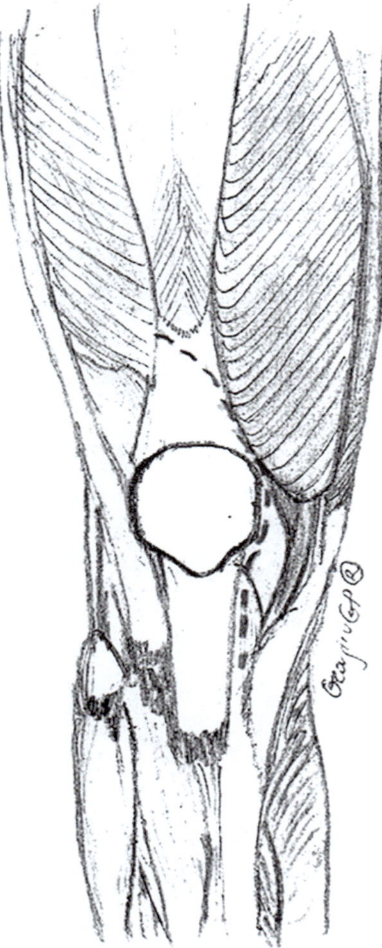

Fig. 14.2 The wandering resident's approach

followed by the removal of prosthesis components. After components removal, posterior synovectomy and posterior release could be made. Precise posterior release might prevent the elevation of the joint line [5].

14.4 Insall's Modification to Medial Parapatellar Approach

Due to the disruption of the extensor mechanism, instability, and damage to the patellar articular surface, a modification of MPA was proposed by Insall [21]. This technique ensures a more lateral

parapatellar arthrotomy and, in that way, allows for easier lateral subluxation or eversion of the patella [22].

In this approach, the division of the quadriceps tendon is 8–10 cm above the patella; the incision is prolonged over the medial one-third of the patella, thus detaching the medial patellofemoral ligament; the quadriceps expansion is sharply detached from the medial third of the bone till the medial part of the patella is clearly revealed; the incision is prolonged around the patella and over the medial one-third of the patellar tendon down to the tibial tuberosity [7, 22]. During wound closure, the medial retinaculum is sutured to the lateral two-thirds of the patella. Vaishya et al. [7], during suture of the extensor apparatus, applied three stitches between the medial retinaculum and the patella in the 90° flexed knee.

The disadvantages of the approach included injury to the infrapatellar branch of the saphenous nerve, patellar dislocation, subluxation, stress fractures, and fragmentation of the patella secondary to avascular necrosis [23, 24].

14.5 Lateral Approach

The lateral approach was published for the first time by Cameron and Fedorkow in 1882 [25]. Later, in 1991, Keblish [26] developed it for use in TKA in valgus knees and considered it as technically demanding. In cases of revision surgery, especially in infection, if a lateral arthrotomy has been previously performed, it should also be used in the subsequent approach; medial arthrotomy could provoke avascular osteonecrosis of the patella [13].

Anterior midline skin incision, a curvilinear midline skin incision, or a laterally placed anterior skin incision could be used [13, 26]. Usually, the skin incision starts around 5 cm proximally to the base of the patella and reaches the tibial tubercle. The incision is deepened through the subcutaneous tissue and the prepatellar bursa, and after reaching the lateral part of the patella, a parapatellar arthrotomy is started from the lateral side of the quadriceps tendon, passing over the

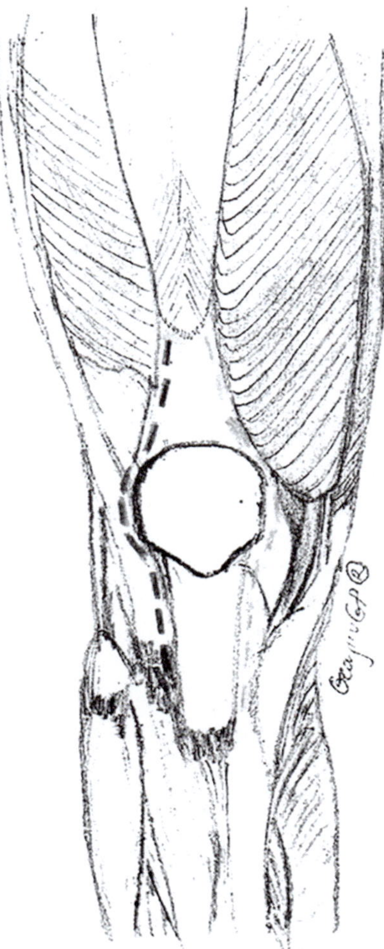

Fig. 14.3 Lateral parapatellar approach

lateral side of the patella to the anterior compartment fascia to the tibial tuberosity (Fig. 14.3). Then, medial eversion of the patella in extended knee is done; thereafter, knee flexion ensures exposure of the joint [7, 13]. Preserving a medial soft-tissue cuff ensures easier closure of the incision of the lateral retinaculum later [26].

14.6 Techniques for Exposure of Difficult TKA

rTKA is commonly performed using MPA. However, revision surgery is not an easy task and sometimes poses real challenges for surgeons. Scars from the previous operations make exposure to the joint difficult. Particular attention should be directed to the insertion site of the patellar tendon during eversion of the patella. In some difficult cases, the need for a more extensive exposure of the joint should be accepted [3–5, 7, 13, 27]. Different options for better exposure of the joint and easier removal of prosthetic components are clearly summarized and explained below. The author hopes this to be of use to revision surgeons and help them in their practice and other surgeons who will perform this surgery in the future.

14.6.1 Rectus Snip

In cases of limited exposure after MPA, a "quadriceps snip" or "rectus snip" is an option. Indications for a rectus snip include failure of adequate exposure after medial gutters debridement and medial release from the tibia together with debridement of the lateral gutters [13].

In 1983, Insall et al. [28] described the rectus snip for quadriceps lengthening, thus releasing the proximal tension of the quadriceps. In this technique, the proximal part of the medial parapatellar arthrotomy is prolonged obliquely and laterally at a 45°-angle to divide the tendon of the rectus femoris muscle from a distal-medial to proximal-lateral direction (Fig. 14.4). The underlying tendinous parts of the vasti muscles should also be cut. It should be pointed out that no detachment from the vastus lateralis should be performed [3–5, 7, 13, 27]. For anatomical repair of the tendon, Abdel and Della Valle [5] recommended putting two nonabsorbable sutures at the corners of where the quadriceps snip is started [5].

The advantages of this technique are its simplicity and effectiveness, ease of performance, no extensor lag, no need for modification of rehabilitation after surgery, protection of the lateral superior genicular artery, and the tendon of vastus lateralis [27, 29, 30]. Barrack et al. [31] and Garvin et al. [29] established no weakness in the strength of quadriceps after this technique.

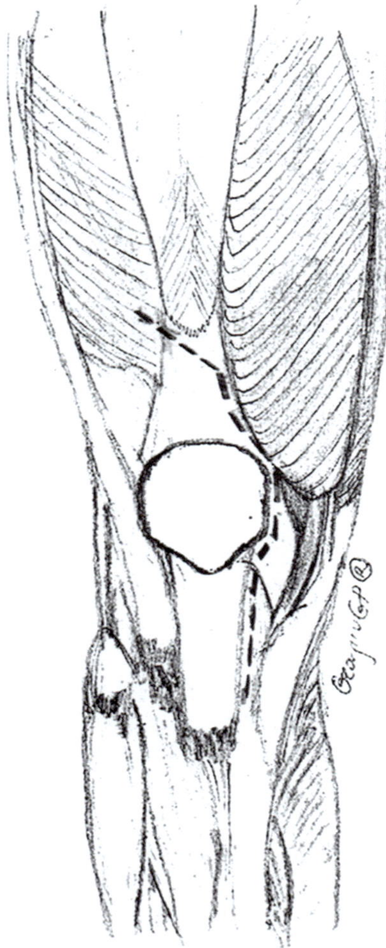

Fig. 14.4 The quadriceps snip

In summary, the rectus snip could be described simply as an oblique apical extension of the knee arthrotomy through the patellar tendon. This technique should not be performed through the muscle because it is difficult to repair, impeding the early postoperative rehabilitation [18].

14.6.2 V-Y Quadricepsplasty

A medial parapatellar retinacular incision can be extended into a V-Y quadricepsplasty procedure through the lateral patellar retinaculum if better exposure of the knee is needed in rTKA

[32]. Abdel and Della Valle [5] point out that a V-Y quadricepsplasty is rarely performed, usually in cases of shortening or contracture of the extensor apparatus when real lengthening is needed and also to facilitate the exposure. It could also be used in cases of degraded local skin conditions over the proximal tibia or with insufficient bone stock after TTO with poor capacity to heal. However, when the exposure is inadequate, and it seems to be due to contracture of the distal part of the extensor apparatus, a TTO is indicated [13].

Coonse and Adams [32] were the first to present a V-shaped turndown of the distal quadriceps for better visualization of the knee joint. Later, Insall used it during MPA; he extended the arthrotomy from the apex, in a distal and lateral direction at a 45° angle, through the vastus lateralis tendon down to the anterior fibers of the iliotibial band. In that way, the formed flap gives an easy approach to the knee [33] (Fig. 14.5). A V-shaped approach can be further changed into Y if the incision is extended proximally to the apex of the V [7].

In this technique, care should be taken to avoid injury of the superior lateral genicular artery. Moreover, excessive thinning of the peripatellar fat pad could lead to loss of blood supply to the patella. Cases of radiographic but asymptomatic patellar osteonecrosis after quadriceps turndown have been reported [34].

The closure of the V-Y quadricepsplasty should be performed at 30° of knee flexion [5]. Postoperatively, for 6 weeks brace protection, restriction of flexion, limited range of motion, and partial weight-bearing are mandatory [5, 35]. A V-Y quadricepsplasty could lead to an extensor lag after revision [5]. Scott and Siliski [36] presented their experience with this technique in 7 patients, and in 4 of them, transient extensor lag was established; in the other three, the lag was permanent. In contrast, Trousdale et al. [37] presented their experience with this technique in revision and primary TKA. They concluded that after V-Y quadricepsplasty, the patients had near to normal extension and moderate extensor weakness. These results were based on 9 revisions and 5 primary TKAs.

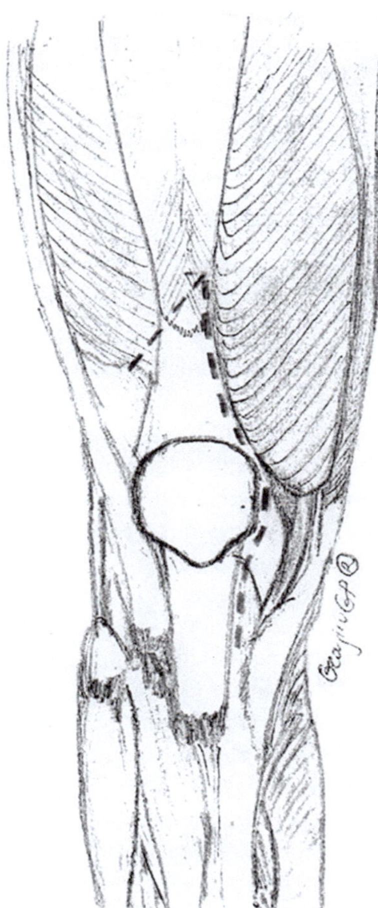

Fig. 14.5 V-Y quadricepsplasty

14.6.3 Tibial Tubercle Osteotomy

A TTO is performed in cases when other techniques cannot ensure adequate visibility of the knee. TTO allows for distal release of the extensor mechanism and is indicated in patients with stable tibial component or second re-implantation with excessive fibrotic tissue, in cases of extraction of a long-stemmed tibial component, in patients with excessive scarring at the anterolateral tibial area or when there is arthrofibrosis or patella baja [4, 5, 27]. A relative contraindication for TTO is the poor bone quality of the tibial tubercle, which impedes adequate fixation of the osteotomized fragment [38].

In 1983, Dolin reported a TTO for the first time [39]. Later, this technique was modified by Whiteside and Ohl [40]. The TTO is made in the coronal plane from the medial side of the tibia. The osteotomized fragment should be 7–10 cm long and should have a thickness of 1 cm proximally tapering to 5 mm distally [41] (Fig. 14.6). According to Tanzer and Burnett [27], the thickness of the osteotomized fragment should be 10–20 mm, because a smaller fragment could be fractured and would have a limited area for healing after fixation. Usually, the length of the fragment is 8–10 cm, but it depends on the needs of the surgical exposure. If the tibial tubercle will not be transferred, pre-drilling of the fragment before osteotomy is preferable. The TTO is made with the knee extended or slightly flexed [27]. After osteotomy, the fragment needs to be reflected laterally on an osteoperiosteal hinge. Preserving the attachments of the muscles of the anterior compartment is crucial for the fragment's vitality [5].

At the end of the procedure, the osteotomy needs to be reduced with the knee extended

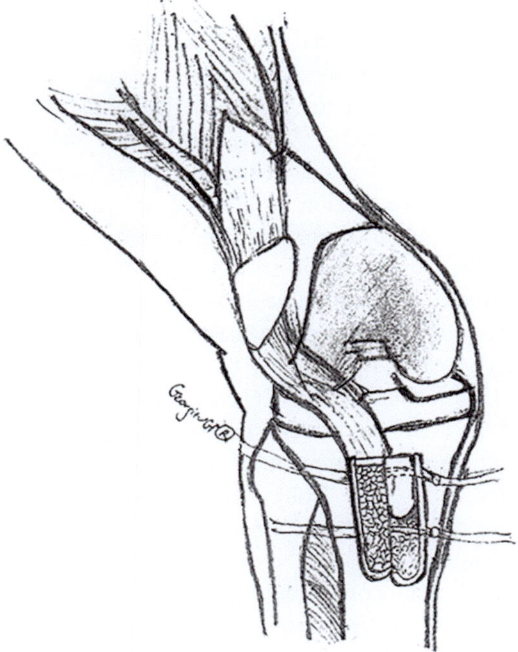

Fig. 14.6 Tibial tubercle osteotomy

and the fragment returned to its anatomical place. In cases of patella baja, the fragment could be transferred and reattached proximally [7]. In addition, autologous bone grafts could be placed around the fragment and in the surrounding free bony areas [27]. The fragment could be reattached by wire/cable fixation, screws, or a combination thereof. Usually, the wire fixation is performed by 2–4 stainless steel #16 g wires [27]. Della Valle et al. [5] prefer to fix the fragment with three 16-gauge wires [16].

According to Tanzer and Burnett [27], in larger fragments and good bone quality, fixation could be performed with two to four screws perpendicular to the cut surface, thus ensuring better compression. In stemmed tibial components, the screws need to be inserted obliquely to avoid the stem of the prosthesis. Usage of titanium screws is preferable, avoiding galvanic corrosion between stainless steel screws and titanium or cobalt-chrome stem.

After fixation of the fragment, the stability of fixation is tested by gentle flexion. This determines the postoperative active range of motion. Passive range of motion and high flexion attempts are not allowed in the first 12–16 weeks. A hinged brace locked in extension ensures weight-bearing [27]. According to Abdel and Della Valle [5], flexion is limited to <90° with a brace for 6 weeks. During mobilization, the brace is locked in extension. Active flexion is allowed, but an active extension and straight leg raises are avoided. Of course, the rehabilitation protocol with an increase of exercises depends on the stability of fixation. The brace could be removed at 12 weeks [27].

The advantages of TTO are excellent visibility of the knee, easy lateral eversion of the patella, sparing the attachment of the patellar tendon, easy and secure fixation of the fragment, and preservation of the blood supply to the extensor apparatus [27].

Different complications of TTO have been reported: non-union or delayed union, displacement of the fragment, iatrogenic fracture, hardware cutout, persistent anterior knee pain, infection, necrosis of the wound, excessive prominence of the hardware, periprosthetic fracture, and restricted physiotherapy protocol [4, 13, 27, 31, 40, 41].

In summary, the TTO could be performed when other techniques have failed. Lower patient satisfaction after TTO was established [31].

14.6.4 Femoral Peel

As its name suggests, in FP, a full subperiosteal release of the distal femur is performed, the so-called femoral skeletonization. This technique violates the stability of the joint and needs to be used only in cases with restriction of flexion due to excessive scar tissue and failure of the other techniques. In rTKA with no excessive scar tissue, additional release of the surrounding knee structures will predispose to instability. In cases of excessive scar formation, this technique ensures stability despite the stripping of the ligaments and joint capsule [3, 13, 27].

In 1988, Windsor and Insall [42] used the FP in a severely ankylosed knee. During its performance, all soft tissues were subperiosteally released from the distal femur. In this technique, the medial collateral ligament and joint capsule are released, which causes knee instability but allows for excision of the fibrotic tissues that do not allow flexion. In case of inadequate release, the dissection is broadened with the detachment of the lateral collateral ligament and joint capsule, and thus real skeletonization of the femur is achieved; this could provoke devascularization of the distal part of the femur. All surrounding tissues should be detached with a scalpel or with electrocautery, as close to the bone as possible. The soft-tissue release should allow for full excision of the scar tissue from the posterior corner of the knee for better flexion. This technique could be extended with disinsertion of the origins of the gastrocnemius muscles. Finally, the surgeon does not reattach the ligaments and only closes the structures layer by layer in an extended knee [3, 13, 27].

With this technique, Lahav and Hofmann [43] had no cases of ruptures of the extensor apparatus or compromised extension of the knee.

The reported complications after femoral peel are iatrogenic vascular injury, tibiofemoral dislocations, infection, rupture of the patellar tendon, and periprosthetic fracture [44].

14.6.5 Medial Epicondylar Osteotomy

MEO is indicated in cases where flexion of the knee is blocked, but there is no excessive scarring of the surrounding structures. The choice between FP and MEO depends on the scarred tissue found during surgery [3, 13, 27].

In 1999, Engh [45] was the first to describe this technique for better visualization and correction of a varus deformity of the knee. The osteotomy is done with the knee flexed at 90°. With an osteotome, the bone cut is started laterally to the origin of the medial collateral ligament and finished above the insertion of the adductor magnus tendon, and thus the osteotomized fragment includes the medial epicondyle and the adductor tubercle (Fig. 14.7). A bone segment around 4 cm long and 1 cm wide is formed and hinged posteriorly, including the insertions of the medial collateral ligament and the tendons of the adductor magnus muscle. After flexion of the joint and eversion of the patella, the knee could be opened by external rotation and a valgus bend. At the end of the procedure, after implantation of the components, the bone segment is reattached by a minimum of three stitches with heavy nonabsorbable sutures, at 90° of knee flexion, or by a single screw. In some cases, this technique could be performed on the lateral epicondyle when lateral exposure is needed [3, 13, 27].

14.7 Conclusion

Knowledge of the clinical anatomy of the knee is crucial for preparing and performing different options for better and atraumatic exposure of the knee. Apart from the gold standard, the MPA with synovectomy in rTKA, the knowledge of other approaches, and better visualization

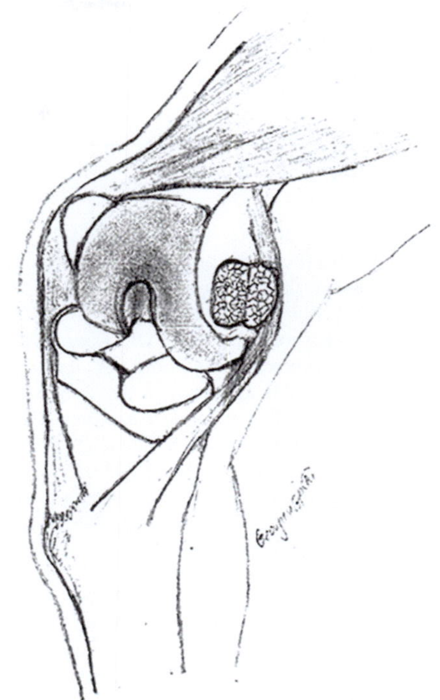

Fig. 14.7 Medial epicondylar osteotomy

options are essential. The aim of the surgical approach in rTKA should be to allow easy removal of components and implants and implantation of others without damaging the extensor apparatus or other surrounding structures. In cases where additional exposure is needed, a quadriceps snip could be performed. Rarely, in difficult revisions, TTO and V-Y quadricepsplasty are excellent options. Finally, the author would like to present the results and experience of Barrack et al. [31] after evaluation of 123 cases of rTKA from three centers. They concluded that the results after a standard MPA were the same with or without the quadriceps snip; patients with quadricepsplasty and a TTO had the same results, but worse than the standard approach. The results of patients with quadricepsplasty were significantly better in terms of a range of motion than the TTO group; patients after TTO had a lower degree of extension lag but a higher degree of difficulties with kneeling and stooping and a high rate of dissatisfaction with surgery.

Acknowledgments The author thanks Assist. Prof. Dr. Svetoslav A. Slavchev (Department of Orthopaedics and Traumatology, Medical University of Sofia, Bulgaria) for his kind proofreading of the English text.

References

1. Postler A, Lützner C, Beyer F, Tille E, Lützner J. Analysis of total knee arthroplasty revision causes. BMC Musculoskelet Disord. 2018;19(1):55. https://doi.org/10.1186/s12891-018-1977-y.
2. Chun KC, Kweon SH, Nam DJ, Kang HT, Chun CH. Tibial tubercle osteotomy vs the extensile medial parapatellar approach in revision total knee arthroplasty: is tibial tubercle osteotomy a harmful approach? J Arthroplasty. 2019;34(12):2999–3003. https://doi.org/10.1016/j.arth.2019.07.015.
3. Engh GA. Exposure options for revision total knee arthroplasty. In: Bono JV, Scott RD, editors. Revision total knee arthroplasty. 1st ed. New York: Springer; 2005. p. 63–75.
4. Thienpont E. Revision knee surgery techniques. EFORT Open Rev. 2017;1(5):233–8. https://doi.org/10.1302/2058-5241.1.000024.
5. Abdel MP, Della Valle CJ. The surgical approach for revision total knee arthroplasty. Bone Joint J. 2016;98-B(1 Suppl A):113–5. https://doi.org/10.1302/0301-620X.98B1.36315.
6. Lazaro LE, Cross MB, Lorich DG. Vascular anatomy of the patella: implications for total knee arthroplasty surgical approaches. Knee. 2014;21(3):655–60. https://doi.org/10.1016/j.knee.2014.03.005.
7. Vaishya R, Vijay V, Demesugh DM, Agarwal AK. Surgical approaches for total knee arthroplasty. J Clin Orthop Trauma. 2016;7(2):71–9. https://doi.org/10.1016/j.jcot.2015.11.003.
8. Johnson DP, Houghton TA, Radford P. Anterior midline or medial parapatellar incision for arthroplasty of the knee. A comparative study. J Bone Joint Surg Br. 1986;68(5):812–4.
9. Aso K, Ikeuchi M, Izumi M, Kato T, Tani T. Transcutaneous oxygen tension in the anterior skin of the knee after minimal incision total knee arthroplasty. Knee. 2012;19(5):576–9. https://doi.org/10.1016/j.knee.2011.10.002.
10. Warren LF, Marshall JL. The supporting structures and layers on the medial side of the knee: an anatomical analysis. J Bone Joint Surg Am. 1979;61(1):56–62.
11. Younger AS, Duncan CP, Masri BA. Surgical exposures in revision total knee arthroplasty. J Am Acad Orthop Surg. 1998;6(1):55–64.
12. Colombel M, Mariz Y, Dahhan P, Kénési C. Arterial and lymphatic supply of the knee integuments. Surg Radiol Anat. 1998;20(1):35–40.
13. Khan M, Green G, Gabr A, Haddad FS. Principles of revision total knee arthroplasty: incisions, approaches, implant removal and debridement. In: Rodríguez-Merchán E, Oussedik S, editors. Total knee arthroplasty. 1st ed. Cham, Heidelberg, New York, Dordrecht, London: Springer; 2015. p. 235–47.
14. Daines BK. Avoiding wound complications in total knee replacement. In: Hirschmann M, Becker R, editors. The unhappy total knee replacement a comprehensive review and management guide. 1st ed. Berlin: Springer; 2015. p. 117–26.
15. Windsor RE, Insall JN, Vince KG. Technical considerations of total knee arthroplasty after proximal tibial osteotomy. J Bone Joint Surg Am. 1988;70(4):547–55.
16. Della Valle CJ, Berger RA, Rosenberg AG. Surgical exposures in revision total knee arthroplasty. Clin Orthop Relat Res. 2006;446:59–68.
17. Gehrke T, Alijanipour P, Parvizi J. The management of an infected total knee arthroplasty. Bone Joint J. 2015;97-B(10 Suppl A):20–9. https://doi.org/10.1302/0301-620X.97B10.36475.
18. Della Valle CJ. Exposure options for the revision knee: getting there safely. Orthopaedic proceedings. Bone Joint J. 2014;96-B(Issue Supp 12):43.
19. Von Langenbeck B. Zur resection des kniegellenks. Verhandlungen der Deutschen Gesellschaft fur Churg. 1878;7:23–30.
20. Stern SH, Moeckel BH, Insall JN. Total knee arthroplasty in valgus knees. Clin Orthop Relat Res. 1991;273:5–8.
21. Insall J. A midline approach to the knee. J Bone Joint Surg Am. 1971;53(8):1584–6.
22. Sanna M, Sanna C, Caputo F, Piu G, Salvi M. Surgical approaches in total knee arthroplasty. Joints. 2013;1(2):34–44.
23. Mochizuki RM, Schurman DJ. Patellar complications following total knee arthroplasty. J Bone Joint Surg Am. 1979;61(6A):879–83.
24. Moreland JR. Mechanisms of failure in total knee arthroplasty. Clin Orthop Relat Res. 1988;226:49–64.
25. Cameron HU, Fedorkow DM. The patella in total knee arthroplasty. Clin Orthop Relat Res. 1982;165:197–9.
26. Keblish PA. The lateral approach to the valgus knee. Surgical technique and analysis of 53 cases with over two-year follow-up evaluation. Clin Orthop Relat Res. 1991;271:52–62.
27. Tanzer M, Burnett S. Technique of revision: surgical approach. In: Bonnin M, Amendola A, Bellemans J, MacDonald S, Ménétrey J, editors. The knee joint. 1st ed. Paris: Springer; 2012. p. 989–1002.
28. Insall JN, Thompson FM, Brause BD. Two-stage reimplantation for the salvage of infected total knee arthroplasty. J Bone Joint Surg Am. 1983;65(8):1087–98.
29. Garvin KL, Scuderi G, Insall JN. Evolution of the quadriceps snip. Clin Orthop Relat Res. 1995;321:131–7.
30. Gooding C, Garbuz D, Masri BA. Extensile surgical exposures for revision total knee replacement. In: Scott W, editor. Surgery of the knee. 5th ed. Philadelphia: Churchill Livingstone; 2011. p. 1320–6.
31. Barrack RL, Smith P, Munn B, Engh G, Rorabeck C. The Ranawat award. Comparison of surgical

approaches in total knee arthroplasty. Clin Orthop Relat Res. 1998;356:16–21.

32. Coonse K, Adams JD. A new operative approach to the knee joint. Surg Gynecol Obstet. 1943;77:344–7.

33. Insall JN. Surgical approaches. In: Insall JN, Windsor RE, Scott WN, Kelly MA, Aglietti P, editors. Surgery of the knee. 2nd ed. New York: Churchill Livingstone; 1993. p. 135–48.

34. Smith PN, Parker DA, Gelinas J, Rorabeck CH, Bourne RB. Radiographic changes in the patella following quadriceps turndown for revision total knee arthroplasty. J Arthroplasty. 2004;19(6):714–9.

35. Kelly MA, Clarke HD. Stiffness and ankylosis in primary total knee arthroplasty. Clin Orthop Relat Res. 2003;416:68–73.

36. Scott RD, Siliski JM. The use of a modified V-Y quadricepsplasty during total knee replacement to gain exposure and improve flexion in the ankylosed knee. Orthopedics. 1985;8(1):45–8.

37. Trousdale RT, Hanssen AD, Rand JA, Cahalan TD. V-Y quadricepsplasty in total knee arthroplasty. Clin Orthop Relat Res. 1993;286:48–55.

38. Ries MD, Richman JA. Extended tibial tubercle osteotomy in total knee arthroplasty. J Arthroplasty. 1996;11(8):964–7.

39. Dolin MG. Osteotomy of the tibial tubercle in total knee replacement. A technical note. J Bone Joint Surg Am. 1983 Jun;65(5):704–6.

40. Whiteside LA, Ohl MD. Tibial tubercle osteotomy for exposure of the difficult total knee arthroplasty. Clin Orthop Relat Res. 1990;260:6–9.

41. Young CF, Bourne RB, Rorabeck CH. Tibial tubercle osteotomy in total knee arthroplasty surgery. J Arthroplasty. 2008;23(3):371–5. https://doi.org/10.1016/j.arth.2007.02.019.

42. Windsor RE, Insall JN. Exposure in revision total knee arthroplasty: the femoral peel. Tech Orthop. 1988;3:1–4.

43. Lahav A, Hofmann AA. The "banana peel" exposure method in revision total knee arthroplasty. Am J Orthop (Belle Mead NJ). 2007;36(10):526–9.

44. Lavernia C, Contreras JS, Alcerro JC. The peel in total knee revision: exposure in the difficult knee. Clin Orthop Relat Res. 2011;469(1):146–53. https://doi.org/10.1007/s11999-010-1431-4.

45. Engh GA. Medial epicondylar osteotomy: a technique used with primary and revision total knee arthroplasty to improve surgical exposure and correct varus deformity. Instr Course Lect. 1999;48:153–6.

DAIR (Debridement, Antibiotics, and Implant Retention) for the Treatment of Periprosthetic Joint Infection of Knee

Nicolaas C. Budhiparama, Asep Santoso, Hendy Hidayat, and Nadia N. Ifran

15.1 Introduction

Prosthetic joint infection (PJI) is one of the most devastating complications following joint replacement. It occurs in approximately 1–2% of all joint replacement [1]. With increase in number of joint replacement procedures performed each year, it can be calculated that the number of PJI will also increase. Revisions for infected knee arthroplasties are complex, expensive, require more surgical time, longer hospitalization, and have higher risk of failure compared to aseptic revisions [1–3]. The primary goal of treatment is eradication of the infection. Maintenance of a pain-free, functional joint is the secondary goal, which is also important [2, 4].

The surgical options include irrigation, debridement, antibiotics, and implant retention with or without polyethylene exchange (DAIR), one-stage or two-stage revision, resection arthroplasty, arthrodesis, and amputation [2, 5–8]. When patients are contraindicated to undergo DAIR treatment, either one stage or multiple stages revision surgery is the preferred option. Resection arthroplasty (without reimplantation), arthrodesis, and amputation remain valid options for difficult to treat and chronic PJI, and these treatment options very rarely have a role in acute PJI cases. Non-surgical medical treatment such as antibiotic suppression therapy should be reserved for patients who are unfit or contraindicated for surgery [1, 3].

DAIR (debridement, antibiotics, and implant retention) remains the treatment of choice for acute PJI. An irrigation and debridement procedure is not a new one and has been performed ever since infected knee arthroplasty cases emerged [9, 10]. The abbreviated term of "DAIR" itself has been first used in a publication by Byren et al. in 2009 [11]. Since then the procedure has been more popular and there have been increasing number of research and reports on the role of DAIR in the acute setting, with special attention given to the topic lately.

N. C. Budhiparama (✉)
Nicolaas Institute of Constructive Orthopaedic Research and Education Foundation for Arthroplasty and Sports Medicine, Jakarta, Indonesia

Department of Orthopaedic and Traumatology, Faculty of Medicine, University of Airlangga, Surabaya, Indonesia

Department of Orthopaedics, Leiden University Medical Center, Leiden, The Netherlands

A. Santoso · H. Hidayat · N. N. Ifran
Nicolaas Institute of Constructive Orthopaedic Research and Education Foundation for Arthroplasty and Sports Medicine, Jakarta, Indonesia

U. G. Longo et al. (eds.), *Infection in Knee Replacement*,
https://doi.org/10.1007/978-3-030-81553-0_15

15.2 Preoperative Considerations

15.2.1 Definition of PJI and Classification

During the past period, various definition criteria for PJI have been described by several organizations and societies. There is no uniform definition for periprosthetic joint infection (PJI). New diagnostic criteria are formulated and updated constantly [12]. The latest diagnostic criteria include the 2018 definition of periprosthetic hip and knee infection, the European Bone and Joint Infection Society (EBJIS) 2018, and the International Consensus Meeting (ICM) 2018 [13–15]. The 2018 definition of periprosthetic hip and knee infection is a scoring system which involves newer laboratory marker including *D-dimer, synovial alpha defensin, synovial CRP, and synovial leukocyte esterase (LE)* [13]. Those markers were not included in the previous diagnostic cri-

teria. These criteria have been proved to increase the diagnostic efficiency of PJI [16]. The scoring system is summarized in Fig. 15.1.

Understanding the classification of PJI is important as one of the factors to determine the appropriate treatment and ensure the best results. There are several classifications that have been proposed to define the onset of PJI [1]. Current guidelines from the ICM on PJI and the pro-implant foundation make a clear distinction between acute and chronic PJI [17, 18]:

1. Acute postoperative infection is considered to occur <4 weeks of the procedure,
2. Acute hematogenous infection is considered as <3 weeks of the development of symptoms.
3. Any infection which develops ≥4 weeks after the index surgery or symptoms duration of acute hematogenous ≥3 weeks considered as chronic PJI.

Major criteria (at least one of the following)	Decision
Two positive cultures of the same organism	Infected
Sinus tract with evidence of communication to the joint or visualization of the prosthesis	Infected

Preoperative Diagnosis

	Minor Criteria	Score	Decision
Serum	Elevated CRP *or* D-Dimer	2	≥6 Infected
Serum	Elevated ESR	1	≥6 Infected
Synovial	Elevated synovial *WBC count or LE*	3	2-5 Possibly Infected [a]
Synovial	Positive alpha-defensin	3	2-5 Possibly Infected [a]
Synovial	Elevated synovial PMN (%)	2	0-1 Not Infected
Synovial	Elevated synovial CRP	1	0-1 Not Infected

Intraoperative Diagnosis

Inconclusive pre-op score *or* dry tap[a]	Score	Decision
Preoperative score	-	≥6 Infected
Positive histology	3	**4-5 Inconclusive [b]**
Positive purulence	3	**4-5 Inconclusive [b]**
Single positive culture	2	≤3 Not Infected

Fig. 15.1 The 2018 definition for periprosthetic joint infection (PJI). (From Parvizi et al. [13]. With kind permission from Elsevier)

15.2.2 Treatment Algorithm

An early infection may be treated with aggressive debridement, antibiotics, exchange of modular parts, and retention of the fixed components, while late infection requires the removal of the components either in one- or two-stage fashion [7]. The fundamental aspects for a successful DAIR are related to tissue, stability of the prosthesis, and susceptibility of the organism. The management strategies of PJI are summarized in Fig. 15.2 [17].

15.2.3 Patients Selection for DAIR

Implant retention without infection is the ideal goal of treatment for an infected knee arthroplasty. If the conditions and criteria are met, DAIR treatment is preferable because it is less invasive, less technical demanding, has lower morbidity, shorter hospitalization, better bone stock preservation, and lower economic burden [7, 19, 20]. However according to Koyonos et al., DAIR treatment is still a source of controversy among orthopedic surgeons because this procedure continues to be performed at relatively high rates despite an inability to consistently control infection, with rates of infection control ranging from 12% to 80% [19].

Microorganisms causing PJI are mainly *S. aureus* and coagulase-negative *Staphylococcus*, which account for up to more than half of the infections. Other microorganisms responsible include *Streptococcus* species, *Enterococcus* species, and Gram-negative bacteria [3, 4, 7, 21, 22]. Acute PJI is more often caused by *S. aureus* and *Streptococcus* species [1, 3]. *Coagulase-negative Staphylococci* are often associated with late chronic or clinically unapparent infection due to high biofilm production [3, 22]. Prolonged infection is associated with increased biofilm forma-

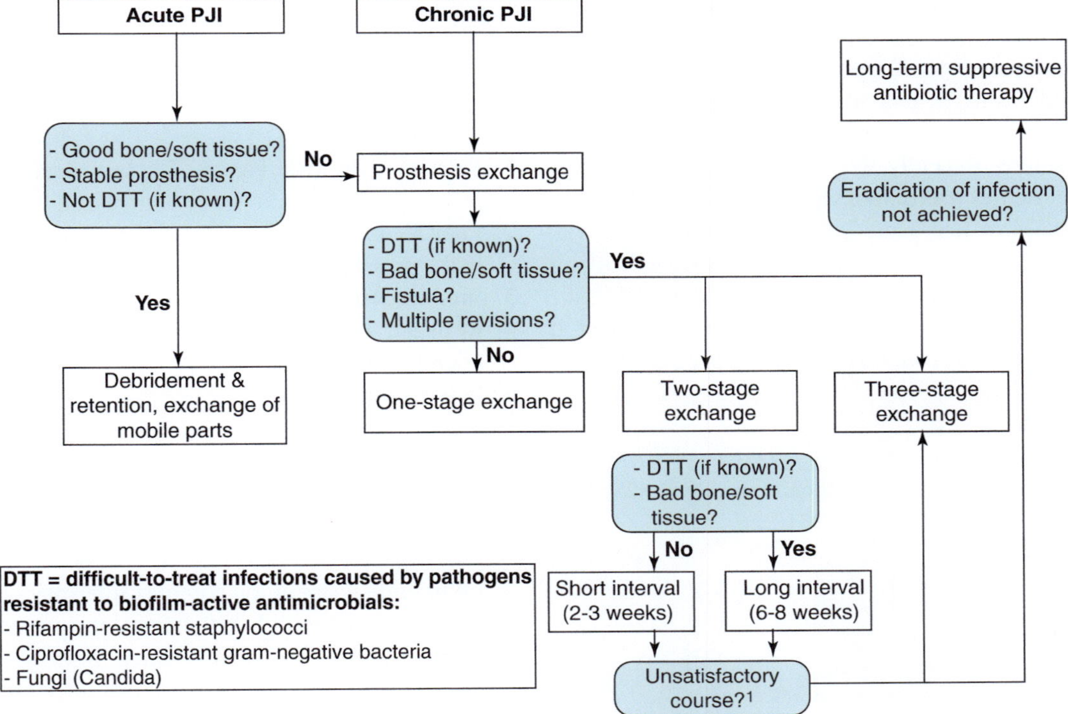

[1] Clinical signs of infection, elevated CRP, intra-operative pus, compromised tissue

Fig. 15.2 Treatment algorithm for PJI. (From Trampuz et al. [17]. With kind permission from PRO-IMPLANT Foundation)

tion and potential deep osteomyelitis [23]. The distinction between early and late PJI is based on the hypothesis that a biofilm was formed within 3 weeks on the surface of the components, thus necessitating their removal [6]. It is crucial to eradicate biofilm within a short time frame before it attaches to the implant [23]. Therefore, DAIR treatment shows better outcome in acute PJI compared to chronic infections [22, 23].

While tempting to perform DAIR on all PJI cases, the procedure is suitable only in selective cases and in recent years there is an emphasis on optimal patient selection. The wide range of success/failure between 10 and 90% emphasized this need. The decision to retain implants should be based on factors related to the host (comorbidities), the implant (stability), and infecting organism (virulence and ability to produce biofilm) [3, 6, 7, 24, 25]. Correct indications lead to higher rates of successful outcomes. Based on the 2018 ICM, the KLIC score is a recommended tool to predict treatment failure after DAIR procedure for early acute PJI (Table 15.1) [18, 26]. Patients with a score $\geq$ 7 are 2 times more likely to fail compared to those with a score < 7 [27]. Interestingly, patients with late acute infections show different characteristics and risk factors for failure. Recently the CRIME80 score was suggested as useful tool for patients stratification in cases of late acute infections (Table 15.2). The CRIME80 score $\geq$ 3 showed as independent predictor of failure for DAIR in late acute PJI [28].

The DAIR procedure is best performed if these criteria are met [1–4, 6, 8, 18, 22, 24]:

Table 15.1 KLIC score (from Tornero et al. [26]. With kind permission from Elsevier)

Variable		Score
K	Chronic renal failure (kidney)	2
L	Liver failure	1.5
I	Index surgery:	1.5
	Revision surgery	
	Or prosthesis to treat femoral neck fracture	
C	Cemented prosthesis	2
C	C-reactive protein (CRP > 115 mg/L)	2.5
	Total	9.5

Table 15.2 CRIME80-score, preoperative risk score for predicting DAIR failure in late acute periprosthetic joint infections. (From Wouthuyzen-Bakker M et al. [28]. With kind permission from Elsevier)

Variable	Description	Score
C	COPD	2
	CRP > 150 mg/dL	1
R	Rheumatoid arthritis	3
I	Index surgery (prosthesis indicated for fracture)	3
M	Male gender	1
E	Exchange of mobile components	−1
80	Age > 80 years	2

1. Patients with an early acute PJI or acute hematogenous infection <3 weeks.
2. Adequate skin coverage conditions.
3. Stable implant.
4. Identified definitive microorganisms, especially Gram-positive infection.
5. Availability of effective antimicrobial agent.
6. Patient with high risk of complication in more aggressive surgery.

The DAIR procedure has a higher rate of failure in below conditions; therefore, it should be contraindicated in [1, 3, 6, 8]:

1. Patients with risk factors for persistent or recurrent infection.
2. Poor local soft tissues conditions, especially in the presence of sinus.
3. Immunocompromised patients.
4. Resistant or unknown pathogens found in microbiology tests.
5. Polymicrobial infection.
6. Sepsis.
7. Prior failed procedures or debridements.
8. Late chronic infections.
9. Loose prosthesis.

Taking into account the complex interplay of factors associated with DAIR failure, the use of machine learning has been recently proposed for patient selection due to its ability to learn from continuous data input. By this means, machine learning models are able to process more complex data and make patient specific predictions. Recently, an algorithm based on such technique was created and validate with promising results. Although such models still needs to be validated in external cohorts they have great potential to be used in daily practice by easily entering patient data in a computer-based software or phone application and may aid in clinical decision making and patient counseling [29].

15.3 Intraoperative Considerations

15.3.1 Surgical Technique

The components of DAIR include arthrotomy, extensive debridement and synovectomy, irrigation, retention of well-fixed implant, and exchange of modular components. The aggressive debridement of the periarticular tissues and the components aims to reduce the bioburden of the pathogens and to improve the efficiency of the patient's immune system and antibiotics against the surviving pathogens [6]. Debridement must be thorough and meticulous and all devitalized tissues must be excised. Various additional treatments have been used to improve local infection control and reduce biofilm, including the use of local antibiotics (e.g., antibiotic beads, sponges, and powder), chemical debridement and irrigation with various antiseptic agents (e.g., povidone iodine, chlorhexidine, peroxide, etc.), and physical treatment to the implants [18, 28, 30, 31].

Based on The International Consensus Group, we suggest the following protocol on how the DAIR procedure should be performed:

1. Debridement is not an emergency procedure in patients without sepsis. General conditions should be optimized prior to surgery [3, 18].
2. Acquire multiple tissue samples to identify the etiology of infection prior to surgery. Antibiotics should be withheld until representative samples are identified [3].
3. Adequate surgical exposure (preferred from the previous incision) to the infected area is mandatory. Including excision of the skin fistula if it is present.
4. Obtain multiple intraoperative tissue culture for further isolation of causal microorganism. No less than 5 cultures should be obtained intraoperatively [6].
5. All non-bleeding soft or osseous tissues should be removed, including excision of sinuses and synovectomy [1, 3, 6].
6. The mobile component (PE liner/insert) must be removed to access all part of the joint, and exchange of the modular component is strongly recommended [1–3, 6, 18, 32].
7. All the components should be inspected for loosening and the interfaces of the components should be exposed [6].
8. Irrigation of the joint with copious amounts of irrigation solution (see irrigation protocol).
9. Switching to a clean patient setup prior to wound closure is also recommended to facilitate more sterile and uncontaminated wound [33].
10. A suction drain should be left in situ until there is minimal output. If drainage persists or if the infection fails to settle, then consideration has to be given to a further debridement procedure. Continuous closed irrigation has not shown any benefit compared to standard procedure with primary closure and in situ drain [3].

15.3.2 Irrigation Protocol

Several protocols for the irrigation have been proposed. The International Consensus Meeting 2018 strongly recommend 6–9 L of irrigation solution as minimum necessary volume [18]. The most commonly used to irrigate the joint is normal saline. Several authors believed that adding some chemical agent to the irrigation solutions could help in reducing pathogen load. Detergents, antiseptics, or even antibiotics have been proposed as adjuvant agent. Adding antibiotics including bacitracin, neomycin, polymyxin/neomycin, and gentamycin to the irrigation solution has been shown to be no beneficial effect compared to saline alone [34, 35]. Recently, there has been increased interest in using chlorhexidine gluconate 0.05%. Studies by Smith et al. and Schwechter et al. showed chlorhexidine gluconate to be the most effective option at decreasing bacterial colony counts when compared to normal saline, povidone iodine, or castile soap [31, 36].

There is little consensus regarding use of low-pressure (<15 pounds per square inch) or high-pressure (>45 pounds per square inch) lavage. High-pressure lavage provides rapid and effective removal of necrotic tissues, but may cause tissue damage or penetration of bacteria into deeper soft-tissue layers [6, 37]. However, both low-pressure or high-pressure lavage can be used and no significant difference has been shown to exist in clinical practice [38].

15.3.3 Modular Component Exchange

Removing the modular components during DAIR (i.e., polyethylene liner/insert, femoral head) provides better access to the joint capsule for extensive debridement and synovectomy. Recent study by Hirsiger et al. showed that mobile component exchange doubled the probability for long-term remission [39]. They found the exchange of mobile parts was protective with hazard ratio 1.9 (95% confidence interval 1.2–2.9) in multivariate Cox regression analysis. These findings were supported by several previous studies. Lora-tamayo et al. showed that the exchange of removable components during debridement stands as an independent predictor of a favorable outcome with hazard ratio 0.6 [32]. In addition, Choi et al. reported that regardless of the causative organisms, lack of mobile component exchange resulted in poor outcome after DAIR treatment for PJI of the knee [9]. Another publications by Tsang et al. reviewed cohort studies published during 38 years period (1977–2015) on the results of DAIR for periprosthetic joint infection (PJI) of the hip. The success rate of DAIR with modular

component exchange was 73.9% (471/637 patients) compared with 60.7% (245/404 patients) in the non-modular component exchange group ($P < 0.0001$) [40]. The modular component exchange also became independent predictors of treatment success in a multicenter cohort study evaluating the outcome of DAIR in hip and knee PJIs caused by methicillin-resistant and methicillin-susceptible *S. aureus* [32]. Further, Grammatopoulos et al. reported a success rate of 93.3% when modular components were exchanged compared to 75.7% when modular components were retained in a series of acute PJI of the hips [41]. The rationale behind these findings might be associated with the evidence that bacterial load detected on polyethylene component is higher compared to the metal components of prostheses [42]. Thus, removing the polyethylene modular components will reduce the amount of bacterial load and biofilm in the infected joints.

15.3.4 Local Antibiotics Administration

Carriers for local antibiotic release include antibiotic loaded bone cement (polymethylmethacrylate, PMMA), beads, and dissolvable sponges. The rationale for using local antibiotic treatment is to achieve a high local concentration of antibiotic agents, thereby killing the causative microorganism, without the side-effects of high systemic concentrations [1]. Beads are usually loaded with gentamicin, but vancomycin and tobramycin are also used [1, 4]. Their use in DAIR treatment has been reported in a few studies, with relatively high success rates (75–83%) [43, 44].

Calcium sulfate beads have recently been reported as an alternative to PMMA beads. The advantages of calcium sulfate beads include a bioabsorbable material which excludes the need for additional surgery. It is also believed to have higher sustained concentration of local antibiotics and higher resistance to biofilm formation compared to PMMA beads. In contrast, the disadvantage of using antibiotic beads includes decrease in local antibiotic concentration that occurs as soon as 24 h after implantation, possible colonization by bacteria and their capability of forming a foreign body on which a biofilm can develop after the antibiotic release (10–14 days) and potential for hypercalcemia [1, 22, 45, 46]. Unfortunately, its beneficial effect was still unpromising. Flierl et al. reported only 52% success rate with antibiotic-impregnated calcium sulfate beads in their retrospective report of 32 patients [45]. Calanna et al. modified surgical technique developed to enhance the classical irrigation and debridement procedure to improve the possibilities of retaining an infected total knee arthroplasty with the use of calcium sulfate beads [47]. This technique, debridement antibiotic pearls and retention of the implant (DAPRI), aims to remove the intra-articular biofilm allowing a higher and prolonged local antibiotic concentration using calcium sulfate beads. The combination of three different surgical techniques (methylene blue staining, argon beam electrical stimulation, and chlorhexidine gluconate brushing) might enhance the identification, disruption, and finally removal of the bacterial biofilm, which is mainly responsible for antibiotics and antibodies resistance. The DAPRI technique might represent a safe and more conservative treatment for acute and early hematogenous periprosthetic joint infection. They reported the success rate of infection eradication as high as 80% [47]. Recently, Gramlich et al. showed that the use of calcium based-antibiotic beads in combination DAIR has improved the 3-year infection-free survival compared to DAIR only which has re-infection rate until 81.8% in salvage procedure for chronic PJI of the knee [48].

Resorbable gentamicin-loaded sponges also have been used as local antibiotic in infection case after total hip arthroplasty, with success rates of 70% in a study reported by Kuiper et al. [49]. Another alternative for local antibiotic treatment is vancomycin powder. Riesgo et al. found that the combination of vancomycin powder and a dilute povidone iodine lavage to DAIR increases the success rates up to 83% [50].

15.4 Postoperative Consideration

15.4.1 Postoperative Antibiotics Regimen

The antimicrobial agent should have bactericidal action, even against slow-growth organisms or biofilm producers. Before starting any treatment, the susceptibility of the organism should be tested and alternative regimens should be discussed, given the growing levels of resistance [4]. A combination of rifampicin with quinolones has been used most often, with good results in vitro, in vivo, and in clinical trials [4, 11, 51]. Rifampin is thought to penetrate the biofilm and is recommended in all cases of Staphylococcal PJI treated with DAIR [1]. Higher success rates were found when rifampin was added with another antibiotic regimen [32, 51]. Options such as linezolid, sulfamethoxazole-trimethoprim, and minocycline are possible, although so far no clinical studies for validating their use have been published [5]. The best option is to discuss the best antimicrobial therapy for each case with the hospital infection control committee [3, 4].

Postoperative long-term combined intravenous (IV) antibiotic treatment of between 4 and 6 weeks followed by oral rifampin for 6 months is recommended [3, 6]. Byren et al. demonstrated that the infection-free survival rate after DAIR treatment was 82%, with a follow-up of 2.3 years. However, there is risk of recurrence following discontinuation of the antibiotics [11]. Some authors have suggested a combined protocol consisting of debridement, antibiotic treatment for >1 year, and implant retention (DAIR) for the treatment of PJI [6]. The risks of this happening are increased fourfold according to Byren et al. suggesting that this form of treatment did not eradicate the pathogen but postpones its reactivation [11]. However, there are also some studies that show short duration antibiotics could be used as effective as the long course administration. A study by Chaussade et al. showed no difference between 6 and 12 weeks of intravenous antibiotics with overall success rates of 69% [52]. A multicenter randomized clinical trial by Lora-Tamayo et al. suggests that 8 weeks of levofloxacin +

rifampicin therapy had similar outcomes to longer standard treatment (3–6 months) for acute PJI managed with DAIR [51]. A cohort studies in Leiden University by Scheper et al. also showed the outcome of acute PJI treated with DAIR and 5 days rifampicin was comparable to the outcomes of 3 months rifampicin combination therapy [53]. Recently, the international consensus meeting 2018 stated that a minimum of 6 weeks of antibiotic therapy seems to be sufficient in most cases of PJIs managed by DAIR-provided surgical treatment [18].

15.4.2 Factors Associated with Outcomes of Dair

The outcome of DAIR procedure varies between studies. The results between studies are highly variable due to many confounding variables such as: host condition, characteristics of the microorganism, implant state, operation history, type of surgery/procedure, surgeon's ability in the various series, lack of consistency in definition of acute infection, different failure criteria among studies, and the absence of randomized, controlled, prospective comparison studies [1, 3, 7, 20, 24]. Recent systematic review and meta-analysis by Kunutsor et al. showed that DAIR resulted in quite a wide range of infection control rate by 11.1–100% [54]. This was no better when compared to two-stage revision procedures which has success rate of 85–100% [7].

Outcome may be adversely affected by the time interval between the initial operation and the development of infection [43, 55]. The success rate of DAIR dropped to 40% when the infection started >6 weeks after the TKA [6]. Löwik et al. reported among 769 patients with acute PJI the treatment failure occurred in 38% (294/769) of the patients after DAIR. The treatment failure rate was almost similar between time intervals from index arthroplasty to DAIR: week 1–2 was 42% (95/226) failure rate, week 3–4 was 38% (143/378) failure rate, week 5–6 was 29% (29/100) failure rate, and week 7–12 was 42% (27/65) failure rate. They reported that DAIR could be viable option for acute PJI which pres-

ents more than 4 weeks after the index surgery as far as performed at least 1 weeks after the symptoms and modular component is exchanged [56]. Trebse et al. applied a DAIR protocol to a series of 24 patients with an 86% success rate over 3 years and defined that the factors for a good prognosis were the presence of a stable implant, absence of fistulas contiguous with the prosthetic component, and duration of symptoms less than 3 weeks [57]. Koyonos et al. performed DAIR in 136 patients and reported higher success rate in acute postoperative (31%) and acute hematogenous infections (44%) compared to chronic late infections (28%) [19]. Tsukayama et al., Segawa et al., Mont et al., Cobo et al., also reported a success rate of 57.3–80% when DAIR performed in early PJI (<4 weeks) [43, 55, 58, 59].

Recently some new evidences support the expansion of DAIR indication for a PJI which has symptoms >3–4 weeks. Zhang et al. in a small series of 24 patients with acute PJI, reported that 5 patients who had symptoms between 4 and 8 weeks have 100% success rate after DAIR treatment [60]. Lesens et al. also reported that failure after DAIR was not associated with time from index arthroplasty to debridement, nor with duration of symptoms (>3 weeks) in a retrospective series of 137 patients with early PJI [61]. Although further study is needed to prove these findings, as another recent evidence showed that late acute PJI still has lower success rate compared to early acute PJI especially when the causative agent is *Staphylococcus* spp [28, 62, 63].

Multiple studies have shown *S. aureus* infection to be a contributing factor for failure to eradicate infection due to more virulent nature than other microorganisms (possibly due to their biofilm production) [3, 7, 19, 20, 64, 65]. MRSA, in particular, has shown high failure rates with DAIR [1, 3]. Several studies reported low success rate of 0–45% when DAIR performed in MRSA infection [66–68]. Gram-negative organisms have shown a variable outcome in failure rates as compared to Gram-positive organisms [3, 65]. The DAIR procedure has also shown promising results in patients who are immunocompetent and with PJI caused by a low virulence organism, e.g., *Coagulase-negative staphylococci* [3, 19].

The international consensus meeting 2018 strongly agreed some factors which possibly associated with treatment success in acute PJIs treated with DAIR [18]:

- Exchanging the modular components during debridement.
- Performing a debridement within at least 7 days, but preferably as soon as possible, after the onset of symptoms.
- Adding rifampin to the antibiotic regimen, particularly when combined with a fluoroquinolone, in cases of susceptible *Staphylococci*.
- Treatment with fluoroquinolones in cases of susceptible Gram-negative bacilli.

The following factors also have been shown to be associated with treatment failure after DAIR in acute PJI [18]:

- Host-related factors: rheumatoid arthritis, old age, male sex, chronic renal failure, liver cirrhosis, and chronic obstructive pulmonary disease.
- Prosthesis indication: fracture as indication for the prosthesis, cemented prostheses, and revised prostheses.
- Clinical presentation representing the severity of the infection: a high C-reactive protein, a high bacterial inoculum, and the presence of bacteremia.
- Causative microorganisms: *S. aureus* and *Enterococci*.

References

1. Kuiper JW, Willink RT, Moojen DJ, van den Bekerom MP, Colen S. Treatment of acute periprosthetic infections with prosthesis retention: review of current concepts. World J Orthop. 2014;5(5):667–76.
2. Kalore NV, Gioe TJ, Singh JA. Diagnosis and management of infected total knee arthroplasty. Open Orthop J. 2011;5:86–91.
3. Qasim SN, Swann A, Ashford R. The DAIR (debridement, antibiotics and implant retention) procedure for infected total knee replacement—a literature review. SICOT J. 2017;3:2.
4. de Carvalho Júnior LH, Temponi EF, Badet R. Infection after total knee replacement: diagnosis and treatment. Rev Bras Ortop (English Ed). 2013;48(5):389–96.
5. Santoso A, Park KS, Shin YR, Yang HY, Choi IS, Yoon TR. Two-stage revision for periprosthetic joint infection of the hip: culture-negative versus culture-positive infection. J Orthop. 2018;15:391–5.
6. Gehrke T, Alijanipour P, Parvizi J. The management of an infected total knee arthroplasty. Bone Joint J. 2015;97-B(10 Suppl A):20–9.
7. Choi HR, von Knoch F, Zurakowski D, Nelson SB, Malchau H. Can implant retention be recommended for treatment of infected TKA? Clin Orthop Relat Res. 2011;469(4):961–9.
8. Santoso A, Yoon TR, Yang HY, Park KS. Internal iliac artery injury due to intrapelvic migration of infected acetabular reconstruction cage with hook: a case report. J Orthop Sci. 2020;25(1):201–4.
9. Schoifet SD, Morrey BF. Treatment of infection after total knee arthroplasty by débridement with retention of the components. J Bone Joint Surg Am. 1990;72(9):1383–90.
10. Burger RR, Basch T, Hopson CN. Implant salvage in infected total knee arthroplasty. Clin Orthop. 1991;273:105–12.
11. Byren I, Bejon P, Atkins BL, Angus B, Masters S, McLardy-Smith P, Gundle R, Berendt A. One hundred and twelve infected arthroplasties treated with 'DAIR' (debridement, antibiotics and implant retention): antibiotic duration and outcome. J Antimicrob Chemother. 2009;63(6):1264–71.
12. Villa JM, Pannu TS, Piuzzi N, Riesgo AM, Higuera CA. Evolution of diagnostic definitions for periprosthetic joint infection in total hip and knee arthroplasty. J Arthroplasty. 2020;35(3S):S9–S13.
13. Parvizi J, Tan TL, Goswami K, Higuera C, Della Valle C, Chen AF, Shohat N. The 2018 definition of periprosthetic hip and knee infection: an Evidence-based and validated criteria. J Arthroplasty. 2018;33(5):1309–1314.e2.
14. Izakovicova P, Borens O, Trampuz A. Periprosthetic joint infection: current concepts and outlook. EFORT Open Rev. 2019;4(7):482–94.
15. Shohat N, Bauer T, Buttaro M, Budhiparama N, Cashman J, Della Valle CJ, Drago L, Gehrke T, Marcelino Gomes LS, Goswami K, Hailer NP, Han SB, Higuera CA, Inaba Y, Jenny JY, Kjaersgaard-Andersen P, Lee M, Llinás A, Malizos K, Mont MA, Jones RM, Parvizi J, Peel T, Rivero-Boschert S, Segreti J, Soriano A, Sousa R, Spangehl M, Tan TL, Tikhilov R, Tuncay I, Winkler H, Witso E, Wouthuyzen-Bakker M, Young S, Zhang X, Zhou Y, Zimmerli W. Hip and Knee Section, What is the definition of a periprosthetic joint infection (PJI) of the knee and the hip? Can the same criteria be used for both Joints?: Proceedings of International Consensus on Orthopedic Infections. J Arthroplasty. 2019;34(2S):S325–7.
16. Guan H, Fu J, Li X, Chai W, Hao L, Li R, Zhao J, Chen J. The 2018 new definition of periprosthetic joint infection improves the diagnostic efficiency in the Chinese

population. J Orthop Surg Res. 2019;14(1):151. https://doi.org/10.1186/s13018-019-1185-y.

17. PRO-IMPLANT Foundation. Pocket guide to diagnosis & treatment of periprosthetic joint infection (PJI). Version 8. 2019.

18. Argenson JN, Arndt M, Babis G, Battenberg A, Budhiparama N, Catani F, Chen F, de Beaubien B, Ebied A, Esposito S, Ferry C, Flores H, Giorgini A, Hansen E, Hernugrahanto KD, Hyonmin C, Kim TK, Koh IJ, Komnos G, Lausmann C, Loloi J, Lora-Tamayo J, Lumban-Gaol I, Mahyudin F, Mancheno-Losa M, Marculescu C, Marei S, Martin KE, Meshram P, Paprosky WG, Poultsides L, Saxena A, Schwechter E, Shah J, Shohat N, Sierra RJ, Soriano A, Stefánsdóttir A, Suleiman LI, Taylor A, Triantafyllopoulos GK, Utomo DN, Warren D, Whiteside L, Wouthuyzen-Bakker M, Yombi J, Zmistowski B. Hip and knee section, treatment, debridement and retention of implant: Proceedings of International Consensus on Orthopedic Infections. J Arthroplasty. 2019;34(2S):S399–419.

19. Koyonos L, Zmistowski B, Della Valle CJ, Parvizi J. Infection control rate of irrigation and debridement for periprosthetic joint infection. Clin Orthop Relat Res. 2011;469(11):3043–8.

20. Gardner J, Gioe TJ, Tatman P. Can this prosthesis be saved?: implant salvage attempts in infected primary TKA. Clin Orthop Relat Res. 2011;469(4):970–6.

21. Moran E, Byren I, Atkins BL. The diagnosis and management of prosthetic joint infections. J Antimicrob Chemother. 2010;65(Suppl 3):iii45–54.

22. Kuiper JW, Vos SJ, Saouti R, Vergroesen DA, Graat HC, Debets-Ossenkopp YJ, et al. Prosthetic joint-associated infections treated with DAIR (debridement, antibiotics, irrigation, and retention): analysis of risk factors and local antibiotic carriers in 91 patients. Acta Orthop. 2013;84(4):380–6.

23. de Vries L, van der Weegen W, Neve WC, Das H, Ridwan BU, Steens J. The effectiveness of debridement, antibiotics and irrigation for periprosthetic joint infections after primary hip and knee arthroplasty. A 15 years retrospective study in two community hospitals in the Netherlands. J Bone Jt Infect. 2016;1:20–4.

24. Van Kleunen JP, Knox D, Garino JP, Lee GC. Irrigation and debridement and prosthesis retention for treating acute periprosthetic infections. Clin Orthop Relat Res. 2010;468(8):2024–8.

25. Moran E, Masters S, Berendt AR, McLardy-Smith P, Byren I, Atkins BL. Guiding empirical antibiotic therapy in orthopaedics: the microbiology of prosthetic joint infection managed by debridement, irrigation and prosthesis retention. J Infect. 2007;55(1):1–7.

26. Tornero E, Morata L, et al. KLIC-score for predicting early failure in prosthetic joint infections treated with debridement implant retention and antibiotics. Clin Microbiol Infect. 2015;21:786.e9–786.e17.

27. Dx Duffy S, Ahearn N, Darley ES, Porteous AJ, Murray JR, Howells NR. Analysis of the KLIC-score; an outcome predictor tool for prosthetic joint infections treated with debridement, antibiotics and implant retention. J Bone Jt Infect. 2018;3(3):150–5.

28. Wouthuyzen-Bakker M, Sebillotte M, Lomas J, Kendrick B, Palomares EB, Murillo O, Parvizi J, Shohat N, Reinoso JC, Sánchez RE, Fernandez-Sampedro M, Senneville E, Huotari K, JMB A, García AB, Lora-Tamayo J, Ferrari MC, Vaznaisiene D, Yusuf E, Aboltins C, Trebse R, Salles MJ, Benito N, Vila A, MDD T, Kramer TS, Petersdorf S, Diaz-Brito V, Tufan ZK, Sanchez M, Arvieux C, Soriano A, ESCMID Study Group for Implant-Associated Infections (ESGIAI). Timing of implant-removal in late acute periprosthetic joint infection: a multicenter observational study. J Infect. 2019;79(3):199–205.

29. Shohat N, Goswami K, Tan T, Yayac M, Soriano A, Sousa R, et al. Who will fail following irrigation and debridement for periprosthetic joint infection: a machine learning based validated tool. Bone Joint J. 2020; in press.

30. Ferry T, Leboucher G, Fevre C, Herry Y, Conrad A, Josse J, Batailler C, Chidiac C, Medina M, Lustig S, Laurent F, Lyon BJI Study Group. Salvage debridement, antibiotics and implant retention ("DAIR") with local injection of a selected cocktail of bacteriophages: is it an option for an elderly patient with relapsing *Staphylococcus aureus* prosthetic-joint infection? Open Forum Infect Dis. 2018;5(11):ofy269.

31. Schwechter EM, Folk D, Varshney AK, Fries BC, Kim SJ, Hirsh DM. Optimal irrigation and debridement of infected joint implants: an in vitro methicillin-resistant *Staphylococcus aureus* biofilm model. J Arthroplasty. 2011;26(6 Suppl):109–13.

32. Lora-Tamayo J, Murillo O, Iribarren JA, Soriano A, Sanchez-Somolinos M, Baraia-Etxaburu JM, et al. A large multicenter study of methicillin-susceptible and methicillin-resistant *Staphylococcus aureus* prosthetic joint infections managed with implant retention. Clin Infect Dis. 2013;56(2):182–94.

33. Choo KJ, Austin M, Parvizi J. Irrigation and debridement, modular exchange, and implant retention for acute periprosthetic infection after total knee arthroplasty. JBJS Essent Surg Tech. 2019;9(4):e38.1–2.

34. Anglen JO, Apostoles S, Christensen G, Gainor B. The efficacy of various irrigation solutions in removing slime-producing Staphylococcus. J Orthop Trauma. 1994;8(5):390–6.

35. Bartoszewicz M, Rygiel A, Krzeminski M, Przondo-Mordarska A. Penetration of a selected antibiotic and antiseptic into a biofilm formed on orthopedic steel implants. Ortop Traumatol Rehabil. 2007;9(3):310–8.

36. Smith DC, Maiman R, Schwechter EM, Kim SJ, Hirsh DM. Optimal irrigation and debridement of infected Total joint implants with chlorhexidine gluconate. J Arthroplasty. 2015;30(10):1820–2.

37. Kalteis T, Lehn N, Schroder H-J, Schubert T, Zysk S, Handel M, et al. Contaminant seeding in bone by different irrigation methods: an experimental study. J Orthop Trauma. 2005;19(9):591–6.

38. Munoz-Mahamud E, Garcia S, Bori G, Martinez-Pastor JC, Zumbado JA, Riba J, et al. Comparison of a low-pressure and a high-pressure pulsatile lavage

during debridement for orthopaedic implant infection. Arch Orthop Trauma Surg. 2011;131(9):1233–8.

39. Hirsiger S, Betz M, Stafylakis D, Götschi T, Lew D, Uçkay I. The benefice of mobile parts' exchange in the management of infected total joint arthroplasties with prosthesis retention (DAIR Procedure). J Clin Med. 2019;8(2):E226.

40. Tsang S-TJ, Ting J, Simpson AHRW, Gaston P. Outcomes following debridement, antibiotics and implant retention in the management of periprosthetic infections of the hip: a review of cohort studies. Bone Joint J. 2017;99-B:1458–66.

41. Grammatopoulos G, Bolduc M-E, Atkins BL, Kendrick BJL, McLardy-Smith P, Murray DW, et al. Functional outcome of debridement, antibiotics and implant retention in periprosthetic joint infection involving the hip: a case- control study. Bone Joint J. 2017;99-B:614–22.

42. Lass R, Giurea A, Kubista B, Hirschl AM, Graninger W, Presterl E, et al. Bacterial adherence to different components of total hip prosthesis in patients with prosthetic joint infection. Int Orthop. 2014;38:1597–602.

43. Tsukayama DT, Estrada R, Gustilo RB. Infection after total hip arthroplasty. A study of the treatment of one hundred and six infections. J Bone Joint Surg Am. 1996;78(4):512–23.

44. Geurts JA, Janssen DM, Kessels AG, Walenkamp GH. Good results in postoperative and hematogenous deep infections of 89 stable total hip and knee replacements with retention of prosthesis and local antibiotics. Acta Orthop. 2013;84(6):509–16.

45. Flierl MA, Culp BM, Okroj KT, Springer BD, Levine BR, Della Valle CJ. Poor outcomes of irrigation and debridement in acute periprosthetic joint infection with antibiotic-impregnated calcium sulfate beads. J Arthroplasty. 2017;32(8):2505–7.

46. Kallala R, Haddad FS. Hypercalcaemia following the use of antibiotic-eluting absorbable calcium sulphate beads in revision arthroplasty for infection. Bone Joint J. 2015;97-B(9):1237–41.

47. Calanna F, Chen F, Risitano S, Vorhies JS, Franceschini M, Giori NJ, Indelli PF. Debridement, antibiotic pearls, and retention of the implant (DAPRI): A modified technique for implant retention in total knee arthroplasty PJI treatment. J Orthop Surg (Hong Kong). 2019;27(3):2309499019874413.

48. Gramlich Y, Johnson T, Kemmerer M, Walter G, Hoffmann R, Klug A. Salvage procedure for chronic periprosthetic knee infection: the application of DAIR results in better remission rates and infection-free survivorship when used with topical degradable calcium-based antibiotics. Knee Surg Sports Traumatol Arthrosc. 2020;28:2823–34.

49. Kuiper JW, Brohet RM, Wassink S, van den Bekerom MP, Nolte PA, Vergroesen DA. Implantation of resorbable gentamicin sponges in addition to irrigation and debridement in 34 patients with infection complicating total hip arthroplasty. Hip Int. 2013;23(2):173–80.

50. Riesgo AM, Park BK, Herrero CP, Yu S, Schwarzkopf R, Iorio R. Vancomycin povidone-iodine protocol improves survivorship of periprosthetic joint infection treated with irrigation and debridement. J Arthroplasty. 2018;33(3):847–50.

51. Lora-Tamayo J, Euba G, Cobo J, Horcajada JP, Soriano A, Sandoval E, et al. Short-versus long-duration levofloxacin plus rifampicin for acute staphylococcal prosthetic joint infection managed with implant retention: a randomised clinical trial. Int J Antimicrob Agents. 2016;48(3):310–6.

52. Chaussade H, Uçkay I, Vuagnat A, Druon J, Gras G, Rosset P, et al. Antibiotic therapy duration for prosthetic joint infections treated by debridement and implant retention (DAIR): similar long-term remission for 6 weeks as compared to 12 weeks. Int J Infect Dis. 2017;63:37–42.

53. Scheper H, Hooven DV, MVD S, Boer SD, Mahdad R, Beek MVD, et al. Treatment of prosthetic joint infection: debridement, antibiotics and implant retention with short duration of rifampicin. Open Forum Infect Dis. 2016;3(suppl_1):1141.

54. Kunutsor SK, Beswick AD, Whitehouse MR, Wylde V, Blom AW. Debridement, antibiotics and implant retention for periprosthetic joint infections: a systematic review and meta-analysis of treatment outcomes. J Infect. 2018;77(6):479–88.

55. Segawa H, Tsukayama DT, Kyle RF, Becker DA, Gustilo RB. Infection after total knee arthroplasty. A retrospective study of the treatment of eighty-one infections. J Bone Joint Surg Am. 1999;81(10):1434–45.

56. Löwik CAM, Parvizi J, Jutte PC, Zijlstra WP, Knobben BAS, Xu C, Goswami K, Belden KA, Sousa R, Carvalho A, Martínez-Pastor JC, Soriano A, Wouthuyzen-Bakker M, Northern Infection Network Joint Arthroplasty (NINJA) and ESCMID Study Group for Implant-Associated Infections (ESGIAI). Debridement, antibiotics and implant retention is a viable treatment option for early periprosthetic joint infection presenting more than four weeks after index arthroplasty. Clin Infect Dis. 2020;71(3):630–6. pii: ciz867.

57. Trebse R, Pisot V, Trampuz A. Treatment of infected retained implants. J Bone Joint Surg Br. 2005;87(2):249–56.

58. Mont MA, Waldman B, Banerjee C, Pacheco IH, Hungerford DS. Multiple irrigation, debridement, and retention of components in infected total knee arthroplasty. J Arthroplasty. 1997;12(4):426–33.

59. Cobo J, Miguel LG, Euba G, Rodriguez D, Garcia-Lechuz JM, Riera M, et al. Early prosthetic joint infection: outcomes with debridement and implant retention followed by antibiotic therapy. Clin Microbiol Infect. 2011;17(11):1632–7.

60. Zhang CF, He L, Fang XY, Huang ZD, Bai GC, Li WB, Zhang WM. Debridement, antibiotics, and implant retention for acute periprosthetic joint infection. Orthop Surg. 2020;12:463–70.

61. Lesens O, Ferry T, Forestier E, Botelho-Nevers E, Pavese P, Piet E, Pereira B, Montbarbon E, Boyer B,

Lustig S, Descamps S, Auvergne-Rhône-Alpes Bone and Joint Infections Study Group. Should we expand the indications for the DAIR (debridement, antibiotic therapy, and implant retention) procedure for *Staphylococcus aureus* prosthetic joint infections? A multicenter retrospective study. Eur J Clin Microbiol Infect Dis. 2018;37(10):1949–56.

62. Wouthuyzen-Bakker M, Sebillotte M, Huotari K, Escudero Sánchez R, Benavent E, Parvizi J, Fernandez-Sampedro M, Barbero-Allende JM, Garcia-Cañete J, Trebse R, Del Toro M, Diaz-Brito V, Sanchez M, Scarborough M, Soriano A, ESCMID Study Group for Implant-Associated Infections (ESGIAI). Lower success rate of débridement and implant retention in late acute versus early acute periprosthetic joint infection caused by Staphylococcus spp. Results from a matched cohort study. Clin Orthop Relat Res. 2020;478(6):1348–55.

63. Wouthuyzen-Bakker M, Sebillotte M, Lomas J, Taylor A, Palomares EB, Murillo O, Parvizi J, Shohat N, Reinoso JC, Sánchez RE, Fernandez-Sampedro M, Senneville E, Huotari K, Barbero JM, Garcia-Cañete J, Lora-Tamayo J, Ferrari MC, Vaznaisiene D, Yusuf E, Aboltins C, Trebse R, Salles MJ, Benito N, Vila A, MDD T, Kramer TS, Petersdorf S, Diaz-Brito V, Tufan ZK, Sanchez M, Arvieux C, Soriano A, ESCMID Study Group for Implant-Associated Infections (ESGIAI). Clinical outcome and risk factors for failure in late acute prosthetic joint infections treated with debridement and implant retention. J Infect. 2019;78(1):40–7.

64. Deirmengian C, Greenbaum J, Lotke PA, Booth RE Jr, Lonner JH. Limited success with open debridement and retention of components in the treatment of acute *Staphylococcus aureus* infections after total knee arthroplasty. J Arthroplasty. 2003;18(7 Suppl 1):22–6.

65. Vilchez F, Martinez-Pastor JC, Garcia-Ramiro S, Bori G, Macule F, Sierra J, et al. Outcome and predictors of treatment failure in early post-surgical prosthetic joint infections due to *Staphylococcus aureus* treated with debridement. Clin Microbiol Infect. 2011;17(3):439–44.

66. Bradbury T, Fehring TK, Taunton M, Hanssen A, Azzam K, Parvizi J, et al. The fate of acute methicillin-resistant *Staphylococcus aureus* periprosthetic knee infections treated by open debridement and retention of components. J Arthroplasty. 2009;24(6 Suppl):101–4.

67. Zurcher-Pfund L, Uckay I, Legout L, Gamulin A, Vaudaux P, Peter R. Pathogen-driven decision for implant retention in the management of infected total knee prostheses. Int Orthop. 2013;37(8):1471–5.

68. Triantafyllopoulos GK, Poultsides LA, Zhang W, Sculco PK, Ma Y, Sculco TP. Periprosthetic knee infections treated with irrigation and debridement: outcomes and preoperative predictive factors. J Arthroplasty. 2015;30(4):649–57.

One-Stage Exchange Arthroplasty of the Infected Knee

16

Mustafa Citak, Sophia-Marlene Busch, Christian Lausmann, Philip Linke, and Thorsten Gehrke

16.1 Introduction

Chronic periprosthetic joint infection (PJI) of the knee joint requires exchange arthroplasty. Worldwide, two-stage exchange arthroplasty has become the "golden standard." In contrast, the ENDO-Klinik follows a distinct one-stage exchange for PJI in over 85% of all our infected cases according to the first implementation of mixing antibiotics into bone cement introduced by Prof. Buchholz in the 1970s.

From a global perspective, the concept of one-stage exchange arthroplasty has become increasingly popular in several specialized centers due to the potential functional benefits for the patients and a decreased burden to their national health-care system [1].

The one-stage exchange offers certain advantages, as mainly based on need for only one operative procedure, displayed in the chapter "clinical results." In order to fulfill a one-stage approach with its potential success, there are obligatory pre-, peri-, and postoperative requirements, which need to be meticulously respected. The following book chapter provides an evidence-based overview in regard to the key points of one-stage exchange arthroplasty of the infected knee.

16.2 Indications for One-Stage Exchange Arthroplasty

The germ has to be known for one-stage exchange arthroplasty based on microbiological diagnostics as well as a distinct patient specific plan for the topic and systemic antibiotic treatment by a multidisciplinary team (Table 16.1). Table 16.1 reveals the indications along with contraindications for the one-stage procedure. In a recent study by Citak et al. [2], risk factors for failure after one-stage exchange TKA in the management of PJI have been identified. According to the study results, the isolation of enterococci and streptococci had significantly higher risk for failure. However, similar results have also been found for the two-stage procedure [3, 4]. Therefore, further comparative studies are required to determine both germs as either indications or contraindications for the one-stage procedure.

M. Citak (✉) · S.-M. Busch · C. Lausmann · P. Linke
T. Gehrke
Department of Orthopedic Surgery, ENDO-Klinik
Hamburg, Hamburg, Germany
e-mail: christian.lausmann@helios-gesundheit.de;
thorsten.gehrke@helios-gesundheit.de

© ISAKOS 2022
U. G. Longo et al. (eds.), *Infection in Knee Replacement*,
https://doi.org/10.1007/978-3-030-81553-0_16

Table 16.1 The indications and contraindications for the one-stage procedure

Indications	Contraindications
• PJI after TKA in which infection is proven, based on the ICM criteria 2018	• Culture-negative PJI
• Late or chronic infection more than 30 days postoperatively	• Non-availability of the required antibiotic
• Hematogenous infection more than 30 days after onset of the symptoms	• Systemic sepsis of the patient
• Known germ with known susceptibility based on microbiological diagnostics	• Failure of 2 or more previous 1-stage procedures
• Possibility of primary wound closure	• Severe soft tissue infection spreading to the nerve-vessel bundle
	• Extensive soft tissue involvement that would prevent closure of the wound

16.3 Endo-Klinik Diagnostic Protocol

Despite the fact that there are no specific symptoms for periprosthetic joint infections, it is recommended that every patient with the following criteria should be further tested to validate or exclude a PJI:

- patient's medical history (e.g. prolonged wound secretion, fever, wound healing disorders),
- painful total joint arthroplasty,
- loosening of the total joint arthroplasty within the first year,
- unspecific symptoms such as night sweat, fatigue, unwanted loss of weight,
- elevated inflammatory markers (e.g. serum C-reactive Protein, erythrocyte sedimentation rate),
- prior elective revision arthroplasty.

The joint aspiration is the most needed and relevant preoperative diagnostic test in any case of a planned one-stage exchange. Hereby, it is highly recommended to respect a prolonged microbiologic culture time of at least 14 days [5]. Furthermore, the antibiotics should be withheld for 14 days prior to the aspiration. The joint aspiration should be performed under operating room conditions with sterile washing and draping. In order to avoid false negative results, local anesthetics or saline rinsing should not be administered.

Synchronous PJI is a rare, but serious complication with an incidence rate of 4% [6]. Therefore, joint aspiration is obligatory for exclusion of the suspicion of PJI after joint arthroplasty.

Several tests for diagnosing PJI are performed in order to differentiate between septic and aseptic failure. At our institution, besides serum CRP, synovial fluid is tested in the following descending order:

1. culture and susceptibility,
2. quantitative alpha defensin test,
3. leukocyte esterase test,
4. cell count,
5. polymorphonuclear leukocytes (PMN%).

The verification of periprosthetic joint infection is made according to the ICM 2018 Criteria [7]. In case of a negative germ detection, a secondary control aspiration is recommended to eliminate suspicion for PJI. If the results of the second aspiration for germ identification remain negative, an open biopsy should be performed (Fig. 16.1).

16.4 Surgical Technique

16.4.1 Preoperative Planning and Surgical Approach

In every case, preoperative plain radiographs (anteroposterior and lateral views of the knee joint and tangential view of the patella) and anteroposterior standing long-leg radiographs are performed. The preoperative identification of the bacteria defines which antibiotic-loaded acrylic cement is required and is the main factor to perform the one-stage exchange arthroplasty.

Fig. 16.1 Flow chart of the Endo-Klinik Treatment Protocol of chronic PJI

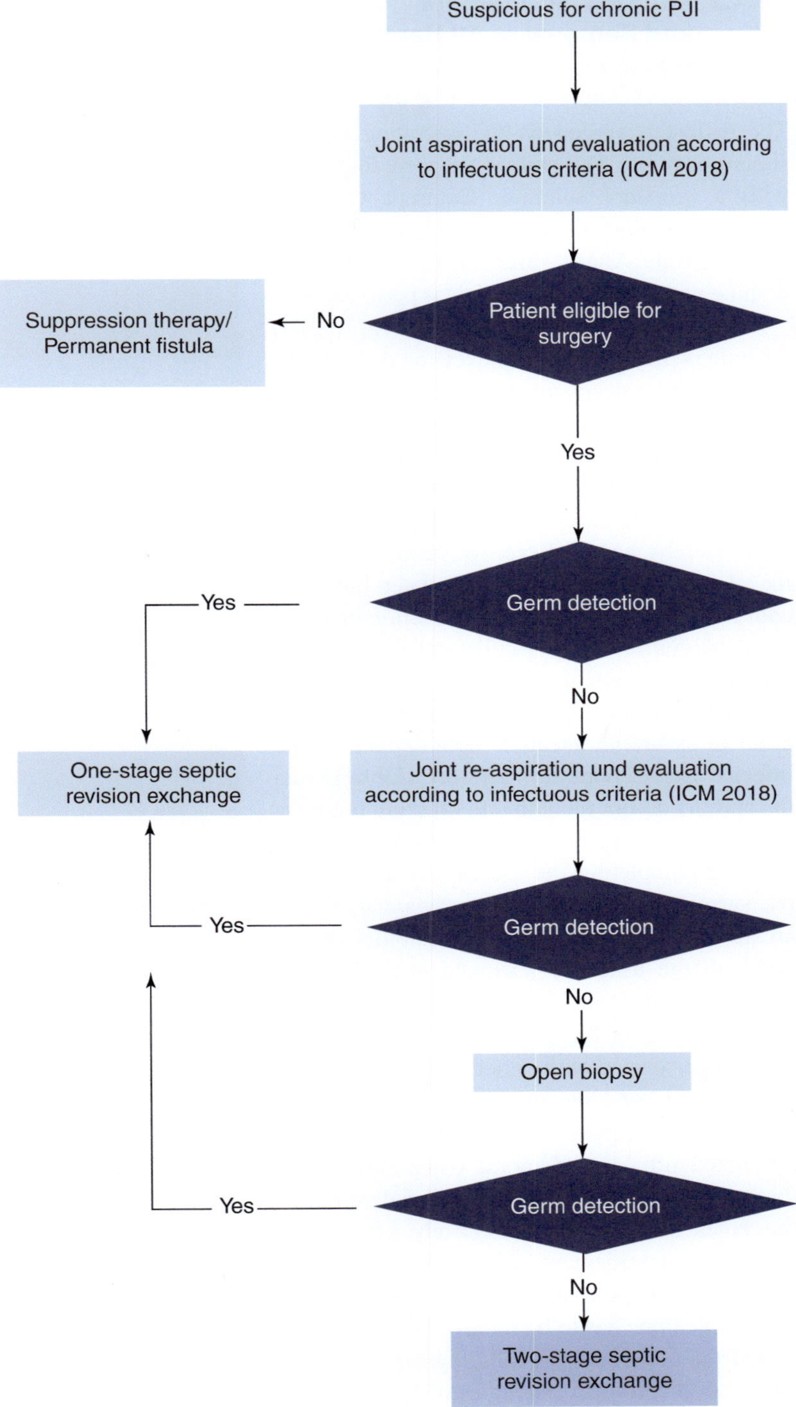

16.4.2 Radical Debridement and Removal of All Hardware Materials

The patient is placed on the operating table in supine position. The skin is prepped four times with a propanol solution (Cutasept G, Bode Chemie, Hamburg, Germany) within at least 2 min of acting time. After disinfection, a standard knee draping with single use materials is performed.

First, the existing scar is excised (Fig. 16.2). If a fistula is present, a radical excision down to the joint capsule is necessary. Second, an extraarticular debridement of the joint capsule and the synovium is carried out. Third, the joint is opened and a radical debridement is performed, including a complete synovectomy (Figs. 16.3 and 16.4). Hereby, a radical excision needs to be done for all non-bleeding tissues and related bones. In addition, the radical soft tissue resection incorporates the debridement of collateral ligaments as well as the excision of each infected tissue around the patella region and in the patella surface. In order to assure an adequate debridement of the infected tissues/bone down to the viable tissue, the authors do not recommend utilizing the tourniquet during the debridement process.

After completing the radical debridement of the surrounding tissues, all hardware materials are removed. To increase the feasibility of the removal, the usage of adequate instruments is crucial. In this case, the implant–cement interface loosening of the femoral and tibial components is performed with either an oscillating saw (Fig. 16.5) or an osteotome (Fig. 16.6). Subsequently, a punch is utilized to remove the mobilized tibial and femoral components with direct blows. After hardware material removal, the cement has to be removed entirely. Afterwards, meticulous debridement of bone and soft-tissues is fundamental including all areas of the knee. All non-viable bone has to be removed (Fig. 16.7).

For the combined microbiological and histological evaluation, five samples of biopsy material are collected during the debridement from all relevant areas of the operation site and sent to the laboratory for further evaluation. After the last

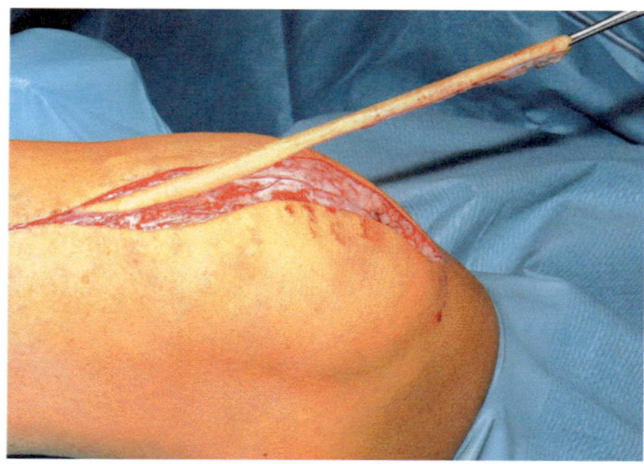

Fig. 16.2 Intraoperative image displays the excision of the persisting scar

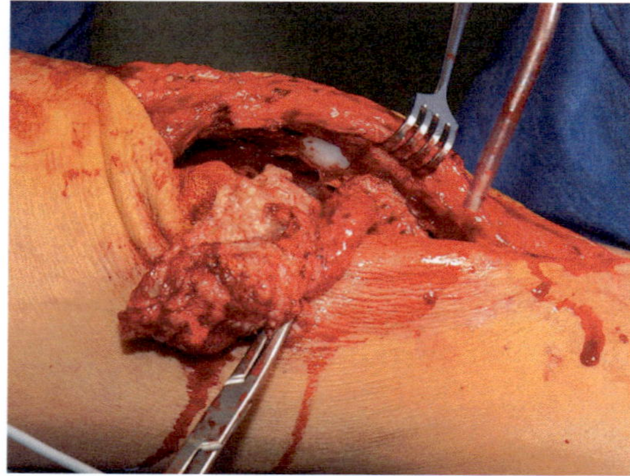

Fig. 16.3 Intraoperative situs showing the synovectomy

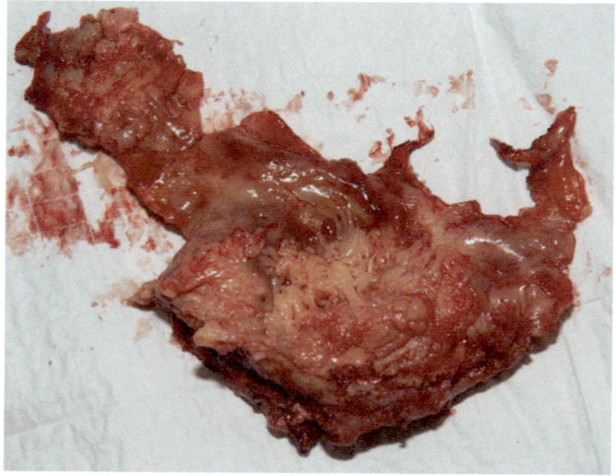

Fig. 16.4 The removal of the infected tissue

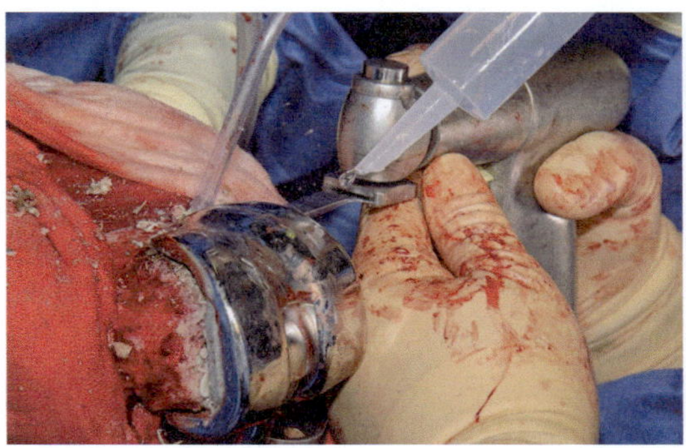

Fig. 16.5 The implant–cement interface loosening of the femoral component utilizing the oscillating saw

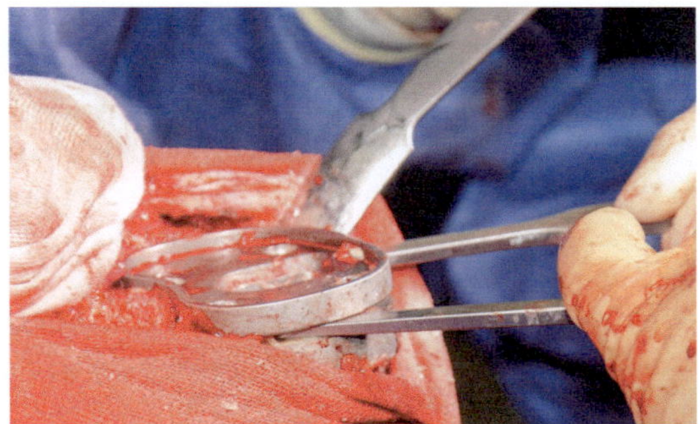

Fig. 16.6 Implant–cement interface loosening of the tibial component utilizing the osteotome

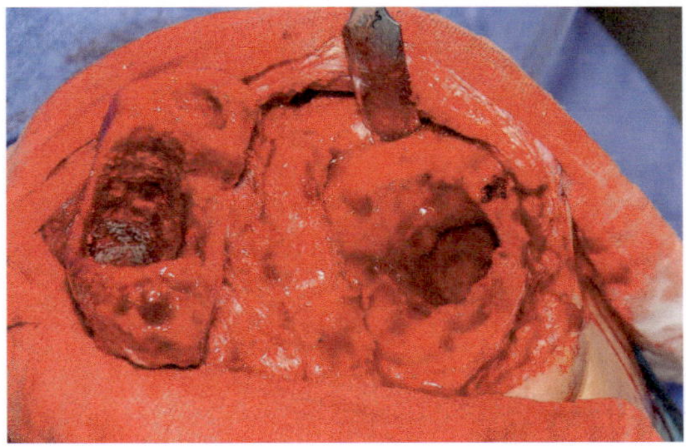

Fig. 16.7 The viable bone and soft tissue after radical debridement

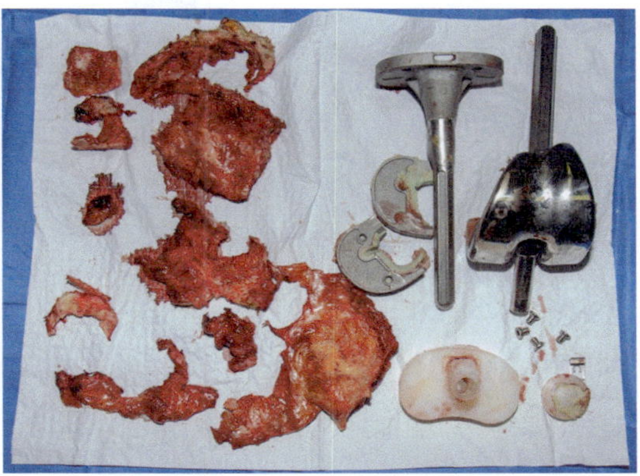

Fig. 16.8 The result of the radical debridement. Every infected tissue or bone and all foreign hardware materials have to be removed

before new operative setup is prepared. The new operative setup includes the re-draping of the surgical field, the change of light handles, suction tips, surgical gowns along with gloves.

16.4.3 Re-Implantation

After the last microbiological sample was taken, the systemic antibiotic therapy is started as recommended by the microbiologist. Then, the reconstruction of the joint is carried out with implantation of a cemented rotating hinge/full hinge knee implant (ENDO-Model, Waldemar Link, Hamburg, Germany) after preparing the tibia and femur with appropriate resection blocks. Antibiotic-loaded cement is utilized for both the fixation of the new implant and the reconstruction of bone defects. Instead of using allograft bone, we recommend to fill the defects either with polymethylmethacrylate (PMMA) bone cement (Copal, Heraeus Medical, Wehrheim, Germany) or trabecular metal cones (Fig. 16.9).

The preparation of antibiotic-loaded cement is followed after a strict protocol. In general, manufactured antibiotic bone cements are used, such as Copal G + C or Copal G + V (Heraeus Medical, Wehrheim, Germany). An admixture of antibiotics might be indicated, based on the preoperative microbiological findings. Finally, a primary soft tissue closure is accomplished, after the harden-

biopsy that was taken and completed radical debridement, the irrigation is performed with pulsatile lavage with 0.02% polyhexanide solution (Lavasept, B. Braun, Melsungen, Germany) (Fig. 16.8). The polyhexanide-soaked swabs are placed over the wound area for at least 10 min

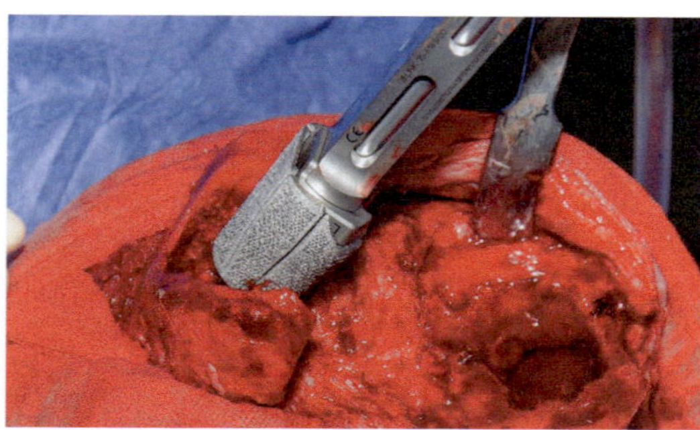

Fig. 16.9 Femoral bone defect filled with trabecular metal cone

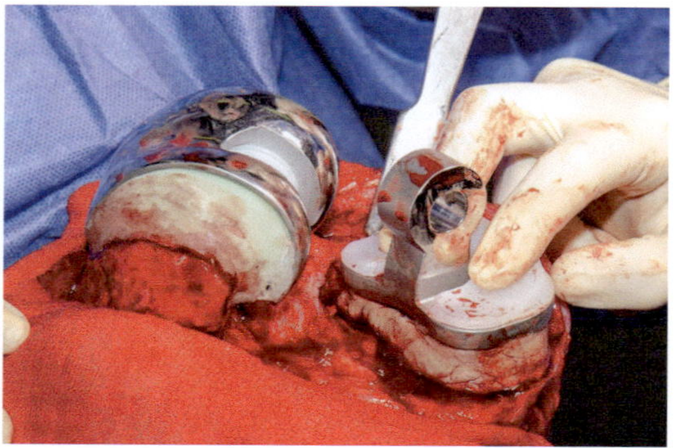

Fig. 16.10 Implantation of the new prosthesis during the hardening process

ing process of the cement and irrigation (Fig. 16.10). Intraarticular suction drainage is strongly recommended.

16.4.4 Postoperative Course

Anteroposterior and lateral plain radiographs of the knee should be carried out instantly after surgery. Although the evidence about the optimal duration of intravenous antibiotic therapy remains scarce, we recommend to administer postoperative systemic antibiotic therapy for 14 days, based on the recommendations by the microbiologist [8]. On the day of surgery, the patient is mobilized with full weight bearing and support by crutches under intensive physiotherapy and sufficient analgesia. The wound drainage is taken off 48 h after surgery.

16.5 Clinical Results

There is a lack of studies on the outcomes after one-stage revision surgery [2, 9–20].

For instance, the reported eradication rates of one-stage revision technique vary between 73.1% and 100%, depending on the time of follow-up (Table 16.2). At our institution, the 10 year infection-free survival rate was 93% [20]. Other long-term studies with 10- or 12 years follow-up present success rates beyond 90% after one-stage revision arthroplasty [18, 21]. According to Citak et al. [2], the risk factors for failure after one-stage exchange TKA in the management of PJI have been identified. The top three causes for failure following one-stage knee exchange were with 51.6% recurrence of infection, followed by aseptic loosening with 40.7%, and finally patella complications with 3.3%. In this study, the mean time to failure after one-stage procedure was 25.2 months [2]. The top three risk factors for reinfection were the isolation of enterococcus, followed by failed one-stage exchange and persistent wound drainage. Isolation of streptococcus was also a significant risk factor for reinfection.

Table 16.2 Overview about the current literature of the one-stage septic knee exchange arthroplasty

	N	Follow-up (in years)	Eradication rate (in %)
Freeman et al. [11]	8	2.2	100
von Foerster et al. [19]	104	Not reported	73.1
Goksan and Freeman [12]	18	5	89
Lu et al. [27]	8	1.7	100
Silva et al. [15]	37	4	89.2
Buechel et al. [10]	21	10.2	90.9
Sofer et al. [17]	15	1.5	93.3
Bauer et al. [9]	30	4.3	Not reported
Singer et al. [16]	63	3	95
Jenny et al. [14]	47	2.75	87
Haddad et al. [13]	28	6.5	100
Tibrewal et al. [18]	50	10.5	98
Zahar et al. [20]	70	10	93

Streptococcus and enterococcus infections have also poor outcomes with the two-stage procedure [3, 4]. In a recently published review article, the one-stage exchange showed similar results in the eradication rate and functional outcomes, compared to the two-stage procedure, and offers the advantage of a unique surgical procedure [22]. Besides performing solely one operation, the one-stage exchange offers five main advantages:

1. higher quality of life [23],
2. lower morbidity/mortality rate [24],
3. lower in-hospital complications [25],
4. lower blood loss and allogeneic blood transfusion rates [26],
5. higher cost-effectiveness [23].

16.6 Conclusions

Based on the authors experience and the literature, the success of one-stage revision surgery is based on the following requirements: Well-defined intra-hospital infrastructure; meticulous preoperative aspiration regime; radical debridement including removal of all hardware materials; multidisciplinary approach (microbiologist, surgeon, etc.); adjusted local antibiotic-loaded bone cement; and postoperative adjusted systemic antibiotic therapy.

References

1. Kildow BJ, Della-Valle CJ, Springer BD. Single vs 2-stage revision for the treatment of periprosthetic joint infection. J Arthroplasty. 2020;35(3S):S24–30. Epub 2020/02/13.
2. Citak M, Friedenstab J, Abdelaziz H, Suero EM, Zahar A, Salber J, et al. Risk factors for failure after 1-stage exchange total knee arthroplasty in the management of periprosthetic joint infection. J Bone Joint Surg Am. 2019;101(12):1061–9. Epub 2019/06/21.
3. Akgun D, Trampuz A, Perka C, Renz N. High failure rates in treatment of streptococcal periprosthetic joint infection: results from a seven-year retrospective cohort study. Bone Joint J. 2017;99-B(5):653–9. Epub 2017/04/30.
4. Ma CY, Lu YD, Bell KL, Wang JW, Ko JY, Wang CJ, et al. Predictors of treatment failure after 2-stage reimplantation for infected total knee arthroplasty: a 2- to 10-year follow-up. J Arthroplasty. 2018;33(7):2234–9. Epub 2018/03/25.
5. Schafer P, Fink B, Sandow D, Margull A, Berger I, Frommelt L. Prolonged bacterial culture to identify late periprosthetic joint infection: a promising strategy. Clin Infect Dis. 2008;47(11):1403–9. Epub 2008/10/22.
6. Thiesen DM, Mumin-Gunduz S, Gehrke T, Klaber I, Salber J, Suero E, et al. Synchronous periprosthetic joint infections: the need for all artificial joints to be aspirated routinely. J Bone Joint Surg Am. 2020;102(4):283–91. Epub 2019/12/20.
7. Shohat N, Bauer T, Buttaro M, Budhiparama N, Cashman J, Della Valle CJ, et al. Hip and knee section, what is the definition of a periprosthetic joint infection (PJI) of the knee and the hip? Can the same criteria be used for both joints?: proceedings of international consensus on orthopedic infections. J Arthroplasty. 2019;34(2S):S325–S7. Epub 2018/10/23.
8. Sandiford NA, McHale A, Citak M, Kendoff D. What is the optimal duration of intravenous antibiotics following single-stage revision total hip arthroplasty for prosthetic joint infection? A systematic review. Hip Int. 2020;27:1120700020922850. Epub 2020/05/28.
9. Bauer T, Piriou P, Lhotellier L, Leclerc P, Mamoudy P, Lortat-Jacob A. Results of reimplantation for infected total knee arthroplasty: 107 cases. Rev Chir Orthop Reparatrice Appar Mot. 2006;92(7):692–700. Epub 2006/11/25.
10. Buechel FF, Femino FP, D'Alessio J. Primary exchange revision arthroplasty for infected total knee replacement: a long-term study. Am J Orthop (Belle Mead NJ). 2004;33(4):190–8; discussion 8. Epub 2004/05/11.
11. Freeman MA, Sudlow RA, Casewell MW, Radcliff SS. The management of infected total knee replacements. J Bone Joint Surg Br. 1985;67(5):764–8. Epub 1985/11/01.
12. Goksan SB, Freeman MA. One-stage reimplantation for infected total knee arthroplasty. J Bone Joint Surg Br. 1992;74(1):78–82. Epub 1992/01/01.
13. Haddad FS, Sukeik M, Alazzawi S. Is single-stage revision according to a strict protocol effective in treatment of chronic knee arthroplasty infections? Clin Orthop Relat Res. 2015;473(1):8–14. Epub 2014/06/14.
14. Jenny JY, Barbe B, Gaudias J, Boeri C, Argenson JN. High infection control rate and function after routine one-stage exchange for chronically infected TKA. Clin Orthop Relat Res. 2013;471(1):238–43. Epub 2012/07/17.
15. Silva M, Tharani R, Schmalzried TP. Results of direct exchange or debridement of the infected total knee arthroplasty. Clin Orthop Relat Res. 2002;404:125–31. Epub 2002/11/20.
16. Singer J, Merz A, Frommelt L, Fink B. High rate of infection control with one-stage revision of septic knee prostheses excluding MRSA and MRSE. Clin Orthop Relat Res. 2012;470(5):1461–71. Epub 2011/11/15.

17. Sofer D, Regenbrecht B, Pfeil J. Early results of one-stage septic revision arthroplasties with antibiotic-laden cement. A clinical and statistical analysis. Orthopade. 2005;34(6):592–602. Epub 2005/04/19.

18. Tibrewal S, Malagelada F, Jeyaseelan L, Posch F, Scott G. Single-stage revision for the infected total knee replacement: results from a single centre. Bone Joint J. 2014;96-B(6):759–64. Epub 2014/06/04.

19. von Foerster G, Kluber D, Kabler U. Mid- to long-term results after treatment of 118 cases of periprosthetic infections after knee joint replacement using one-stage exchange surgery. Orthopade. 1991;20(3):244–52. Epub 1991/06/01.

20. Zahar A, Kendoff DO, Klatte TO, Gehrke TA. Can good infection control be obtained in one-stage exchange of the infected TKA to a rotating hinge design? 10-year results. Clin Orthop Relat Res. 2016;474(1):81–7. Epub 2015/06/24.

21. Macheras GA, Kateros K, Galanakos SP, Koutsostathis SD, Kontou E, Papadakis SA. The long-term results of a two-stage protocol for revision of an infected total knee replacement. J Bone Joint Surg. 2011;93(11):1487–92.

22. Pangaud C, Ollivier M, Argenson JN. Outcome of single-stage versus two-stage exchange for revision knee arthroplasty for chronic periprosthetic infection. EFORT Open Rev. 2019;4(8):495–4502. Epub 2019/09/21.

23. Srivastava K, Bozic KJ, Silverton C, Nelson AJ, Makhni EC, Davis JJ. Reconsidering strategies for managing chronic periprosthetic joint infection in total knee arthroplasty: using decision analytics to find the optimal strategy between one-stage and two-stage total knee revision. J Bone Joint Surg Am. 2019;101(1):14–24. Epub 2019/01/03.

24. Leta TH, Lygre SHL, Schrama JC, Hallan G, Gjertsen JE, Dale H, et al. Outcome of revision surgery for infection after total knee arthroplasty: results of 3 surgical strategies. JBJS Rev. 2019;7(6):e4. Epub 2019/06/13.

25. Thiesen DM, Sobhani H, Gehrke T, Suero EM, Klatte TO, Citak M. A comparison of short term complication rate between 44 two- and 385 one-stage septic exchange arthroplasties in chronic periprosthetic joint infections. Orthop Traumatol Surg Res. 2021;107:102668. Epub 2020/08/17.

26. Sharqzad AS, Cavalheiro C, Zahar A, Lausmann C, Gehrke T, Kendoff D, et al. Blood loss and allogeneic transfusion for surgical treatment of periprosthetic joint infection: a comparison of one- vs. two-stage exchange total hip arthroplasty. Int Orthop. 2019;43(9):2025–30. Epub 2018/09/07.

27. Lu H, Kou B, Lin J. One-stage reimplantation for the salvage of total knee arthroplasty complicated by infection. Zhonghua Wai Ke Za Zhi. 1997;35(8):456–8. Epub 1997/08/01.

Two-Stage Revision Arthroplasty for Periprosthetic Knee Infection

Umile Giuseppe Longo, Sergio De Salvatore, Vincenzo Candela, Giovanna Stelitano, Calogero Di Naro, Carlo Casciaro, Laura Risi Ambrogioni, and Vincenzo Denaro

17.1 Introduction

Periprosthetic joint infection (PJI) is one of the most catastrophic complications following joint arthroplasty. The complexity of treatment of PJI leads to dramatic physical, emotional, and financial costs. Despite advances in the prevention, diagnosis, and treatment of PJI, it remains the most commonly reported cause of early failure in total knee arthroplasty (TKA). The goal of PJI treatment is to eradicate the infection and restore a functional and stable joint [1]. Treatment of PJI includes surgical interventions such as irrigation and debridement, one-stage reimplantation, two-stage reimplantation, resection arthroplasty, or amputations. The choice of the treatment depends upon the type of infection and the type of the organism responsible, the general conditions of the patient and his life expectancy. Treatment of periprosthetic joint infections with a two-stage revision arthroplasty remains a widely used treatment strategy. The potential advantages of one-stage exchange arthroplasty are multiple, including a decrease in surgical morbidity and

mortality, earlier functional return, and lower costs. One-stage revision has a lower risk of mortality and morbidity compared to two-stage revision, which exposes the patient to the risks of an additional procedure. However, several authors demonstrated a reduced rate of recurrent infection after two-stage revision in comparison to one-stage revision [2–5]. The reinfection rate after two-stage revision is between 9 and 20% of cases [6]. Two-stage revision is the most used procedure for prosthetic joint infection treatment in North America [7].

17.2 History

Insall was the first to describe a two-stage reimplantation procedure for the management of infected total knee arthroplasties [8, 9]. Two-stage revision arthroplasty consists of removing all foreign materials from the joint, making an extensive debridement of periarticular tissues and inserting a static or articulating spacer.

The use of an impregnated antibiotic cement spacer block maintains the joint space, prevents retraction of the collateral ligaments, and provides a local antibiotic release. However, static spacers present several disadvantages, such as restriction of knee movement, tissue adherence formation, and quadriceps shortening. To overcome the problems of block spacers and to facilitate reimplantation surgery, articulating spacers

U. G. Longo (✉) · S. De Salvatore · V. Candela
G. Stelitano · C. Di Naro · C. Casciaro
L. Risi Ambrogioni · V. Denaro
Department of Orthopaedic and Trauma Surgery,
Campus Bio-Medico University, Via Alvaro del
Portillo, Rome, Trigoria, Italy
e-mail: g.longo@unicampus.it

© ISAKOS 2022
U. G. Longo et al. (eds.), *Infection in Knee Replacement*,
https://doi.org/10.1007/978-3-030-81553-0_17

were introduced. The implantation of the cement spacer is followed by systemic antibiotic therapy for an extended period. When the eradication of the infection is completed and the wound is healed, reimplantation could be considered. Patients report instability, pain, and limited function during this period, mainly if the non-articulating spacer is used. Reimplantation consists of removing the spacer, repeating debridement, and implanting revision arthroplasty components. There is a lack of high-quality evidence on the ideal type of spacer.

In our clinical practice, two-stage revision is the primary choice for the majority of PJI.

17.3 Timing for Reimplantation

There is not a consensus on the optimal timing for reimplantation [1]. The authors reported an interval between few weeks and several months [10–14]. The range of infection's eradication after two-stage revision is between 70 and 100%, without a clear correlation to the time of reimplantation [11–13, 15].

Several variables can be associated with unsuccessful eradication of infection following a two-stage revision knee procedure, including an increased duration between resection and reimplantation [16, 17]. On the other side, Babis et al. [18, 19] found a high rate of success with a mean 9-month interval in patients with multiresistant bacteria.

In our opinion, the timing for reimplantation must be decided based on clinical evaluations, wound healing, and serologic tests after a period of antibiotic therapy and subsequent antibiotic washout period. Our consideration finds its reason in the current literature. The most recent review about two-stage revision, realized by Tozun et al. in 2020, explains that a precise timing for the interval between the two stages still does not exist. In case of optimal local tissue conditions and quick time of recovery after the first stage, a short interval of 2–4 weeks should be considered. Conversely, when the culture in the first stage identifies a difficult-to-treat microorganisms, a longer interval of 4–6 weeks should

be preferred. Longer time intervals of over 8 weeks should be avoided as the antibiotic bone cement spacer misses its antibiotic concentration. The prolonged duration among resection and reimplantation seems to be associated with a greater risk of reinfection [20].

17.4 Non-Articulating Vs. Articulating Spacers

Periprosthetic joint infections could be managed with two-stage revision using non-articulating (Fig. 17.1) or articulating spacers (Fig. 17.2).

There is a lack of high-quality evidence on the ideal type of spacer [21–23]. Some authors reported the superiority of articulating spacers when compared to non-articulating spacers in terms of functional outcomes, time of hospital, and range of motion [24]. However, complications of spacers include fractures and dislocations. Surgeon-made articulating spacers are reported to have more risk of fracture when compared to preformed spacers.

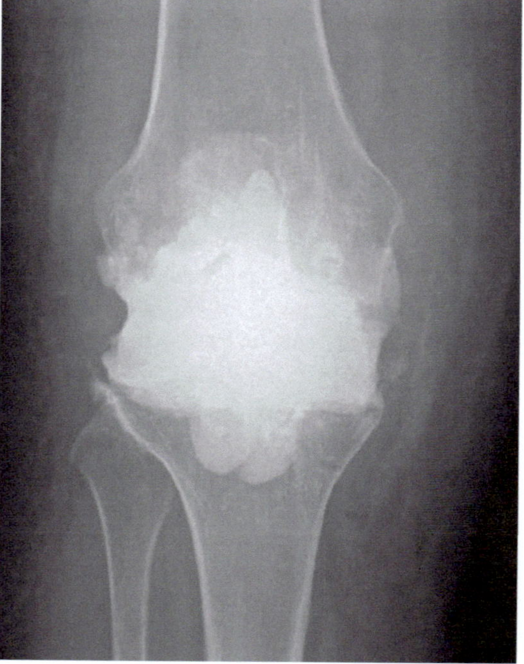

Fig. 17.1 Non-articulating knee spacer

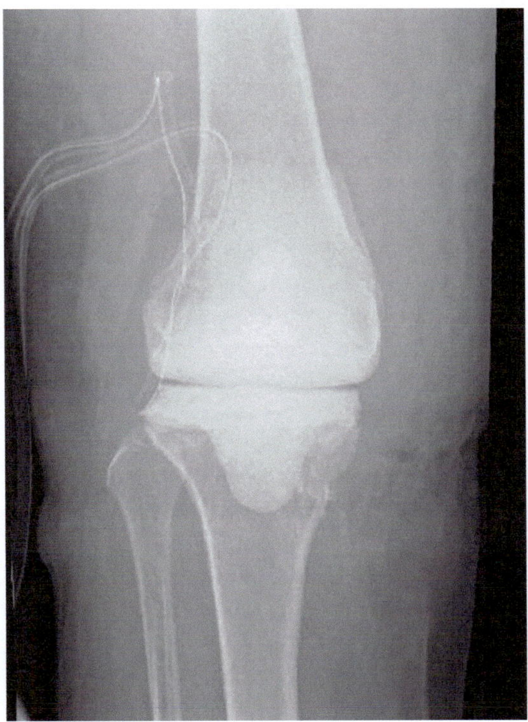

Fig. 17.2 Articulating knee spacer

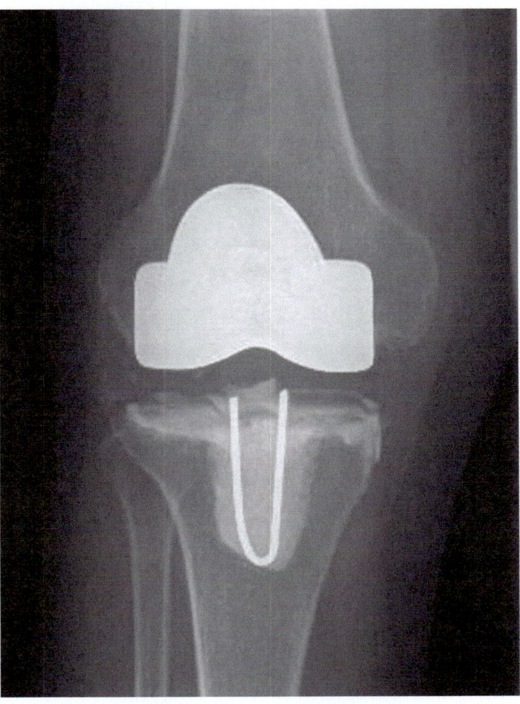

Fig. 17.3 Hofmann reported the use of the original, resterilized femoral component fixed with antibiotic-loaded cement and a new polyethylene insert cemented to the tibia for the knee

Hofmann reported the use of the original, resterilized femoral component fixed with antibiotic-loaded cement and a new polyethylene insert cemented to the tibia for the knee with good outcomes (Fig. 17.3) [25].

Patients may be candidates for non-articulating spacers if they have major bone loss, ligamentous, or muscles injuries that cause a probability of dislocation or periprosthetic fractures or soft tissue defects. In these patients, a reduction in motion allows wound healing. On the other side, articulating spacers provide a better range of motion and less functional limitations but are indicated only in selected patients.

Emerson et al. [26] compared static block spacers with articulating spacers and reported an improvement in post-operative ROM with no significant difference in the reinfection rate.

However, antibiotic cement spacers should be used for a limited period: bacterial colonization of spacers can occur with increasing in situ time [27, 28].

17.5 Local Antibiotics

Local antibiotics added to cement have a higher concentration and duration in comparison to systemic antibiotic [29]. They should be tailored based on preoperative cultures and patients medical conditions, particularly renal function [27, 30]. If the infective organism is not isolated from preoperative cultures, a broad-spectrum empiric combination of antibiotics can be used [31, 32]. An ideal antibiotic should be safe, thermostable, hypoallergenic, water-soluble, with a high bacterial spectrum and available as sterile [33]. Antibiotics like gentamicin, vancomycin, ampicillin, clindamycin, and meropenem can be used as a combination based on organism susceptibility. Vancomycin is usually used for methicillin-resistant *Staphylococcus aureus* (MRSA) or methicillin-resistant *Staphylococcus epidermidis* (MRSE) [34], usually in combination with an aminoglycoside, such as gentamicin or tobramycin.

Third-generation cephalosporins, carbapenems, and monobactam antibiotics are used with success for susceptible gram-negative bacteria [35–38].

A rare complication of local antibiotic is the systemic toxicity as a result of elution of antibiotics from cement spacers. To prevent this complication renal clearance of the patients and viscosity of the cement must be checked. The optimal antibiotic dosage per 40-g bag of bone cement has not yet been determined. The reported doses range from 2 to 5 g for gentamicin, from 2.4 to 9.6 g for tobramycin, and from 3 to 9 g for vancomycin [39].

17.6 Systemic Antimicrobial Therapy

Systemic antimicrobial therapy should be tailored based on isolated bacteria and patients characteristics. Patients treated without bacteria isolation have 4.5 times increased risk of reinfection when compared to those patients where an organism was identified by culture [40, 41]. There is not a consensus on the optimal length of antibiotic treatment after resection arthroplasty. However, antibiotic therapy administrated for more than 6 weeks may increase the rate of antibiotic-related complications [42–44]. Excellent results are obtained with a combination of oral and intravenous antibiotic administration for 6 weeks or less [31, 45, 46]. Antimicrobial treatment is usually started with intravenous antibiotics to obtain the appropriate concentrations locally and after are switched to oral antibiotics.

17.7 Surgical Tips and Tricks

- During revision foreign materials, including cement, must be removed. These materials can act as a nidus for biofilm and persistence of infection [29, 47].
- Complete debridement of the joint and removal of all hardware is ideal during the surgical treatment.
- Is desirable to remove accessible heterotopic ossification if this procedure does not compromise future reconstruction.

- Allograft for management of bone defects during reimplantation seems not to increase the risk of reinfection [48, 49].
- The two-stage revision of unicompartmental knee arthroplasty requires the resection of all the compartments and of the fat pad.
- Soft tissue defects could be managed with a reconstructive flap at the time of explant or at the time of reimplantation. Medial gastrocnemius rotational flaps are usually used to manage soft tissue defects in knee arthroplasty revision. However, lateral gastrocnemius, latissimus dorsi, quadriceps, sartorius, and rectus abdominus could be alternatively used [50–52].
- During reimplantation cemented or cementless prosthesis could be alternatively used. No differences were demonstrated in terms of success rate of infection treatment. The choice between cemented or cementless components must be made based on classical factors such as bone quality or body mass. If cemented prostheses are used, consideration should be given to the addition of antibiotics active on the isolated bacteria [53].

17.8 Cement Spacer Exchange

Cement spacer exchange (Figs. 17.4 and 17.5) gives a new load of local antibiotics when the infection is not under control [54]. However, there is a lack of evidence on the benefit of this procedure. Indications for spacer exchange

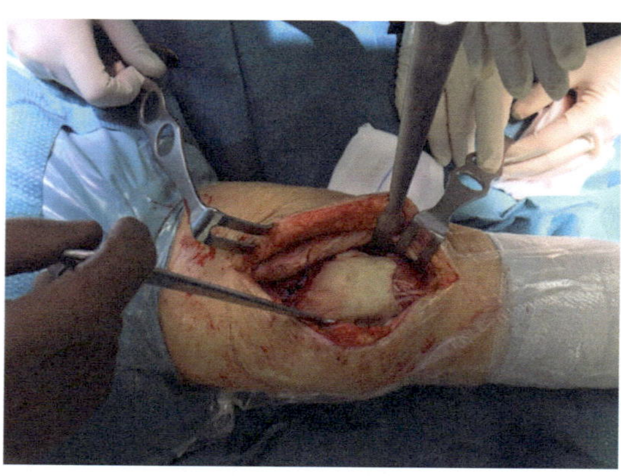

Fig. 17.4 In situ non-articulating knee spacer

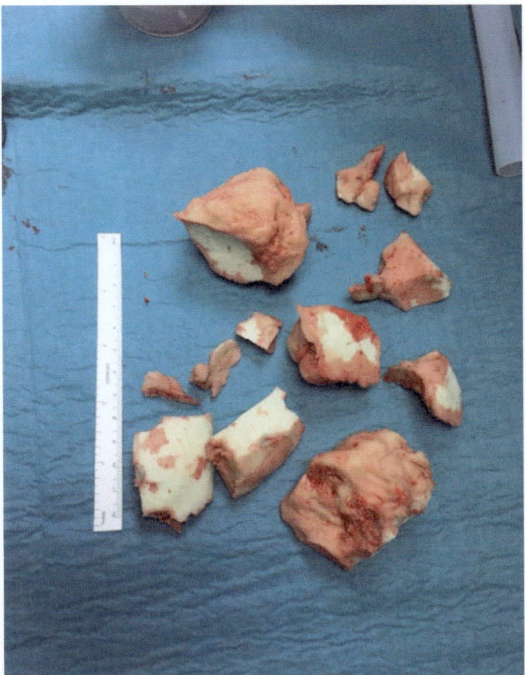

Fig. 17.5 Removal of the knee spacer

Table 17.1 Advantages and disadvantages of one-stage vs. two-stage PJI revision procedures

	One-stage	Two-stage
Advantages	• Lower morbidity and higher functional outcomes • Higher quality of life • Lower recovery rates • Lower cost • Technically easier • Quicker rehabilitation	• Targeted micro-organism eradication • Lower rate of reinfection • Extensive debridement
Disadvantages	• Unable to direct antibiotic in cement to specific organism • Unable to observe response to antibiotic therapy • Higher reinfection rate • Only one debridement • Able to eradicate distant sites of infection	• Higher morbidity and mortality • High complexity of the surgical technique • Higher rate of recovery • Lower quality of life • Higher surgical risks • Higher cost • Slower rehabilitation

include persistent infection, wound-related problems, draining sinus, or mechanical complications such as spacer dislocation or fracture [55, 56].

17.9 Cement Spacer Irrigation and Debridement

Cement spacer irrigation and debridement is an alternative to cement spacer exchange to reduce the microbial bioburden. However, for this procedure, there is a lack of evidence on the practical benefits. Moreover, repeated cement spacer irrigation, without antibiotic spacer exchange, does not seem to have any evidence [57].

17.10 Infected Bilateral Knee Arthroplasties

Limited evidence is available to recommend a single-stage or two-stage revision procedure for infected bilateral knee arthroplasties [58–60]. Two-stage revision is made placing an antibiotic-impregnated cement spacer for at least 6–8 weeks before reimplantation. The authors reported that patients could wait for several days between each side reimplantation or perform a simultaneous bilateral revision surgery [58–60]. The decision to perform simultaneous bilateral revision surgery should consider several factors, such as the patient's comorbidities and functional status. Wolff et al. [61] demonstrated improved outcomes with a simultaneous two-staged revision when compared with irrigation, debridement, and prosthetic salvage. However, concerns exist about the morbidity of a two-stage revision and the immobility on both extremities during the antibiotic spacer period (Table 17.1).

17.11 Conclusion

Limited evidence is available on the superiority of two-stage over one-stage revision in terms of success, eradication of infection, or patient satisfaction [2–4]. Future studies are necessary to delineate the superiority of a one- or two-stage revision approach.

References

1. Papalia R, Vespasiani-Gentilucci U, Longo UG, Esposito C, Zampogna B, Antonelli Incalzi R, et al. Advances in management of periprosthetic joint infections: an historical prospective study. Eur Rev Med Pharmacol Sci. 2019;23(2 Suppl):129–38.
2. Haddad FS, Sukeik M, Alazzawi S. Is single-stage revision according to a strict protocol effective in treatment of chronic knee arthroplasty infections? Clin Orthop Relat Res. 2015;473(1):8–14.
3. Wolf M, Clar H, Friesenbichler J, Schwantzer G, Bernhardt G, Gruber G, et al. Prosthetic joint infection following total hip replacement: results of one-stage versus two-stage exchange. Int Orthop. 2014;38(7):1363–8.
4. Azzam K, McHale K, Austin M, Purtill JJ, Parvizi J. Outcome of a second two-stage reimplantation for periprosthetic knee infection. Clin Orthop Relat Res. 2009;467(7):1706–14.
5. Longo UG, Candela V, Pirato F, Hirschmann MT, Becker R, Denaro V. Midflexion instability in total knee arthroplasty: a systematic review. Knee Surg Sports Traumatol Arthrosc. 2020;29(2):370–80.
6. Zahar A, Gehrke TA. One-stage revision for infected total hip arthroplasty. Orthop Clin North Am. 2016;47(1):11–8.
7. Engesaeter LB, Dale H, Schrama JC, Hallan G, Lie SA. Surgical procedures in the treatment of 784 infected THAs reported to the Norwegian arthroplasty register. Acta Orthop. 2011;82(5):530–7.
8. Insall JN, Thompson FM, Brause BD. Two-stage reimplantation for the salvage of infected total knee arthroplasty. J Bone Joint Surg Am. 1983;65(8):1087–98.
9. Longo UG, Ciuffreda M, Mannering N, D'Andrea V, Locher J, Salvatore G, et al. Outcomes of posterior-stabilized compared with cruciate-retaining total knee arthroplasty. J Knee Surg. 2018;31(4):321–40.
10. Lange J, Troelsen A, Soballe K. Chronic periprosthetic hip joint infection. a retrospective, observational study on the treatment strategy and prognosis in 130 non-selected patients. PLoS One. 2016;11(9):e0163457.
11. Sakellariou VI, Poultsides LA, Vasilakakos T, Sculco P, Ma Y, Sculco TP. Risk factors for recurrence of periprosthetic knee infection. J Arthroplasty. 2015;30(9):1618–22.
12. Vielgut I, Sadoghi P, Wolf M, Holzer L, Leithner A, Schwantzer G, et al. Two-stage revision of prosthetic hip joint infections using antibiotic-loaded cement spacers: when is the best time to perform the second stage? Int Orthop. 2015;39(9):1731–6.
13. Triantafyllopoulos GK, Memtsoudis SG, Zhang W, Ma Y, Sculco TP, Poultsides LA. Periprosthetic infection recurrence after 2-stage exchange arthroplasty: failure or fate? J Arthroplasty. 2017;32(2):526–31.
14. Longo UG, Ciuffreda M, D'Andrea V, Mannering N, Locher J, Denaro V. All-polyethylene versus metal-backed tibial component in total knee arthroplasty. Knee Surg Sports Traumatol Arthrosc. 2017;25(11):3620–36.
15. Longo UG, Loppini M, Trovato U, Rizzello G, Maffulli N, Denaro V. No difference between unicompartmental versus total knee arthroplasty for the management of medial osteoarthtritis of the knee in the same patient: a systematic review and pooling data analysis. Br Med Bull. 2015;114(1):65–73.
16. Sabry FY, Buller L, Ahmed S, Klika AK, Barsoum WK. Preoperative prediction of failure following two-stage revision for knee prosthetic joint infections. J Arthroplasty. 2014;29(1):115–21.
17. Kubista B, Hartzler RU, Wood CM, Osmon DR, Hanssen AD, Lewallen DG. Reinfection after two-stage revision for periprosthetic infection of total knee arthroplasty. Int Orthop. 2012;36(1):65–71.
18. Babis GC, Sakellariou VI, Pantos PG, Sasalos GG, Stavropoulos NA. Two-stage revision protocol in multidrug resistant periprosthetic infection following total hip arthroplasty using a long interval between stages. J Arthroplasty. 2015;30(9):1602–6.
19. Longo UG, Maffulli N, Denaro V. Minimally invasive total knee arthroplasty. N Engl J Med. 2009;361(6):633–4; author reply 4.
20. Tözün IR, Ozden VE, Dikmen G, Karaytuğ K. Trends in the treatment of infected knee arthroplasty. EFORT Open Rev. 2020;5(10):672–83.
21. Park SJ, Song EK, Seon JK, Yoon TR, Park GH. Comparison of static and mobile antibiotic-impregnated cement spacers for the treatment of infected total knee arthroplasty. Int Orthop. 2010;34(8):1181–6.
22. Chiang ER, Su YP, Chen TH, Chiu FY, Chen WM. Comparison of articulating and static spacers regarding infection with resistant organisms in total knee arthroplasty. Acta Orthop. 2011;82(4):460–4.
23. Van Thiel GS, Berend KR, Klein GR, Gordon AC, Lombardi AV, Della Valle CJ. Intraoperative molds to create an articulating spacer for the infected knee arthroplasty. Clin Orthop Relat Res. 2011;469(4):994–1001.
24. Citak M, Masri BA, Springer B, Argenson JN, Kendoff DO. Are preformed articulating spacers superior to surgeon-made articulating spacers in the treatment of PJI in THA? A literature review. Open Orthop J. 2015;9:255–61.
25. Hofmann AA, Kane KR, Tkach TK, Plaster RL, Camargo MP. Treatment of infected total knee arthroplasty using an articulating spacer. Clin Orthop Relat Res. 1995;321:45–54.
26. Emerson RH Jr, Muncie M, Tarbox TR, Higgins LL. Comparison of a static with a mobile spacer in total knee infection. Clin Orthop Relat Res. 2002;404:132–8.

27. Aeng ES, Shalansky KF, Lau TT, Zalunardo N, Li G, Bowie WR, et al. Acute kidney injury with tobramycin-impregnated bone cement spacers in prosthetic joint infections. Ann Pharmacother. 2015;49(11):1207–13.

28. Cabo J, Euba G, Saborido A, Gonzalez-Panisello M, Dominguez MA, Agullo JL, et al. Clinical outcome and microbiological findings using antibiotic-loaded spacers in two-stage revision of prosthetic joint infections. J Infect. 2011;63(1):23–31.

29. Kini SG, Gabr A, Das R, Sukeik M, Haddad FS. Two-stage revision for periprosthetic hip and knee joint infections. Open Orthop J. 2016;10:579–88.

30. Luu A, Syed F, Raman G, Bhalla A, Muldoon E, Hadley S, et al. Two-stage arthroplasty for prosthetic joint infection: a systematic review of acute kidney injury, systemic toxicity and infection control. J Arthroplasty. 2013;28(9):1490–8e1.

31. Hsieh PH, Huang KC, Lee PC, Lee MS. Two-stage revision of infected hip arthroplasty using an antibiotic-loaded spacer: retrospective comparison between short-term and prolonged antibiotic therapy. J Antimicrob Chemother. 2009;64(2):392–7.

32. Fowler NO, McCall D, Chou TC, Holmes JC, Hanenson IB. Electrocardiographic changes and cardiac arrhythmias in patients receiving psychotropic drugs. Am J Cardiol. 1976;37(2):223–30.

33. Sukeik M, Haddad FS. Two-stage procedure in the treatment of late chronic hip infections—spacer implantation. Int J Med Sci. 2009;6(5):253–7.

34. Kuzyk PR, Dhotar HS, Sternheim A, Gross AE, Safir O, Backstein D. Two-stage revision arthroplasty for management of chronic periprosthetic hip and knee infection: techniques, controversies, and outcomes. J Am Acad Orthop Surg. 2014;22(3):153–64.

35. Nordmann P, Mammeri H. Extended-spectrum cephalosporinases: structure, detection and epidemiology. Future Microbiol. 2007;2(3):297–307.

36. Samuel S, Mathew BS, Veeraraghavan B, Fleming DH, Chittaranjan SB, Prakash JA. In vitro study of elution kinetics and bio-activity of meropenem-loaded acrylic bone cement. J Orthop Traumatol. 2012;13(3):131–6.

37. Solomon AW, Stott PM, Duffy K, Kumar PG, Holliman RE, Bridle SH. Elution and antibacterial activity of meropenem from implanted acrylic bone cement. J Antimicrob Chemother. 2010;65(8):1834–5.

38. Hsieh PH, Chang YH, Chen SH, Ueng SW, Shih CH. High concentration and bioactivity of vancomycin and aztreonam eluted from simplex cement spacers in two-stage revision of infected hip implants: a study of 46 patients at an average follow-up of 107 days. J Orthop Res. 2006;24(8):1615–21.

39. Joseph TN, Chen AL, Di Cesare PE. Use of antibiotic-impregnated cement in total joint arthroplasty. J Am Acad Orthop Surg. 2003;11(1):38–47.

40. Mortazavi SM, Vegari D, Ho A, Zmistowski B, Parvizi J. Two-stage exchange arthroplasty for infected total knee arthroplasty: predictors of failure. Clin Orthop Relat Res. 2011;469(11):3049–54.

41. Parvizi J, Erkocak OF, Della Valle CJ. Culture-negative periprosthetic joint infection. J Bone Joint Surg Am. 2014;96(5):430–6.

42. Duggal A, Barsoum W, Schmitt SK. Patients with prosthetic joint infection on IV antibiotics are at high risk for readmission. Clin Orthop Relat Res. 2009;467(7):1727–31.

43. Bernard L, Legout L, Zurcher-Pfund L, Stern R, Rohner P, Peter R, et al. Six weeks of antibiotic treatment is sufficient following surgery for septic arthroplasty. J Infect. 2010;61(2):125–32.

44. Esposito S, Esposito I, Leone S. Considerations of antibiotic therapy duration in community- and hospital-acquired bacterial infections. J Antimicrob Chemother. 2012;67(11):2570–5.

45. Castelli CC, Gotti V, Ferrari R. Two-stage treatment of infected total knee arthroplasty: two to thirteen year experience using an articulating preformed spacer. Int Orthop. 2014;38(2):405–12.

46. Hart WJ, Jones RS. Two-stage revision of infected total knee replacements using articulating cement spacers and short-term antibiotic therapy. J Bone Jt Surg. 2006;88(8):1011–5.

47. Gehrke T, Zahar A, Kendoff D. One-stage exchange: it all began here. Bone Jt J. 2013;95-B(11 Suppl A):77–83.

48. Berry DJ, Chandler HP, Reilly DT. The use of bone allografts in two-stage reconstruction after failure of hip replacements due to infection. J Bone Joint Surg Am. 1991;73(10):1460–8.

49. Bauman RD, Lewallen DG, Hanssen AD. Limitations of structural allograft in revision total knee arthroplasty. Clin Orthop Relat Res. 2009;467(3):818–24.

50. Tetreault MW, Della Valle CJ, Bohl DD, Lodha SJ, Biswas D, Wysocki RW. What factors influence the success of medial gastrocnemius flaps in the treatment of infected TKAs? Clin Orthop Relat Res. 2016;474(3):752–63.

51. Corten K, Struelens B, Evans B, Graham E, Bourne RB, MacDonald SJ. Gastrocnemius flap reconstruction of soft-tissue defects following infected total knee replacement. Bone Jt J. 2013;95-B(9):1217–21.

52. Young K, Chummun S, Wright T, Darley E, Chapman TW, Porteous AJ, et al. Management of the exposed total knee prosthesis, a six-year review. Knee. 2016;23(4):736–9.

53. Fehring TK, Calton TF, Griffin WL. Cementless fixation in 2-stage reimplantation for periprosthetic sepsis. J Arthroplasty. 1999;14(2):175–81.

54. Anagnostakos K, Meyer C. Antibiotic elution from hip and knee acrylic bone cement spacers: a systematic review. Biomed Res Int. 2017;2017:4657874.

55. Zmistowski BM, Clyde CT, Ghanem ES, Gotoff JR, Deirmengian CA, Parvizi J. Utility of synovial white blood cell count and differential before reimplantation surgery. J Arthroplasty. 2017;32(9):2820–4.

56. Kusuma SK, Ward J, Jacofsky M, Sporer SM, Della Valle CJ. What is the role of serological testing between stages of two-stage reconstruction of the

infected prosthetic knee? Clin Orthop Relat Res. 2011;469(4):1002–8.

57. Gomez MM, Tan TL, Manrique J, Deirmengian GK, Parvizi J. The fate of spacers in the treatment of periprosthetic joint infection. J Bone Joint Surg Am. 2015;97(18):1495–502.

58. Dauty M, Dubois C, Coisy M. Bilateral knee arthroplasty infection due to *Brucella melitensis*: a rare pathology? Joint Bone Spine. 2009;76(2):215–6.

59. David J, Nasser RM, Goldberg JW, Reed KD, Earll MD. Bilateral prosthetic knee infection by *Campylobacter fetus*. J Arthroplasty. 2005;20(3):401–5.

60. Rajgopal A, Panda I, Gupta A. Unusual *Salmonella typhi* periprosthetic joint infection involving bilateral knees: management options and literature review. BMJ Case Rep. 2017;2017.

61. Wolff LH 3rd, Parvizi J, Trousdale RT, Pagnano MW, Osmon DR, Hanssen AD, et al. Results of treatment of infection in both knees after bilateral total knee arthroplasty. J Bone Joint Surg Am. 2003;85(10):1952–5.

The Use of Static Spacers in Periprosthetic Knee Infections

Thomas Barnavon, Cécile Batailler, John Swan,
Frédéric Laurent, Tristan Ferry, Sébastien Lustig,
and on Behalf of the Lyon Bji Study Group

18.1 Introduction

The increasing number of total knee arthroplasty (TKA) being performed has led to a corresponding increase in the overall number of TKA infections. Periprosthetic knee infection is a severe and not infrequent complication, with an incidence ranging from 0.4 to 2.5% for primary TKA and 4 to 8% for revision surgery.

The surgical treatment differs depending on the duration of the infection. The aim is to eradicate infection and maintain satisfactory knee function (range of motion, stability, no pain). For acute infection, prosthesis removal is not necessary and a simple DAIR (debridement, antibiotics, implant retention) should be performed in association with replacement of the polyethylene insert. For subacute or chronic infection, prosthetic replacement is necessary, and two methods of management can be discussed: single-stage or two-stage exchange arthroplasty.

Single-stage exchange arthroplasty involves implant removal with debridement, followed by reimplantation of a new prosthesis during the same operation. Although single-stage exchange knee arthroplasty is possible in certain specific cases, prosthetic replacement in two stages is currently considered as standard treatment. The indications of single-stage exchange are absence of systemic sepsis, minimal bone loss and soft tissue defects, absence of difficulties related to the skin, and preoperative isolation of a pathogenic organism which is sensitive to bactericidal treatment.

During two-stage exchange arthroplasty, the first stage is to remove all prosthetic materials with thorough debridement of the periprosthetic tissues. Multiple tissue samples are collected during the first stage debridement. An antibiotic-

on Behalf of the Lyon Bji Study Group

T. Barnavon · J. Swan
Arthritis and Joint Replacement Unit, Orthopaedic
Department, Knee and Hip Arthroplasty Surgery,
Hospices Civils de Lyon, Lyon North University
Hospital, Lyon, France

C. Batailler · S. Lustig (✉)
Arthritis and Joint Replacement Unit, Orthopaedic
Department, Knee and Hip Arthroplasty Surgery,
Hospices Civils de Lyon, Lyon North University
Hospital, Lyon, France

Univ Lyon Claude Bernard Lyon I University,
IFSTTA, LBMC_UMRT9406, Lyon, France

F. Laurent
Institut des agents infectieux, Laboratoire de
bactériologie, Centre National de référence des
staphylocoques, Hôpital de la Croix-Rousse,
Lyon, France
e-mail: frederic.laurent@chu-lyon.fr

T. Ferry
Service des maladies infectieuses et tropicales,
Hospices Civils de Lyon, Hôpital de la Croix-Rousse,
Lyon, France
e-mail: tristan.ferry@chu-lyon.fr

© ISAKOS 2022
U. G. Longo et al. (eds.), *Infection in Knee Replacement*,
https://doi.org/10.1007/978-3-030-81553-0_18

impregnated cement spacer is positioned in place of the TKA implants. Later, once the infection is controlled, prosthesis reimplantation is performed during the second stage. The optimal delay before the second surgery is still debated. The use of a cement spacer is practically systematic in the treatment of TKA infection, because it allows the preservation of sufficient joint space during the intermediate period without a prosthesis, which allows maintenance of the space for reimplantation of the new prosthesis during the second stage surgery. There are two types of spacer commonly used: static spacer or dynamic spacer. Both types of spacer have advantages and disadvantages. A good understanding of the spacer function and indications is critical for appropriate management of the two-stage exchange knee arthroplasty.

In this chapter, we will discuss the characteristics and use of a static spacer, the surgical technique, and outcomes using a static spacer.

18.2 General Spacer Properties

A spacer is a temporary piece of organic cement. After removal of the infected implant and tissue, the principle is to create a cement-based replacement prosthesis, shaping them manually or using moulds.

18.2.1 Mechanical Properties

The role of the spacer is to stabilize the femorotibial joint during the intermediate time between surgical stages, to prevent knee dislocation and avoid pain. Adequate knee stability during this period protects the periarticular soft tissue, such as the extensor mechanism and avoids additional tissue injuries. It also limits fibrosis filling the joint space and limits ligament and tendon retraction. Thus, using a spacer facilitates reimplantation surgery during the second stage. Without the use of a spacer, the knee ligaments significantly retract, possibly necessitating further bone resection, and therefore leg shortening, to create space for reimplantation of a new prosthesis or necessitating ligament release and implantation of a highly constrained or hinged prosthesis.

18.2.2 Anti-Microbial Properties

Whilst the patient is receiving appropriate systemic antibiotic therapy, spacers are also delivering high doses of antibiotics directly within the knee. The local diffusion of antibiotics contained within the spacer facilitates the eradication of the microbes and limits the development of secondary infection. The antibiotics present in cement are usually aminoglycosides such as gentamycin or tobramycin and or glycopeptide such as vancomycin. The dose delivered locally is ten times greater than the critical minimum inhibitory concentration (CMI) for antibiotic activity. In addition, the spacer fills the femorotibial space and reduces the risk of secondary infection by limiting the volume of intra-articular dead space.

18.2.3 Two Types of Cement Spacer

Antibiotic-impregnated cement spacers are static or dynamic.

The static spacer consists of a single block of cement inserted between the femur and the tibia (Fig. 18.1). It is not articulated and constitutes a temporary knee arthrodesis keeping the knee in full extension. This temporary immobilization leads, among other things, to joint stiffness and exposure difficulties at the time of reimplantation.

As a result, dynamic spacers have been developed to solve these problems. The dynamic spacer consists of a femoral component articulated on a tibial baseplate. It is effectively a temporary prosthesis made out of cement. With a smooth and congruent interface, the articulated spacers are designed to allow knee range of motion. Thus, it allows passive mobilization of the knee during the intermediate phase. The dynamic spacer reduces the risk of muscular atrophy and retraction of the peripheral soft tissues.

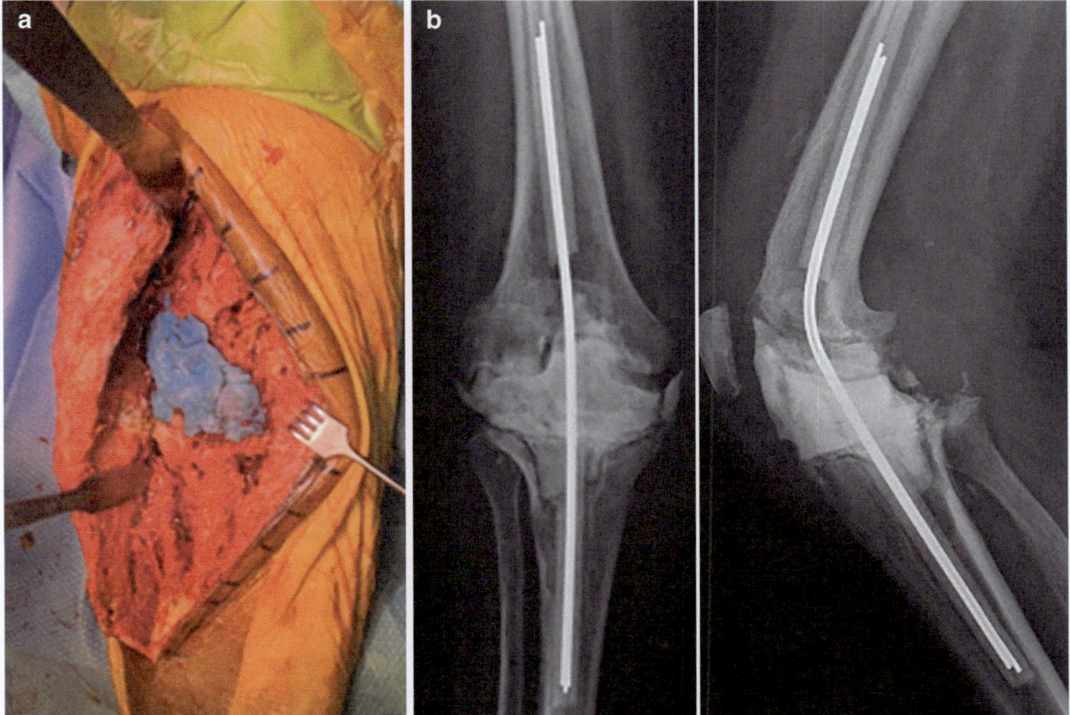

Fig. 18.1 (**a**) Perioperative photo of a static spacer with methylene blue denatured cement. (**b**) Postoperative radiograph after insertion of the static spacer reinforced with Kirschner wires

18.3 Indications for a Static Spacer in TKA Infections

The use of a spacer is indicated for subacute or chronic TKA infections requiring a two-stage revision. In the absence of contraindications, the dynamic spacer should be preferred, because it improves the knee function, as well as postoperative mobility and facilitates the exposure during the reimplantation.

The indications for a static spacer correspond to the contraindications of the dynamic spacer, specifically:

- Major bone loss, which is associated with a high risk of fracture, as well as a lack of fixation for a dynamic spacer (Figs. 18.2 and 18.3).
- An incompetence of the collateral ligaments or of the extensor mechanism, which can cause femoro-tibial dislocation with a dynamic spacer (Fig. 18.3).
- A skin condition at high risk of complications, needing a limitation of flexion or even an immobilization of the knee to promote healing.

18.4 Surgical Technique

Knee exposure can be performed via a preexisting scar or as per surgeon preference. After knee exposure, the level of the joint line is identified and measured relative to a drill hole which is made on the femur and the tibia at a safe distance from the joint level. The prosthesis is carefully explanted, and the surrounding contaminated tissues are excised. The femoral and tibial intramedullary canals are reamed and cleaned. After multiple tissue samples are taken, a thorough knee joint lavage is performed.

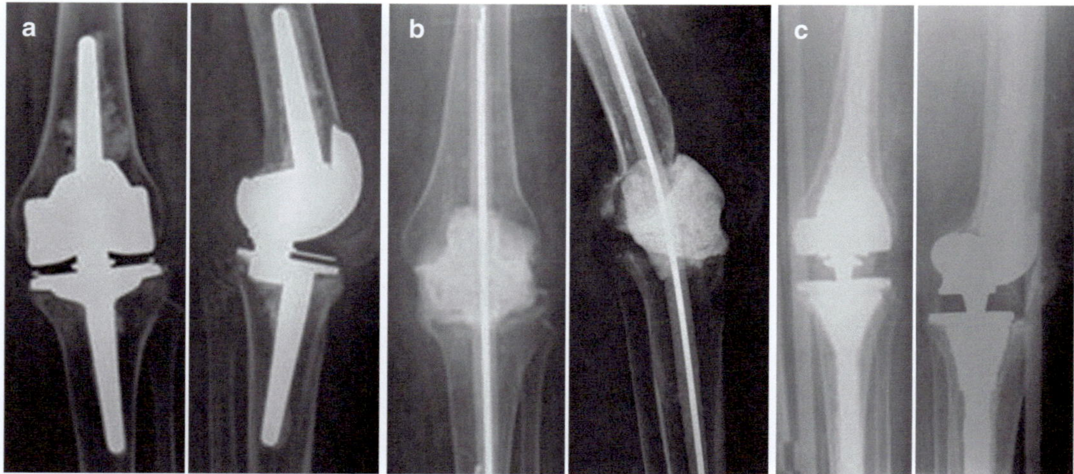

Fig. 18.2 Case report: A 57-year-old man had septic loosening of his revision TKA and chronic rupture of the quadriceps tendon. After removal of the TKA, there was major femoral and tibial bone loss. (**a**) Radiograph before revision showing loosening. (**b**) Radiograph after insertion of the static spacer. (**c**) Radiograph after reimplantation of a hinge knee prosthesis, associated with reconstruction of extensor mechanism using the Hanssen technique

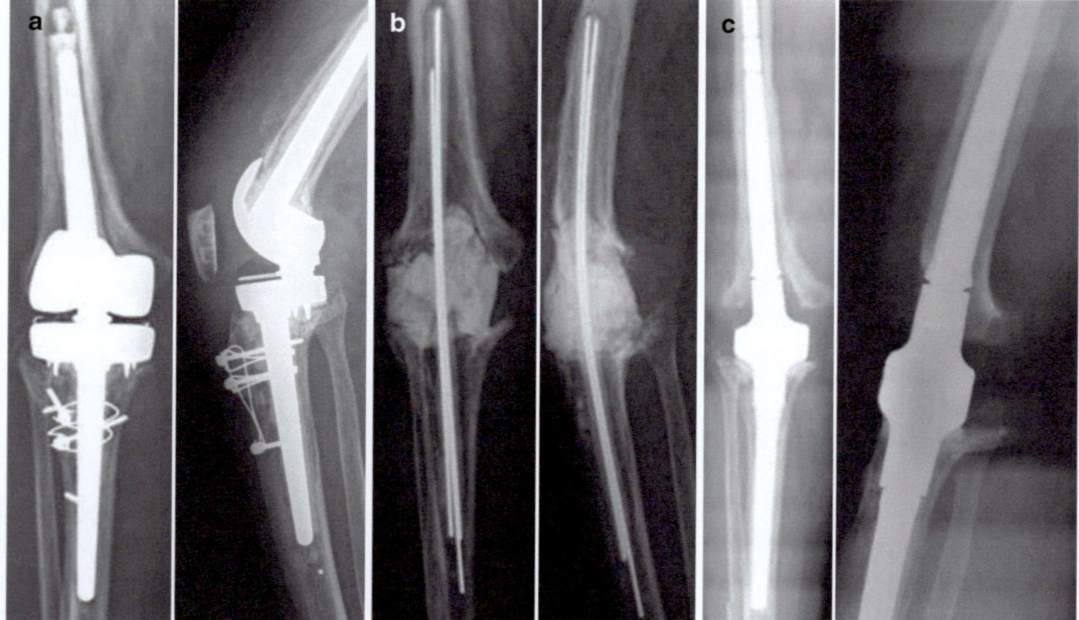

Fig. 18.3 Case report: A 69-year-old man had chronic sepsis of his revision TKA and rupture of the allograft extensor mechanism. (**a**) Radiograph before revision. (**b**) Radiograph after insertion of the static spacer with reinforcement Kirschner wires. (**c**) Radiograph after reimplantation of an arthrodesis prosthesis at the second stage revision

Static cement spacers must be reinforced with wires. Without reinforcement, the risk of spacer fracture is very high.

The first step is to create a rod of cement around Kirschner wires that will go into the intramedullary canal. The surgeon should use 3 or 4 wires of approximately 2 mm diameter and high-viscosity antibiotic cement. Manually, the surgeon fashions a rod of cement with the wires inside. The length must be long enough to have at least 6 cm of rod in each femoral and tibial canal, plus the length of the joint space. Once set, this rod, marked at its centre, is introduced back and forth into the femoral and tibial canals until the centre mark is at the midpoint of the joint space.

During the second step, high-viscosity antibiotic cement, with the addition of methylene blue, is prepared. This second cementation will fill the joint space, to maintain the native leg length. At 2 min after the mixing of the second cement mixture, the joint is opened with traction in leg extension, in order to fill any bone defects and the articular space. All of the knee joint space is filled with the second cementation. The size of the spacer should be appropriate, and not so large as to cause excessive skin tension during wound closure.

This second cementation stabilizes the construct and prevents spacer migration. The methylene blue is used to facilitate cement removal during the second stage surgery and causes poor fixation between bone and cement, which also aids removal. The joint capsule, subcutaneous tissues, and the skin are closed in layers.

Postoperatively, patients are kept in a brace without range of motion and locked in extension. Weight bearing is forbidden.

During the second stage surgery, the surgeon removes the cement spacer by breaking the spacer and removing the rod spacer (with wires inside). An osteotome and mallet can be used to carefully crack the fragment of the cement spacer. Another thorough debridement is performed prior to implantation of the new definitive prosthesis.

18.5   Results and Complications of Static Spacers (Table 18.1)

In the context of chronic TKA infections, several studies have compared infection management using articulated and static spacers. A meta-analysis published in 2017, including 10 studies, compared the effectiveness of static and dynamic spacers according to several criteria, specifically: rate of infection eradication, range of motion and functional scores, and soft tissue release during prosthetic reimplantation [1].

18.5.1 Rate of Infection Eradication

In a study of 81 static spacers and 34 dynamic spacers, Johnson et al. [2] found that the rate of infection eradication was 88% for the static spacer group and 82% for the dynamic spacer

Table 18.1 Literature review of the use of static and dynamic spacers during two-stage prosthesis exchanges

	Date	Type of study	Number of static spacer	Infection eradication	Range of motion	Mean KSS function score	Mean HSS score	Lengthening of the femoral quadriceps	TTO
Brunnekreef et al. [4]	2013	Retrospective	9	100%	73.8°	–	–	–	55%
Chiang et al. [6]	2011	Prospective	21	90%	85°	–	82	33%	–
Choi et al. [2]	2012	Retrospective	33	67%	97°	–	–	18%	57%
Emerson et al. [13]	2002	Retrospective	26	92%	93.7°	–	–	–	–
Fehring et al. [7]	2000	Retrospective	25	88%	98°	–	83	8%	–
Freeman et al. [8]	2007	Retrospective	28	89%	–	45	–	–	–
Hsu et al. [9]	2006	Retrospective	7	85%	78°	57.8	–	28%	–
Johnson et al. [3]	2012	Retrospective	81	82%	95°	–	–	–	–
Jämsen et al. [14]	2006	Retrospective	8	75%	92°	53	–	–	–
Park et al. [5]	2010	Retrospective	20	85%	92°	50	80	35%	4%

group. This rate was comparable in the two groups. Choi et al. [3] found lower, but comparable, infection eradication rates with 67% for the static spacer group and 71% for the dynamic spacer group. In a study by Brunnekreef et al. [4] 35 patients underwent two-stage revision surgery for chronic infection on TKA. The infection eradication rates were 100% for both the static and dynamic spacer groups.

Thus, the rate of eradication of infection using a static spacer is between 67% [2] and 100% [3]. There is no significant difference between static and dynamic spacers.

18.5.2 Range of Motion

Regarding range of motion, Park et al. [5] compared the clinical results of static and dynamic cement spacers for the treatment of infected TKA in 36 patients. They found a significant difference between groups: an average flexion at the last follow-up of 92° in the static spacer group versus 108° in the dynamic spacer group. In a study of 45 patients, Chiang et al. [6] reported similar results, with 85° of flexion in the static spacer group versus 113° in the dynamic spacer group.

In the literature review by Hai Ding et al. [1], the average flexion at the last follow-up is between 74° and 98°. Flexion was significantly lower after static spacer use compared to dynamic spacer use.

18.5.3 Knee Society Score (KSS) and Hospital for Special Surgery Knee Score (HSS)

Park et al. [5] and Freeman et al. [8] found an average KSS functional score of 50 and 45 points, respectively, in the static spacer group versus 76 and 70 points in the dynamic spacer group. Chiang et al. [6] and Park et al. [5], respectively, found an average HSS score of 82 and 80 points for the static spacer group against 90 and 87 points for the dynamic spacer group.

The functional scores at the last follow-up are comparable between different studies. These scores are significantly lower in the static spacer groups compared to the dynamic spacer groups.

18.5.4 Rate of Surgical Soft Tissue Release

Several authors have sought to assess the retraction of peripheral soft tissues during prosthetic reimplantation and particularly the need to perform quadriceps tendon release or tibial tuberosity osteotomy (TTO).

In a study of 28 patients, Hsu et al. [9] performed two rectus femoris snips and one Y-plasty of the quadriceps tendon during prosthetic reimplantation. They found that 29% of patients in the static group required a more extensive approach compared to only 5% of patients in the articulated group. Choi et al. [2] found that a more extensive approach was more frequently required in the static spacer group than in the dynamic spacer group (5 rectus femoris snips, 1 Y-plasty of the quadriceps tendon and 19 TTO in the static spacer group versus 3 rectus femoris snips and 1 TTO in the dynamic spacer group).

Therefore, the use of articulated spacers facilitates the surgical exposure during the prosthetic reimplantation stage. The mobilization of the knee between the two surgeries avoids the retraction of the extensor mechanism and the articular capsule [10].

18.5.5 Complications

Johnson et al. [3] described complications requiring surgical revision due to dynamic spacers. Four of the 34 patients with dynamic spacers presented with mechanical failure and there were no failures of the 81 static spacers. Two patients with dynamic spacer failure who admitted to having resumed full weight bearing presented with fractures of the femoral component. The other patients presented with a dislocation of the femoral component and a subluxation of the tibial component with skin breakdown who needed flap coverage. In a study by Streulens et al. [11], the dynamic spacer dislocated and caused significant knee subluxation in 7% of the patients.

Wilson et al. [12] described a series of 3 complicated cases of anterior migration of the cement with partial or even total rupture of the patellar tendon following the implantation of dynamic spacers.

Thus, static spacers have less risk of complications than dynamic spacers (Figs. 18.4, 18.5, and 18.6).

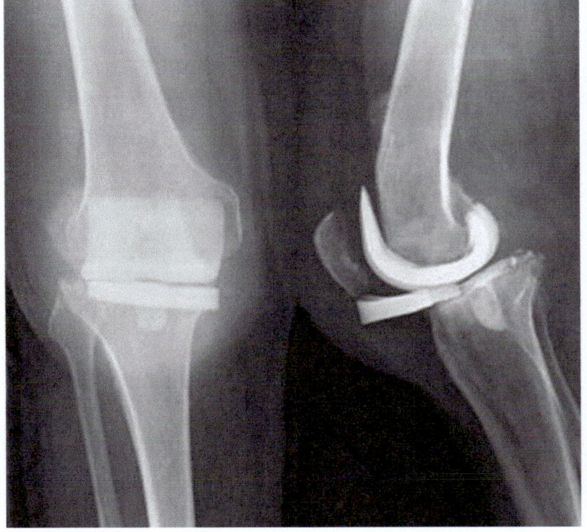

Fig. 18.4 Case report: Radiographs of the knee of a 69-year-old man showing an anterior subluxation of the tibial cement spacer

18.6 Conclusion

Two-stage prosthetic replacement, with the use of a cement spacer during the intermediate phase, is currently considered as the gold standard treatment for chronic prosthetic knee infections.

During prosthetic reimplantation, static spacers are associated with retraction of peripheral soft tissue and greater difficulty in surgical exposure. This difficulty in exposure is related to the immobilization of the knee during the intermediate phase and may require an important soft tissue release. The use of a static spacer impacts the functional knee results of patients.

Articulated spacers allow limited knee mobilization between the two surgical stages and can facilitate the ease of prosthesis reimplantation during the second stage. However, the dynamic spacers are associated with a greater number of complications compared with static spacers, particularly in cases of improper use. When there are contraindications for the use of a dynamic spacer, a static cement spacer is preferred, such as when there is major bone loss, knee instability with collateral ligament or extensor mechanism incompetence, or when there is a precarious skin condition.

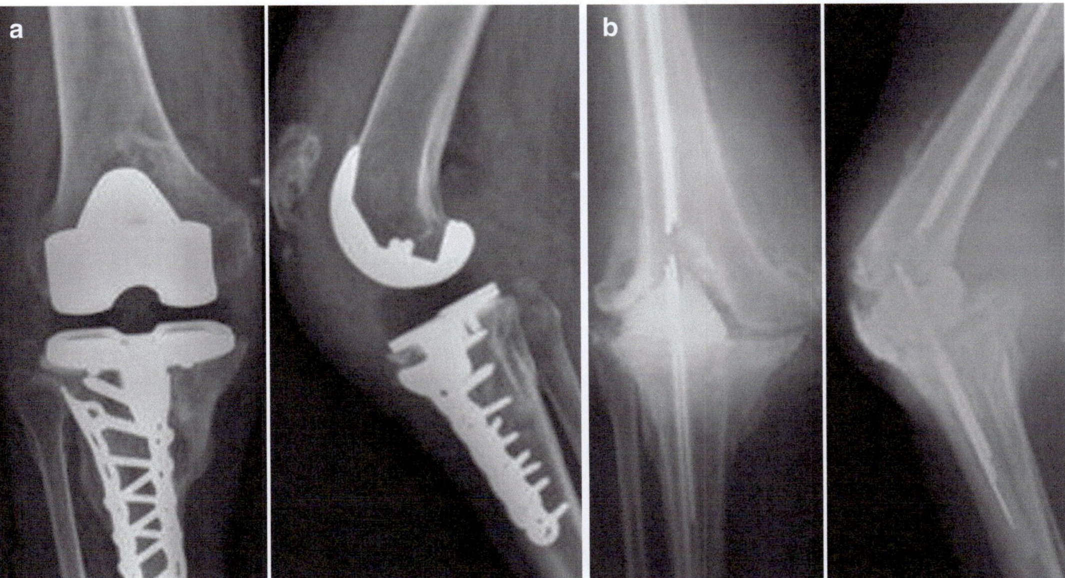

Fig. 18.5 Case report: A 69-year-old man had chronic sepsis of his TKA with chronic rupture of the patellar tendon. (**a**) Radiograph before revision. (**b**) Radiograph after the first stage revision showing a broken static cement spacer

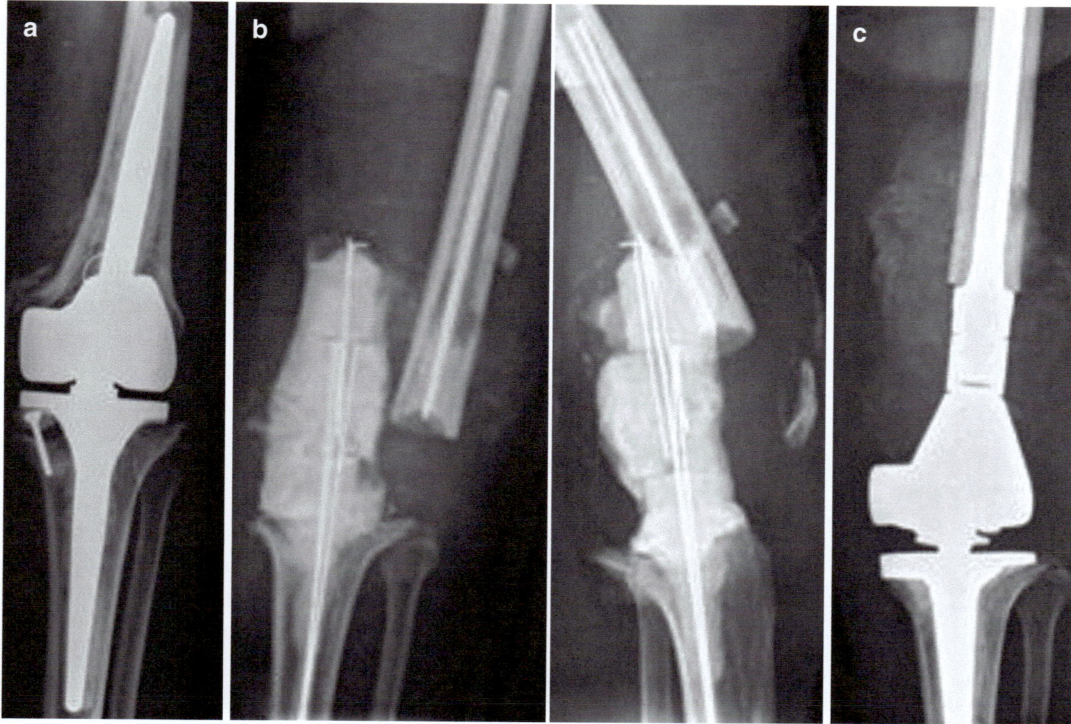

Fig. 18.6 Case report: A 75-year-old man had chronic sepsis of his TKA with major femoral bone loss. (**a**) Radiograph before revision. (**b**) Radiograph showing a broken massive static cement spacer. (**c**) Radiograph after reimplantation of rotating hinge distal femoral replacement prosthesis during the second stage revision

In order to minimize the risk of complications of spacers during the intermediate phase, the surgical technique and the indications of each type of spacer must be well known and understood.

Acknowledgments   Lyon bone and joint study group (list of collaborators)

Coordinator: *Tristan Ferry*; **Infectious diseases specialists:** *Tristan Ferry, Florent Valour, Thomas Perpoint, Patrick Miailhes, Florence Ader, Sandrine Roux, Agathe Becker, Claire Triffault-Fillit, Anne Conrad, Cécile Pouderoux, Nicolas Benech, Pierre Chauvelot, Marielle Perry, Fatiha Daoud, Johanna Lippman, Evelyne Braun, Christian Chidiac;* **Surgeons:** *Elvire Servien, Cécile Batailler, Stanislas Gunst, Axel Schmidt, Matthieu Malatray, Eliott Sappey-Marinier, Michel-Henry Fessy, Anthony Viste, Jean-Luc Besse, Philippe Chaudier, Lucie Louboutin, Quentin Ode, Adrien Van Haecke, Marcelle Mercier, Vincent Belgaid, Arnaud Walch, Sébastien Martres, Franck Trouillet, Cédric Barrey, Ali Mojallal, Sophie Brosset, Camille Hanriat, Hélène Person, Nicolas Sigaux, Philippe Céruse, Carine Fuchsmann;* **Anesthesiologists:** *Frédéric Aubrun, Mikhail Dziadzko, Caroline Macabéo;* **Microbiologists:** *Frédéric Laurent, Laetitia Beraud, Tiphaine Roussel-Gaillard, Céline Dupieux, Camille Kolenda, Jérôme Josse;* **Pathology:** *Marie Brevet, Alexis Trecourt;* **Imaging:** *Fabien Craighero, Loic Boussel, Jean-Baptiste Pialat, Isabelle Morelec;* **PK/PD specialists:** *Michel Tod, Marie-Claude Gagnieu, Sylvain Goutelle;* **Clinical research assistant and database manager:** *Eugénie Mabrut.*

References

1. Ding H, et al. Comparison of the efficacy of static versus articular spacers in two-stage revision surgery for the treatment of infection following total knee arthroplasty: a meta-analysis. J Orthop Surg Res. 2017;12(1):151.
2. Choi HR, Malchau H, Bedair H. Are prosthetic spacers safe to use in 2-stage treatment for infected total knee arthroplasty? J Arthroplasty. 2012;27(8):1474–9. e1.
3. Johnson AJ, Sayeed SA, Naziri Q, Khanuja HS, Mont MA. Minimizing dynamic knee spacer complications in infected revision arthroplasty. Clin Orthop Relat Res. 2012;470(1):220–7.

4. Brunnekreef J, Hannink G, Malefijt MW. Recovery of knee mobility after a static or mobile spacer in total knee infection. Acta Orthop Belg. 2013;79(1):83–9.
5. Park SJ, Song EK, Seon JK, Yoon TR, Park GH. Comparison of static and mobile antibiotic-impregnated cement spacers for the treatment of infected total knee arthroplasty. Int Orthop. 2010;34(8):1181–6.
6. Chiang ER, Su YP, Chen TH, Chiu FY, Chen WM. Comparison of articulating and static spacers regarding infection with resistant organisms in total knee arthroplasty. Acta Orthop. 2011;82(4):460.
7. Fehring TK, Odum S, Calton TF, Mason JB. Articulating versus static spacers in revision total knee arthroplasty for sepsis. The Ranawat Award. Clin Orthop Relat Res. 2000;(380):9–16.
8. Freeman MG, Fehring TK, Odum SM, Fehring K, Griffin WL, Mason JB. Functional advantage of articulating versus static spacers in 2-stage revision for total knee arthroplasty infection. J Arthroplasty. 2007;22(8):1116.
9. Hsu YC, Cheng HC, Ng TP, Chiu KY. Antibiotic-loaded cement articulating spacer for 2-stage reim-plantation in infected total knee arthroplasty: a simple and economic method. J Arthroplasty. 2007;22(7):1060–6.
10. Thabe H, Schill S. Two-stage reimplantation with an application spacer and combined with delivery of anti-biotics in the management of prosthetic joint infec-tion. Oper Orthop Traumatol. 2007;19(1):78–100.
11. Struelens B, Claes S, Bellemans J. Spacer-related problems in two-stage revision knee arthroplasty. Acta Orthop Belg. 2013;79(4):422.
12. Wilson K, Kothwal R, Khan WS, Williams R, Morgan-Jones R. Patella tendon injuries secondary to cement spacers used at first-stage revision of infected total knee replacement. Front Surg. 2015;2:11.
13. Emerson RH Jr, Muncie M, Tarbox TR, Higgins LL. Comparison of a static with a mobile spacer in total knee infection. Clin Orthop Relat Res. 2002;(404):132.
14. Jämsen PSE, Halonen P, Lehto MUK, Moilanen T, Pajamäki J, Puolakka T, Konttinen YT. Spacer pros-theses in two-stage revision of infected knee arthro-plasty. Int Orthop. 2006;30(4):257–61.

Dynamic (Mobile) Spacers in Infected Total Knee Arthroplasty

M. Enes Kayaalp and Roland Becker

19.1 Introduction

Two-stage exchange for infected knee arthroplasty is the most common method for prosthetic joint infection [1]. During the interim following removal of implants, the resection area is supported by implantation of spacers. There are two kinds of options: dynamic or static spacers.

Articulating spacers are called dynamic or mobile spacers, or simply articulating spacers. These spacers are assumed to provide some advantages over the static, i.e., non-articulating ones, in selected patients. This chapter will focus on the historical aspects and current scientific evidence on dynamic spacers.

The first reported two-stage treatment of prosthetic joint infection was in 1983 by Insall [2]. During the course of following clinical applications, it was revealed that the use of antibiotic-impregnated cement following removal of implants and until reimplantation significantly increased the success rate of revision due to infection. Followingly, placement of antibiotic-impregnated cement rather than leaving the joint empty became a routine procedure. However, as experience gathered, it was revealed that static spacers caused unexpected bone loss due to migration of unstable spacer [3]. This led to introduction of dynamic spacers, which would theoretically decrease complications occurring when static spacers are used, such as bone loss, immobility-related problems, and adhesions around the operation site.

Currently, reliable scientific evidence in favor of neither type exists in the literature [4]. This is mainly caused by the multifactorial setting between cases and studies.

19.2 Types and Properties of Dynamic Spacers

Dynamic all cement spacers were shown to provide similar eradication rates as static spacers [1]. Lack of apparent disadvantages and quest for betterment in terms of range of motion and interim mobility by maintaining muscle activity lead to their widespread use. However, almost synchronously, different types were reported in the literature.

Dynamic spacers can be handmade by the operating surgeon, or re-sterilized components might be used during the interim. The first applied dynamic spacer was shaped antibiotic-

M. E. Kayaalp
Department of Orthopedics and Traumatology,
Istanbul Taksim Training and Research Hospital,
Istanbul, Turkey
e-mail: mek@mek.md

R. Becker (✉)
Department of Orthopaedics and Traumatology,
Center of Joint Replacement, Medical Director of the
University Hospital, University of Brandenburg an
der Havel, Brandenburg, Germany

© ISAKOS 2022
U. G. Longo et al. (eds.), *Infection in Knee Replacement*,
https://doi.org/10.1007/978-3-030-81553-0_19

impregnated cement by surgeon, either manually or using molds. This handmade facsimile of a knee replacement was followed by a molded prosthesis and commercially available pre-shaped and posterior stabilized designs [5].

Essentially, three types of dynamic spacers might be distinguished:

1. intraoperatively prepared cement spacers (either handmade or using molds) (Fig. 19.1),
2. re-sterilized components,
3. commercially available pre-shaped components (with or without metal or polyethylene components) [4, 6].

Regarding the contact area properties of articulating parts, one can also classify the dynamic spacers as:

1. cement on cement
2. cement on polyethylene
3. metal-on-polyethylene.

Although variations exist regarding the preparation technique of handmade or molded spacers, there seems to be a consensus on using antibiotic-impregnated cement for their preparation [7].

Various authors reported good eradication rates of infection using dynamic cement spacers compared to static ones, wherefore the use of dynamic spacers became widespread [8–10].

Conversely, Hofmann et al. [11] used re-sterilized components in the interim, and many authors also reported successful results with this technique [1]. Chen et al. reported good results with autoclaved metal-on-cement spacer with satisfactory interim ROM without additional costs [12]. Regarding autoclaving of used components, potential legal implications and lack of standards were the primary concerns of operating surgeons, so this method lost interest. This method is now reserved for restricted conditions, where economic or logistic considerations do not allow for cement or commercially available spacers [13].

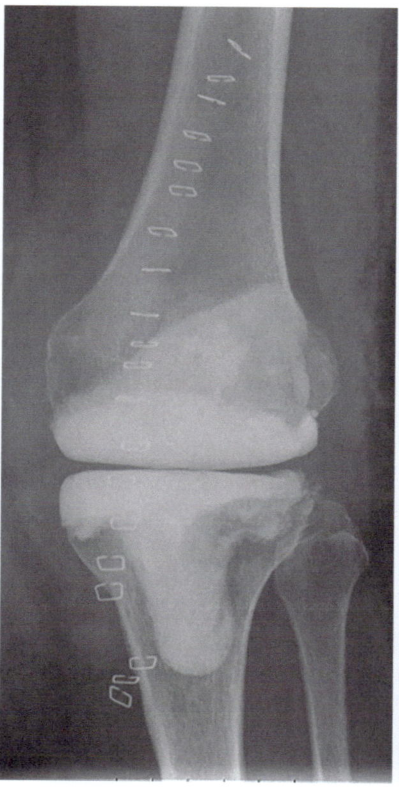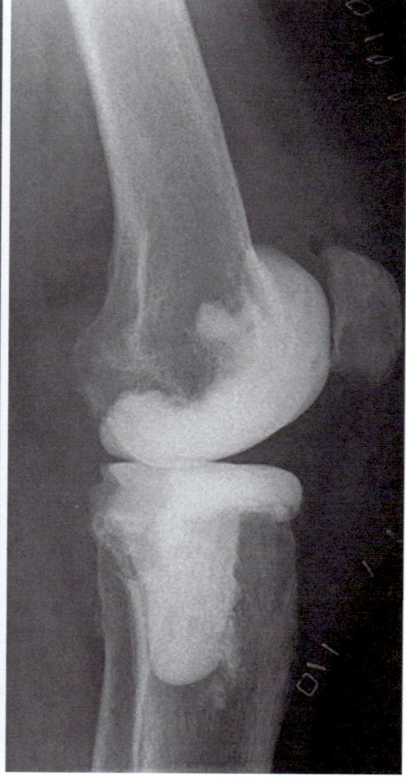

Fig. 19.1 Postoperative images of a patient implanted with handmade dynamic cement-on-cement spacer following stage one

As experience gathered, different authors proposed modified techniques. Akhtar et al. proposed using intramedullary pedestals. Their arguments consisted of obtaining a more stable spacer to prevent dynamic cement spacer-related complications such as fractures, dislocations, and malalignment, which were reportedly found at a level above expectations [7, 14].

Shen et al. proposed to use molded cement spacers created intraoperatively using prosthesis trials to overcome issues such as lack of proper antibiotic amount and type when commercially available spacers are used and shape and congruency related problems when hand-molded spacers are implanted. The authors reported promising results with their technique [15].

Functional demands and increasing expectations from patients, together with surgical tendency to ease and standardize the procedure, commercially available spacers found more recognition and area of use. As a result, the production of commercially available pre-shaped, ready to implant dynamic spacers, which include limited polyethylene and metal components, got more widespread [5].

One of the concerns about handmade cement spacers would be the mechanical fatigue strength of these spacers. Hand-molded spacers were compared with commercially available spacers in terms of mechanical strength [16]. The authors concluded that hand-molded spacers provide sufficient strength and that their use will be cost-effective in revision total knee arthroplasty. Similar functional results with handmade dynamic spacers compared to expensive, industrial spacers have been reported by others [17].

No difference in terms of eradication rate has been reported between the usage of a handmade spacer with 92.2% (84 reinfections) and an industry-made spacer with 90.5% [7].

However, Citak et al. observed that surgeon-made dynamic spacers were more likely to fracture than industry-made spacers despite having equivalent functional outcomes and infection eradication rates [18]. Similarly, other authors reported no increase in infection rates when industrial spacers with metal and polyethylene components were used [5].

An analysis of 1525 infected TKA cases showed no difference in functional outcome when manufactured versus surgeon-made dynamic spacers are used in the knee. The mean flexion at latest follow-up was tendentially higher with a mean of 102° using a handmade spacer compared to a mean of 90° using a manufactured spacer [7]. However, the clinical relevance of the difference in terms of range of motion remains questionable.

As of today, no conclusive evidence favors any of these methods one over another [10]. Preformed spacers have the disadvantages of fixed antibiotic dose and type, and whereas using cement and antibiotics, surgeons can prepare hand-molded spacers intraoperatively. The disadvantages of this method are less congruent contact and more fragile cement due to mixture with antibiotics [4].

19.3 Advantages of Dynamic Spacers

The claimed advantages of dynamic spacers are various. However, as will be seen, there are also contradictory results within the literature. Due to the heterogeneity of studies and cases, a clear deduction in terms of advantages cannot be made with a high level of evidence.

Expert opinions and case series mostly report several advantages of dynamic spacers, consisting of maintaining joint motion, facilitating surgical exposure at the time of reimplantation, and an enhanced postoperative function [1, 5, 7, 13]. Conversely, selection bias and case-related restrictions and selections may hinder objective deductions on this issue.

The first and most important argument in favor of dynamic spacers is the comparable infection eradication rates as with the static spacers [6].

Dynamic spacers were shown to constitute a safe alternative to fixed spacers in two-stage revision for infected total knee arthroplasty, which equally preserves ligament balancing and has equal infection eradication rates. However, the authors did not observe a long-term improvement of the range of motion following reimplantation of the new joint [19].

Other authors also did not report any significant difference in ROM at a minimum of 2 years follow-up between dynamic and static spacers. Citak et al. showed that published studies reported a 96.4° of knee ROM after an average follow-up of 44.3 months using dynamic spacers, compared to 91.2° at an average follow-up of 52 months using static spacers. However, experts seem to favor dynamic spacers, despite the lack of significant difference [7].

In contrast, some studies found better ranges of motion not only during the interim but also following reimplantation of revision components after the usage of dynamic spacers. Park et al. compared 36 consecutive patients, 20 of whom received static and 16 received dynamic spacers. The authors concluded that dynamic spacers appear to provide a better range of motion and less functional limitations to the patients, wherefore they should be used whenever possible. The reported knee ROM at a mean follow-up time of 36 months following revision surgery was 92° (range 65–140°) in patients with a static spacer in the interim versus 108° (range 85–140°) in patients with a dynamic spacer [20].

Villanueva-Martinez et al. stated that a mobile and functional joint is a key factor related to a successful outcome with a two-stage reimplantation procedure. Moreover, they have the advantages of preserving bone stock, delivering high concentrations of antibiotics, facilitating patient comfort, and early hospital discharge [17]. The ease of reimplantation and ease of rehabilitation was the most important argument for some surgeons favoring dynamic spacers [5].

It has been stated that selection bias in the majority of studies comparing static and dynamic spacers exists, wherefore no clear conclusion can be drawn on the ideal type of spacer. However, the authors proposed to use dynamic spacers whenever possible, as a result of clinical evidence on dynamic spacers suggesting improved function, better satisfaction, reduced hospital stays, and better ROM [13].

A systemic review also showed no differences regarding infection control between static and dynamic spacers in the treatment of infected TKA [21].

19.4 Contraindication of Dynamic Spacers

Although there are no clear contraindications for the application of dynamic spacers, technical feasibility problems, lack of soft tissues or ligaments around the knee, or extensive bone deficiency are the major concerns that redirect surgeons to static spacers.

Pivec et al. draw attention to the differences between case series and questioned the quasi advantages of dynamic spacers over static ones due to the fact that more simple cases are mostly implanted with dynamic spacers for the interim, whereas complex cases with soft tissue or bone stock problems get static spacers. The authors also underlined the differences between former and modern static spacers, indicating a need for higher-level evidence for future clinical applications [9].

It was shown that as an expert preference, in patients with soft tissue compromise, surgeons tend to implant a static spacer to prevent motion and obtain a better healing environment for the soft tissue [7, 13].

19.5 Antibiotic Properties of Dynamic Spacers

Locally applied antibiotics far outweighs the concentration and effect of systemic antibiotics and are therefore preferred. This is done by mixing a powder form of antibiotic with the cement. There is also commercially available antibiotic-impregnated cement. However, the elution of antibiotics from the cement decreases over time, and bacterial colonization can occur on the spacers [22–25]. Supporting this argument, Nelson et al. showed that sonication of antibiotic spacers at the time of second stage operation predicted revision arthroplasty failures due to another infection [24]. Therefore, the interim length should be limited up to 6 weeks. After that time, the risk of colonization of the spacer becomes higher than its antibiotic effect itself.

For an antibiotic to be mixed into the cement, the first and most important requirement is to be thermostable. Further desired properties of antibiotics are broad-spectrum, efficiency at low concentrations, and low risk of allergy [1]. Antibiotics are suggested to be mixed by hand in a bowl without a vacuum. Some fillers such as Xylitol, sugar alcohol, or Ancef were proposed to improve the elution of active antibiotics [7].

The most commonly used antibiotics are gentamicin, tobramycin, and vancomycin [1]. Antibiotics such as vancomycin, gentamicin, ampicillin, clindamycin, and meropenem can be used as a combination based on the causative organism and its susceptibility [26, 27].

The higher dose of antibiotics mixed with cement is a concerning issue. However, the commonly accepted limit of 5%–10% antibiotic for the whole cement mass is reliably exceeded in the clinical practice when spacers in two-stage revision are concerned [6]. Although it is a known fact that higher mixing rates decrease the fatigue strength of the cement, the desired antibiotic effect far outweighs this flaw. Even so, it must be remembered that the addition of more than 4.5 g of powder substantially weakens the cement [7].

Reported doses for selected antibiotics from various clinical studies are listed in Table 19.1. Although different antibiotics are recommended, the best choice of treatment depends on the antibiogram result obtained from the individual patient's samples prior to revision surgery.

Table 19.1 Reported doses of selected antibiotics from clinical studies

Antibiotic type	Dose in g per 40 g cement
Vancomycin	0.5–4
Gentamicin	0.25–4.8
Tobramycin	1–4.8
Cefazolin (first generation cephalosporin)	1–2
Cefuroxime (second generation cephalosporin)	1.5–2
Ceftazidime (third generation cephalosporin)	2
Cefotaxime (fourth generation cephalosporin)	2
Ciprofloxacin	0.2–3
Clindamycin	1–2
Tazobactam	0.5
Meropenem	0.5–4

Gentamycin and/or vancomycin are the most frequently used antibiotics [28]. Gentamycin is a bactericide against gram-negative coccus and vancomycin against gram-positive microorganisms.

Infection caused by methicillin-resistant staphylococcus aureus (MRSA) or methicillin-resistant staphylococcus epidermidis (MRSE) should be treated with vancomycin added to the cement. Infections with vancomycin-resistant enterococcus (VRE) or multidrug-resistant organisms should be treated with individual decision-making with consultation with infectious disease specialist [13].

Kuzyk et al. stated that they used 4 g of vancomycin and 4 g of ceftazidime per 40 g of cement when the infecting organism is unknown. The authors detail that they use three packs of 40 g cement bags to make their spacers [29].

Besides the antibiotic-loaded cement, appropriate IV antibiotic management is compulsory. A management plan should be discussed with the microbiologist and infectious disease specialist of the hospital.

Antifungal agents, such as amphotericin B and voriconazole, have also been reported to be mixed with cement [4].

19.6 Interim Period Length and Mobilization with Dynamic Spacers

19.6.1 Length of the Interim

Regarding the length of the interim, different approaches exist. A mainstream approach is to wait for 6 weeks with parenteral antibiotics until the reimplantation [30].

However, different studies report different intervals for reimplantation. Villanueva-Martinez et al. reported an average time of 14 (8–130) weeks [17]. Pitto et al. reported a shorter cement spacer period with mobile spacers than with static spacers (3.3 months vs. 4.2 months) [6]. Kuzyk et al. stated they prescribe intravenous antibiotics for a total of 6 to 8 weeks, ceasing antibiotics for 2 weeks before reoperation. The authors prolong this treatment for patients, who are immunocompromised, whose soft tissue envelopes are poor, or who have a large draining sinus, or whose infecting organism is especially virulent (e.g., MRSA or MRSE). In these situations, the authors stated that the prolongation with continuous intravenous antibiotics exceeds for a total of 3 to 4 months before reimplantation and consider the use of oral antibiotics for 4 to 6 weeks after reimplantation [29].

Other authors reported a mean interval between stages for their entire cohort to be 15.5 weeks (3.6 to 96.7) using a commercially available dynamic spacer [5]. Another study reported even an interim time of 128.2± 80.8 days [31]. In contrast, Fink et al. reported reimplantation after 6 weeks. During this period, antibiotics were given intravenously, followed by 4 weeks of oral treatment [32]. Winkler et al. investigated the effect of interim length on reinfection rate and functional outcome. Taking 4 weeks as a cut-off value, the authors concluded that an interim length of less than 4 weeks had similar results in terms of controlling infection with those of more than 4 weeks of an interval. Moreover, patient inconvenience and care costs were found to be less in patients with a shorter interim. All patients in the study had received antimicrobial treatment for the first 7–10 days, vancomycin or daptomycin combined with ampicillin/sulbactam. Patients received i.v. antibiotics for 2 weeks following explantation and 1–2 weeks following reimplantation. After discharge, they were given oral antibiotics [33].

Pro-Implant Foundation from Germany (https://pro-implant.org/) proposed a treatment algorithm for patients undergoing a revision surgery due to an infection. The research group suggested that patients undergoing a two-stage revision with a short interim should be given a total of 3 weeks of i.v. antibiotics treatment, i.e., 2 weeks within the interval, followed by the revision surgery at the second week, and a week of i.v. antibiotics following reimplantation. The group proposed to use 2 weeks of i.v. antibiotics after explantation, followed by 4 weeks of oral antibiotics and reimplantation surgery at the sixth week, followed by a week of i.v. antibiotics, and

5 weeks of oral antibiotics in patients undergoing a two-stage revision with a long interim [34].

Although numerous suggestions exist, there is currently a lack of high-level evidence for the length of interim and antibiotic treatment.

19.6.2 Mobility During the Interim

One of the main advantages of dynamic spacers is the ability to maintain movement during the interim. However, different approaches exist in terms of weight-bearing due to the mechanical susceptibility of the cement spacer caused by mixing of antibiotics and inherently unstable mounting into the resected joint.

Some authors allow partial weight-bearing with the aid of crutches or a cane as tolerated and let patients wore an extension or hinge orthosis of the knee until soft tissue healing had occurred. If slight or mild laxity remained, the brace was worn until reimplantation, the authors stated [17].

Others use preformed cement spacer (InterSpace; Exactech) and wait for a short period of time to allow wound healing, followed by weight-bearing with one or two supports and active range of motion [4].

The limitation of hand-molded spacers in terms of mechanical strength has been highlighted [16]. The authors defined these spacers as potentially unstable and proposed to use an extension brace or orthosis to be worn during ambulation.

Fink et al. used dynamic cement spacers, and the patient was mobilized with crutches, and partial weight-bearing of 20 kg on the surgically treated leg was allowed [32].

19.7 Complications Related to the Use of Dynamic Spacers

Potential disadvantages of dynamic spacers were reported to be related to wound healing, cement fracture, and dislocation of the spacer [1].

Mobile spacers show cement abrasion causing fibrosis of the articular tissue already within

6 weeks [32]. An increase in immunomodulation of synovial tissue has also been reported [35]. Because of these findings, total synovectomy and extensive lavage are recommended at the second stage of surgery to decrease the number of particles and any retained bacteria.

Lanting et al. investigated dynamic spacer-related complications, more specifically coronal and sagittal subluxation, and their effect on postoperative outcome following the second stage of revision. They found that subluxated knees of more than one standard deviation from the mean in the sagittal plane had lower Knee Society Function Scores ($p = 0.045$). The authors suggested that the operating surgeons who used dynamic spacers as part of a staged revision protocol should be aware that subluxation may affect on outcome following second stage revision [31]. The risk of subluxation might be reduced when both the femoral and tibial components are molded with a stem to gain stability [14].

According to an expert survey, a strong consensus exists not to revise or reduce dislocated dynamic antibiotic spacers, except for circumstances such as pressure against the skin with imminent necrosis/ulceration, resulting in severe, progressive loss of essential soft tissue or bone, neurovascular compromise, or notable pain and disability for the patient [13].

Chen et al. found less favorable results for static spacers, which resulted in a higher incidence of patella baja and decreased ROM [36].

19.8 Conclusion

Dynamic spacers are recommended whenever possible in two-stage revision for infected total knee arthroplasty. Although the evidence level is low, some benefits were reported favoring dynamic spacers, such as better ROM, shorter hospital stay, and better eventual outcome following the second stage revision.

Handmade cement spacers constitute an important option for these operations at a low cost, providing the possibility of tailoring antibiotic mixture with cement at the desired dose with the desired types, which should be culture and antibiogram specific, whenever possible.

Mobility and weight-bearing should be closely monitored, taking into account the added antibiotic dose to the cement, which would decrease the mechanical properties of the spacer.

The length of the interim period should be carefully planned, and it must be remembered that the elution of antibiotics decreases over time with an increased risk of bacterial colonization on the spacer.

Careful selection of patients to be implanted with dynamic spacers can decrease spacer-related complications and early address of spacer subluxations might be beneficial for better outcome following the second stage revision.

References

1. Jacobs C, Christensen CP, Berend ME. Static and mobile antibiotic-impregnated cement spacers for the management of prosthetic joint infection. J Am Acad Orthop Surg. 2009;17(6):356–68. https://doi.org/10.5435/00124635-200906000-00004.
2. Insall JN, Thompson FM, Brause BD. Two-stage reimplantation for the salvage of infected total knee arthroplasty. J Bone Joint Surg Am. 1983;65(8):1087–98.
3. Calton TF, Fehring TK, Griffin WL. Bone loss associated with the use of spacer blocks in infected total knee arthroplasty. Clin Orthop Relat Res. 1997;345:148–54.
4. Lachiewicz PF, Wellman SS, Peterson JR. Antibiotic cement spacers for infected total knee arthroplasties. J Am Acad Orthop Surg. 2020;28(5):180–8. https://doi.org/10.5435/JAAOS-D-19-00332.
5. Haddad FS, Masri BA, Campbell D, McGraw RW, Beauchamp CP, Duncan CP. The PROSTALAC functional spacer in two-stage revision for infected knee replacements. Prosthesis of antibiotic-loaded acrylic cement. J Bone Joint Surg Br. 2000;82(6):807–12. https://doi.org/10.1302/0301-620x.82b6.10486.
6. Pitto RP, Spika IA. Antibiotic-loaded bone cement spacers in two-stage management of infected total knee arthroplasty. Int Orthop. 2004;28(3):129–33. https://doi.org/10.1007/s00264-004-0545-2.
7. Citak M, Argenson JN, Masri B, Kendoff D, Springer B, Alt V, Baldini A, Cui Q, Deirmengian GK, del Sel H, Harrer MF, Israelite C, Jahoda D, Jutte PC, Levicoff E, Meani E, Motta F, Pena OR, Ranawat AS, Safir O, Squire MW, Taunton MJ, Vogely C, Wellman SS. Spacers. J Orthop Res. 2014;32(Suppl 1):S120–9. https://doi.org/10.1002/jor.22555.
8. Voleti PB, Baldwin KD, Lee GC. Use of static or articulating spacers for infection following total knee arthroplasty: a systematic literature review. J Bone

Joint Surg Am. 2013;95(17):1594–9. https://doi.org/10.2106/JBJS.L.01461.

9. Pivec R, Naziri Q, Issa K, Banerjee S, Mont MA. Systematic review comparing static and articulating spacers used for revision of infected total knee arthroplasty. J Arthroplasty. 2014;29(3):553–557e551. https://doi.org/10.1016/j.arth.2013.07.041.

10. Becker R, Clauss M, Rotigliano N, Hirschmann MT. Periprosthetic joint infection treatment in total hip and knee arthroplasty. Oper Tech Orthop. 2016;26(1):20–33. https://doi.org/10.1053/j.oto.2016.01.001.

11. Hofmann AA, Kane KR, Tkach TK, Plaster RL, Camargo MP. Treatment of infected total knee arthroplasty using an articulating spacer. Clin Orthop Relat Res. 1995;(321):45–54.

12. Chen YP, Wu CC, Ho WP. Autoclaved metal-on-cement spacer versus static spacer in two-stage revision in periprosthetic knee infection. Indian J Orthop. 2016;50(2):146–53. https://doi.org/10.4103/0019-5413.177587.

13. Abdel MP, Barreira P, Battenberg A, Berry DJ, Blevins K, Font-Vizcarra L, Frommelt L, Goswami K, Greiner J, Janz V, Kendoff DO, Limberg AK, Manrique J, Moretti B, Murylev V, O'Byrne J, Petrie MJ, Porteous A, Saleri S, Sandiford NA, Sharma V, Shubnyakov I, Sporer S, Squire MW, Stockley I, Tibbo ME, Turgeon T, Varshneya A, Wellman S, Zahar A. Hip and knee section, treatment, two-stage exchange spacer-related: proceedings of international consensus on orthopedic infections. J Arthroplasty. 2019;34(2S):S427–38. https://doi.org/10.1016/j.arth.2018.09.027.

14. Akhtar A, Mitchell C, Assis C, Iranpour F, Kropelnicki A, Strachan R. Cement pedestal spacer technique for infected two-stage revision knee arthroplasty: description and comparison of complications. Indian J Orthop. 2019;53(6):695–9. https://doi.org/10.4103/ortho.IJOrtho_90_19.

15. Shen H, Zhang X, Jiang Y, Wang Q, Chen Y, Wang Q, Shao J. Intraoperatively-made cement-on-cement antibiotic-loaded articulating spacer for infected total knee arthroplasty. Knee. 2010;17(6):407–11. https://doi.org/10.1016/j.knee.2009.11.007.

16. Chong SY, Shen L, Frantz S. Loading capacity of dynamic knee spacers: a comparison between hand-moulded and COPAL spacers. BMC Musculoskelet Disord. 2019;20(1):613. https://doi.org/10.1186/s12891-019-2982-5.

17. Villanueva-Martinez M, Rios-Luna A, Pereiro J, Fahandez-Saddi H, Villamor A. Hand-made articulating spacers in two-stage revision for infected total knee arthroplasty: good outcome in 30 patients. Acta Orthop. 2008;79(5):674–82. https://doi.org/10.1080/17453670810016704.

18. Citak M, Masri BA, Springer B, Argenson JN, Kendoff DO. Are preformed articulating spacers superior to surgeon-made articulating spacers in the treatment of PJI in THA? A literature review. Open Orthop J. 2015;9:255–61. https://doi.org/10.2174/1874325001509010255.

19. Skwara A, Tibesku C, Paletta RJ, Sommer C, Krodel A, Lahner M, Daniilidis K. Articulating spacers compared to fixed spacers for the treatment of infected knee arthroplasty: a follow-up of 37 cases. Technol Health Care. 2016;24(4):571–7. https://doi.org/10.3233/THC-161152.

20. Park SJ, Song EK, Seon JK, Yoon TR, Park GH. Comparison of static and mobile antibiotic-impregnated cement spacers for the treatment of infected total knee arthroplasty. Int Orthop. 2010;34(8):1181–6. https://doi.org/10.1007/s00264-009-0907-x.

21. Citak M, Citak M, Kendoff D. Dynamic versus static cement spacer in periprosthetic knee infection: a meta-analysis. Orthopade. 2015;44(8):599–606. https://doi.org/10.1007/s00132-015-3091-2.

22. Cabo J, Euba G, Saborido A, Gonzalez-Panisello M, Dominguez MA, Agullo JL, Murillo O, Verdaguer R, Ariza J. Clinical outcome and microbiological findings using antibiotic-loaded spacers in two-stage revision of prosthetic joint infections. J Infect. 2011;63(1):23–31. https://doi.org/10.1016/j.jinf.2011.04.014.

23. Sorli L, Puig L, Torres-Claramunt R, Gonzalez A, Alier A, Knobel H, Salvado M, Horcajada JP. The relationship between microbiology results in the second of a two-stage exchange procedure using cement spacers and the outcome after revision total joint replacement for infection: the use of sonication to aid bacteriological analysis. J Bone Joint Surg Br. 2012;94(2):249–53. https://doi.org/10.1302/0301-620X.94B2.27779.

24. Nelson CL, Jones RB, Wingert NC, Foltzer M, Bowen TR. Sonication of antibiotic spacers predicts failure during two-stage revision for prosthetic knee and hip infections. Clin Orthop Relat Res. 2014;472(7):2208–14. https://doi.org/10.1007/s11999-014-3571-4.

25. Aeng ES, Shalansky KF, Lau TT, Zalunardo N, Li G, Bowie WR, Duncan CP. Acute kidney injury with tobramycin-impregnated bone cement spacers in prosthetic joint infections. Ann Pharmacother. 2015;49(11):1207–13. https://doi.org/10.1177/1060028015600176.

26. Koo KH, Yang JW, Cho SH, Song HR, Park HB, Ha YC, Chang JD, Kim SY, Kim YH. Impregnation of vancomycin, gentamicin, and cefotaxime in a cement spacer for two-stage cementless reconstruction in infected total hip arthroplasty. J Arthroplasty. 2001;16(7):882–92. https://doi.org/10.1054/arth.2001.24444.

27. Fink B, Grossmann A, Fuerst M, Schafer P, Frommelt L. Two-stage cementless revision of infected hip endoprostheses. Clin Orthop Relat Res. 2009;467(7):1848–58. https://doi.org/10.1007/s11999-008-0611-y.

28. Emerson RH Jr, Muncie M, Tarbox TR, Higgins LL. Comparison of a static with a mobile spacer in total knee infection. Clin Orthop Relat Res. 2002;404:132–8. https://doi.org/10.1097/00003086-200211000-00023.

29. Kuzyk PR, Dhotar HS, Sternheim A, Gross AE, Safir O, Backstein D. Two-stage revision arthroplasty for management of chronic periprosthetic hip and knee infection: techniques, controversies, and outcomes. J

Am Acad Orthop Surg. 2014;22(3):153–64. https://doi.org/10.5435/JAAOS-22-03-153.

30. Charette RS, Melnic CM. Two-stage revision arthroplasty for the treatment of prosthetic joint infection. Curr Rev Musculoskelet Med. 2018;11(3):332–40. https://doi.org/10.1007/s12178-018-9495-y.

31. Lanting BA, Lau A, Teeter MG, Howard JL. Outcome following subluxation of mobile articulating spacers in two-stage revision total knee arthroplasty. Arch Orthop Trauma Surg. 2017;137(3):375–80. https://doi.org/10.1007/s00402-017-2630-1.

32. Fink B, Rechtenbach A, Buchner H, Vogt S, Hahn M. Articulating spacers used in two-stage revision of infected hip and knee prostheses abrade with time. Clin Orthop Relat Res. 2011;469(4):1095–102. https://doi.org/10.1007/s11999-010-1479-1.

33. Winkler T, Stuhlert MGW, Lieb E, Muller M, von Roth P, Preininger B, Trampuz A, Perka CF. Outcome of short versus long interval in two-stage exchange for periprosthetic joint infection: a prospective cohort study. Arch Orthop Trauma Surg. 2019;139(3):295–303. https://doi.org/10.1007/s00402-018-3052-4.

34. Pocket Guide to Diagnosis & Treatment of Periprosthetic Joint Infection (PJI). Pro-implant foundation. 2019. https://pro-implant.org/tools/pocket-guide. Accessed 1 Dec 2020.

35. Singh G, Deutloff N, Maertens N, Meyer H, Awiszus F, Feuerstein B, Roessner A, Lohmann CH. Articulating polymethylmethacrylate (PMMA) spacers may have an immunomodulating effect on synovial tissue. Bone Joint J. 2016;98-B(8):1062–8. https://doi.org/10.1302/0301-620X.98B8.36663.

36. Chen AF, Tetreault MW, Levicoff EA, Fedorka CJ, Rothenberg AC, Klatt BA. Increased incidence of patella Baja after total knee arthroplasty revision for infection. Am J Orthop (Belle Mead, NJ). 2014;43(12):562–6.

Knee Arthrodesis

20

Claire Bolton and David Parker

20.1 Introduction

Knee arthrodesis is an option for limb salvage in complex periprosthetic joint infections for which revision knee arthroplasty cannot be considered. John Key first described compression knee arthrodesis in 1932 in the treatment for tuberculosis of the knee joint [1]. He used a turnbuckle applied across transtibial and transfemoral pins that could be tightened to maintain pressure across the arthrodesis site, with the addition of a circular plaster. He achieved union in 4 out of 5 patients, with the fifth dying of sepsis prior to union. Charnley [2] further expanded on this technique using special screw-clamps and wing-nuts to tighten across the construct until the Steinmann pins bent. His results showed successful arthrodesis in a total of 15 knees: 6 with old tuberculosis and 9 for osteoarthritis.

While knee arthrodesis usually provides good pain relief, it is associated with specific functional limitations and is not usually considered an attractive option for patients. It is therefore seen as a salvage procedure, and the decision as to when to proceed to a knee arthrodesis in the setting of a failed periprosthetic joint infection is a difficult one. Repeating a failed 2-stage revision procedure can lead to further bone loss and may compromise the soft tissue envelope, both of which may cause difficulties with salvage procedures in the future. Kheir et al. [3] found that 38.4% of patients failed to have their infection controlled after a repeated 2-stage revision. Wu et al. [4] in a systematic review looked at the utility of different treatment options after failure of a 2-stage revision TKA for periprosthetic joint infection. The treatment options included repeat 2-stage revision, knee arthrodesis, above knee amputation, or suppressive antibiotics. Knee arthrodesis was found to be the intervention that was most likely to give the highest quality of life. Knee arthrodesis therefore does have a role, albeit a very limited one, in the salvage of the failed TKR when other reconstructive options are not viable.

20.2 Indications and Contraindications for Arthrodesis

Knee fusion was initially introduced as a treatment for septic arthritis, tuberculosis and poliomyelitis [1, 2, 5, 6]. Before the development of total knee arthroplasty, knee arthrodesis was also used to treat osteoarthritis and rheumatoid arthritis. These days the most common indication for knee arthrodesis is for failure of a total knee arthroplasty, for which revision is not an option due to presence of a persistent periprosthetic joint infection, extensor mechanism defect that is irreparable, or massive soft tissue or bone loss [7,

C. Bolton · D. Parker (✉)
Sydney Orthopaedic Research Institute, Sydney, NSW, Australia
e-mail: dparker@sydneyortho.com.au

© ISAKOS 2022
U. G. Longo et al. (eds.), *Infection in Knee Replacement*,
https://doi.org/10.1007/978-3-030-81553-0_20

8]. Persistence of periprosthetic joint infection in knees that have undergone implantation of an antibiotic spacer is reported in the literature as 9–12% [9]. Knee arthrodesis is also used outside of arthroplasty for treatment of extensive bone or tissue loss, weakness or loss of the extensor mechanism, for the treatment of tumours, and post traumatic arthritis.

Traditional contraindications are a contralateral knee fusion or an ipsilateral hip arthrodesis [10]. The ipsilateral hip and ankle should be supple and free from significant arthritis due to the increased load that will be transferred to these joints post arthrodesis.

20.3 Limitations of Knee Arthrodesis

Knee arthrodesis imparts several physical and psychological limitations to the patient. The inability to bend the knee can cause issues with sitting, climbing stairs and taking public transportation.

A study undertaken on healthy subjects to simulate knee arthrodesis using a brace assessed gait kinematics and kinetics affected by knee arthrodesis [11]. The results showed that compensations for knee immobilisation include (1) increased spinal movement of the lumbosacral spine, (2) increase in vertical excursion (hip-hiking) and transverse rotation of the pelvis on the involved side, (3) increase in extension of the contralateral hip, (4) increased peak flexion in the contralateral knee during swing phase, and (5) a decrease in plantarflexion of the ipsilateral ankle at toe off to help assist with foot clearance. This study looked at the effect of acclimation time, which did not alter the braced gait kinematics, and hence the authors felt the results support a model of longer-term knee rigidity. Marshall et al. [12] found similar results in their study on 2 postoperative knee arthrodesis patients who had achieved union.

Other studies have shown energy expenditure to be higher by 30% than for normal walking in experimental models of knee arthrodesis [13, 14]. In contrast, the increase in energy expenditure for a transfemoral amputation is higher at 50–60%.

20.4 Principles of Knee Arthrodesis

In order to improve the chances of successful knee arthrodesis and infection clearance, the host must be optimised preoperatively systemically. Infection needs to be controlled as much as possible, and the preoperative planning for the knee fusion should optimise available bone contact and required leg length.

20.4.1 Host Optimisation

The patient should be managed in a multidisciplinary team. Modifiable risk factors for infection that may contribute to problems with wound healing should be addressed, such as smoking, diabetic control, cessation of relevant medications, and the nutritional status of the patient. The periprosthetic infection should be managed with antibiotics while also ensuring any treatment of systemic or more widespread infection. If wound issues or soft tissue defects exist, then it is wise to consult a plastic surgeon.

20.4.2 Knee Fusion Position

The ideal position for knee fusion is in 5–7° of anatomical valgus and 10° of flexion, which shortens the limb to help with foot clearance during ambulation and is more practical for sitting than with the knee extended [14]. The aim for limb shortening is 1 cm; however, it is often significantly more than this when performed for failed total knee replacement due to bone loss.

20.4.3 One-Stage Versus Two-Stage Arthrodesis

Arthrodesis may be done as a single-stage procedure or a 2-stage procedure post failure for infection of a total knee replacement. A one-stage arthrodesis involves removal of total knee replacement prosthesis, thorough debridement and lavage, followed by completion of the knee arthrodesis using the surgeon's preferred technique. Several studies have shown a one-stage procedure to increase the risk of a subsequent deep infection of the arthrodesis if internal implants are used [7, 13, 15]. However, this has been disputed by other studies that have shown a one-stage arthrodesis to be effective in low virulence organisms and in the absence of polymicrobial infections, when either an external fixator or intramedullary device is used [16–20].

A 2-stage arthrodesis involves removal of the total knee implants and thorough debridement and lavage of the joint, followed by application of an antibiotic-impregnated cement spacer and a period of intravenous antibiotics to allow the infection to clear prior to proceeding to the arthrodesis. At the second stage the spacer is removed, and the knee arthrodesis is then performed via the surgeon's preferred technique.

20.5 Techniques for Arthrodesis

Multiple techniques for arthrodesis of the knee have been described in the literature. The two more commonly used procedures are the external fixator and the fusion intramedullary nail.

20.5.1 External Fixator

External fixators include uniplanar and biplanar fixators as well as circular fixators. Circular frames are ideal in that multiplanar deformity correction as well as length can be adjusted through the frame. Circular frames also provide better stability to the fusion construct than the uniplanar and biplanar frames.

There are several advantages of using external fixators for arthrodesis. Blood loss is minimised as only small incisions are needed. Shortening of the limb can be achieved progressively with circular frames, in the setting of large bone defects, where immediate shortening may compromise soft tissues and neurovascular structures. Circular frames can also be used to perform a limb lengthening procedure concurrently with the knee arthrodesis, either through a separate site on the tibia or femur. External fixation also minimises the presence of internal hardware, which is a potential advantage in cases of established infection.

Complications of external fixators include a high rate of pin-site infections, stress fractures through pin sites, and neurovascular injuries. Disadvantages to the technique, particularly for circular frames, is that it may not be a familiar procedure for many surgeons, and it requires specialist training to be performed successfully.

20.5.2 Fusion Nail

A variety of intramedullary nails (IMNs) have been used to achieve knee arthrodesis. Short nails are inserted through the knee joint and are either modular or non-modular. The modular nails have a coupling device that connects the two components, which are inserted into the femoral and tibial canals separately. The coupling device also allows for compression at the arthrodesis site. Short IMNs are ideal when there is an ipsilateral hip replacement.

Long IMNs are inserted through the piriformis fossa and interlocked both proximally and distally, following preparation of the knee fusion site via the knee incision. This technique can be more challenging to control the position of the knee fusion, mainly due to the involvement of the entire length of the femur in the fixation.

Disadvantages of IMNs are the increased operative time and increased perioperative blood loss. The position of fusion is limited by the relationship of the geometry of the nail with the patient's anatomy. The position achieved with an IMN is also fixed at the time of the procedure, unlike external fixation which can allow for ongoing adjustments. IMN may also not be able to be used when there is large deformity in the tibia or femur, or significant bone loss that would cause unacceptable substantial shortening of the limb. Newer technology with IMNs can however potentially facilitate limb lengthening at a further surgical procedure via "lengthening over the nail" or by exchange nailing to an adjustable intramedullary nail. An example of modular short intramedullary nail is reported in Fig. 20.1.

Fig. 20.1 AP radiograph (**a**) and lateral radiograph (**b**) of a modular short intramedullary nail (Witchita® Nail Stryker) placed for knee arthrodesis post periprosthetic joint infection with successful fusion

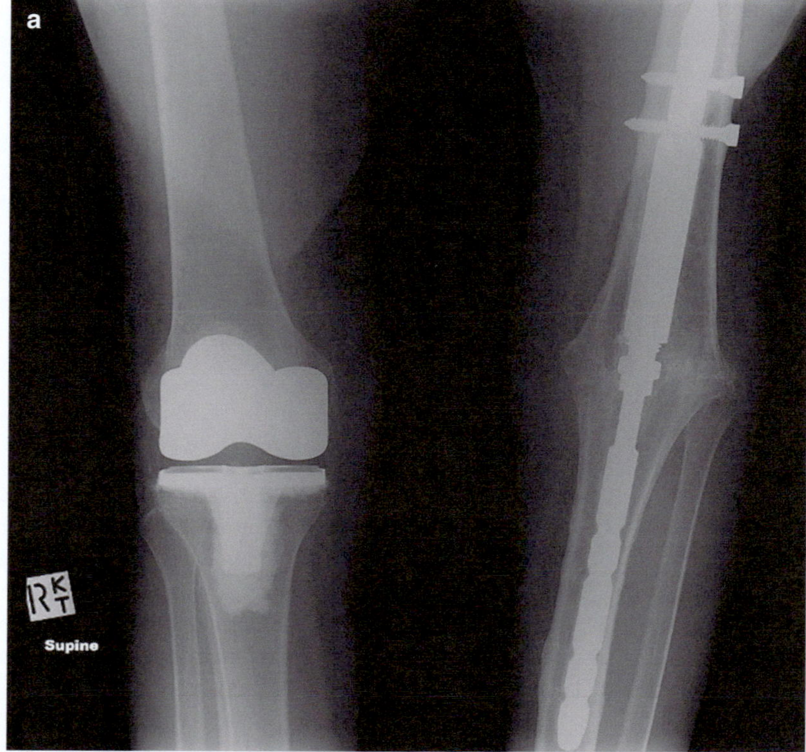

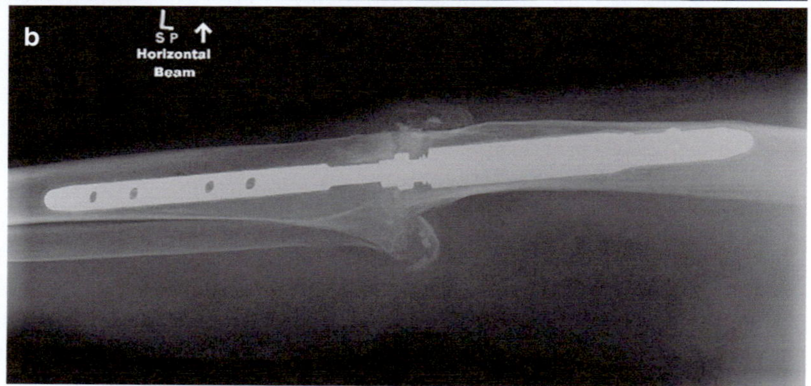

20.5.3 Combined Surgical Techniques

The use of a circular frame until the fusion site begins to consolidate, and then removing the frame and placing an intramedullary device is an example of a combined technique. The advantages of doing this are that no hardware is placed at the area of infection, which has the theoretical advantage of increasing clearance rates for the prosthetic infection. Removal of the frame prior to complete fusion minimises the risk of pin-site infections from long-term frame use, while the intramedullary nail allows stability and protection of the fusion site to prevent against fusion site fracture. This is particularly useful when bone quality at the fusion site is poor [20].

20.5.4 Dealing with Massive Bone Defects

After prosthesis removal in infected total knee arthroplasty it is not uncommon to have large volumes of bone loss [21, 22]. If arthrodesis is performed at the residual bone ends, then a large leg length discrepancy is the outcome. In an attempt to minimise further surgery on patients who have multiple comorbidities, while maintaining leg length, several techniques have been described in the literature.

Vascularised fibular bone graft (VFBG) can be used to bridge the bone defect. This procedure must be done in a staged fashion for infected total knee arthroplasty so that the graft does not fail due to infection. Other disadvantages include the increase in operative time, donor site morbidity, and the graft itself offers little stability. Rasmussen et al. [23] used this technique in 13 patients, 4 of whom had a failed infected total knee replacement and achieved successful fusion in all patients.

Voss [24] described a technique using a long IMN combined with a cement spacer used to fill the bone defect at the knee site. Similar techniques have been reported using a short modular IMN and antibiotic-impregnated cement spacer [7, 25, 26]. Alt et al. [27] reported on the use of a modular IMN coated with silver and connected with a central spacer, also coated in silver, in an 86-year-old woman for treatment of failed infected total knee arthroplasty. The arthrodesis was done as a 2-stage procedure with cement spacer and cement coated rods placed in the first stage, and the modular IMN with central spacer all coated in silver. There was no recurrence of infection within 26 months follow-up.

Peterson et al. [28] described the use of trabecular metal cones (Zimmer, Biomet) together with a long IMN and autograft to bridge the massive bone loss during the knee arthrodesis for failure of infected total knee arthroplasty. In their series of 6 patients, 5 patients achieved a solid fusion, but one patient required an above knee amputation for a septic non-union.

20.6 Arthrodesis Outcomes

Rates of fusion following knee arthrodesis depend on the mode of fixation [29–33]. External fixation rates of fusion range from 50% to 99% [34], 88% to 100% for intramedullary nails [15], 90% to 95% for modular nails and 85% to 100% where a combined nail and external fixator is applied [15].

Fusion rate following conversion of total knee arthroplasty to arthrodesis is lower than in those knees where joint replacement has not been undertaken. This is theorised to be due to persistence of any infection, poorer bone stock and poorer bone apposition. Knutson et al. showed that after treating 91 failed total knee replacements with conversion to arthrodesis, 82 who had a form of external fixation and the remaining 9 with either intramedullary nail or plate osteosynthesis, only 50% achieved fusion [15].Robinson et al. [9] showed in their study of 23 knees, a fusion rate of 87% using either intramedullary nail, external fixation or compression plating. Persistent infection has been shown to be high post knee arthrodesis [35–39]. In a study by Rohner et al. [39], the rate of persistent infection was 50%, with persistent infection resulting in patients either undergoing above knee amputation, exchange intramedullary nailing, or developing an established sinus overlying the fusion site [40].

Carr II et al. [40] compared outcomes of patients who underwent above knee amputation (AKA) with those who had a knee arthrodesis for the treatment of failed periprosthetic total knee arthroplasty. The arthrodesis cohort had significantly higher rates of postoperative infection as well as blood transfusion. The AKA patients had a higher rate of systemic complications and in-hospital mortality (3.7% vs. 2.1%). Rohner et al. reported a 50% rate of persistent infection after conversion of TKA to knee fusion [39]. AKA after failed infected TKA is also associated with infection rates reported at 20% [41]. Ambulation after AKA is dependent on a prosthesis, and in a study by Sierra et al. a prosthesis was only fitted in 9 out of 25 patients with limited ambulation achieved in 5 of those patients [41].

Patient reported outcome measures (PROMs) in patients converted from an infected total knee replacement to a knee arthrodesis have been shown to be comparable to patients who have undergone total knee arthroplasty [22]. This study on 8 patients, 7 of whom achieved a successful fusion, was assessed with the Japanese knee osteoarthritis measurement (JKOM) and the Knee Society score (KSS). The JKOM scored comparably to normative data for total knee arthroplasty patients, while the KSS, which has a significant component assessing range of motion, was not surprisingly worse when compared to normative data for total knee arthroplasty. Benson et al. [42] compared 9 patients who underwent a knee arthrodesis for failed total knee arthroplasty (8 for periprosthetic infection) to 9 total knee arthroplasty patients. The SF-36 score and arthritis impact measurement score (AIMS) were assessed, with the SF-36 score being similar between the 2 groups, while the AIMS was better in the TKA group. De Vil et al. also showed comparable SF-36 scores in physical functioning and role-emotional scores between knee arthrodesis and total knee arthroplasty cohorts, with the knee arthrodesis group having better scores for bodily pain and general health; however, the knee arthrodesis group scored worse on mental health and social functioning [35]. Therefore, although outcome scores are reasonable for knee arthrodesis, particularly secondary to good pain relief, they do not function as well as a successful total knee arthroplasty.

20.7 Arthrodesis Complications

Non-union is the most common complication of knee arthrodesis surgery [7]. Factors that affect this are persistence of infection, adequacy of bone stock, and deficiency in fixation construct or bony apposition. The treatment of the non-union is done via fracture principles. In an atrophic non-union, the host biology and any nutritional deficiency should be addressed, as well as optimisation of control of conditions such as diabetes. Once the patient is optimised the non-union should be taken down and bone grafted with either iliac crest or the addition of a vascularised fibular graft. Hypertrophic non-unions can be treated by revision of fixation to increase rigidity and provide adequate stability to achieve union. Treatment of the infected non-union is difficult. Debridement of the non-union and revision fixation, with repeated cultures taken and antibiotics targeted at the infective organism may be performed as a single-stage or two-stage procedure. While intramedullary nails can be used as the fixation method, this is a situation for which there is a clear advantage of an external fixator to avoid the presence of hardware at the site of infection. Alternatively, if the surgeon believes that the chances of achieving union are unacceptably low, or a patient wouldn't tolerate multiple further procedures, then AKA would be indicated.

Leg length discrepancy of greater than 2 cm has been reported in several studies [37, 43, 44]. Other studies have suggested an average LLD of greater than 5 cm [21, 22]. A small LLD of less than 2 cm is of some advantage in achieving ground clearance during walking in the absence of knee flexion, and generally does not require treatment. If the LLD is between 2 and 5 cm, a shoe raise can be used. LLD greater than 5 cm are difficult to manage with a shoe raise as balance issues tend to occur, and so surgical intervention with distraction osteogenesis may be warranted. Techniques to achieve lengthening include lengthening over an IMN and exchange nailing to a lengthening nail [45].

Other complications include intraoperative fracture, persistent infection, additional superinfection, deep vein thrombosis, wound dehiscence and peroneal nerve palsy. Intraoperative fracture has been described to have an incidence of 6–12% [43, 44]. As previously discussed, persistence in infection is a problem when revising an infected TKA to a knee fusion. The rates reported in the literature for persistent infection range from 6–50% [16, 17, 19, 21, 44, 46–49]. Peroneal nerve palsy has an incidence in the literature of 6–12% [17, 43, 44].

20.8 Conclusion

Knee arthrodesis is a rarely used salvage procedure for failed infected total knee arthroplasty that has significant functional limitations for the patient. The benefits are that it may allow the patient to continue to ambulate independently on a pain-free, stable extremity, which is the main advantage in comparison to transfemoral amputation. Good results have been achieved with the use of IMN, both long and coupled devices, as well as with circular external fixators, and also when using a combined technique. The surgeon must choose whether to proceed with a one- or two-stage procedure and utilise the best surgical technique based on their expertise and a thorough assessment of the features of each individual patient.

References

1. Key JA. Positive pressure in arthrodesis for tuberculosis of the knee joint. 1932. South Med J. 1932;25:909. https://doi.org/10.1097/BLO.0b013e318123eb6e.
2. Charnley JC. Positive pressure in arthrodesis of the knee joint. J Bone Jt Surg. 1948;30B(3):478–86.
3. Kheir MM, Tan TL, Gomez MM, Chen AF, Parvizi J. Patients with failed prior two-stage exchange have poor outcomes after further surgical intervention. J Arthroplasty. 2017;32(4):1262–5. https://doi.org/10.1016/j.arth.2016.10.008.
4. Wu CH, Gray CF, Lee GC. Arthrodesis should be strongly considered after failed two-stage Reimplantation TKA. Clin Orthop Relat Res. 2014;472(11):3295–304. https://doi.org/10.1007/s11999-014-3482-4.
5. Hibbs R. The treatment of tuberculosis of the joints of the lower extremities by operative fusion. J Bone Jt Surg. 1930;12:749.
6. Soto-Hall R. Fusion in charcots disease of the knee: new technique for arthrodesis. Ann Surg. 1938;108:124.
7. MacDonald J, Agarwal S, Lorei M, Johanson N, Frieberg A. Knee arthrodesis. J Am Acad Orthop Surg. 2006;14:154–63.
8. Somayaji HS, Tsaggerides P, Ware HE, Dowd GSE. Knee arthrodesis-a review. Knee. 2008;15(4):247–54. https://doi.org/10.1016/j.knee.2008.03.005.
9. Robinson M, Piponov HI, Ormseth A, Helder CW, Schwartz B, Gonzalez MH. Knee arthrodesis outcomes after infected Total knee arthroplasty and failure of two-stage revision with an antibiotic cement spacer. JAAOS Glob Res Rev. 2018;2(1):e077. https://doi.org/10.5435/jaaosglobal-d-17-00077.
10. Nelson C, Evarts C. Arthroplasty and arthrodesis of the knee joint. Orthop Clin North Am. 1971;2(1):245–64.
11. Hutchison RE, Lucas EM, Marro J, Gambon T, Bruneau KN, DesJardins JD. The effects of simulated knee arthrodesis on gait kinematics and kinetics. Proc Inst Mech Eng H J Eng Med. 2019;233(7):723–34. https://doi.org/10.1177/0954411919850028.
12. Marshall R, Nade S. Effects of arthrodeses on walking: kinematic and kinetic studies of subtalar and knee arthrodesis. Clin Biomech. 1991;6:51–9.
13. Conway JD, Mont MA, Bezwada HP. Arthrodesis of the knee. J Bone Joint Surg Am. 2004;86:835–48.
14. Chakravarty R, Kapadia B, Jauregui J, Mont M. Knee arthrodesis. In: Wiesel SW, editor. Operative techniques in orthopaedic surgery. 2nd ed. Philadelphia: Wolters Kluwer; 2016. p. 1268–79.
15. Knutson K, Hovelius L, Lindstrand A, Lidgren L. Arthrodesis after failed knee arthroplasty: a nationwide multicenter investigation of 91 cases. Clin Orthop Relat Res. 1984;191:202–11.
16. Kuchinad R, Fourman MS, Fragomen AT, Rozbruch SR. Knee arthrodesis as limb salvage for complex failures of total knee arthroplasty. J Arthroplasty. 2014;29(11):2150–5. https://doi.org/10.1016/j.arth.2014.06.021.
17. Gallusser N, Goetti P, Luyet A, Borens O. Knee arthrodesis with modular nail after failed TKA due to infection. Eur J Orthop Surg Traumatol. 2015;25(8):1307–12. https://doi.org/10.1007/s00590-015-1707-1.
18. Gottfriedsen TB, Schroder HM, Odgaard A. Knee arthrodesis after failure of knee arthroplasty: a nationwide register-based study. J Bone Joint Surg (Am Vol). 2016;98(16):1370–7. https://doi.org/10.2106/JBJS.15.01363.
19. Friedrich MJ, Schmolders J, Wimmer MD, et al. Two-stage knee arthrodesis with a modular intramedullary nail due to septic failure of revision total knee arthroplasty with extensor mechanism deficiency. Knee. 2017;24(5):1240–6. https://doi.org/10.1016/j.knee.2017.05.019.
20. Makhdom AM, Fragomen A, Rozbruch SR. Knee arthrodesis after failed total knee arthroplasty. J Bone Joint Surg (Am Vol). 2019;101(7):650–60. https://doi.org/10.2106/JBJS.18.00191.
21. Bargiotas K, Wohlrab D, Sewecke JJ, Lavinge G, Demeo PJ, Sotereanos NG. Arthrodesis of the knee with a long intramedullary nail following the failure of a total knee arthroplasty as the result of infection. J Bone Joint Surg Am. 2006;88(3):553–8.
22. Watanabe K, Minowa T, Takeda S, et al. Outcomes of knee arthrodesis following infected total knee arthroplasty: a retrospective analysis of 8 cases. Mod Rheumatol. 2013;19:243–9. https://doi.org/10.1007/s10165-013-0862-7.

23. Rasmussen MRMD, Bishop AT, Wood MB. Arthrodesis of the knee with a vascularized fibular rotatory graft. J Bone Joint Surg Am. 1995;77(5):751–9.

24. Voss FR. A new technique of limb salvage after infected revision total knee arthroplasty: artificial fusion. J Arthroplasty. 2001;16(4):524–8. https://doi.org/10.1054/arth.2001.23624.

25. Iacono F, Bruni D, Lo Presti M, et al. Knee arthrodesis with a press-fit modular intramedullary nail without bone-on-bone fusion after an infected revision TKA. Knee. 2012;19(5):555–9. https://doi.org/10.1016/j.knee.2012.01.005.

26. Hawi N, Kendoff D, Citak M, Gehrke T, Haasper C, Hawi VN. Septic single-stage knee arthrodesis after failed total knee arthroplasty using a cemented coupled nail. Bone Jt J. 2015;97-B(5):645–53. https://doi.org/10.1302/0301-620X.97B5.

27. Alt V, Heiss C, Rupp M. Treatment of a recurrent periprosthetic joint infection with an intramedullary knee arthrodesis system with low-amount metallic silver coating. J Bone Jt Infect. 2019;4(3):111–4. https://doi.org/10.7150/jbji.34484.

28. Peterson BE, Bal S, Aggarwal A, Crist BD. Novel technique: knee arthrodesis using trabecular metal cones with intramedullary nailing and intramedullary autograft. J Knee Surg. 2016;29(6):510–5. https://doi.org/10.1055/s-0035-1566738.

29. John Charnley K, Lowe HG. A study of the end-results of compression arthrodesis of the knee. J Bone Joint Surg Br Vol. 1958;40B(4):633–5.

30. Knutson K, Lindstrand A, Lidgren L. Arthrodesis for failed knee arthroplasty: a report of 20 cases. J Bone Jt Surg. 1985;67-B(1):47–52.

31. Rand JA, Bryan RS. The outcome of failed knee arthrodesis following total knee arthroplasty. Clin Orthop Relat Res. 1986;205(April):86–92.

32. Figgie H, Brody G, Inglis A, Sculco T, Goldberg V, Figgie M. Knee arthrodesis following total knee arthroplasty in rheumatoid arthritis. Clin Orthop Relat Res. 1987;224:237–43.

33. Hak DJ, Lieberman JR, Finerman GAM. Single plane and biplane external fixators for knee arthrodesis. Clin Orthop Relat Res. 1995;316:134–44.

34. Vlasak R, Gearen P, Petty W. Knee arthrodesis in the treatment of failed total knee replacement. Clin Orthop Relat Res. 1995;321:138–44.

35. de Vil J, Almqvist KF, Vanheeren P, Boone B, Verdonk R. Knee arthrodesis with an intramedullary nail: a retrospective study. Knee Surg Sports Traumatol Arthrosc. 2008;16(7):645–50. https://doi.org/10.1007/s00167-008-0525-y.

36. Senior CJ, Assunção RE, Barlow IW. Knee arthrodesis for limb salvage with an intramedullary coupled nail. Arch Orthop Trauma Surg. 2008;128(7):683–7. https://doi.org/10.1007/s00402-007-0386-8.

37. Francesco I, Francesco RG, Danilo B, et al. Arthrodesis after infected revision TKA: retrospective comparison of intramedullary nailing and external fixation. HSS J. 2013;9(3):229–35. https://doi.org/10.1007/s11420-013-9349-5.

38. Scarponi S, Drago L, Romanò D, et al. Cementless modular intramedullary nail without bone-on-bone fusion as a salvage procedure in chronically infected total knee prosthesis: long-term results. Int Orthop. 2014;38(2):413–8. https://doi.org/10.1007/s00264-013-2232-7.

39. Röhner E, Windisch C, Nuetzmann K, Rau M, Arnhold M, Matziolis G. Unsatisfactory outcome of arthrodesis performed after septic failure of revision total knee arthroplasty. J Bone Joint Surg (Am Vol). 2015;97(4):298–301. https://doi.org/10.2106/JBJS.N.00834.

40. Carr JB, Werner BC, Browne JA. Trends and outcomes in the treatment of failed septic total knee arthroplasty: comparing arthrodesis and above-knee amputation. J Arthroplasty. 2016;31(7):1574–7. https://doi.org/10.1016/j.arth.2016.01.010.

41. Sierra RJ, Trousdale RT, Pagnano MW. Above-the-knee amputation after a total knee replacement: prevalence, etiology and functional outcome. J Bone Joint Surg Am. 2003 Jun;85(6):1000–4. https://doi.org/10.2106/00004623-200306000-00003.

42. Benson E, Resine S, Lewis C. Functional outcome of arthrodesis for failed total knee arthroplasty. Orthopedics. 1998;21(8):875–9.

43. Garcia-Lopez I, Aguayo M, Cuevas A, Navarro P, Prieto C, Carpintero P. Knee arthrodesis with the Vari-Wall nail for treatment of infected total knee arthroplasty. Acta Orthop Belg. 2008;74(6):809–15.

44. Leroux B, Aparicio G, Fontanin N, et al. Arthrodesis in septic knees using a long intramedullary nail: 17 consecutive cases. Orthop Traumatol Surg Res. 2013;99(4):399–404. https://doi.org/10.1016/j.otsr.2013.03.011.

45. Wood JH, Conway JD. Advanced concepts in knee arthrodesis. World J Orthop. 2015;6(2):202–10. https://doi.org/10.5312/wjo.v6.i2.202.

46. Domingo LJ, Caballero MJ, Cuenca J, Herrera A, Sola A, Herrero L. Knee arthrodesis with the Wichita fusion nail. Int Orthop. 2004;28(1):25–7. https://doi.org/10.1007/s00264-003-0514-1.

47. Mabry TM, Jacofsky DJ, Haidukewych GJ, Hanssen AD. The Chitranjan Ranawat award: comparison of intramedullary nailing and external fixation knee arthrodesis for the infected knee replacement. Clin Orthop Relat Res. 2007;464:11–5. https://doi.org/10.1097/BLO.0b013e31806a9191.

48. Yeoh D, Goddard R, Macnamara P, et al. A comparison of two techniques for knee arthrodesis: the custom made intramedullary mayday nail versus a monoaxial external fixator. Knee. 2008;15(4):263–7. https://doi.org/10.1016/j.knee.2008.02.011.

49. Bruno AAM, Kirienko A, Peccati A, et al. Knee arthrodesis by the Ilizarov method in the treatment of total knee arthroplasty failure. Knee. 2017;24(1):91–9. https://doi.org/10.1016/j.knee.2016.11.002.

Outcomes

Vincenzo Candela, Giovanna Stelitano,
Sergio De Salvatore, Carlo Casciaro,
Calogero Di Naro, Laura Risi Ambrogioni,
Umile Giuseppe Longo, and Vincenzo Denaro

21.1 Introduction

Periprosthetic joint infection (PJI) is an important cause of failure after total knee replacement. Treatment of PJI aims to eradicate the infection, improve joint motion, improve patients' satisfaction and independence during the activity of daily living, and avoid medical and surgical complications. Treatment options include long-term suppressive antibiotics (in patients who are not suitable for surgery), debridement, antibiotics and implant retention (DAIR), one- or two-stage revision, resection arthroplasty, arthrodesis and amputation. However, there is not a univocal definition of success or failure after treatment of PJI [1, 2]. Volin et al. [3] define the success after two-stage revision as the absence of disease at the latest follow-up. Bradbury et al. [4] consider successful not only the clinical resolution of infection and lack of further surgery but also the clinical resolution of infection under suppressive oral antibiotics. Treatment response is defined as post-debridement period free from periprosthetic

joint infections relapse during the time of follow-up by Waagsbo et al. [5]. The absence of symptoms and signs of infection until the date of the last follow-up is the definition of success for Azzam et al. [2]. Success is considered as infection control with serum inflammatory markers (ESR and CRP) normalized and no clinical signs or symptoms of infection by Estes et al. [6]. Parvizi et al. [7] consider success the eradication of infection. Remission is defined by the absence of local or systemic signs of infection assessed during the most recent contact with the patient and lack of the need to reoperation or to administer antibiotic therapy directed to the first infected site from the end of treatment to the most recent contact by Senneville et al. [8]. The Delphi-based International Multidisciplinary Consensus definition of a successfully treated periprosthetic joint infections is infection eradication, no subsequent surgical intervention, no mortality related to periprosthetic joint infection. The Delphi-based International Multidisciplinary Consensus agrees on the definition of midterm follow-up defining the time of 5 or more years after the definitive surgery, and of long-term results determining the time of 10 or more years after surgery [9–11]. Summarizing, the outcomes reported are: infection control without antibiotic therapy; infection control with antibiotic treatment; aseptic revision longer than 1 year from initiation treatment; septic revision longer than 1 year from initiation of treatment; aseptic revision inferior or equal to

V. Candela · G. Stelitano · S. De Salvatore
C. Casciaro · C. Di Naro · L. Risi Ambrogioni
U. G. Longo (✉) · V. Denaro
Department of Orthopaedic and Trauma Surgery,
Campus Bio-Medico University, Via Alvaro del
Portillo, Rome, Trigoria, Italy
e-mail: g.longo@unicampus.it

© ISAKOS 2022
U. G. Longo et al. (eds.), *Infection in Knee Replacement*,
https://doi.org/10.1007/978-3-030-81553-0_21

1 year from initiation of treatment; septic revision inferior or equal to 1 year from initiation of treatment; amputation, resection arthroplasty, or fusion; retained spacer; death inferior or equal to 1 year from initiation of treatment; death longer than 1 year from initiation of treatment.

21.2 Debridement, Antibiotics and Implant Retention (DAIR)

DAIR consists of debridement, antibiotics and implant retention. Open DAIR is considered a less disruptive intervention that seeks to preserve a functional implant minimizing the significant morbidity of implant removal. DAIR approach is indicated in early postoperative periprosthetic joint infections and acute hematogenous periprosthetic joint infections, defined as symptoms existing for no longer than 4 weeks.

The infection control rate of DAIR ranges from 11.1% to 100% [12–14]. An infection control rate of 32.6% is reported in a review of 23 studies with 530 infected total knee arthroplasties using an open DAIR approach [15, 16]. The overall success rate after DAIR is reported to be 47% in a review of 28 studies involving 599 cases [13]. Infection control after DAIR is influenced by several factors, such as patient's age, type of infection, involved joint, and duration of antibiotic therapy [17]. Several studies report no differences in infection control rate comparing DAIR performed during the 3 weeks following the onset of symptoms or later [18, 19]. However, on the other side, other authors report that a longer duration between onset of symptoms and DAIR is associated with lower infection control [17, 20]. Several studies demonstrate a high treatment success rate when DAIR is performed within 1 week after the onset of symptoms [21–23].

Recommendations suggest that the DAIR approach is indicated in early postoperative periprosthetic joint infections and acute hematogenous periprosthetic joint infections. Chronic periprosthetic joint infections should be considered an absolute contraindication to perform a DAIR procedure [24]. Other contraindications are severe and extensive infections, long duration of symptoms, any possibility to exchange the modular components, hard to eradicate causative microorganism [25, 26]. DAIR success is reported to be 73.9% in patients who undergo modular component exchange, compared to 60.7% in patients who don't do modular component exchange [25]. The great success obtained with modular component exchange is confirmed by several authors [21, 27]. Other factors associated with a poor outcome are rheumatoid arthritis, old age, male sex, chronic renal failure, liver cirrhosis, chronic obstructive pulmonary disease, fractures, especially in early acute periprosthetic joint infections, revision arthroplasty; high C-reactive protein, high bacterial inoculums, infections caused by *S. aureus* and Enterococci [28]. Patients with rheumatoid arthritis have a failure rate of DAIR of 74% in the case of late acute periprosthetic joint infections, versus 43% in patients without rheumatoid arthritis. Patients older than 80 years old with late acute periprosthetic joint infections have a significantly higher risk of failure of DAIR. Failure rates following DAIR for acute periprosthetic joint infections range from 20% to 70%, with higher failure seen in acute hematogenous periprosthetic joint infections. The failure rate at 2-year follow-up following DAIR for acute hematogenous infections is 52% [29]. Other authors report a success rate of 82.1% of DAIR for early postoperative infections and 57.1% for acute hematogenous infections [30]. On the other side, Bryan et al. report no significantly different outcomes between early postoperative infection versus acute hematogenous infection [30]. Factors associated with DAIR failure are the presence of a sinus, impaired immune response, short antibiotic therapy, and delayed DAIR [31].

In conclusion, the DAIR procedure has shown diminished morbidity and superior functional outcomes compared to one- or two-stage revision, reducing bone loss and soft tissue trauma. Despite its advantages, the outcome of DAIR must be balanced against the reduced eradication rates compared to more invasive revision surgery. Nevertheless, even if a failed previous DAIR could tend towards more formal one- or two-stage revision because of the possible increased physical or psychological impairment for the patient with delay in definitive treatment, it does not appear to negatively impact eventual infection eradication [32]. Due to the lack of conclusive evidence, further large-scale prospective study or randomized controlled trials are required.

21.3 One-Stage Exchange Arthroplasty

One-stage exchange arthroplasty aims to decrease surgical morbidity and mortality of patients with periprosthetic joint infections, decrease economic costs, and increase patients' quality of life. One-stage revision procedures have a success rate between 75% and 95% [15, 33–45].

Good outcomes are observed in patients with strict selection criteria. A reinfection rate of 0% is documented in a series of 28 patients with infected knee arthroplasties at a minimum of 3 years follow-up [41]. Preoperative bacterial identification is required to delineate antibiotic therapy. Excellent results are reported in patients in which microbiological susceptibility is preoperatively known [41]. However, the lack of preoperative microbiological diagnosis is considered by several authors a relative, rather than absolute, contraindication for one-stage exchange arthroplasty [44, 46, 47].

Contraindications to one-stage exchange arthroplasty are failure of prior one-stage revision, unclear causative pathogen, lack of susceptibility to available antibiotics, extensive infections, systemic sepsis, gross tissue inflammation, and severe immunosuppression.

Infections caused by polymicrobial organisms, atypical and gram-negative organisms, methicillin-resistant *S. aureus* (MRSA), and methicillin-resistant *Staphylococcus epidermidis* (MRSE) are associated with a higher failure rate (44%) [48–50].

Confounding results are obtained by analyzing the impact of soft tissue defects and sinus tracts on outcomes. Jenny et al. [51] report a negative effect, with a reinfection rate of 27%. On the other side, in an earlier series of 47 patients, is documented an 87% infection-free survival period at 3 years even though 43% of patients presented a sinus tract [52]. For Raut et al., a fistula is not an absolute contraindication to one-stage exchange arthroplasty [53].

Soft tissue debridement, removal of foreign material, and the use of antibiotic-loaded cement for reimplantation are recommended for success.

Two recent meta-analyses show equivalent reinfection (8.2%) comparing one-stage versus two-stage procedures for periprosthetic total knee infections [54]. Wolf et al. underline the superiority of a two-stage protocol in term of infection recurrence; on the other side, the same authors show the superiority of one-stage protocol in terms of quality of life [55]. One-stage mortality range from 4.4% to 11.4% [39, 55]. Loty et al. [56] report mortality of 4.4% analyzing 90 patients with a mean follow-up of 47 months. Miley et al. [57] found a mortality of 11% analyzing 100 patients with a mean follow-up of 48.5 months. Wolf et al. [55] after a Markov cohort simulation decision analysis report a mortality rate of 0.52% (3 of 576) for single-stage and 2.5% (8 of 321) for two-stage revision, based on 18 published papers. Haddad et al. have conducted a proper study on the analysis of functional outcomes after a one-stage revision procedure, considering patient's preoperative functions, evaluated by the Knee Society Score (KSS), and their postoperative status. This research has shown a statistically significant difference in the improvement of functional scores, supporting the one-stage procedure. The mean increase in KSS scores was +56 for one-stage and + 45 for two-stage, which takes into account a patient's anatomical stability postoperatively, but also their self-reported functional status and pain levels [58]. These findings are, however, limited: future studies are necessary to delineate the superiority of a one- or two-stage revision approach.

21.4 Two-Stage Exchange Arthroplasty

Two-stage revision is the most used procedure for prosthetic joint infection treatment. It consists of removing all foreign material from the joint, making an extensive debridement of periarticular tissues and inserting a static or articulating spacer in the joint. This surgical procedure is followed by antibiotic therapy for an extended period. Finally, reimplantation is made when the infection is eradicated.

The two-stage revision procedure is mostly used for patients with an unclear causative pathogen, bacteria unsusceptible to available antibiotics, patients with signs of systemic sepsis, and patients with extensive comorbidities.

Two-stage revision is traditionally considered the gold standard for the management of periprosthetic joint infections. However, compared to the one-stage revision, it exposes patients to the risks of an additional surgical procedure. The success of treatment with two-stage revision arthroplasty is between 70% and 100%. The reinfection rate after two-stage revision is between 9% and 20% of cases [54]. Citak et al. [59] reported superior functional outcomes with the use of articulating spacers when compared to static spacers. Articulating spacers are associated with a little time of hospitalization and improved range of motion. Kim et al. have shown the optimal functional outcomes of 20 patients treated by two-stage revision arthroplasty using an articulating spacer under the diagnosis of infected TKA, considering a follow-up period of about 22 months. The results obtained are described below. ROM increasing from 69.8° (range, 50° to 100°) before first stage surgery to 102.8° (range, 80° to 130°) following second stage surgery. KSKS (Knee Society knee score) increases from 33.8 points (range, 28 to 52 points) before first stage surgery to 85.3 points (range, 77 to 94 points) following second stage surgery. The mean KSFS (Knee Society function score) increases from 35.0 points (range, 20 to 55 points) before first stage surgery to 87.5 points (range, 70 to 100 points) following second stage surgery. Partial weight-bearing granted at 6 days after first stage surgery. There is no sign of infection recurrence in more than 90% of patients. No complications (e.g., medial collateral ligament tears and periprosthetic fractures) observed. These data confirm the advantage of the articulating spacer in terms of infection eradication and recovery of joint mobility and function [60]. An overall 15% complications rate, including reinfection rate, lower joint mobility, painful symptoms, [61], and

a 9.1% fractures rate are reported for static knee spacers [62]. No significant differences in terms of infection eradication and complications between articulating and non-articulating spacers for periprosthetic knee are found [63, 64]. Two-stage revision mortality ranges from 2.9% to 25.7% [65–70]. Chen et al. [65] report a mortality of 8.7% analyzing 57 patients with a mean follow-up of 67.2 months. Haddad et al. [66] report a mortality of 4.0% analyzing 50 patients with a mean follow-up of 5.8 years. Hsieh et al. [67], evaluating 99 patients at mean 43 months of follow-up, report attributable mortality of 3.0%. Romanò et al. [68] record mortality of 2.9% analyzing 102 patients with a mean follow-up of 48 months. Toulson et al. [69] report mortality of 25.7% analyzing 132 patients with a mean follow-up of 64.8 months. Finally, Ibrahim et al. report a mortality of 15.2% analyzing 125 patients with a mean follow-up of 5.8 years [70]. Currently, an interesting summarization about two-stage TKA revision complications rate and functional outcomes has been realized by Claassen et al. They reviewed study patient's charts including demographics, prior surgeries, comorbidities, incidence of persistent infection, and revisions. At the final follow-up examination, they evaluated patient's satisfaction, pain level, and disorders. A successful clinical outcome was defined as a functioning prosthesis without wound healing disorders, no sinuses tracts, or other clinical evidence of a persistent infection, which resulted in about 86% of patients. Reimplantation of prosthesis was performed in 95% of patients; only three patients received a septic arthrodesis. Two-stage reimplantation has resulted in a success rate of 76.0%. Only one patient needed to be treated with knee amputation [71]. Due to the lack of conclusive evidence, further large-scale prospective study or randomized controlled trials are required.

21.5 Conclusion

There is not a univocal definition of success or failure after treatment of PJIs. Treatment of PJI aims to eradicate the infection, improve patients' satisfaction, and avoid medical and surgical complications. The successful treatment of PJI depends largely on multiple factors, including the causing microorganisms, soft tissue and bone stock, host factors, prior treatments, and chronicity of infection. Treatment options for PJI include long-term suppressive antibiotics (in patients who are not suitable for surgery), DAIR, one- or two-stage revision, resection arthroplasty, arthrodesis and amputation. DAIR approach is indicated in early postoperative PJI and acute hematogenous PJI. Chronic PJI should be considered an absolute contraindication to perform a DAIR procedure. One-stage exchange arthroplasty has good outcomes in patients with strict selection criteria. Contraindications to one-stage exchange arthroplasty are failure of prior one-stage revision, unclear causative pathogen, lack of susceptibility to available antibiotics, extensive infections, systemic sepsis, gross tissue inflammation, and severe immunosuppression. Two-stage revision is the most used procedure for prosthetic joint infection treatment. The reinfection rate after two-stage revision is between 9% and 20% of cases. Undoubtedly, in the setting of chronic PJI, two-stage exchange arthroplasty is a safe and efficacious treatment. As widely already discussed, an absolute gold standard for the choice of PJI treatment doesn't still exist. However, we can assume that in carefully selected cases the DAIR protocol allows a non-invasive treatment of the patient with a low morbidity rate, even if the one-stage revision guarantees recovery times and superior functionality. The two-stage treatment remains the best procedure in terms of targeted and definitive eradication of the infection, despite elevated morbidity rates persist. However, the choice of the most suitable treatment must take into account the all patient's characteristics in their complexity.

References

1. Mahmud T, Lyons MC, Naudie DD, Macdonald SJ, McCalden RW. Assessing the gold standard: a review of 253 two-stage revisions for infected TKA. Clin Orthop Relat Res. 2012;470(10):2730–6.
2. Azzam KA, Seeley M, Ghanem E, Austin MS, Purtill JJ, Parvizi J. Irrigation and debridement in the management of prosthetic joint infection: traditional indications revisited. J Arthroplasty. 2010;25(7):1022–7.
3. Volin SJ, Hinrichs SH, Garvin KL. Two-stage reimplantation of total joint infections: a comparison of resistant and non-resistant organisms. Clin Orthop Relat Res. 2004;427:94–100.
4. Bradbury T, Fehring TK, Taunton M, Hanssen A, Azzam K, Parvizi J, et al. The fate of acute methicillin-resistant Staphylococcus aureus periprosthetic knee infections treated by open debridement and retention of components. J Arthroplasty. 2009;24(6 Suppl):101–4.
5. Waagsbo B, Sundoy A, Martinsen TM, Nymo LS. Treatment results with debridement and retention of infected hip prostheses. Scand J Infect Dis. 2009;41(8):563–8.
6. Estes CS, Beauchamp CP, Clarke HD, Spangehl MJ. A two-stage retention debridement protocol for acute periprosthetic joint infections. Clin Orthop Relat Res. 2010;468(8):2029–38.
7. Parvizi J, Saleh KJ, Ragland PS, Pour AE, Mont MA. Efficacy of antibiotic-impregnated cement in total hip replacement. Acta Orthop. 2008;79(3):335–41.
8. Senneville E, Joulie D, Legout L, Valette M, Dezeque H, Beltrand E, et al. Outcome and predictors of treatment failure in total hip/knee prosthetic joint infections due to Staphylococcus aureus. Clin Infect Dis. 2011;53(4):334–40.
9. Diaz-Ledezma C, Higuera CA, Parvizi J. Success after treatment of periprosthetic joint infection: a Delphi-based international multidisciplinary consensus. Clin Orthop Relat Res. 2013;471(7):2374–82.
10. Longo UG, Maffulli N, Denaro V. Minimally invasive total knee arthroplasty. N Engl J Med. 2009;361(6):633–4; author reply 4.
11. Longo UG, Loppini M, Trovato U, Rizzello G, Maffulli N, Denaro V. No difference between unicompartmental versus total knee arthroplasty for the management of medial osteoarthtritis of the knee in the same patient: a systematic review and pooling data analysis. Br Med Bull. 2015;114(1):65–73.
12. Achermann Y, Sahin F, Schwyzer HK, Kolling C, Wust J, Vogt M. Characteristics and outcome of 16 periprosthetic shoulder joint infections. Infection. 2013;41(3):613–20.
13. Zurcher-Pfund L, Uckay I, Legout L, Gamulin A, Vaudaux P, Peter R. Pathogen-driven decision for implant retention in the management of infected total knee prostheses. Int Orthop. 2013;37(8):1471–5.
14. Longo UG, Candela V, Pirato F, Hirschmann MT, Becker R, Denaro V. Midflexion instability in total knee arthroplasty: a systematic review. Knee Surg Sports Traumatol Arthrosc. 2021;29(2):370–80.
15. Silva M, Tharani R, Schmalzried TP. Results of direct exchange or debridement of the infected total knee arthroplasty. Clin Orthop Relat Res. 2002;404:125–31.
16. Longo UG, Ciuffreda M, D'Andrea V, Mannering N, Locher J, Denaro V. All-polyethylene versus metal-backed tibial component in total knee arthroplasty. Knee Surg Sports Traumatol Arthrosc. 2017;25(11):3620–36.
17. Kunutsor SK, Beswick AD, Whitehouse MR, Wylde V, Blom AW. Debridement, antibiotics and implant

retention for periprosthetic joint infections: a systematic review and meta-analysis of treatment outcomes. J Infect. 2018;77(6):479–88.

18. Achermann Y, Stasch P, Preiss S, Lucke K, Vogt M. Characteristics and treatment outcomes of 69 cases with early prosthetic joint infections of the hip and knee. Infection. 2014;42(3):511–9.

19. Longo UG, Ciuffreda M, Mannering N, D'Andrea V, Locher J, Salvatore G, et al. Outcomes of posterior-stabilized compared with cruciate-retaining total knee arthroplasty. J Knee Surg. 2018;31(4):321–40.

20. Zimmerli W, Trampuz A, Ochsner PE. Prosthetic-joint infections. N Engl J Med. 2004;351(16):1645–54.

21. Grammatopoulos G, Bolduc ME, Atkins BL, Kendrick BJL, McLardy-Smith P, Murray DW, et al. Functional outcome of debridement, antibiotics and implant retention in periprosthetic joint infection involving the hip: a case-control study. Bone Jt J. 2017;99-B(5):614–22.

22. Kuiper JW, Vos SJ, Saouti R, Vergroesen DA, Graat HC, Debets-Ossenkopp YJ, et al. Prosthetic joint-associated infections treated with DAIR (debridement, antibiotics, irrigation, and retention): analysis of risk factors and local antibiotic carriers in 91 patients. Acta Orthop. 2013;84(4):380–6.

23. Hsieh PH, Lee MS, Hsu KY, Chang YH, Shih HN, Ueng SW. Gram-negative prosthetic joint infections: risk factors and outcome of treatment. Clin Infect Dis. 2009;49(7):1036–43.

24. Lebeaux D, Ghigo JM, Beloin C. Biofilm-related infections: bridging the gap between clinical management and fundamental aspects of recalcitrance toward antibiotics. Microbiol Mol Biol Rev MMBR. 2014;78(3):510–43.

25. Tsang SJ, Ting J, Simpson A, Gaston P. Outcomes following debridement, antibiotics and implant retention in the management of periprosthetic infections of the hip: a review of cohort studies. Bone Jt J. 2017;99-B(11):1458–66.

26. Byren I, Bejon P, Atkins BL, Angus B, Masters S, McLardy-Smith P, et al. One hundred and twelve infected arthroplasties treated with 'DAIR' (debridement, antibiotics and implant retention): antibiotic duration and outcome. J Antimicrob Chemother. 2009;63(6):1264–71.

27. Choi HR, von Knoch F, Zurakowski D, Nelson SB, Malchau H. Can implant retention be recommended for treatment of infected TKA? Clin Orthop Relat Res. 2011;469(4):961–9.

28. Lora-Tamayo J, Murillo O, Iribarren JA, Soriano A, Sanchez-Somolinos M, Baraia-Etxaburu JM, et al. A large multicenter study of methicillin-susceptible and methicillin-resistant Staphylococcus aureus prosthetic joint infections managed with implant retention. Clin Infect Dis. 2013;56(2):182–94.

29. Rodriguez D, Pigrau C, Euba G, Cobo J, Garcia-Lechuz J, Palomino J, et al. Acute haematogenous prosthetic joint infection: prospective evaluation of medical and surgical management. Clin Microbiol Infect. 2010;16(12):1789–95.

30. Fink B, Schuster P, Schwenninger C, Frommelt L, Oremek D. A standardized regimen for the treatment of acute postoperative infections and acute hematogenous infections associated with hip and knee arthroplasties. J Arthroplasty. 2017;32(4):1255–61.

31. Qasim SN, Swann A, Ashford R. The DAIR (debridement, antibiotics and implant retention) procedure for infected total knee replacement—a literature review. Sicot J. 2017;3:2.

32. Vaz K, Scarborough M, Bottomley N, Kendrick B, Taylor A, Price A, et al. Debridement, antibiotics and implant retention (DAIR) for the management of knee prosthetic joint infection. Knee. 2020;27(6):2013–5.

33. Selmon GP, Slater RN, Shepperd JA, Wright EP. Successful 1-stage exchange total knee arthroplasty for fungal infection. J Arthroplasty. 1998;13(1):114–5.

34. von Foerster G, Kluber D, Kabler U. Mid- to long-term results after treatment of 118 cases of periprosthetic infections after knee joint replacement using one-stage exchange surgery. Der Orthopade. 1991;20(3):244–52.

35. Buechel FF, Femino FP, D'Alessio J. Primary exchange revision arthroplasty for infected total knee replacement: a long-term study. Am J Orthop. 2004;33(4):190–8; discussion 8.

36. Zeller V, Lhotellier L, Marmor S, Leclerc P, Krain A, Graff W, et al. One-stage exchange arthroplasty for chronic periprosthetic hip infection: results of a large prospective cohort study. J Bone Joint Surg Am. 2014;96(1):e1.

37. Hansen E, Tetreault M, Zmistowski B, Della Valle CJ, Parvizi J, Haddad FS, et al. Outcome of one-stage cementless exchange for acute postoperative periprosthetic hip infection. Clin Orthop Relat Res. 2013;471(10):3214–22.

38. Winkler H, Stoiber A, Kaudela K, Winter F, Menschik F. One stage uncemented revision of infected total hip replacement using cancellous allograft bone impregnated with antibiotics. J Bone Jt Surg. 2008;90(12):1580–4.

39. Raut VV, Siney PD, Wroblewski BM. One-stage revision of total hip arthroplasty for deep infection. Long-term followup. Clin Orthop Relat Res. 1995;321:202–7.

40. Zahar A, Gehrke TA. One-stage revision for infected total hip arthroplasty. Orthop Clin North Am. 2016;47(1):11–8.

41. Haddad FS, Sukeik M, Alazzawi S. Is single-stage revision according to a strict protocol effective in treatment of chronic knee arthroplasty infections? Clin Orthop Relat Res. 2015;473(1):8–14.

42. Choi HR, Kwon YM, Freiberg AA, Malchau H. Comparison of one-stage revision with antibiotic cement versus two-stage revision results for infected total hip arthroplasty. J Arthroplasty. 2013;28(8 Suppl):66–70.

43. Wolf M, Clar H, Friesenbichler J, Schwantzer G, Bernhardt G, Gruber G, et al. Prosthetic joint infection following total hip replacement: results of one-stage versus two-stage exchange. Int Orthop. 2014;38(7):1363–8.

44. Castellani L, Daneman N, Mubareka S, Jenkinson R. Factors associated with choice and success of one-

versus two-stage revision arthroplasty for infected hip and knee prostheses. HSS J. 2017;13(3):224–31.

45. Gehrke T, Zahar A, Kendoff D. One-stage exchange: it all began here. Bone Jt J. 2013;95-B(11 Suppl A):77–83.

46. Lange J, Troelsen A, Solgaard S, Otte KS, Jensen NK, Soballe K, et al. Cementless one-stage revision in chronic periprosthetic hip joint infection. Ninety-one percent infection free survival in 56 patients at minimum 2-year follow-up. J Arthroplasty. 2018;33(4):1160–5e1.

47. Bori G, Navarro G, Morata L, Fernandez-Valencia JA, Soriano A, Gallart X. Preliminary results after changing from two-stage to one-stage revision arthroplasty protocol using cementless arthroplasty for chronic infected hip replacements. J Arthroplasty. 2018;33(2):527–32.

48. Laudermilch DJ, Fedorka CJ, Heyl A, Rao N, McGough RL. Outcomes of revision total knee arthroplasty after methicillin-resistant *Staphylococcus aureus* infection. Clin Orthop Relat Res. 2010;468(8):2067–73.

49. Buchholz HW, Elson RA, Engelbrecht E, Lodenkamper H, Rottger J, Siegel A. Management of deep infection of total hip replacement. J Bone Jt Surg. 1981;63-B(3):342–53.

50. Jackson WO, Schmalzried TP. Limited role of direct exchange arthroplasty in the treatment of infected total hip replacements. Clin Orthop Relat Res. 2000;381:101–5.

51. Jenny JY, Lengert R, Diesinger Y, Gaudias J, Boeri C, Kempf JF. Routine one-stage exchange for chronic infection after total hip replacement. Int Orthop. 2014;38(12):2477–81.

52. Jenny JY, Barbe B, Gaudias J, Boeri C, Argenson JN. High infection control rate and function after routine one-stage exchange for chronically infected TKA. Clin Orthop Relat Res. 2013;471(1):238–43.

53. Raut VV, Siney PD, Wroblewski BM. One-stage revision of infected total hip replacements with discharging sinuses. J Bone Jt Surg. 1994;76(5):721–4.

54. Kunutsor SK, Whitehouse MR, Blom AW, Beswick AD, Team I. Re-infection outcomes following one- and two-stage surgical revision of infected hip prosthesis: a systematic review and meta-analysis. PLoS One. 2015;10(9):e0139166.

55. Wolf CF, Gu NY, Doctor JN, Manner PA, Leopold SS. Comparison of one and two-stage revision of total hip arthroplasty complicated by infection: a Markov expected-utility decision analysis. J Bone Joint Surg Am. 2011;93(7):631–9.

56. Loty B, Postel M, Evrard J, Matron P, Courpied JP, Kerboull M, et al. One stage revision of infected total hip replacements with replacement of bone loss by allografts. Study of 90 cases of which 46 used bone allografts. Int Orthop. 1992;16(4):330–8.

57. Miley GB, Scheller AD Jr, Turner RH. Medical and surgical treatment of the septic hip with one-stage revision arthroplasty. Clin Orthop Relat Res. 1982;170:76–82.

58. Nagra NS, Hamilton TW, Ganatra S, Murray DW, Pandit H. One-stage versus two-stage exchange arthroplasty for infected total knee arthroplasty: a systematic review. Knee Surg Sports Traumatol Arthrosc. 2016;24(10):3106–14.

59. Citak M, Masri BA, Springer B, Argenson JN, Kendoff DO. Are preformed articulating spacers superior to surgeon-made articulating spacers in the treatment of PJI in THA? A literature review. Open Orthop J. 2015;9:255–61.

60. Kim YS, Bae KC, Cho CH, Lee KJ, Sohn ES, Kim BS. Two-stage revision using a modified articulating spacer in infected total knee arthroplasty. Knee Surg Relat Res. 2013;25(4):180–5.

61. Nahhas CR, Chalmers PN, Parvizi J, Sporer SM, Berend KR, Moric M, et al. A randomized trial of static and articulating spacers for the treatment of infection following total knee arthroplasty. J Bone Joint Surg Am. 2020;102(9):778–87.

62. Faschingbauer M, Reichel H, Bieger R, Kappe T. Mechanical complications with one hundred and thirty eight (antibiotic-laden) cement spacers in the treatment of periprosthetic infection after total hip arthroplasty. Int Orthop. 2015;39(5):989–94.

63. Pivec R, Naziri Q, Issa K, Banerjee S, Mont MA. Systematic review comparing static and articulating spacers used for revision of infected total knee arthroplasty. J Arthroplasty. 2014;29(3):553–7. e1

64. Voleti PB, Baldwin KD, Lee GC. Use of static or articulating spacers for infection following total knee arthroplasty: a systematic literature review. J Bone Joint Surg Am. 2013;95(17):1594–9.

65. Chen WS, Fu TH, Wang JW. Two-stage reimplantation of infected hip arthroplasties. Chang Gung Med J. 2009;32(2):188–97.

66. Haddad FS, Muirhead-Allwood SK, Manktelow AR, Bacarese-Hamilton I. Two-stage uncemented revision hip arthroplasty for infection. J Bone Jt Surg. 2000;82(5):689–94.

67. Hsieh PH, Huang KC, Lee PC, Lee MS. Two-stage revision of infected hip arthroplasty using an antibiotic-loaded spacer: retrospective comparison between short-term and prolonged antibiotic therapy. J Antimicrob Chemother. 2009;64(2):392–7.

68. Romano CL, Romano D, Logoluso N, Meani E. Long-stem versus short-stem preformed antibiotic-loaded cement spacers for two-stage revision of infected total hip arthroplasty. Hip Int. 2010;20(1):26–33.

69. Toulson C, Walcott-Sapp S, Hur J, Salvati E, Bostrom M, Brause B, et al. Treatment of infected total hip arthroplasty with a 2-stage reimplantation protocol: update on "our institution's" experience from 1989 to 2003. J Arthroplasty. 2009;24(7):1051–60.

70. Ibrahim MS, Raja S, Khan MA, Haddad FS. A multidisciplinary team approach to two-stage revision for the infected hip replacement: a minimum five-year follow-up study. Bone Jt J. 2014;96-B(10):1312–8.

71. Claassen L, Plaass C, Daniilidis K, Calliess T, von Lewinski G. Two-stage revision total knee arthroplasty in cases of periprosthetic joint infection: an analysis of 50 cases. Open Orthop J. 2015;9: 49–56.

Complications 22

Warran Wignadasan, Justin Chang, Mark Roussot, and Sam Oussedik

22.1 Introduction

A prosthetic joint infection (PJI) following primary total knee arthroplasty (TKA) is a devastating complication for both the patient and the surgeon. Fortunately, PJI is relatively rare, with pooled international registry data suggesting a 1.03% risk following primary TKA [1]. The demand for TKA is projected to rise by 400% from the early 2000s to 2030 due to an aging and increasingly active population [2, 3]. This will inevitably result in an increased number of prosthetic joint infections and subsequent revision arthroplasties, which have higher complication rates and worse functional outcomes. Revision arthroplasty for PJI has a significantly higher risk of mortality compared to revision surgery for aseptic failure; there is evidence suggesting that the risk of 1-year mortality for PJI is comparable to a number of common cancers [4]. Considerable efforts and resources have been expended in attempting to decrease the burden of PJI. Treatment requires a multidisciplinary approach with specialized microbiologists, physiotherapists, and revision arthroplasty specialists. There is increasing evidence that treatment of infected TKAs at specialized arthroplasty centers with high volume surgeons leads to improved outcomes [5–7].

Despite the improvements in preventing PJI, a proportion of patients will unfortunately, still develop a deep infection. Management of these patients ultimately involves both antibiotics and surgical intervention. Appropriate surgical intervention may consist of a DAIR (debridement, antibiotics, implant retention) procedure, single-stage revision, or two-stage revision depending on the organism and host factors. Revision TKA in the setting of infection is technically challenging and has a higher risk of complications compared to aseptic revisions [8].

Complications of infected total knee arthroplasty can arise during the procedure (intraoperative), early in the postoperative recovery (early), and later once recovery from the initial procedure is complete (late). It is imperative that surgeons recognize and appreciate the potential complications associated with revision TKA in the setting of infection. This will subsequently lead to a decreased risk of complications and an improved understanding of how to appropriately manage specific complications when they do occur.

W. Wignadasan
Chelsea and Westminster Hospital, London, UK

University College London Hospital, London, UK
e-mail: w.wignadasan@nhs.net

J. Chang
University College London Hospital, London, UK

Humber River Hospital, Toronto, ON, Canada
e-mail: justin.chang@mail.utoronto.ca

M. Roussot · S. Oussedik (✉)
University College London Hospital, London, UK
e-mail: mark.roussot@nhs.net

© ISAKOS 2022
U. G. Longo et al. (eds.), *Infection in Knee Replacement*,
https://doi.org/10.1007/978-3-030-81553-0_22

22.2 Intraoperative Complications

22.2.1 Surgical Exposure

Adequate surgical exposure and careful handling of the soft tissue envelope are critical for any revision arthroplasty procedure. Previous incisions should be employed in order to minimize wound complications and breakdown. In situations with multiple incisions, the most lateral incision should be used to preserve blood supply to the skin, ensuring that this allows access to the joint without creating large skin flaps. Sinus tracts should be excised to prevent ongoing and recurrent infection (Fig. 22.1), and this must be considered when planning incisions. Incisions should be of sufficient length to prevent any excess tension on the skin edges. Full-thickness fasciocutaneous flaps should be created to maintain vascular integrity. Any necrotic or infected subcutaneous tissue should be debrided to bleeding, healthy tissue.

Patients are often stiff with a thickened and inflamed soft tissue envelope. In the setting of infection, thorough and systematic debridement and complete synovectomy are necessary to eradicate infection and adequate exposure of the previous implants. Often after thorough debridement, adequate exposure of the implants is possible. However, extensile approaches may be required to prevent iatrogenic injury to the extensor mechanism. Surgeons should be prepared to perform a quadriceps snip, VY turndown, or tibial tubercle osteotomy if exposure is not adequate for implant removal or subsequent reconstruction.

22.2.2 Extensor Mechanism Rupture

Protection of the extensor mechanism is imperative when performing revision TKA for prosthetic joint infection; extensor mechanism injury or failure significantly worsens functional outcomes even with successful eradication of infection. The extensor mechanism can be disrupted as a result of infection or iatrogenic injury. This is a devastating complication that makes the restoration of knee function much more difficult. A study involving 60 patients with concomitant periprosthetic joint infection and extensor mechanism disruption has shown low success rates, regardless of treatment. Of these, 53 patients underwent extensor mechanism repair or replacement, with 41 of these considered failures, recurrent infection being the most common cause of failure [9].

Treatment of an extensor mechanism disruption typically involves a 2-stage revision with a subsequent extensor mechanism allograft or mesh reconstruction. Articulating spacers are preferred in order to allow for movement in the affected knee and facilitate recovery of knee function [10]. However, significant damage to the extensor mechanism or surrounding soft tissue envelope may necessitate the use of a static spacer [11, 12]. Spacers should be monitored for any impingement or translation of the extensor mechanism, and any problems should be appropriately addressed to prevent further complications. Extensor mechanism allograft reconstruction has shown good survivorship. A single-center study showed that 69% of knees retained their initial allograft at final follow-up. However, patients had consistently worse functional outcomes and high reoperation rates [13]. At the time of definitive revision TKA, it is crucial to ensure that the femoral and tibial components are well-positioned to optimize patellar tracking. Failure to do so may lead to early failure.

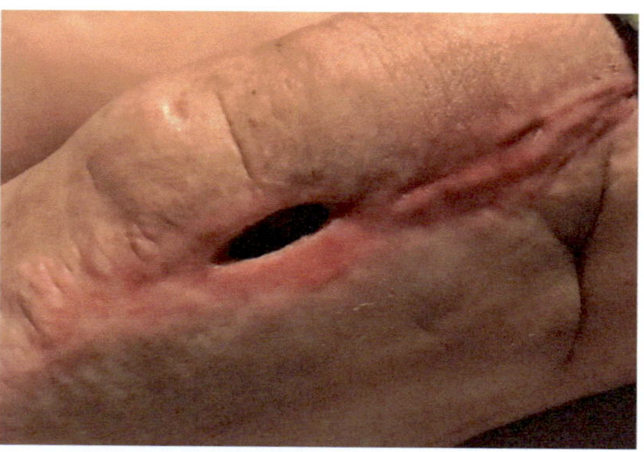

Fig. 22.1 Sinus tract developed as a result of prosthetic joint infection

22.2.3 Increased Operative Time

Debridement, antibiotics, and implant retention (DAIR), one-stage, or two-stage revision procedures are the mainstay of surgical treatment options for periprosthetic knee joint infections. These operations are technically challenging and generally require increased operative time compared to primary TKA. Prolonged operating times have been shown to increase the risk of a surgical site infection, which in turn can lead to disastrous consequences for an already infected joint. It has been suggested that operative length over two and a half hours increases the risk of infection [14, 15]. As revision TKA procedures can often be time-consuming, these cases are subsequently at greater risk of infection compared to primary TKA. A nationwide study involving over 10,000 revision TKAs concluded that operative times had the greatest effect on length of stay in hospital postoperatively compared to other variables, including age, sex, and BMI [16]. There is growing evidence that treatment of prosthetic joint infections should be managed in specialized centers by experienced, high volume revision surgeons in order to minimize operative time and decrease complication rates [3, 5].

22.2.4 Intraoperative Fracture

An intraoperative fracture is a potential risk during revision knee arthroplasty. A North American study reported an intraoperative peri-prosthetic fracture incidence of 0.78% in 645 revision total knee replacements [17]. Surgeons should be conscious of the risk of fracture during explantation of previous components, preparation of the medullary canal, and insertion of stemmed revision components [18]. This risk of peri-prosthetic fracture during revision arthroplasty increases in the setting of infection due to poor bone quality and loss of bone stock. A study that analyzed 894 infected TKA patients treated with 2-stage revision demonstrated an intraoperative fracture rate of 2.3% [19]. Of these, 17% of fractures occurred during removal of components and 82% during reimplantation. 56% of fractures were femoral fractures, 30% were tibial fractures, and 13% were patella fractures.

Fractures identified intraoperatively should be anatomically reduced and stabilized appropriately. Stemmed components should bypass the fracture site by a minimum of two cortical diameters. Fractures of the femoral and tibial condyles often require screw or plate fixation. The fracture should be sufficiently stable to allow an immediate range of motion postoperatively. However, weight-bearing may need to be delayed, which can further hinder the rehabilitation process [20]. An intraoperative fracture also significantly increases operative time; this may further increase the risk of complications, including reinfection.

22.2.5 Instability

The stability of the joint is at risk following a prosthetic knee infection. Surgeons must ensure that the knee is stable intraoperatively; it is often necessary to use revision components with an increased varus-valgus constraint or a rotating hinge design. The stability of the knee joint depends on intact collateral ligaments and balanced load distribution over the medial and lateral condyles. In order to successfully eradicate infection, aggressive debridement of the joint and surrounding soft tissue envelope is required. This may include important ligamentous and capsular structures, which subsequently would compromise stability. A semi-constrained or hinged implant is necessary after resection of the collateral ligaments following debridement [21].

It has been reported that the incidence of instability following revision knee surgery is 22% [22]. It is likely that the incidence of instability following revision TKA for PJI is significantly higher given the degree of necessary debridement. Instability can be divided into coronal and sagittal plane instability. Instability in extension results from an insufficient filling of the extension gap and can arise due to inadequate release of fixed deformity. A flexion instability comes as a result of a flexion gap greater than an extension gap. A femoral component that is undersized or a steep tibial slope can give rise to this form of instability [23].

Consequently, during revision surgery for PJI, surgeons should endeavor to extract components with minimal bone loss, balance the knee ligaments, use stable components that restore the joint line, and also achieve good soft tissue coverage. Varying landmarks have been described in the literature to assist in the precise reproduction of the joint line in revision TKA procedures: 1.5–2 cm proximal to the fibular head, the "meniscal scar," 2–2.5 cm distal to the lateral femoral epicondyle, 2.5–3 cm distal to the medial femoral epicondyle, 2 cm proximal to the tibial tubercle, and 2 cm below the inferior pole of the patella in extension [24–26]. Radiographs of the contralateral knee and then measuring the size of the resected prosthesis is often helpful. Careful preoperative planning and anticipation of potential instability are essential when undertaking revision TKA for infection.

22.2.6 Neurovascular Injury

The neurovascular structures surrounding the knee joint are at increased risk of iatrogenic injury during a revision procedure. The common peroneal nerve is the most commonly injured nerve during revision TKA procedures. While direct nerve injury is rare, compression, traction, and ischemia are the most common mechanisms of injury [27]. The incidence of common peroneal injury ranges from 0.58% to 1.8% in primary TKA [28]. Risk is increased in a preoperative valgus knee, fixed flexion of >20°, previous laminectomy, and the use of a spinal anesthetic [29]. A prolonged tourniquet time is also associated with an increased risk of neural damage. This is especially important in revision procedures, which can often be more technically challenging and therefore longer operations. A retrospective study reported a 7.7% incidence of neural injury (common peroneal or tibial nerve) involving 1001 patients who underwent primary or revision

TKA with a tourniquet time of greater than 120 min [30].

Vascular injury, albeit less common than neural injury, can result in disastrous complications. Furthermore, the incidence of arterial damage in the revision TKA setting is greater than twice that of in primary TKAs (0.36% vs. 0.15%) [31]. A greater exposure is required during revision TKA for infection to enable adequate debridement of infected tissue, including the often thickened posterior capsule. The neurovascular bundle can be adherent to the posterior capsule, which increases the risk of injury during debridement. Vascular injury can be direct, for example, from a sharp object such as a scalpel or drill, or indirect, such as from the tourniquet or traction. Direct injury of the artery can result in a massive hemorrhage, which may be visualized intraoperatively or manifest as a significant drop in blood pressure. Surgeons should seek immediate vascular consultation for surgical treatment, a bypass graft, or direct repair of the artery. Indirect arterial injury, leading to ischemia, can easily be missed in the immediate postoperative phase due to a lack of bleeding and the masking of pain by analgesic agents commonly used postoperatively. These patients are at an increased risk of compartment syndrome, leading to fasciotomy, neural injury, and muscle necrosis [31]. Doppler ultrasound and an ankle-brachial pressure index (ABPI) should be immediately considered in patients suspected of having indirect arterial injury following revision TKA. An immediate vascular opinion and possible vascular studies should be requested if there is any clinical suspicion.

22.3 Early Complications

22.3.1 Venous Thromboembolism

Venous thromboembolism (VTE) is a potential early complication following revision TKA for PJI. Preoperative risk assessment and appropriate use of both mechanical and pharmacological prophylaxis are of the utmost importance when treating these patients. The prevalence of proximal deep vein thrombosis (DVT) and distal DVT following primary TKA has been reported between 0% and 16% and 1% and 67%, respectively [32]. Moreover, the prevalence of symptomatic pulmonary embolism (PE) ranges from 1% to 1.9%, with fatal PE being reported as between 0.2% and 0.7% [32].

There is limited evidence on the prevalence of VTE in revision TKAs when compared to primary TKAs. A large multi-center study in Illinois involving 2986 revision TKA patients showed a reported DVT rate of 1.4% and PE rate of 1.6% [33]. Another study involving 645 revision TKAs reported rates of DVT and PE of 0.16% and 2.02%, respectively [17]. Careful soft tissue handling and minimization of excessive knee hyperflexion has been suggested to reduce venous stasis and ultimately decrease the risk of VTE [34].

Nonpharmacological prophylaxis includes using compressive stockings, intermittent pneumatic devices, and early mobilization with ankle exercises. Additionally, epidural anesthetics have a lower associated risk of DVT compared to a general anesthetic (4% and 9%, respectively) [35]. There is an ongoing debate as to the most effective form of pharmacological VTE prophylaxis. Low molecular weight heparin is thought to be more effective than warfarin in the prevention of symptomatic thrombosis [32, 36]. However, there is an increased risk of minor bleeding found with pharmacological prophylaxis [37], which can complicate revision surgery. The combined use of pharmacological and nonpharmacological VTE prophylaxis has been found to reduce the rate of VTE even further post TKA [38]. Surgeons should, therefore, consider a combined pharmacological and nonpharmacological approach to VTE prophylaxis for revision knee surgery for an infected joint, with careful, regular monitoring to assess for bleeding.

22.3.2 Hematoma and Wound Complications

Hematoma can develop postoperatively, resulting from increased bleeding from thorough debridement and pharmacological VTE prophylaxis. Hematoma can lead to persistent draining, wound complications, and dehiscence; this can increase the risk of recurrent infection [39]. A retrospective review study involving 17,784 patients who underwent TKA showed that the patients who underwent an evacuation of hematoma within 30 days of the procedure had a 5-year risk of deep infection of 6% compared to 0.8% for patients who did not have a reoperation [40]. Due to the extensive debridement of soft tissue in PJI revision cases, there is an increased risk of persistent venous bleeding. The use of drains, while controversial, may help decrease hematoma formation postoperatively.

Furthermore, the use of negative pressure wound therapy has also been shown to be beneficial in treating wounds treated for infection after TKA [41, 42]. Wound dehiscence is a devastating complication that can act as a gateway for microbes to enter the joint and increase the risk of recurrent infection. This is especially true in patients with comorbidities such as diabetes mellitus, obesity, hypertension, arteriosclerosis, neuropathy, and smoking. Therefore, it is crucial to ensure that medical treatments of chronic conditions are optimized to promote wound healing [43]. In the presence of wound dehiscence, plastic surgery consultation, and soft tissue coverage with a rotational or free muscle flap may be necessary for wound closure.

22.3.3 Recurrent Infection

Recurrent infection is another devastating early complication associated with the treatment of a PJI. Both surgical and patient factors can contribute to the risk of persistent or recurrent infection. A multidisciplinary approach ensuring that patients have adequate surgical debridement, optimization of medical comorbidities, and appropriate antibiotics is essential in preventing recurrence. Despite this, a proportion of patients will still develop an ongoing infection. DAIR has a variable success rate, from 18% in treating PJI with MRSA to 100% in another arthroscopic study [44, 45]. A literature review on the efficacy of DAIR concluded that it could be an effective method of eradicating PJI. It is recommended to be carried out in the acute postoperative period, within 4 weeks of surgery, and that the procedure should be done in an open fashion rather than arthroscopically [46]. A systematic review article comparing the results of 687 patients who underwent a single-stage exchange arthroplasty to 1086 patients who underwent a two-stage exchange arthroplasty for chronic PJI showed that the eradication rate was 87.1% and 84.8%, respectively [47].

A retrospective study examining 548 patients that received a two-stage exchange arthroplasty for an infected hip or knee prosthesis showed that female gender, psychiatric illness, and heart disease all increased the likelihood of recurrent infection [48]. Moreover, an Italian study concluded that continuing with antibiotic therapy between the two stages of exchange arthroplasty, without an antibiotic-free "holiday period" reduced the prospect of a recurrence of PJI and provided better outcomes in immunocompromised patients [49].

22.4 Late Complications

22.4.1 Stiffness

Stiffness is a common complication after an infected knee PJI and revision surgery. A study conducted looking at the range of motion post revision TKA surgery showed that 4% of patients presented with stiffness, which was defined by a range of motion of <90° at the 3-month postoperative follow-up appointment [50]. A further German study which involved 867 primary TKAs and 176 revision TKAs found that 4.54% of pri-

mary TKAs and 5.11% of revision TKAs were deemed stiff (<90° flexion) [51].

Predicting stiffness after revision surgery for an infected implant is challenging. However, preoperative range of motion has been shown to be the greatest determinant [43, 44]. A shorter duration between primary and revision TKA has also been shown to increase the risk of recurrent stiffness [50]. A high BMI is a modifiable risk factor linked to postoperative stiffness in revision TKAs [52].

Conservative approaches, such as physical therapy, can be used initially. Early manipulation under anesthetic, within 3 months of the surgery, has proven successful in improving stiffness [53]. More invasive procedures such as open arthrolysis and revision surgery should be considered in more resistant cases [53].

22.4.2 Peri-Prosthetic Fracture

Peri-prosthetic fractures can occur both intraoperatively and postoperatively secondary to trauma. They are particularly difficult to treat in the setting of a periprosthetic joint infection. Goals of treatment include restoration of length, alignment, and rotation, stable fixation and/or reconstruction, and eradication of infection [54].

Peri-prosthetic distal femoral fractures around the femoral component of a TKA are extremely challenging to deal with. The Su classification divides fractures into 3 types (I–III) according to the location relative to the proximal aspect of the femoral component. Type I fractures are proximal to the femoral component, type II originates at the proximal aspect of the femoral component and extends proximally, and type III extends distal to the proximal border of the femoral component [55]. The Lewis and Rorabeck classification divides fracture into 3 types (I–III). Type I describes an undisplaced fracture with the intact prosthesis, type II is a displaced fracture with an intact prosthesis, and type III is a displaced or undisplaced fracture with loosening of the femoral component [56].

Tibial PPFs can be classified using the Felix classification [57]. This system divides fractures around the tibial component into 4 types (I–IV). Type I represents a fracture of the tibial plateau, type II fractures are adjacent to the prosthetic stem, type III fractures are of the tibial shaft, distal to the tibial component and type IV fractures represent a fracture of the tibial tubercle. Additionally, peri-prosthetic fractures can be classified using the Unified classification system, which recognizes 6 types (A-F). Type A is an apophyseal fracture, B represents fractures at the bed of the implant, C are fractures clear of the implant, D is a fracture in between two prosthesis, E is a fracture of each of two bones supporting one joint replacement, and F is a fracture articulating or facing an implant [58].

PPFs around a revision knee prosthesis can occur early or late postoperatively. The risk factors include poor bone stock, which is often seen in infected cases, multiple re-revisions, osteopenia, certain comorbidities, such as inflammatory arthritis and anterior cortical stress risers [59]. The risk of a PPF around the implant post-revision TKA is twice that of the risk post primary TKA [60, 61]. The Scottish registry showed that the incidence of a PPF was 0.6% and 1.7% in primary and revision TKAs, respectively [60]. The review also found that the only risks that significantly increased the likelihood of PPFs around a TKA were female gender, age over 70, and revision surgery.

The treatment of fractures around a revision component is much more challenging as orthodox treatment options for PPFs around a primary implant such as an intramedullary nail or a periarticular locking plate are often unsuitable. Unstable fractures with a stable prosthesis require open reduction and internal fixation (ORIF). Displaced fractures with a loose component should be revised with a longer stem that bypasses the fracture site [57]. In the case of non-union due to comminution, bone loss or failure of ORIF around a PFF of the distal femur, a distal femoral replacement can be considered as a limb salvaging procedure [62].

Patella fractures post TKA are less common and can generally be managed non-operatively in the absence of extensor mechanism disruption and patella component instability [63]. If patella component instability is present, treatment should be based on the bone stock available. If there is adequate bone stock, ORIF with or without component revision should be attempted; however, if bone stock is poor, partial or complete patellectomy may be an alternative [64].

22.4.3 Stem Tip Pain

Stem tip pain is a common cause of discomfort expressed by patients following revision surgery. The poor bone stock that frequently coincides with PJI makes maintaining accurate component alignment difficult. A tibial stem extension is often employed to improve component fixation [65]. Pain in the region of the stem tip has been described in 14% of patients who had undergone revision TKA [66]. Also, stem design does not seem to influence the incidence of stem tip pain post revision [67]. Placement of a tibial plate in the region of the stem tip has been found to reduce the incidence of pain [48]; however, the use of additional metalwork in the treatment of PJI can increase risks further. For this reason, a fixation strategy that gains purchase in the metaphyseal regions of femur or tibia in conjunction with short, cemented stems may be a more successful strategy [68].

22.5 Conclusion

In conclusion, the mainstay of treatment for an infected knee prosthesis involves the eradication of the infection and the provision of a pain-free, stable and functioning knee joint that allows sufficient range of motion. The process of achieving this is often difficult and can seem interminable due to complexities that surround a PJI. Treatment must to be tailored to patients on an individual and carefully planned basis in a specialized arthroplasty center where the input from a revision knee specialist, microbiologist, and specialist physiotherapists are available in order to achieve a satisfactory outcome and decrease the risks of further devastating complications [5].

Case Presentation

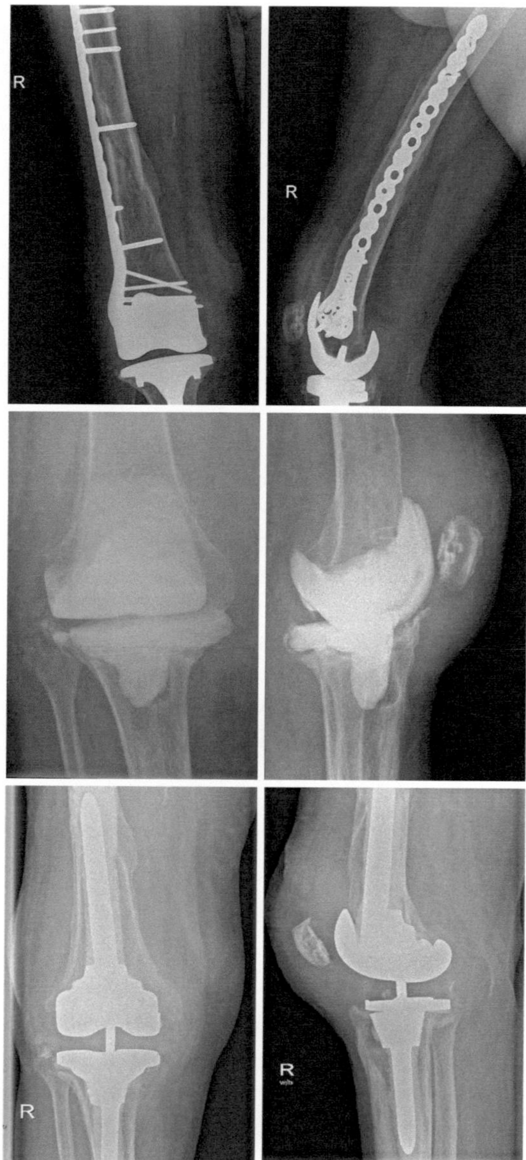

This 65-year-old patient sustained a distal femur peri-prosthetic fracture that was managed with an open reduction and internal fixation with a lateral locking plate. He subsequently developed a prosthetic joint infection and underwent a two-stage revision with an articulating spacer followed by a constrained revision prosthesis.

References

1. Springer BD, Cahue S, Etkin CD, Lewallen DG, McGrory BJ. Infection burden in total hip and knee arthroplasties: an international registry-based perspective. Arthroplast Today. 2017;3(2):137–40.
2. Neufeld ME, Masri BA. Can the Oxford Knee and Hip Score identify patients who do not require total knee or hip arthroplasty? Bone Joint J. 2019;101-B(6_Supple_B):23–30.
3. Ahmed SS, Haddad FS. Prosthetic joint infection. Bone Joint Res. 2019;8(11):570–2.
4. Zmistowski B, Karam JA, Durinka JB, Casper DS, Parvizi J. Periprosthetic joint infection increases the risk of one-year mortality. J Bone Joint Surg Am. 2013;95(24):2177–84.
5. Garceau S, Warschawski Y, Dahduli O, Alshaygy I, Wolfstadt J, Backstein D. The effect of patient institutional transfer during the interstage period of two-stage treatment for prosthetic knee infection. Bone Joint J. 2019;101-B(9):1087–92.
6. Katz JN, Mahomed NN, Baron JA, et al. Association of hospital and surgeon procedure volume with patient-centered outcomes of total knee replacement in a population-based cohort of patients age 65 years and older. Arthritis Rheum. 2007;56(2):568–74.
7. Katz JN, Barrett J, Mahomed NN, Baron JA, Wright RJ, Losina E. Association between hospital and surgeon procedure volume and the outcomes of total knee replacement. J Bone Joint Surg Am. 2004;86(9):1909–16.
8. Dai WL, Lin ZM, Shi ZJ, Wang J. Outcomes following revision total knee arthroplasty septic versus aseptic failure: a National Propensity-Score-Matched Comparison. J Knee Surg. 2020.
9. Anderson LA, Culp BM, Della Valle CJ, et al. High failure rates of concomitant periprosthetic joint infection and extensor mechanism disruption. J Arthroplasty. 2018;33(6):1879–83.
10. Charette RS, Melnic CM. Two-stage revision arthroplasty for the treatment of prosthetic joint infection. Curr Rev Musculoskelet Med. 2018;11(3):332–40.
11. Abdel MP, Barreira P, Battenberg A, et al. Hip and knee section, treatment, two-stage exchange spacer-related: proceedings of international consensus on orthopedic infections. J Arthroplasty. 2019;34(2S):S427–38.
12. Haddad FS, Masri BA, Campbell D, McGraw RW, Beauchamp CP, Duncan CP. The PROSTALAC functional spacer in two-stage revision for infected knee replacements. Prosthesis of antibiotic-loaded acrylic cement. J Bone Joint Surg Br. 2000;82(6):807–12.
13. Ricciardi BF, Oi K, Trivellas M, Lee YY, Della Valle AG, Westrich GH. Survivorship of extensor mechanism allograft reconstruction after total knee arthroplasty. J Arthroplasty. 2017;32(1):183–8.

14. Illingworth KD, Mihalko WM, Parvizi J, et al. How to minimize infection and thereby maximize patient outcomes in total joint arthroplasty: a multicenter approach: AAOS exhibit selection. J Bone Joint Surg Am. 2013;95(8):e50.

15. Rezapoor M, Parvizi J. Prevention of periprosthetic joint infection. J Arthroplasty. 2015;30(6):902–7.

16. Garbarino LJ, Gold PA, Sodhi N, et al. The effect of operative time on in-hospital length of stay in revision total knee arthroplasty. Ann Transl Med. 2019;7(4):66.

17. Vince K. Modes of failure in total knee arthroplasty. In: Advanced reconstruction knee AAOS; 2011. p. 3141–55.

18. Hipfl C, Winkler T, Janz V, Perka C, Müller M. Management of chronically infected total knee arthroplasty with severe bone loss using static spacers with intramedullary rods. J Arthroplasty. 2019;34(7):1462–9.

19. Sassoon AA, Nelms NJ, Trousdale RT. Intraoperative fracture during staged total knee reimplantation in the treatment of periprosthetic infection. J Arthroplasty. 2014;29(7):1435–8.

20. Gross AE. Periprosthetic fractures of the knee: puzzle pieces. J Arthroplasty. 2004;19(4 Suppl 1):47–50.

21. Haddad F. The Hinge: prerequisite solution for the infected TKA—opposes. In: Orthopaedic proceedings, vol. 100-B. London: Bone and Joint Publishing; 2018. p. 111.

22. Azzam K, Parvizi J, Kaufman D, Purtill JJ, Sharkey PF, Austin MS. Revision of the unstable total knee arthroplasty: outcome predictors. J Arthroplasty. 2011;26(8):1139–44.

23. Chang MJ, Lim H, Lee NR, Moon YW. Diagnosis, causes and treatments of instability following total knee arthroplasty. Knee Surg Relat Res. 2014;26(2):61–7.

24. Mason M, Belisle A, Bonutti P, Kolisek FR, Malkani A, Masini M. An accurate and reproducible method for locating the joint line during a revision total knee arthroplasty. J Arthroplasty. 2006;21(8):1147–53.

25. Hoeffel DP, Rubash HE. Revision total knee arthroplasty: current rationale and techniques for femoral component revision. Clin Orthop Relat Res. 2000;380:116–32.

26. Hofmann AA, Kurtin SM, Lyons S, Tanner AM, Bolognesi MP. Clinical and radiographic analysis of accurate restoration of the joint line in revision total knee arthroplasty. J Arthroplasty. 2006;21(8):1154–62.

27. Rose HA, Hood RW, Otis JC, Ranawat CS, Insall JN. Peroneal-nerve palsy following total knee arthroplasty. A review of The Hospital for Special Surgery experience. J Bone Joint Surg Am. 1982;64(3):347–51.

28. Saleh KJ, Hoeffel DP, Kassim RA, Burstein G. Complications after revision total knee arthroplasty. J Bone Joint Surg Am. 2003;85-A(Suppl 1):S71–4.

29. Idusuyi OB, Morrey BF. Peroneal nerve palsy after total knee arthroplasty. Assessment of predisposing and prognostic factors. J Bone Joint Surg Am. 1996;78(2):177–84.

30. Horlocker TT, Hebl JR, Gali B, et al. Anesthetic, patient, and surgical risk factors for neurologic complications after prolonged total tourniquet time during total knee arthroplasty. Anesth Analg. 2006;102(3):950–5.

31. Calligaro KD, Dougherty MJ, Ryan S, Booth RE. Acute arterial complications associated with total hip and knee arthroplasty. J Vasc Surg. 2003;38(6):1170–7.

32. Brookenthal KR, Freedman KB, Lotke PA, Fitzgerald RH, Lonner JH. A meta-analysis of thromboembolic prophylaxis in total knee arthroplasty. J Arthroplasty. 2001;16(3):293–300.

33. Feinglass J, Koo S, Koh J. Revision total knee arthroplasty complication rates in northern Illinois. Clin Orthop Relat Res. 2004;429:279–85.

34. Jimenez MA, Trousdale RT. Thromboembolic disease in total knee arthroplasty. Instr Course Lect. 2001;50:415–9.

35. Sharrock NE, Go G, Williams-Russo P, Haas SB, Harpel PC. Comparison of extradural and general anaesthesia on the fibrinolytic response to total knee arthroplasty. Br J Anaesth. 1997;79(1):29–34.

36. Howard AW, Aaron SD. Low molecular weight heparin decreases proximal and distal deep venous thrombosis following total knee arthroplasty. A meta-analysis of randomized trials. Thromb Haemost. 1998;79(5):902–6.

37. Eikelboom JW, Quinlan DJ, Douketis JD. Extended-duration prophylaxis against venous thromboembolism after total hip or knee replacement: a meta-analysis of the randomised trials. Lancet. 2001;358(9275):9–15.

38. Kakkos SK, Warwick D, Nicolaides AN, Stansby GP, Tsolakis IA. Combined (mechanical and pharmacological) modalities for the prevention of venous thromboembolism in joint replacement surgery. J Bone Joint Surg Br. 2012;94(6):729–34.

39. Patel VP, Walsh M, Sehgal B, Preston C, DeWal H, Di Cesare PE. Factors associated with prolonged wound drainage after primary total hip and knee arthroplasty. J Bone Joint Surg Am. 2007;89(1):33–8.

40. Galat DD, McGovern SC, Larson DR, Harrington JR, Hanssen AD, Clarke HD. Surgical treatment of early wound complications following primary total knee arthroplasty. J Bone Joint Surg Am. 2009;91(1):48–54.

41. Helito CP, Bueno DK, Giglio PN, Bonadio MB, Pécora JR, Demange MK. Negative-pressure wound therapy in the treatment of complex injuries after total knee arthroplasty. Acta Ortop Bras. 2017;25(2):85–8.

42. Siqueira MB, Ramanathan D, Klika AK, Higuera CA, Barsoum WK. Role of negative pressure wound ther-

apy in total hip and knee arthroplasty. World J Orthop. 2016;7(1):30–7.

43. Ackermann PW, Hart DA. Influence of comorbidities: neuropathy, vasculopathy, and diabetes on healing response quality. Adv Wound Care (New Rochelle). 2013;2(8):410–21.

44. Bradbury T, Fehring TK, Taunton M, et al. The fate of acute methicillin-resistant *Staphylococcus aureus* periprosthetic knee infections treated by open debridement and retention of components. J Arthroplasty. 2009;24(6 Suppl):101–4.

45. Chung JY, Ha CW, Park YB, Song YJ, Yu KS. Arthroscopic debridement for acutely infected prosthetic knee: any role for infection control and prosthesis salvage? Arthroscopy. 2014;30(5):599–606.

46. Qasim SN, Swann A, Ashford R. The DAIR (debridement, antibiotics and implant retention) procedure for infected total knee replacement—a literature review. SICOT J. 2017;3:2.

47. Pangaud C, Ollivier M, Argenson JN. Outcome of single-stage versus two-stage exchange for revision knee arthroplasty for chronic periprosthetic infection. EFORT Open Rev. 2019;4(8):495–502.

48. Triantafyllopoulos GK, Memtsoudis SG, Zhang W, Ma Y, Sculco TP, Poultsides LA. Periprosthetic infection recurrence after 2-stage exchange arthroplasty: failure or fate? J Arthroplasty. 2017;32(2):526–31.

49. Ascione T, Balato G, Mariconda M, Rotondo R, Baldini A, Pagliano P. Continuous antibiotic therapy can reduce recurrence of prosthetic joint infection in patients undergoing 2-stage exchange. J Arthroplasty. 2019;34(4):704–9.

50. Kim GK, Mortazavi SM, Purtill JJ, Sharkey PF, Hozack WJ, Parvizi J. Stiffness after revision total knee arthroplasty. J Arthroplasty. 2010;25(6):844–50.

51. Ipach I, Schäfer R, Lahrmann J, Kluba T. Stiffness after knee arthrotomy: evaluation of prevalence and results after manipulation under anaesthesia. Orthop Traumatol Surg Res. 2011;97(3):292–6.

52. Kasmire KE, Rasouli MR, Mortazavi SM, Sharkey PF, Parvizi J. Predictors of functional outcome after revision total knee arthroplasty following aseptic failure. Knee. 2014;21(1):264–7.

53. Rodríguez-Merchán EC. The stiff total knee arthroplasty: causes, treatment modalities and results. EFORT Open Rev. 2019;4(10):602–10.

54. Müller M, Winkler T, Märdian S, et al. The worst-case scenario: treatment of periprosthetic femoral fracture with coexistent periprosthetic infection-a prospective and consecutive clinical study. Arch Orthop Trauma Surg. 2019;139(10):1461–70.

55. Su ET, DeWal H, Di Cesare PE. Periprosthetic femoral fractures above total knee replacements. J Am Acad Orthop Surg. 2004;12(1):12–20.

56. Lewis P, Rorabeck C. Periprosthetic fractures. In: Engh G, Rorabeck C, editors. Revision total knee arthroplasty. Philadelphia: Lippincott Williams and Wilkins; 1997. p. 275–95.

57. Felix NA, Stuart MJ, Hanssen AD. Periprosthetic fractures of the tibia associated with total knee arthroplasty. Clin Orthop Relat Res. 1997;345:113–24.

58. Duncan CP, Haddad FS. The unified classification system (UCS): improving our understanding of periprosthetic fractures. Bone Joint J. 2014;96-B(6):713–6.

59. Kempshall PJSH, Morgan-Jones RL. Revision total knee arthroplasty: complications. Orthop Trauma. 2012;26:2.

60. Meek RM, Norwood T, Smith R, Brenkel IJ, Howie CR. The risk of peri-prosthetic fracture after primary and revision total hip and knee replacement. J Bone Joint Surg Br. 2011;93(1):96–101.

61. Kim KI, Egol KA, Hozack WJ, Parvizi J. Periprosthetic fractures after total knee arthroplasties. Clin Orthop Relat Res. 2006;446:167–75.

62. Freedman EL, Hak DJ, Johnson EE, Eckardt JJ. Total knee replacement including a modular distal femoral component in elderly patients with acute fracture or nonunion. J Orthop Trauma. 1995;9(3):231–7.

63. Ortiguera CJ, Berry DJ. Patellar fracture after total knee arthroplasty. J Bone Joint Surg Am. 2002;84(4):532–40.

64. Yoo JD, Kim NK. Periprosthetic fractures following total knee arthroplasty. Knee Surg Relat Res. 2015;27(1):1–9.

65. Kimpton CI, Crocombe AD, Bradley WN, Gavin Huw Owen B. Analysis of stem tip pain in revision total knee arthroplasty. J Arthroplasty. 2013;28(6):971–7.

66. Barrack RL, Rorabeck C, Burt M, Sawhney J. Pain at the end of the stem after revision total knee arthroplasty. Clin Orthop Relat Res. 1999;367:216–25.

67. Barrack RL, Stanley T, Burt M, Hopkins S. The effect of stem design on end-of-stem pain in revision total knee arthroplasty. J Arthroplasty. 2004;19(7 Suppl 2):119–24.

68. Morgan-Jones R, Oussedik SI, Graichen H, Haddad FS. Zonal fixation in revision total knee arthroplasty. Bone Joint J. 2015;97-B(2):147–9.

Part VI

Current Evidence on Prevention of Knee Replacement Infections

Treatment of Periprosthetic Joint Infections with Resistant Organisms

Kevin A. Sonn and R. Michael Meneghini

23.1 Introduction

The successful eradication of periprosthetic joint infection (PJI) depends on various host factors, treatment modalities, and infection characteristics. Infections caused by antibiotic-resistant organisms have been increasing in recent years [1, 2]. Studies have clearly demonstrated the difficulty of treating PJI caused by organisms including methicillin-resistant *Staphylococcus epidermidis* (MRSE), methicillin-resistant *Staphylococcus aureus* (MRSA), and *enterococcus* [1, 3–6]. It is vital to understand the treatment ramifications of the various resistant organisms when treating PJI.

23.1.1 *Staphylococcus epidermidis*

Staphylococcus epidermidis (*S. epidermidis*) was previously thought of as an innocuous bacterial colonizer on human skin. However, it is now recognized as an opportunistic pathogen that is responsible for the greatest proportion of

infections on all indwelling medical devices [7]. *S. epidermidis* falls into the broader category of coagulase-negative staphylococci which causes 30–43% of all PJIs [8]. *S. epidermidis* first non-specifically binds to implanted prostheses, then subsequent biofilm formation occurs via a polysaccharide intercellular adhesin [9]. It is this ability to develop a strong glycocalyx that accounts for the difficulty of eradication of this low-virulent organism [1]. For these reasons, aggressive treatment of *S. epidermidis* is recommended (especially when methicillin resistance is encountered).

23.1.2 *Staphylococcus aureus*

Staphylococcus aureus (*S. aureus*) is a Gram-positive human commensal organism that has shown persistent nasal colonization in 20–25% of adults and intermittent colonization in up to 60% [10]. *S. aureus* infection causes 10–23% of all PJIs. *S. aureus* interacts with host fibronectin, fibrinogen, and collagen to cover a prosthesis immediately after implantation [8, 11]. A subcutaneous foreign body reduces the minimum infection causing inoculum with *S. aureus* more than 100,000×. The susceptibility to PJI caused by *S. aureus* combined with emerging and worsening resistance has increased recurrent infection rates [1]. Successful infection eradication of PJIs

K. A. Sonn · R. M. Meneghini (✉)
Department of Orthopaedic Surgery, Indiana University School of Medicine,
Indianapolis, IN, USA

IU Health Hip & Knee Center, IU Health Saxony Hospital, Fishers, IN, USA
e-mail: ksonn2@iuhealth.org; rmeneghi@iuhealth.org

© ISAKOS 2022
U. G. Longo et al. (eds.), *Infection in Knee Replacement*,
https://doi.org/10.1007/978-3-030-81553-0_23

caused by methicillin-resistant *S. aureus* (MRSA) with debridement and implant retention (DAIR) is reported as low as 20% and is generally not recommended [12]. Even two-stage revision for MRSA infections has demonstrated low rates of infection eradication, thus highlighting the difficulty in managing this virulent and resistant organism [3].

23.1.3 *Enterococcus*

Enterococcus is a Gram-positive, facultative anaerobe which has been reported to cause 2–3% of all PJIs [4, 13]. El Helou et al. reported 94% success with two-stage exchange for enterococcal infections; however, 46% of their cohort were treated with definitive resection while only 34% underwent two-stage revision. Rasouli et al. achieved successful eradication of enterococcal PJIs in only 20% of cases treated with DAIR and only 44% treated with two-stage revision [4]. An additional challenge treating enterococcal PJIs occurs when the bacteria are resistant. Vancomycin-resistant *enterococcus* (VRE) infections remain exceptionally difficult to treat with reimplantation rather than salvage options such as definitive resection, fusion, or above-knee amputation [4, 14].

23.2 Debridement and Implant Retention

Debridement and implant retention (DAIR) is commonly utilized for the treatment of acute periprosthetic joint infections as discussed in previous sections. The success rates vary widely in the literature and largely depend on the infecting organism. Duque et al. report successful infection eradication with DAIR in only 20% of MRSA and 33.3% of *Pseudomonas aeruginosa* infections compared to 85.3% for all other bacteria [12]. Other authors have reported on similar difficulties and comparable failure rates when treating staphylococcal infections with DAIR

[15–17]. Chung et al. have recently reported on improved success of a planned two-stage DAIR [18]. In their protocol, the first stage consists of a thorough debridement with placement of antibiotic cement beads, while the second stage (occurring 5 days later) involves an additional debridement with exchange of modular components. They report successful infection eradication in 89.6% of TKAs (93.5% in primary TKAs), including overall successful treatment of 70% of MRSA infections [18].

The addition of rifampin to targeted intravenous (IV) antibiotic therapy is recommended for all cases of DAIR, especially those caused by staphylococcal species [19–24]. The successful results of adding rifampin are thought to result from its ability to penetrate biofilm when used in DAIR [8].

23.3 Two-Stage Revision

Two-stage revision remains the gold standard for treatment of chronic periprosthetic joint infection. Overall success rates between 80% and 100% are commonly quoted for infection eradication utilizing a two-stage approach [25–29]. However, when stratifying these results based on type of organism, treatment outcomes worsen with resistant bacteria. Kilgus et al. report 89% success treating methicillin-sensitive *S. aureus* (MSSA) compared to only 18% infection eradication of MRSA and MRSE infections utilizing a two-stage approach [3]. Mittal et al. found 24% reinfection rate when treating MRSA and MRSE in a two-staged fashion [1]. However, 14% were reinfected with new organisms rather than recurrence, therefore they recommend two-stage revision as a viable treatment option in this setting [1]. Rasouli et al. successfully eradicated enterococcal PJIs with two-stage revision in only 7 of 16 patients. Six patients were treated with definitive resection and 3 had either knee fusion or above-knee amputation [4].

Case Example

This is a 61-year-old male with a complex history starting with right total knee arthroplasty, subsequent revision for polyethylene wear, and then complete revision TKA. This was complicated by subsequent hematogenous MRSA PJI which was treated with a single-stage revision. Four years subsequent to that he was found to have an MSSA PJI which was treated with two-stage exchange which was complicated by a traumatic wound dehiscence. At this time he presented to our practice with a draining sinus and chronic extensor mechanism disruption with revision components in place (Fig. 23.1). He underwent resection and placement of a static antibiotic cement spacer with multiple intraoperative cultures demonstrating enterococcus. This required 2 additional repeat debridements with 1 spacer exchange before the infection was cleared and the knee was reimplanted (Fig. 23.2). At most recent follow-up 2 years after reimplantation, he demonstrated no evidence of infection and was off all antibiotics.

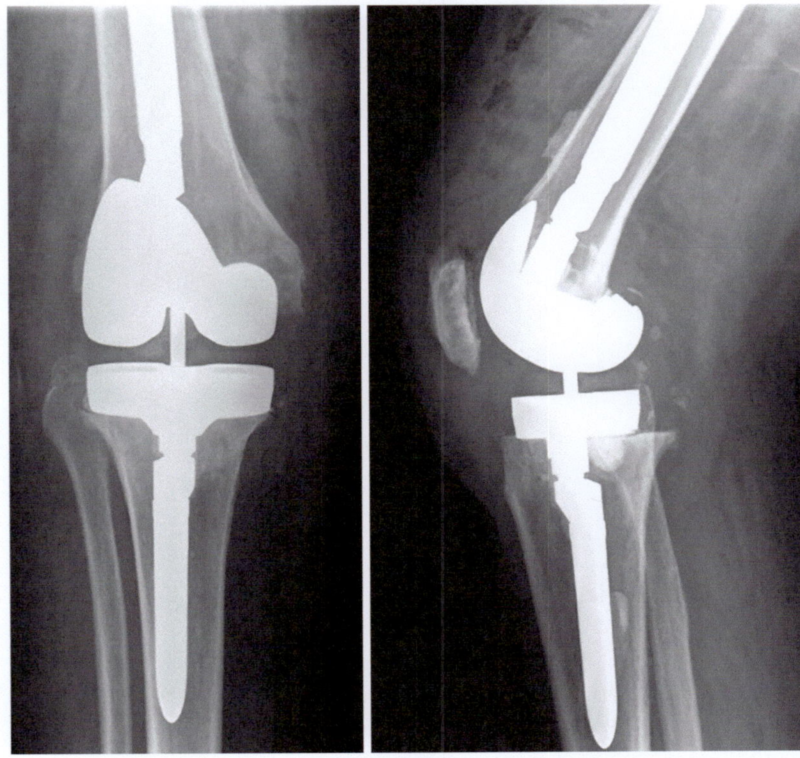

Fig. 23.1 Anteroposterior (AP) and lateral radiographs at presentation demonstrating revision components without evidence of implant loosening

Fig. 23.2 Anteroposterior (AP) and lateral radiographs after reimplantation demonstrating sleeved revision components

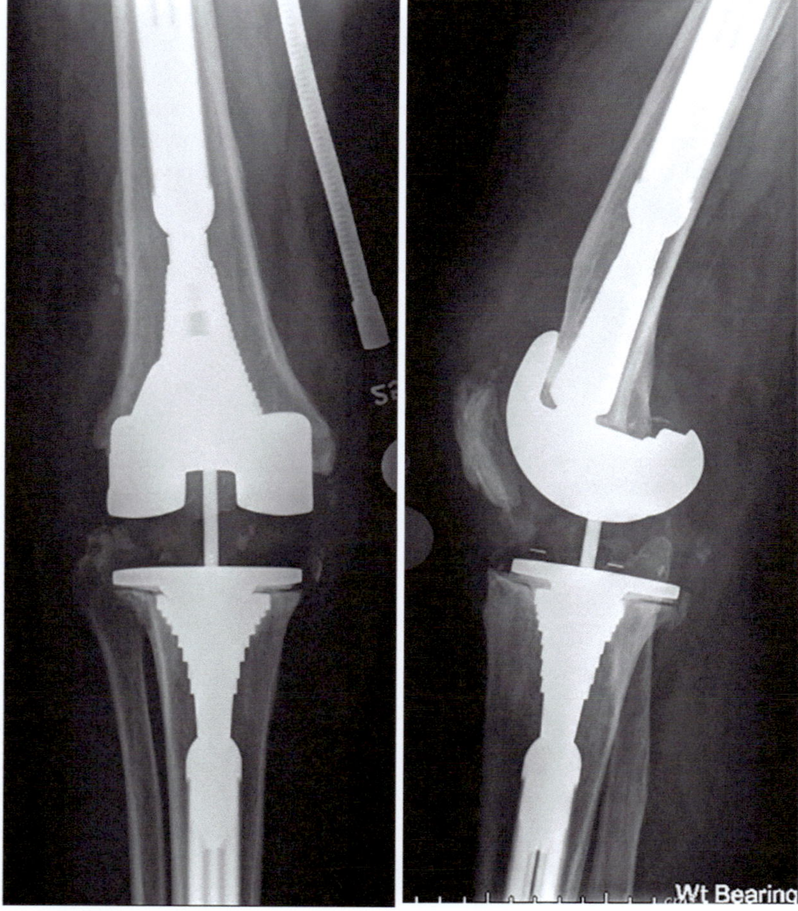

23.4 Conclusion

Treatment of knee PJI with resistant organisms remains a challenge with high complication and reinfection rates. Two-stage revision is often the best approach to maximize chances of successful infection eradication. If DAIR is chosen, consideration should be given to performing a planned two-staged DAIR as described by Chung et al. [18]. Further, the addition of 6 months of oral rifampin to targeted IV antibiotic therapy when treating staphylococcal knee PJI with DAIR has demonstrated improved results. Regardless of treatment approach, infection recurrence remains high and salvage procedures such as fusion, definitive resection, and above-knee amputation are realistic outcomes despite best attempts to retain or reimplant prostheses.

References

1. Mittal Y, Fehring TK, Hanssen A, Marculescu C, Odum SM, Osmon D. Two-stage reimplantation for periprosthetic knee infection involving resistant organisms. J Bone Joint Surg Am. 2007;89(6):1227–31. https://doi.org/10.2106/JBJS.E.01192.
2. Garvin KL, Hinrichs SH, Urban JA. Emerging antibiotic-resistant bacteria. Their treatment in total joint arthroplasty. Clin Orthop Relat Res. 1999;369:110–23.
3. Kilgus DJ, Howe DJ, Strang A. Results of periprosthetic hip and knee infections caused by resistant bacteria. Clin Orthop Relat Res. 2002;404(404):116–24. https://doi.org/10.1097/00003086-200211000-00021.
4. Rasouli MR, Tripathi MS, Kenyon R, Wetters N, Valle Della CJ, Parvizi J. Low rate of infection control in enterococcal periprosthetic joint infections. Clin Orthop Relat Res. 2012;470(10):2708–16. https://doi.org/10.1007/s11999-012-2374-8.

5. Parvizi J, Azzam K, Ghanem E, Austin MS, Rothman RH. Periprosthetic infection due to resistant staphylococci: serious problems on the horizon. Clin Orthop Relat Res. 2009;467(7):1732–9. https://doi.org/10.1007/s11999-009-0857-z.

6. Hirakawa K, Stulberg BN, Wilde AH, Bauer TW, Secic M. Results of 2-stage reimplantation for infected total knee arthroplasty. J Arthroplasty. 1998;13(1):22–8. https://doi.org/10.1016/s0883-5403(98)90071-7.

7. Otto M. *Staphylococcus epidermidis*—the "accidental" pathogen. Nat Rev Microbiol. 2009;7(8):555–67. https://doi.org/10.1038/nrmicro2182.

8. Zimmerli W, Trampuz A, Ochsner PE. Prosthetic-joint infections. N Engl J Med. 2004;351(16):1645–54. https://doi.org/10.1056/NEJMra040181.

9. Darouiche RO. Device-associated infections: a macroproblem that starts with microadherence. Clin Infect Dis. 2001;33(9):1567–72. https://doi.org/10.1086/323130.

10. Lister JL, Horswill AR. *Staphylococcus aureus* biofilms: recent developments in biofilm dispersal. Front Cell Infect Microbiol. 2014;4(37):178. https://doi.org/10.3389/fcimb.2014.00178.

11. Foster TJ, Höök M. Molecular basis of adherence of *Staphylococcus aureus* to biomaterials. Hoboken, NJ: Wiley; 2000. p. 27–39. https://doi.org/10.1128/9781555818067.ch2.

12. Duque AF, Post ZD, Lutz RW, Orozco FR, Pulido SH, Ong AC. Is there still a role for irrigation and debridement with liner exchange in acute periprosthetic total knee infection? J Arthroplasty. 2017;32(4):1280–4. https://doi.org/10.1016/j.arth.2016.10.029.

13. Helou El OC, Berbari EF, Marculescu CE, et al. Outcome of enterococcal prosthetic joint infection: is combination systemic therapy superior to monotherapy? Clin Infect Dis. 2008;47(7):903–9. https://doi.org/10.1086/591536.

14. Ries MD. Vancomycin-resistant Enterococcus infected total knee arthroplasty. J Arthroplasty. 2001;16(6):802–5. https://doi.org/10.1054/arth.2001.24951.

15. Brandt CM, Sistrunk WW, Duffy MC, et al. *Staphylococcus aureus* prosthetic joint infection treated with debridement and prosthesis retention. Clin Infect Dis. 1997;24(5):914–9. https://doi.org/10.1093/clinids/24.5.914.

16. Marculescu CE, Berbari EF, Hanssen AD, et al. Outcome of prosthetic joint infections treated with debridement and retention of components. Clin Infect Dis. 2006;42(4):471–8. https://doi.org/10.1086/499234.

17. Kuiper JW, Willink RT, Moojen DJF, van den Bekerom MP, Colen S. Treatment of acute periprosthetic infections with prosthesis retention: review of current concepts. World J Orthop. 2014;5(5):667–76. https://doi.org/10.5312/wjo.v5.i5.667.

18. Chung AS, Niesen MC, Graber TJ, et al. Two-stage debridement with prosthesis retention for acute periprosthetic joint infections. J Arthroplasty. 2019;34(6):1207–13. https://doi.org/10.1016/j.arth.2019.02.013.

19. Osmon DR, Berbari EF, Berendt AR, et al. Diagnosis and management of prosthetic joint infection: clinical practice guidelines by the Infectious Diseases Society of America. Clin Infect Dis. 2013;56(1):e1–e25. https://doi.org/10.1093/cid/cis803.

20. Drancourt M, Stein A, Argenson JN, Roiron R, Groulier P, Raoult D. Oral treatment of Staphylococcus spp. infected orthopaedic implants with fusidic acid or ofloxacin in combination with rifampicin. J Antimicrob Chemother. 1997;39(2):235–40. https://doi.org/10.1093/jac/39.2.235.

21. Aboltins CA, Page MA, Buising KL, et al. Treatment of staphylococcal prosthetic joint infections with debridement, prosthesis retention and oral rifampicin and fusidic acid. Clin Microbiol Infect. 2007;13(6):586–91. https://doi.org/10.1111/j.1469-0691.2007.01691.x.

22. Berdal J-E, Skråmm I, Mowinckel P, Gulbrandsen P, Bjørnholt JV. Use of rifampicin and ciprofloxacin combination therapy after surgical debridement in the treatment of early manifestation prosthetic joint infections. Clin Microbiol Infect. 2005;11(10):843–5. https://doi.org/10.1111/j.1469-0691.2005.01230.x.

23. Zimmerli W, Widmer AF, Blatter M, Frei R, Ochsner PE. Role of rifampin for treatment of orthopedic implant-related staphylococcal infections: a randomized controlled trial. Foreign-body infection (FBI) study group. JAMA. 1998;279(19):1537–41. https://doi.org/10.1001/jama.279.19.1537.

24. Helou El OC, Berbari EF, Lahr BD, et al. Efficacy and safety of rifampin containing regimen for staphylococcal prosthetic joint infections treated with debridement and retention. Eur J Clin Microbiol Infect Dis. 2010;29(8):961–7. https://doi.org/10.1007/s10096-010-0952-9.

25. Insall JN, Thompson FM, Brause BD. Two-stage reimplantation for the salvage of infected total knee arthroplasty. J Bone Joint Surg Am. 1983;65(8):1087–98.

26. Borden LS, Gearen PF. Infected total knee arthroplasty. A protocol for management. J Arthroplasty. 1987;2(1):27–36. https://doi.org/10.1016/s0883-5403(87)80028-1.

27. Rosenberg AG, Haas B, Barden R, Marquez D, Landon GC, Galante JO. Salvage of infected total knee arthroplasty. Clin Orthop Relat Res. 1988;226:29–33.

28. Wilde AH, Ruth JT. Two-stage reimplantation in infected total knee arthroplasty. Clin Orthop Relat Res. 1988;236:23–35.

29. Windsor RE, Insall JN, Urs WK, Miller DV, Brause BD. Two-stage reimplantation for the salvage of total knee arthroplasty complicated by infection. Further follow-up and refinement of indications. J Bone Joint Surg Am. 1990;72(2):272–8.

Medical Optimization of the Patient Prior to Surgery

24

Claire Bolton, Vikram Kandhari, and Myles Coolican

24.1 Introduction

Periprosthetic joint infection (PJI) after total knee arthroplasty (TKA) is a cause of major concern for the health systems and patients and remains the most common cause for early revision in practically every joint registry [1–3]. It is associated with an increased financial burden, inferior clinical outcomes and increased morbidity. Although the incidence of PJI is relatively low at 1.1–2.2% [4, 5], it adds significantly to the healthcare costs, as these patients have increased hospital stays, require readmissions and additional surgical procedures [6, 7]. It is estimated that the number of primary TKAs performed annually is likely to increase by 673% between 2005 and 2030 [8–10]. A similar increase is anticipated in the number of revision TKAs performed for PJI which will see additional financial strain on the already overburdened healthcare systems the world over [11]. Strategies to prevent the occurrence of PJI after TKA have clear benefits.

Many risk factors associated with the PJI after TKA have been identified and can broadly be categorized into preoperative, intraoperative and post-operative factors [12]. The mortality rate of a two-stage revision arthroplasty done for PJI approaches 25–33% at 5 years [13, 14]. Surgeons should attempt to decrease this risk by managing the modifiable risk factors. In this chapter, we will present a summary of current practice and provide evidence for improved outcomes following the medical optimization of the patient prior to surgery.

24.2 Preoperative Risk Factors

24.2.1 Inflammatory Arthritis

Patients who suffer from inflammatory arthritis such as rheumatoid disease (RD), spondyloarthritis (SpA) including ankylosing spondylitis and psoriasis, and systemic lupus erythematosus (SLE) are at an increased risk of post-operative wound complications and PJI after TKA [15–18]. Many of these patients require chronic management with nonbiologic disease modifying anti-rheumatic medications (DMARDs), glucocorticoids, immunosuppressive medication or biologic agents, some of which puts them at higher risk of acquiring PJI. Consultation with the patients' rheumatologist to alter the medical management of inflammatory arthritis can help diminish wound complications without severely affecting the inflammatory process in other joints.

Rheumatoid disease has been reported as increasing the risk of PJI after TKA [15, 17–19]. The PJI rate in patients with rheumatoid arthritis

C. Bolton · V. Kandhari · M. Coolican (✉)
Sydney Orthopaedic and Research Institute,
Sydney, Australia
e-mail: myles@mylescoolican.com.au

© ISAKOS 2022
U. G. Longo et al. (eds.), *Infection in Knee Replacement*,
https://doi.org/10.1007/978-3-030-81553-0_24

was 1.6 times greater than those with osteoarthritis in a study by Schrama et al. [18] Ravi et al. reported 71,793 patients who had TKA, 4% whom had RD, and found an adjusted hazard ratio of 1.47 ($p = 0.03$) for increased rate of infection with the RD cohort having a rate of 1.26% and the OA group 0.84% [15]. Jämsen et al. [19] reviewed the Finnish Arthroplasty Register with a total of 43,149 primary and revision TKAs, and found an increased risk of PJI in seropositive rheumatoid disease with a hazard ratio of 1.7. This risk for PJI normalized to the same as the primary osteoarthritis cohort after 1-year post procedure.

Patients with psoriasis have been shown to have increased concentrations of bacteria on skin plaques than normal skin [20]. Routine perioperative preparation of these plaques has been found to be successful at sterilization of them with the use of an iodine and alcohol preparation [21]. Reports of PJI in patients with psoriasis are limited and mixed in outcomes for PJI. A deep infection rate of 16.6% and mild skin necrosis in 8.4% out of 24 patients who underwent TKA was reported in one study [22]. Another study of 50 patients undergoing primary TKA only had one (2.0%) deep infection at over 2 years post-surgery, and this patient also had alcoholic cirrhosis which may have contributed to this [23]. Both of these papers had low sample sizes and were retrospective in nature. Menon and Wroblewski [24] reviewed the results of Charnley low-friction hip arthroplasty patients with psoriasis and found a deep infection rate of 5.5% (3 patients); however, one of those patients also had rheumatoid disease.

The evidence for the perioperative management of antirheumatic medication is sparse [25–27]. In 2017, the American College of Rheumatology combined with American Association of Hip and Knee Surgeons to develop evidence-based guidelines on the preoperative management of antirheumatic medications [28]. Each recommendation was graded for strength of evidence with the advice, based on low- to moderate-quality evidence being to continue nonbiologic DMARDs such as methotrexate, sulfasalazine, hydroxychloroquine, leflunomide and

doxycycline through surgery. Biologic agents are recommended to be withheld prior to surgery, with the timing of surgery selected around the dosing regimen for that specific medication. These agents should be restarted once the wound shows evidence of healing, all sutures/staples are removed and there is no wound drainage. Tofacitinib should be withheld for at least 7 days prior to surgery based on non-surgical studies showing an increased incidence of generalized infection. Patients with severe SLE should continue their usual doses of methotrexate, mycophenolate mofetil, azathioprine, cyclosporine or tacrolimus. Patients' with non-severe SLE may have mycophenolate mofetil, azathioprine, cyclosporine or tacrolimus withheld for a week preceding surgery. Stress dosing of glucocorticoids was not recommended, rather the patients treated on glucocorticoids are advised to continue on their usual dose during the perioperative period. The Canadian Rheumatology Association recommendations from 2012 also suggest continuing methotrexate but withholding biologic agents [29].

24.2.1.1 Diabetes Mellitus

Diabetes mellitus is associated with an increased risk of PJI and wound complications in patients undergoing TKA [30–32]. HbA1c levels relate to control of blood glucose levels in the past 1–3 months. Tarabichi et al. showed that HbA1c > 7.7% is associated with increased infection risk of PJI, rather than the often quoted HbA1c of 7% [33]. In a paper by Stryker et al., a HbA1c of >6.7% was associated with an increased risk of wound complications; however, none of the 30 patients in their study developed a PJI [32]. Preoperative hyperglycaemia has also been shown to be associated with increased risk of PJI after TKA [31]. Jämsen et al. showed that PJI risk was more than doubled by the patient having diabetes, but also showed a trend toward a higher rate of PJI if the patient did not have a diagnosis of diabetes but had a preoperative glucose level of ≥6.9 mmol/L (124 mg/dL) in contrast to those with <6.9 mmol/L. [31] The infection rate after TKA in this study was 1.59% in the diabetic cohort vs. 0.66% in the non-diabetic group. In contrast to these studies,

Adams et al. [34] demonstrated no increased risk of PJI in patients with diabetes, regardless of HbA1c. Charstil et al. showed in their 2015 study that perioperative hyperglycaemia was associated with an increased risk of PJI, but HbA1c > 7% was not, with the risk increasing from a preoperative glucose level of ≥194 g/dL (10.6 mmol/L) [35]. Regardless of the discrepancy in the literature of the risk of PJI associated with HbA1c, it is advisable for diabetic control to be optimized prior to surgery with the assistance of an endocrinologist and diabetes educator.

24.2.1.2 Smoking

Smoking is a well-documented cause of PJI and wound healing issues after TKA in the literature [36–42]. Nicotine causes microvascular constriction and increases the level of carboxyhemoglobin, which further decreases the delivery of oxygen at the tissue level [36, 43]. Thus, nicotine is associated with decreased blood and oxygen supply at the microvascular level increasing the risk of wound healing problems and PJI after TKA. To further compound these issues, collagen synthesis is also impaired by nicotine [36, 43].

Duchman et al. found a higher rate of wound complications in a cohort of smokers at 1.8% vs. former smokers at 1.3% and non-smokers at 1.1% in a retrospective study on 78,191 patients who had undergone primary total hip or total knee arthroplasty [38]. Deep wound infections were present in a statistically greater number in the current smoker group at a rate of 0.7%. The increased incidence of surgical site infection in a smoking cohort undergoing THA or TKA was supported in Singh et al. in a study that had a 2.4% surgical site infection rate vs. 1.6% in life-long non-smokers and 1.7% in prior smokers [41]. Unfortunately this paper did not delineate between deep and superficial surgical site infections. A hazard ratio of 2.37 (95% CI 1.19, 4.72; $p = 0.01$) for developing a deep infection was found in current tobacco users in a separate publication by Singh et al. [37].

Recommendations for a smoke-free period vary from 4 to 8 weeks prior to surgery [39, 44]. There are few publications on the effectiveness of smoking cessation programmes prior to total joint arthroplasty. Akhavan et al. conducted a study on 30 patients who were eligible for either total hip arthroplasty (THA) or TKA [45]. The patients were instructed that they needed to cease smoking prior to their surgery. They were given referrals for counselling, telephone support programmes and advised to see their general practitioner for nicotine replacement therapy (NRT). At 8 weeks they were reviewed in clinic and assessed for smoking cessation by an expired carbon monoxide breath test. Of the 70% of patients who passed this test, 62% quit "cold turkey", 24% with NRT and 14% with outpatient treatment programmes. Importantly, 64% continued their smoking abstinence at 6 months post-operatively.

Compliance with smoking cessation can be tested by assessing the patients' cotinine level in a blood test. Cotinine is a metabolite of nicotine and is found in the saliva, urine and blood of smokers. The half-life of cotinine is about 20 h and so a serum cotinine level of <10 ng/mL has been shown to reflect a patient's compliance with non-smoking [39, 44].

24.2.1.3 Obesity

Obese patients appear to be at increased risk for deep joint infection following primary or revision total knee arthroplasty [46–49]. Potential causes included the longer surgical time, greater soft tissue dissection and the presence of thick layer of poorly vascularized subcutaneous tissue [50–52]. In addition, obesity is associated with the presence of comorbidities such as diabetes mellitus and immunosuppression and malnutrition [50–54]. Peterson et al. in 2016 showed an array of nutritional deficiencies in patients who were due to undergo bariatric surgery [53]. Of the 58 obese patients, 15.6% had hypoalbuminemia, 92.9% vitamin D deficiency and 36.2% iron deficiency.

Although many surgeons advocate for weight loss in patients with elevated BMI prior to surgery, the evidence on outcomes of patients who have lost weight prior to TKA is limited. Inacio et al. showed that patients that had a decrease of body weight by 5% had no difference in rate of surgical site infection than a cohort that did not lose weight [55] In contrast to this, Malinzak et al. demonstrated an increased risk of PJI by approximately three times for obese patients with a BMI > 40 and by 21 times for patients with a BMI > 50 [56]. This study was supported by another study that showed increased PJI in patients weighing over 120 kg [57].

Bariatric surgery (a lap band or gastric bypass) may be performed to help morbidly obese patients lose weight; however, having had prior bariatric surgery does not seem to decrease the incidence of PJI, but might decrease the incidence of superficial surgical site infection [54, 58–60]. Bariatric surgery prior to TKA, as opposed to after TKA is advocated due to overall decrease in complications from TKA [58].

Prophylactic antibiotics should be dosed based on the patients' weight. Rondon et al. showed that in their cohort of patients 95.9% of patients who weighed over 120 kg were underdosed at time of primary total joint arthroplasties, and that his cohort also had a significant increase in incidence of PJI by 1 year than patients who weighed less than 120 kg. The current recommendation for cefazolin weight-based dosing protocols is to give 1 g if the patient weighs <60 kg, 2 g if the patient weighs 60–120 kg, and 3 g if the patient weighs >120 kg [61, 62].

24.2.1.4 Malnutrition

Recent studies have suggested malnutrition is associated with an increased risk of infection resulting in more screening for malnutrition. Tests for malnutrition include total leukocyte count <1500 mm^3, serum albumin <3.5 g/dL and transferrin level <200 mg/dL [63]. The prevalence of malnutrition is higher than is often acknowledged and paradoxically, some obese patients requiring TKA tend to suffer from malnutrition despite large deposits of body fat.

Green et al. reported an increased risk of infection in malnourished patients who underwent THA or TKA [64]. Adequate preoperative nutritional status was defined as a total lymphocyte count of ≥1500 cells/mm^3, and albumin level of ≥3.5 g/dL. Of the 217 patients included in the study, 57 had low preoperative lymphocyte counts and 4 low albumin levels, with 2 patients low with both parameters. Major wound complications were defined as either a superficial infection (3.7%), deep infection (1.8%), or wound dehiscence (0.9%). The major wound complication cohort had significantly ($p = 0.002$) lower preoperative lymphocyte count than those who did not have a complication with a mean lymphocyte count of 1553 vs. 1995 cells/mm^3. The albumin level trended lower in the major wound complication group but did not reach significance.

Jaberi et al. did a retrospective review of 300 patients who underwent a TKA or THA and who had persistent wound drainage [63]. Malnutrition as defined by total leukocyte count <1500 mm^3, serum albumin <3.5 g/dL and transferrin level <200 mg/dL was associated with increased risk of developing an infection. Peersman et al. found an association with poor nutrition, obesity and diabetes mellitus and risk of PJI in a retrospective review of 97 PJI in 6489 TKAs, although this paper did not define what constituted poor nutrition [65].

Anthropometric parameters of malnutrition, specifically the triceps skinfold (TSF) was studied in 213 patients undergoing TKA, as well as biochemical measures of nutrition such as the total lymphocyte count and albumin levels [66]. This study found that none of the preoperative biochemical markers was associated with infection; however, there was a statistically significant inverse relationship between TSF and infection. Anthropometric parameters are thought to be a better measure of long-term nutrition than biochemical markers as biochemical markers can be affected by chronic and acute diseases such as renal failure, liver diseases, cancer, and conditions associated with stress and inflammation [66].

From this literature it could be suggested that preoperative management of arthroplasty patients should involve biochemical screening for malnutrition, and further management of any nutritional deficiencies in conjunction with advice from a dietician.

24.2.1.5 Urinary Tract Infection

Patients who are to undergo TKA should be screened for urinary tract infections (UTI). Wang et al. [67] recently showed in a meta-analysis of primary joint replacements that the relative risk for developing PJI when a patient had a perioperative UTI was 3.17. They also showed that the microorganism causing the UTI and PJI were the same in the same patient, supporting the notion that the PJI is caused by haematogenous spread from the genitourinary tract [67]. Pulido et al. [5]. showed an increased risk of PJI in patients with a urinary tract infection. In contrast to these studies, Schmitt et al. [68] showed that the postoperative UTI was associated with both SSI and PJI, but not preoperative UTI. Regardless of the controversy as to the risk of PJI from preoperative UTI, it seems low risk to at least instigate treatment for any preoperative UTI prior to proceeding to TKA.

24.2.1.6 Dental Procedures

The issue of dental surgery following TKA is controversial. The American Academy of Orthopaedic Surgeons (AAOS) and the American Dental Association released a report in 2012 that reviewed the literature around prophylactic antibiotics with dental procedures and joint replacements in situ. Recommendation one from this report is that "the practitioner might consider discontinuing the practice of routinely prescribing prophylactic antibiotics for patients with hip and knee prosthetic joint implants undergoing dental procedures" [69]. The Arthroplasty Society of Australia released a position statement in 2016 that echoes the recommendation from AAOS. The recommendation from this report is that "no routine antibiotic prophylaxis be given to patients with joint prostheses undergoing dental procedures" [70]. The second recommendation of this report is that patients who are immunocompromised or who have poor oral hygiene should be assessed on a case-by-case basis. A large study from Taiwan with a cohort of 255,568 patients who underwent THA or TKA were divided into dental and nondental cohorts based on whether the patients had undergone a dental procedure within the first 2 years following arthroplasty. There was no difference in the incidence of PJI between the cohorts, with a rate of 0.57% in the dental cohort and 0.61% in the nondental cohort [71]. Cost-effectiveness modelling has also been done to compare the benefits, harms and cost of prophylactic antibiotic dosing with dental proce-

dures, and has shown that routine antibiotic prophylaxis is not cost-effective for dental procedures, but might be in the higher risk population [72].

Common sense suggests that any dental issues should be dealt with prior to arthroplasty surgery. Vuorinen et al. showed that 29.4% of patients who underwent dental screening prior to joint arthroplasty did not pass dental clearance and proceeded to dental procedures prior to their arthroplasty [73]. Sonn et al., however, showed in a retrospective review that patients with poor oral hygiene do not have an increased risk of PJI, and so concluded that routine dental clearance was not necessary [74].

24.2.1.7 Hypothyroidism

Hypothyroidism has recently been shown to be associated with an increased risk of PJI [75, 76]. Buller et al. [75] found an odds ratio of 1.502 for developing a PJI in the first 90 days post TKA in patients with hypothyroidism. This study had 98,555 gender and age matched cohorts retrospectively reviewed from US Medicare patients who underwent a primary TKA. This study is supported by a paper by Tan et al. [76] who looked at 32,289 patients who underwent primary or revision TKA or THA and found hypothyroidism to be an independent risk factor for PJI with an adjusted odds ratio of 2.46 ($p < 0.0001$). Thyroid stimulating hormone (TSH) levels were also significantly higher in the patients who developed PJI [76]. We recommend consultation of an endocrinologist to optimize a patients' serum thyroid stimulating hormone levels prior to surgery.

24.2.1.8 Preoperative Anaemia

Preoperative pathology is routinely recommended including haematology and biochemistry. Included in these studies should be evaluation of iron levels as well as haemoglobin. Anaemia is defined as haemoglobin level of less than 12 g/dL in women and less than 13 g/dL in men by the World Health Organization. The rate of preoperative anaemia in patients undergoing THA or TKA is 15–33% [77]. Preoperative anaemia has been associated with both an increased risk for developing a PJI, as well as failure of a debridement and polyethylene exchange (DAIR) in acute haematogenous PJI [77–80]. Allogenic blood transfusion has been shown to increase the risk of post-operative infections [81] and PJI [5]. Greenky et al. [77] found 19.6% of 15,222 patients undergoing a total joint arthroplasty (TJA) had anaemia, and the incidence of PJI in this group was 4.3% vs. 2% in the non-anaemic cohort. Allogenic blood transfusions were required in 44% of the anaemic cohort and 13.4% in the non-anaemic cohort [77]. Swenson et al. demonstrated that a preoperative haematocrit $\leq$32.1 had an odds ratio of 6.7% in predicting failure for open debridement and polyethylene exchange in THA or TKA with PJI from acute haematogenous spread [80]. Some centres prefer to optimize patients' level of haemoglobin and any iron deficiency prior to TKA.

24.2.1.9 Drug and Alcohol Abuse

Substance abuse disorder and alcohol abuse disorder have been shown to be independent risk factors for PJI [82]. In a study looking at 11,403 TKA, multivariate analyses showed the odds ratio was 19.419 for alcohol abuse disorder and 3.693 for substance abuse disorder and the development of PJI. When substance abuse disorder and depression were present in the same patient, the odds ratio for PJI increased to 13.639, a fourfold increase [82]. Bauer et al. [83] retrospectively reviewed 18 TKA performed in 12 patients who had a history of intravenous opioid abuse. An alarmingly high rate of PJI was found at 50%, nine knees in seven patients, with three knees requiring above knee amputation and a further three knees ending with arthrodesis [83].

24.2.1.10 Human Immunodeficiency Virus

The literature on whether a human immunodeficiency virus (HIV) positive patient has an increased risk of PJI is mixed. Parvizi et al. in a 2003 study showed an alarmingly high rate of post-operative complications, including six deep joint infections (29%) [84]. In this study, the average CD4 count was 239 cells/mm^3 for patients who had a PJI compared to 523 cells/

mm^3 in the overall study population. Only 3 patients out of the 15 in the study were on highly active antiretroviral therapy (HAART) at the time of arthroplasty [84]. A similarly high deep infection rate of 14.3% was found in a 2001 study in HIV positive patients, but the CD4 counts and whether the patients were on HAART were not disclosed [85]. A systematic review by Dimitriou et al. [86] of 6,516,186 TKA and THA revealed an elevated risk of complications but no difference in long-term survivorship of the implants. It is unfortunate that this review did not analyse infection risk but rather overall complication rate. Boylan et al. [87] showed that survivorship of TKR in a HIV cohort in comparison to a non-HIV cohort was no different, and importantly showed no deep infections in either cohort. These findings were supported by Roof et al. [88] PJI was found to be higher in patients who had both HIV and haemophilia than in patients who had HIV and no haemophilia with an odds ratio of 5.28 [89]. Issa et al. [90] showed that patients with HIV infection have TKA survivorship similar to that of patients who do not suffer from HIV infection. Patients in their study cohort had CD4 count >200 at the time of surgery and were on active treatment with two nucleotide reverse transcriptase inhibitors and one protease or integrase inhibitor which was continued in the perioperative and post-operative period along with the usual prophylactic antibiotic cover. It is possible that the earlier papers found a higher rate of PJI simply due to the lack of HAART treatment in their cohort of patients, as HAART only began to be used in 1997 [91]. Ensuring that a HIV positive patient has appropriate CD4 count prior to surgery may be a useful strategy to avoid post-operative complications particularly PJI after TKA in patients suffering from HIV infections.

24.2.1.11 Hepatitis C Infection

Patients with hepatitis C virus (HCV) have a higher risk of complications, including PJI, when undergoing TKA [92–95]. Schwarzkopf et al. [96] in their recent study showed that patients with hepatitis C infection should receive perioperative treatment for the infection to decrease the chance of PJI after TKA. This retrospective review of patients with either cured HCV infection or untreated HCV infection showed that the untreated cohort had significantly higher infection rate (15.5% vs. 4.3% with odds ratio 4.1; $p = 0.03$) [96]. This study is supported by another two studies published in 2019 [97, 98]. Bedair et al. studied the effect of treated HCV compared to untreated HCV in THA and demonstrated the rate of PJI was 14.3% in patients who had untreated HCV and 0% in those who had been treated [97]. Bendich et al. did a similar study looking at treated compared to untreated HCV in patients undergoing either THA or TKA and showed an odds ratio of 3.30 for PJI in untreated patients at 90 days post-operative and 2.16 at 1 year post-operative [98]. These studies suggest that treatment of HCV should be undertaken prior to proceeding with TKA to decrease the risk of PJI.

24.2.1.12 Nasal colonization with S. aureus

Various studies have reported the benefits for screening patients for asymptomatic colonization with methicillin resistant (MRSA) or methicillin sensitive staphylococcus aureus (MSSA) organisms [99–106]. Anterior nares serve as the reservoir for staphylococcus organisms as well as the groin and axillae. Methicillin sensitive staphylococcus organisms are present in anterior nares of 20–30% of orthopaedic patients and methicillin resistant staphylococcus organisms are present in 2–6% of pre-op patients for TKA [103]. Surgical site infection after TJA is caused by MSSA or MRSA in >60% of patients [107]. Nasal decolonization of MSSA and MRSA can be done through twice daily application of mupirocin for 5 days prior to surgery [108]. Decolonizing patients who are positive with staphylococcus aureus helps to decrease the incidence of surgical site complications in total arthroplasty patients [99, 101, 102, 104–106]. Another added benefit for the preoperative screening is that it acts as a guide for choice of prophylactic antibiotic for surgery. If the patient is colonized with MSSA, routine antibiotics may be used. If a patient is colonized with MRSA, weight-based vancomycin is the appropriate choice [109]. Some centres provide nasal decolonization empirically to all the preoperative patients undergoing TKA and do not rely on the results of the swab analyses. Patients may also be prescribed with betadine shower and chlorhexidine wipes or shower prior to surgery, which is an additional useful strategy if patients have skin or axillary/groin colonization with staphylococcus aureus.

24.2.1.13 Immunosuppression

Organ transplantation patients are known to require immunosuppression after receiving their transplantation and so are thought to be an at-risk group for developing PJI if they go on to require an arthroplasty. Palmisano et al. [110] did a retrospective review looking at patients who had had a solid organ transplantation and subsequently went on to have a THA or TKA. These patients were on different combinations of anti-rejection medications including azathioprine, mycophenolate, cyclosporine, prednisone and tacrolimus. There were three deep infections recorded out of the seven TKAs that were performed, giving a deep infection rate of 42.9% [110].

24.3 Conclusion

There are many potentially modifiable host risk factors which should be identified and addressed prior to TKA to minimize the risk of PJI. Screening should be performed 4–6 weeks prior to planned surgery to avoid the difficult decision for the clinician and the patient to postpone surgery in the anaesthetic bay. The time to identify a potentially modifiable risk factor is well prior to TKA. Involving the patient in the decision-making process by making the patient aware of the available options to optimize the risk factors prior to TKA is appropriate and to proceed with TKA when the patient is in as good a condition as is possible. Patients should be made aware that without optimization there is an increased chance of suffering from a PJI. The surgeon has an important role to identify the potentially modifiable risk factors of PJI prior to TKA and make every effort to optimize before surgery. A balanced clinical decision requires respect for the patients' autonomy at the same time acting in their best interests to do no harm (Non-maleficence). This will minimize length of stay and additional surgical procedures for wound problems after joint arthroplasty and reduce readmission rates to avoid financial constraints on the healthcare providers.

References

1. Australian Orthopaedic Association National Joint Replacement Registry; 2019. www.aoa.org.au.
2. 16th Annual report. 2019. www.njrreports.org.uk.
3. The New Zealand Joint Registry: twenty year report January 1999 to December 2019. 2020. www.nzoa.org.nz/nz-joint-registry.
4. Kurtz SM, Ong KL, Lau E, Bozic KJ, Berry D, Parvizi J. Prosthetic joint infection risk after TKA in the medicare population. In: Clinical orthopaedics and related research, vol. 468. New York: Springer; 2010. p. 52–6. https://doi.org/10.1007/s11999-009-1013-5.
5. Pulido L, Ghanem E, Joshi A, Purtill JJ, Parvizi J. Periprosthetic joint infection: the incidence, timing, and predisposing factors. Clin Orthop Relat Res. 2008;466(7):1710–5. https://doi.org/10.1007/s11999-008-0209-4.
6. Ong KL, Lau E, Suggs J, Kurtz SM, Manley MT. Risk of subsequent revision after primary and revision total joint arthroplasty. Clin Orthop Relat Res. 2010;468(11):3070–6. https://doi.org/10.1007/s11999-010-1399-0.
7. Bozic KJ, Kamath AF, Ong K, et al. Comparative epidemiology of revision arthroplasty: failed THA poses greater clinical and economic burdens than failed TKA. Clin Orthop Relat Res. 2015;473(6):2131–8. https://doi.org/10.1007/s11999-014-4078-8.
8. Kurtz SM, Ong KL, Lau E, Bozic KJ. Impact of the economic downturn on total joint replacement demand in the United States: updated projections to 2021. J Bone Joint Surg (Am Vol). 2014;96(8):624–30. https://doi.org/10.2106/JBJS.M.00285.
9. Kurtz SM, Lau E, Ong K, Zhao K, Kelly M, Bozic KJ. Future young patient demand for primary and revision joint replacement: national projections from 2010 to 2030. In: Clinical orthopaedics and related research, vol. 467. New York: Springer; 2009. p. 2606–12. https://doi.org/10.1007/s11999-009-0834-6.
10. Kurtz S, Ong K, Lau E, Mowat F, Halpern M. Projections of primary and revision hip and knee arthroplasty in the United States from 2005 to 2030. J Bone Joint Surg A. 2007;89(4):780–5. https://doi.org/10.2106/JBJS.F.00222.
11. Bozic KJ, Kurtz SM, Lau E, et al. The epidemiology of revision total knee arthroplasty in the United States. In: Clinical orthopaedics and related research, vol. 468. New York: Springer; 2010. p. 45–51. https://doi.org/10.1007/s11999-009-0945-0.
12. Tan TL, Maltenfort MG, Chen AF, et al. Development and evaluation of a preoperative risk calculator for periprosthetic joint infection following total joint arthroplasty. J Bone Joint Surg (Am Vol). 2018;100(9):777–85. https://doi.org/10.2106/JBJS.16.01435.
13. Zmistowski B, Karam JA, Durinka JB, Casper DS, Parvizi J. Periprosthetic joint infection increases the risk of one-year mortality. J Bone Joint Surg Am. 2013;95(24):2177–84. https://doi.org/10.2106/JBJS.L.00789.
14. Choi HR, Bedair H. Mortality following revision total knee arthroplasty: a matched cohort study of septic versus aseptic revisions. J Arthroplasty. 2014;29(6):1216–8. https://doi.org/10.1016/j.arth.2013.11.026.
15. Ravi B, Croxford R, Hollands S, et al. Increased risk of complications following total joint arthroplasty in patients with rheumatoid arthritis. Arthritis Rheumatol. 2014;66(2):254–63. https://doi.org/10.1002/art.38231.
16. Lin JA, Liao CC, Lee YJ, Wu CH, Huang WQ, Chen TL. Adverse outcomes after major surgery in patients with systemic lupus erythematosus: a nationwide population-based study. Ann Rheum Dis. 2014;73(9):1646–51. https://doi.org/10.1136/annrheumdis-2012-202758.
17. Singh JA, Inacio MCS, Namba RS, Paxton EW. Rheumatoid arthritis is associated with higher ninety-day hospital readmission rates compared to osteoarthritis after hip or knee arthroplasty: a cohort study. Arthritis Care Res. 2015;67(5):718–24. https://doi.org/10.1002/acr.22497.
18. Schrama JC, Espehaug B, Hallan G, et al. Risk of revision for infection in primary total hip and knee arthroplasty in patients with rheumatoid arthritis compared with osteoarthritis: a prospective, population-based study on 108,786 hip and knee joint arthroplasties from the Norwegian Arthroplasty Register. Arthritis Care Res. 2010;62(4):473–9. https://doi.org/10.1002/acr.20036.
19. Jämsen E, Huhtala H, Puolakka T, Moilanen T. Risk factors for infection after knee arthroplasty a register-based analysis of 43,149 cases. J Bone Joint Surg Am. 2009;91(1):38–47. https://doi.org/10.2106/JBJS.G.01686.
20. Aly R, Maibach HI, Mandel A. Bacterial flora in psoriasis. Br J Dermatol. 1976;95(6):603–6.
21. Lynfield YL. Bacteria, skin sterilization, and wound healing in psoriasis. N Y State J Med. 1972;72(11):1247–50.
22. Stern SH, Insall JN, Windsor RE, Inglis AE, Dines DM. Total knee arthroplasty in patients with psoriasis. Clin Orthop Relat Res. 1989;248:108–10.
23. Beyer CA, Hanssen AD, Lewallen D, Pittelkow MR. Primary total knee arthroplasty patients with psoriasis. J Bone Joint Surg Br. 1991;73:258–9.

24. Menon T, Wroblewski B. Charnley low-friction arthroplasty in patients with psoriasis. Clin Orthop Relat Res. 1983;176(June):127–8.

25. Goodman SM, Johnson B, Zhang M, et al. Patients with rheumatoid arthritis have similar excellent outcomes after total knee replacement compared with patients with osteoarthritis. J Rheumatol. 2016;43(1):46–53. https://doi.org/10.3899/jrheum.150525.

26. LoVerde ZJ, Mandl LA, Johnson BK, et al. Rheumatoid arthritis does not increase risk of short-term adverse events after total knee arthroplasty: a retrospective case-control study. J Rheumatol. 2015;42(7):1123–30. https://doi.org/10.3899/jrheum.141251.

27. Johnson BK, Goodman SM, Alexiades MM, Figgie MP, Demmer RT, Mandl LA. Patterns and associated risk of perioperative use of anti-tumor necrosis factor in patients with rheumatoid arthritis undergoing total knee replacement. J Rheumatol. 2013;40(5):617–23. https://doi.org/10.3899/jrheum.121171.

28. Goodman SM, Springer B, Guyatt G, et al. 2017 American College of Rheumatology/American Association of hip and Knee Surgeons Guideline for the perioperative management of antirheumatic medication in patients with rheumatic diseases undergoing elective total hip or total knee arthroplasty. Arthritis Rheumatol. 2017;69(8):1538–51. https://doi.org/10.1002/art.40149.

29. Bombardier C, Hazlewood GS, Akhavan P, et al. Canadian rheumatology association recommendations for the pharmacological management of rheumatoid arthritis with traditional and biologic disease-modifying antirheumatic drugs: part II safety. J Rheumatol. 2012;39(8):1583–602. https://doi.org/10.3899/jrheum.120165.

30. Iorio R, Williams KM, Marcantonio AJ, Specht LM, Tilzey JF, Healy WL. Diabetes mellitus, hemoglobin A1C, and the incidence of total joint arthroplasty infection. J Arthroplasty. 2012;27(5):726. https://doi.org/10.1016/j.arth.2011.09.013.

31. Jämsen E, Nevalainen P, Eskelinen A, Huotari K, Kalliovalkama J, Moilanen T. Obesity, diabetes, and preoperative hyperglycemia as predictors of periprosthetic joint infection: A single-center analysis of 7181 primary hip and knee replacements for osteoarthritis. J Bone Joint Surg Am. 2012;94(14):e101(1). https://doi.org/10.2106/JBJS.J.01935.

32. Stryker LS, Abdel MP, Morrey ME, Morrow MM, Kor DJ, Morrey BF. Elevated postoperative blood glucose and preoperative hemoglobin a1c are associated with increased wound complications following total joint arthroplasty. J Bone Joint Surg Am. 2013;95(9):808–14. https://doi.org/10.2106/JBJS.L.00494.

33. Tarabichi M, Shohat N, Kheir MM, et al. Determining the threshold for HbA1c as a predictor for adverse outcomes after total joint arthroplasty: a multicenter, retrospective study. J Arthroplasty. 2017;32(9):S263–S267.e1. https://doi.org/10.1016/j.arth.2017.04.065.

34. Adams AL, Paxton EW, Wang JQ, et al. Surgical outcomes of total knee replacement according to diabetes status and glycemic control, 2001 to 2009. J Bone Joint Surg Am. 2013;95(6):481–7. https://doi.org/10.2106/JBJS.L.00109.

35. Chrastil J, Anderson MB, Stevens V, Anand R, Peters CL, Pelt CE. Is hemoglobin A1c or perioperative hyperglycemia predictive of periprosthetic joint infection or death following primary total joint arthroplasty? J Arthroplasty. 2015;30(7):1197–202. https://doi.org/10.1016/j.arth.2015.01.040.

36. Springer BD. Modifying risk factors for total joint arthroplasty: strategies that work nicotine. J Arthroplasty. 2016;31(8):1628–30. https://doi.org/10.1016/j.arth.2016.01.071.

37. Singh JA, Schleck C, Harmsen WS, Jacob AK, Warner DO, Lewallen DG. Current tobacco use is associated with higher rates of implant revision and deep infection after total hip or knee arthroplasty: a prospective cohort study. BMC Med. 2015;13(1):283. https://doi.org/10.1186/s12916-015-0523-0.

38. Duchman KR, Gao Y, Pugely AJ, Martin CT, Noiseux NO, Callaghan JJ. The effect of smoking on short-term complications following total hip and knee arthroplasty. J Bone Joint Surg (Am Vol). 2014;97(13):1049–58. https://doi.org/10.2106/JBJS.N.01016.

39. Jørgensen CC, Kehlet H. Outcomes in smokers and alcohol users after fast-track hip and knee arthroplasty. Acta Anaesthesiol Scand. 2013;57(5):631–8. https://doi.org/10.1111/aas.12086.

40. Kapadia BH, Johnson AJ, Naziri Q, Mont MA, Delanois RE, Bonutti PM. Increased revision rates after total knee arthroplasty in patients who smoke. J Arthroplasty. 2012;27(9):1690. https://doi.org/10.1016/j.arth.2012.03.057.

41. Singh JA, Houston TK, Ponce BA, et al. Smoking as a risk factor for short-term outcomes following primary total hip and total knee replacement in veterans. Arthritis Care Res. 2011;63(10):1365–74. https://doi.org/10.1002/acr.20555.

42. Fini M, Giavaresi G, Salamanna F, et al. Harmful lifestyles on orthopedic implantation surgery: a descriptive review on alcohol and tobacco use. J Bone Miner Metab. 2011;29(6):633–44. https://doi.org/10.1007/s00774-011-0309-1.

43. Porter S, Hanley E. The musculoskeletal effects of smoking. J Am Acad Orthop Surg. 2001;9(1):9–17.

44. Velicer WF, Prochaska JO, Rossi JS, Snow MG. Assessing outcome in smoking cessation studies. Psychol Bull. 1992;Ill(1):23–41.

45. Benowitz NL, Bernert JT, Caraballo RS, Holiday DB, Wang J. Optimal serum cotinine levels for distinguishing cigarette smokers and nonsmokers within different racial/ethnic groups in the United States between 1999 and 2004. Am J Epidemiol. 2009;169(2):236–48. https://doi.org/10.1093/aje/kwn301.

46. Friedman RJ, Hess S, Berkowitz SD, Homering M. Complication rates after hip or knee arthroplasty in morbidly obese patients. Clin Orthop Relat Res.

2013;471(10):3358–66. https://doi.org/10.1007/s11999-013-3049-9.

47. Alvi HM, Mednick RE, Krishnan V, Kwasny MJ, Beal MD, Manning DW. The effect of BMI on 30 day outcomes following total joint arthroplasty. J Arthroplasty. 2015;30(7):1113–7. https://doi.org/10.1016/j.arth.2015.01.049.

48. Watts CD, Wagner ER, Houdek MT, Lewallen DG, Mabry TM. Morbid obesity: increased risk of failure after aseptic revision TKA. Clin Orthop Relat Res. 2015;473(8):2621–7. https://doi.org/10.1007/s11999-015-4283-0.

49. Ward DT, Metz LN, Horst PK, Kim HT, Kuo AC. Complications of morbid obesity in total joint arthroplasty: risk stratification based on BMI. J Arthroplasty. 2015;30(9):42–6. https://doi.org/10.1016/j.arth.2015.03.045.

50. Wagner ER, Kamath AF, Fruth K, Harmsen WS, Berry DJ. Effect of body mass index on reoperation and complications after total knee arthroplasty. J Bone Joint Surg (Am Vol). 2016;98(24):2052–60. https://doi.org/10.2106/JBJS.16.00093.

51. Liabaud B, Patrick DA, Geller JA. Higher body mass index leads to longer operative time in total knee arthroplasty. J Arthroplasty. 2013;28(4):563–5. https://doi.org/10.1016/j.arth.2012.07.037.

52. Ghanim H, Aljada A, Hofmeyer D, Syed T, Mohanty P, Dandona P. Circulating mononuclear cells in the obese are in a proinflammatory state. Circulation. 2004;110(12):1564–71. https://doi.org/10.1161/01.CIR.0000142055.53122.FA.

53. Peterson LA, Cheskin LJ, Furtado M, et al. Malnutrition in bariatric surgery candidates: multiple micronutrient deficiencies prior to surgery. Obes Surg. 2016;26(4):833–8. https://doi.org/10.1007/s11695-015-1844-y.

54. Inacio MCS, Paxton EW, Fisher D, Li RA, Barber TC, Singh JA. Bariatric surgery prior to total joint arthroplasty may not provide dramatic improvements in post-arthroplasty surgical outcomes. J Arthroplasty. 2014;29(7):1359–64. https://doi.org/10.1016/j.arth.2014.02.021.

55. Inacio MCS, Kritz-Silverstein D, Raman R, et al. The impact of pre-operative weight loss on incidence of surgical site infection and readmission rates after total joint arthroplasty. J Arthroplasty. 2014;29(3):458. https://doi.org/10.1016/j.arth.2013.07.030.

56. Malinzak RA, Ritter MA, Berend ME, Meding JB, Olberding EM, Davis KE. Morbidly obese, diabetic, younger, and unilateral joint arthroplasty patients have elevated total joint arthroplasty infection rates. J Arthroplasty. 2009;24(6 Suppl):84–8. https://doi.org/10.1016/j.arth.2009.05.016.

57. Rondon AJ, Kheir MM, Tan TL, Shohat N, Greenky MR, Parvizi J. Cefazolin prophylaxis for total joint arthroplasty: obese patients are frequently under-dosed and at increased risk of periprosthetic joint infection. J Arthroplasty. 2018;33(11):3551–4. https://doi.org/10.1016/j.arth.2018.06.037.

58. Kulkarni A, Jameson SS, James P, Woodcock S, Muller S, Reed MR. Does bariatric surgery prior to lower limb joint replacement reduce complications? Surgeon. 2011;9(1):18–21. https://doi.org/10.1016/j.surge.2010.08.004.

59. Severson EP, Singh JA, Browne JA, Trousdale RT, Sarr MG, Lewallen DG. Total knee arthroplasty in morbidly obese patients treated with bariatric surgery. A comparative study. J Arthroplasty. 2012;27(9):1696–700. https://doi.org/10.1016/j.arth.2012.03.005.

60. Parvizi J, Trousdale RT, Sarr MG. Total joint arthroplasty in patients surgically treated for morbid obesity. J Arthroplasty. 2000;15(8):1003–8. https://doi.org/10.1054/arth.2000.9054.

61. Hansen E, Belden K, Silibovsky R, et al. Perioperative antibiotics. J Arthroplasty. 2014;29(2 SUPPL):29–48. https://doi.org/10.1016/j.arth.2013.09.030.

62. Bratzler DW, Dellinger EP, Olsen KM, et al. Clinical practice guidelines for antimicrobial prophylaxis in surgery. Surg Infect. 2013;14(1):73–156. https://doi.org/10.1089/sur.2013.9999.

63. Jaberi FM, Parvizi J, Haytmanek CT, Joshi A, Purtill J. Procrastination of wound drainage and malnutrition affect the outcome of joint arthroplasty. Clin Orthop Relat Res. 2008;466(6):1368–71. https://doi.org/10.1007/s11999-008-0214-7.

64. Greene KA, Wilde AH, Stulberg BN. Preoperative nutritional status of total joint patients relationship to postoperative wound complications. J Arthroplasty. 1991;6(4):321–5.

65. Peersman G, Laskin R, Davis J, Peterson M. Infection in Total Knee Replacement: A Retrospective Review Of 6489 Total Knee Replacements. Clin Orthop Relat Res. 2001;392:15–23.

66. Font-Vizcarra L, Lozano L, Ríos J, Forga MT, Soriano A. Preoperative nutritional status and postoperative infection in total knee replacements: a prospective study of 213 patients. Int J Artif Organs. 2011;34(9):876–81. https://doi.org/10.5301/ijao.5000025.

67. Wang C, Huang W, Gu Y, et al. Effect of urinary tract infection on the risk of prosthetic joint infection: a systematic review and meta-analysis. Surgeon. 2020; https://doi.org/10.1016/j.surge.2020.04.010.

68. Schmitt DR, Schneider AM, Brown NM. Impact of perioperative urinary tract infection on surgical site infection in patients undergoing primary hip and knee arthroplasty. J Arthroplasty. 2020; https://doi.org/10.1016/j.arth.2020.05.025.

69. Watters III W, Rethman MP, et al., American Academy of Orthopaedic Surgeons and American Dental Association. Prevention of orthopaedic implant infection in patients undergoing dental procedures. Evidence based guideline and evidence report; 2013. AAOS Clinical Practice Guideline Unit v0.2 2.2012.

70. Australian Arthroplasty Society Position Statement on the use of prophylactic antibiotics for dental procedures in patients with prosthetic joints. https://www.aoa.org.au/about-aoa/subspecialties/arthroplasty.

71. Kao FC, Hsu YC, Chen WH, Lin JN, Lo YY, Tu YK. Prosthetic joint infection following invasive dental procedures and antibiotic prophylaxis in patients with hip or knee arthroplasty. Infect Control Hosp Epidemiol. 2017;38(2):154–61. https://doi.org/10.1017/ice.2016.248.

72. Skaar DD, Park T, Swiontkowski MF, Kuntz KM. Is antibiotic prophylaxis cost-effective for dental patients following total knee arthroplasty? JDR Clin Transl Res. 2019;4(1):9–18. https://doi.org/10.1177/2380084418808724.

73. Vuorinen M, Mäkinen T, Rantasalo M, Leskinen J, Välimaa H, Huotari K. Incidence and risk factors for dental pathology in patients planned for elective total hip or knee arthroplasty. Scand J Surg. 2019;108(4):338–42. https://doi.org/10.1177/1457496918816911.

74. Sonn KA, Larsen CG, Adams W, Brown NM, McAsey CJ. Effect of preoperative dental extraction on postoperative complications after total joint arthroplasty. J Arthroplasty. 2019;34(9):2080–4. https://doi.org/10.1016/j.arth.2019.04.056.

75. Buller LT, Rosas S, Sabeh KG, Roche MW, McLawhorn AS, Barsoum WK. Hypothyroidism increases 90-day complications and costs following primary total knee arthroplasty. J Arthroplasty. 2018;33(4):1003–7. https://doi.org/10.1016/j.arth.2017.10.053.

76. Tan TL, Rajeswaran H, Haddad S, Shahi A, Parvizi J. Increased risk of periprosthetic joint infections in patients with hypothyroidism undergoing total joint arthroplasty. J Arthroplasty. 2016;31(4):868–71. https://doi.org/10.1016/j.arth.2015.10.028.

77. Greenky M, Gandhi K, Pulido L, Restrepo C, Parvizi J. Preoperative anemia in total joint arthroplasty: is it associated with periprosthetic joint infection? Hip Clin Orthop Relat Res. 2012;470(10):2695–701. https://doi.org/10.1007/s11999-012-2435-z.

78. Lee Q, Mak W, Wong Y. Risk factors for periprosthetic joint infection in total knee arthroplasty. J Orthop Surg. 2015;23(3):282–6.

79. Marmor S, Kerroumi Y. Patient-specific risk factors for infection in arthroplasty procedure. Orthop Traumatol Surg Res. 2016;102(1):S113–9. https://doi.org/10.1016/j.otsr.2015.05.012.

80. Swenson RD, Butterfield JA, Irwin TJ, Zurlo JJ, Davis CM. Preoperative anemia is associated with failure of open debridement polyethylene exchange in acute and acute hematogenous prosthetic joint infection. J Arthroplasty. 2018;33(6):1855–60. https://doi.org/10.1016/j.arth.2018.01.042.

81. Marik P. The hazards of blood transfusion. Br J Hosp Med. 2009;70(1):12–5.

82. Gold PA, Garbarino LJ, Anis HK, et al. The cumulative effect of substance abuse disorders and depression on postoperative complications after primary total knee arthroplasty. J Arthroplasty. 2020;35(6):S151–7. https://doi.org/10.1016/j.arth.2020.01.027.

83. Bauer DE, Hingsammer A, Ernstbrunner L, et al. Total knee arthroplasty in patients with a history of illicit intravenous drug abuse. Int Orthop. 2018;42(1):101–7. https://doi.org/10.1007/s00264-017-3655-3.

84. Parvizi J, Sullivan TA, Pagnano MW, Trousdale RT, Bolander ME. Total joint arthroplasty in human immunodeficiency virus-positive patients: an alarming rate of early failure. J Arthroplasty. 2003;18(3):259–64. https://doi.org/10.1054/arth.2003.50094.

85. Lehman CR, Ries MD, Paiement GD, Davidson AB. Infection after total joint arthroplasty in patients with human immunodeficiency virus or intravenous drug use. J Arthroplasty. 2001;16(3):330–5. https://doi.org/10.1054/arth.2001.21454.

86. Dimitriou D, Ramokgopa M, Pietrzak JRT, van der Jagt D, Mokete L. Human immunodeficiency virus infection and hip and knee arthroplasty. JBJS Rev. 2017;5(9):e8. https://doi.org/10.2106/JBJS.RVW.17.00029.

87. Boylan MR, Basu N, Naziri Q, Issa K, Maheshwari AV, Mont MA. Does HIV infection increase the risk of short-term adverse outcomes following total knee arthroplasty? J Arthroplasty. 2015;30(9):1629–32. https://doi.org/10.1016/j.arth.2015.03.018.

88. Roof MA, Anoushiravani AA, Chen KK, et al. Outcomes of total knee arthroplasty in human immunodeficiency virus-positive patients. J Knee Surg. 2020;33(8):754–61. https://doi.org/10.1055/s-0039-1684011.

89. Enayatollahi MA, Murphy D, Maltenfort MG, Parvizi J. Human immunodeficiency virus and total joint arthroplasty: the risk for infection is reduced. J Arthroplasty. 2016;31(10):2146–51. https://doi.org/10.1016/j.arth.2016.02.058.

90. Issa K, Pierce TP, Harwin SF, Scillia AJ, Festa A, Mont MA. No decrease in knee survivorship or outcomes scores for patients with HIV infection who undergo TKA. Clin Orthop Relat Res. 2017;475(2):465–71. https://doi.org/10.1007/s11999-016-5122-7.

91. Shah KN, Truntzer JN, Romo FT, Rubin LE. Total joint arthroplasty in patients with human immunodeficiency virus. JBJS Rev. 2016;4(11):e1. https://doi.org/10.2106/JBJS.RVW.15.00117.

92. Kildow BJ, Politzer CS, DiLallo M, Bolognesi MP, Seyler TM. Short and long-term postoperative complications following total joint arthroplasty in patients with human immunodeficiency virus, hepatitis B, or hepatitis C. J Arthroplasty. 2018;33(7):S86–S92.e1. https://doi.org/10.1016/j.arth.2017.10.061.

93. Orozco F, Post ZD, Baxi O, Miller A, Ong A. Fibrosis in hepatitis c patients predicts complications after elective total joint arthroplasty. J Arthroplasty. 2014;29(1):7–10. https://doi.org/10.1016/j.arth.2013.03.023.

94. Cancienne JM, Kandahari AM, Casp A, et al. Complication rates after total hip and knee arthro-

plasty in patients with hepatitis C compared with matched control patients. J Am Acad Orthop Surg. 2017;25(12):e275–81. https://doi.org/10.5435/JAAOS-D-16-00920.

95. Chowdhury R, Chaudhary MA, Sturgeon DJ, et al. The impact of hepatitis C virus infection on 90-day outcomes following major orthopaedic surgery: a propensity-matched analysis. Arch Orthop Trauma Surg. 2017;137(9):1181–6. https://doi.org/10.1007/s00402-017-2742-7.

96. Schwarzkopf R, Novikov D, Anoushiravani AA, et al. The preoperative management of hepatitis C may improve the outcome after total knee arthroplasty. Bone Joint J. 2019;101-B:667–74. https://doi.org/10.1302/0301-620X.101B6.

97. Bedair HS, Schurko BM, Dwyer MK, Novikov D, Anoushiravani AA, Schwarzkopf R. Treatment for chronic hepatitis C prior to total hip arthroplasty significantly reduces periprosthetic joint infection. J Arthroplasty. 2019;34(1):132–5. https://doi.org/10.1016/j.arth.2018.09.036.

98. Bendich I, Takemoto S, Patterson JT, Monto A, Barber TC, Kuo AC. Preoperative treatment of hepatitis C is associated with lower prosthetic joint infection rates in US veterans. J Arthroplasty. 2019;34(7):S319–S326.e1. https://doi.org/10.1016/j.arth.2019.02.052.

99. Stambough JB, Nam D, Warren DK, et al. Decreased hospital costs and surgical site infection incidence with a universal decolonization protocol in primary total joint arthroplasty. J Arthroplasty. 2017;32(3):728–734.e1. https://doi.org/10.1016/j.arth.2016.09.041.

100. Ramos N, Stachel A, Phillips M, Vigdorchik J, Slover J, Bosco JA. Prior staphylococcus aureus nasal colonization: a risk factor for surgical site infections following decolonization. J Am Acad Orthop Surg. 2016;24(12):880–5. https://doi.org/10.5435/JAAOS-D-16-00165.

101. Goyal N, Aggarwal V, Parvizi J. Methicillin-resistant Staphylococcus Aureus screening in total joint arthroplasty: a worthwhile endeavor. J Knee Surg. 2011;25(1):37–44. https://doi.org/10.1055/s-0031-1286194.

102. Romero-Palacios A, Petruccelli D, Main C, Winemaker M, de Beer J, Mertz D. Screening for and decolonization of Staphylococcus aureus carriers before total joint replacement is associated with lower S aureus prosthetic joint infection rates.

Am J Infect Control. 2020;48(5):534–7. https://doi.org/10.1016/j.ajic.2019.09.022.

103. Kerbel YE, Sunkerneni AR, Kirchner GJ, Prodromo JP, Moretti VM. The cost-effectiveness of preoperative Staphylococcus aureus screening and decolonization in total joint arthroplasty. J Arthroplasty. 2018;33(7):S191–5. https://doi.org/10.1016/j.arth.2018.01.032.

104. Pelfort X, Romero A, Brugués M, García A, Gil S, Marrón A. Reduction of periprosthetic Staphylococcus aureus infection by preoperative screening and decolonization of nasal carriers undergoing total knee arthroplasty. Acta Orthop Traumatol Turc. 2019;53(6):426–31. https://doi.org/10.1016/j.aott.2019.08.014.

105. Sporer SM, Rogers T, Abella L. Methicillin-resistant and methicillin-sensitive Staphylococcus aureus screening and decolonization to reduce surgical site infection in elective total joint arthroplasty. J Arthroplasty. 2016;31(9):144–7. https://doi.org/10.1016/j.arth.2016.05.019.

106. Hacek DM, Robb WJ, Paule SM, Kudrna JC, Stamos VP, Peterson LR. Staphylococcus aureus nasal decolonization in joint replacement surgery reduces infection. Clin Orthop Relat Res. 2008;466(6):1349–55. https://doi.org/10.1007/s11999-008-0210-y.

107. Walsh AL, Fields AC, Dieterich JD, Chen DD, Bronson MJ, Moucha CS. Risk factors for Staphylococcus aureus nasal colonization in joint arthroplasty patients. J Arthroplasty. 2018;33(5):1530–3. https://doi.org/10.1016/j.arth.2017.12.038.

108. Kim DH, Spencer M, Davidson SM, et al. Institutional prescreening for detection and eradication of methicillin-resistant Staphylococcus aureus in patients undergoing elective orthopaedic surgery. J Bone Joint Surg Am. 2010;92(9):1820–6. https://doi.org/10.2106/JBJS.I.01050.

109. Iorio R, Osmani FA. Strategies to prevent periprosthetic joint infection after total knee arthroplasty and lessen the risk of readmission for the patient. J Am Acad Orthop Surg. 2017;25:S13–6. https://doi.org/10.5435/JAAOS-D-16-00635.

110. Palmisano AC, Kuhn AW, Urquhart AG, Pour AE. Post-operative medical and surgical complications after primary total joint arthroplasty in solid organ transplant recipients: a case series. Int Orthop. 2017;41(1):13–9. https://doi.org/10.1007/s00264-016-3265-5.

Antibiotic Prophylaxis in Primary and Revision Total Knee Arthroplasty

Francesco Giron

25.1 Introduction

Total knee arthroplasty (TKA) is one of the most successful surgical procedures for the treatment of end-stage arthritis of the knee and the number of primary TKAs will continue to increase because the arthritis is an age-related disease and the life expectancy is increased. It has been estimated that, by 2030, more than four million primary total hip arthroplasty (THA) and TKA procedures will be performed annually in the United States [1, 2]. Despite advances in surgical techniques and infection control efforts, surgical site infection (SSI) following TKA remains an unsolved catastrophic complication. Infection after TKA is one of the major problems that have not been solved during the last 30 years. It can be devastating, and although rarely causing death, infection is associated with increased morbidity and hospitalization. The deep infection rate after primary TKA has been reported between 0.86 and 2.5% [3–6]. If these rates remain constant, by 2030, the estimated number of deep infections following joint arthroplasty will be 40,000–80,000 per year. Along with additional risk for the patient, infection after TKA can bring on a huge financial burden. Patients with an infection are twice as likely to die, twice as likely to spend time in an intensive care unit, and five times more likely to be readmitted after discharge [7].

Development of an infection depends on the number and virulence of the bacteria introduced into a wound, the host's ability to eliminate these bacteria, and the status or viability of the wound environment. Various measures can be adopted to prevent this devastating complication in TKA patients, including optimizing medical comorbidities and patient risk factors, managing the operating room environment (e.g., laminar flow, body exhaust suits, minimizing operating room traffic), using proper skin preparation, and carefully selecting and effectively using antibiotic prophylaxis [8–10].

The majority of early postoperative infections results from intraoperative contamination of the surgical site [11]. Even with a strict aseptic technique, bacterial contamination occurs in most if not all arthroplasty procedures [12].

Antimicrobial prophylaxis is considered beneficial for preventing surgical site infections in clean orthopedic surgery. It is probably the single most effective method for reducing the prevalence of postoperative wound infection. Prophylactic antibiotics have been described as antibiotics given for the purpose of preventing infection when infection is not present but the risk of postoperative infection is present [13]. The goal of antimicrobial prophylaxis is to achieve serum and tissue drug levels that exceed, for the duration of the operation, the minimum

F. Giron (✉)
SOD Traumatologia e Ortopedia Generale, Azienda
Ospedaliera Universitaria Careggi, Florence, Italy

© ISAKOS 2022
U. G. Longo et al. (eds.), *Infection in Knee Replacement*,
https://doi.org/10.1007/978-3-030-81553-0_25

inhibitory concentration for the organisms likely to be encountered during the operation [14].

While the benefits of preventing surgical infections are apparent, one must also keep in mind the disadvantages of excess antimicrobial use. All infections cannot be prevented by the use of prophylactic antibiotics. Each patient has a unique set of immune defenses against, and risks of, infection. The goal of surgical prophylaxis is to decrease the bacterial load at the surgical site, not to sterilize the patient. Essentially, prophylaxis augments the host's natural immune defense mechanisms by increasing the amount of bacterial contamination needed to cause an infection [15].

Antimicrobial prophylaxis is considered helpful for preventing surgical site infections (SSIs) in orthopedic surgery [11]. The World Health Organization (WHO) [7] and the Centers for Disease Control and Prevention (CDC) [16] specified that microbial contamination during a surgical procedure is a precursor of a SSI. Use of prophylactic antibiotics with an antimicrobial spectrum that is effective against the pathogens likely to contaminate the procedure therefore is recommended for use in any clean surgical case. Conversely, the use of broad-spectrum antibiotics promotes the development of multi-drug-resistant organisms. Infections due to resistant organisms are associated with a worse clinical outcome for each individual patient. There must be a delicate balance between the use of antimicrobial agents to prevent infection and the overuse of antimicrobial agents, which is associated with the development of multi-drug-resistant organisms.

The effectiveness of prophylactic antibiotics administered shortly before skin incision to avoid microbial contamination during the procedure was established in the 1960s [17, 18], and it has been recommended in current guidelines for surgical prophylaxis. The ideal prophylactic antimicrobial agent should have excellent in vitro activity against bacteria, penetrate tissue well, have a relatively long serum half-life to provide coverage for the duration of the entire operative procedure, be relatively nontoxic, and be inexpensive.

The choice of antibiotics used as prophylaxis requires an understanding of the common micro-organisms that cause surgical site infections associated with TKA.

25.2 Common Microorganism Involved in Surgical Site Infection

The identification of organisms most frequently involved in SSI is the most important factor for the appropriate decision on what could be the proper drug to be adopted in antibiotic prophylaxis before TKA. Early infections (within 1 year postoperatively) and infections in patients with persistent pain and discomfort since the index surgery are commonly thought to be caused by direct inoculation during the perioperative period, whereas late infections are thought to occur via hematogenous seeding of the prosthesis or through compromised local tissues [19].

Wound infections following clean surgical procedures are primarily caused by skin or exogenous airborne microorganisms since other reservoirs of bacteria, such as the gastrointestinal tract, are not entered. Numerous studies have documented that gram-positive organisms are the most common bacteria causing infections associated with joint arthroplasty.

The most frequent pathogenic organisms causing deep wound infections in clean orthopedic surgery are *methicillin-sensitive Staphylococcus aureus* (MSSA) and *coagulase-negative Staphylococci (CoNS)*, such as *Staphylococcus Epidermidis* [11, 19]. CoNS in particular are recognized as the most common contaminant obtained in cultures taken from surgical sites other than MSSA [20], and generally are accepted as being one of the most resistant pathogens worldwide [21]. Other gram-positive organisms, including *Streptococcus* and *Enterococcus* species, can cause infections, as well. Furthermore, the increasing frequency of infection caused by organism such as *methicillin-resistant Staphylococcus aureus* (MRSA) and *vancomycin-resistant Enterococcus species*, which are generally resistant to more than one antibiotic, provides a dilemma with regard to prophylaxis and treatment. In some cases, infections surrounding a joint replacement can be very difficult to eradicate due to the bacteria's ability to adhere to orthopedic implants and form a local biofilm [22]. This glycocalyx layer, which is formed on the surface of the orthopedic devices, creates a complex environment for the bacteria. This self-produced matrix of extracellular polymeric substance creates a favorable environment for bacterial replication, accelerates mutation rates, confers a relative resistance to host defenses, and impairs effective penetration of antibiotics [23]. Antibiotic treatment can suppress the symptoms of the infection, but eradication usually requires removal of the device and its associated glycocalyx layer.

Other possible sources of infection can be Gram-negative organism such as *Escherichia coli*, *Pseudomonas species*, and *Klebsiella species*. Gram-negative infections are less common and reportedly account for 10–20% of infections [24]. Approximately 20% of periprosthetic joint infections (PJIs) are polymicrobial [25].

All of these microorganisms can be part of normal skin flora. Therefore, direct infection from the patient's skin or airborne contamination from surgical team personnel and the operating room environment is the most probable route of infection. Hare and Thomas [26] described staphylococcal "dispersers" as people who are Staphylococcus aureus carriers and lose the organism in vast numbers. Ritter [27] also recognized the importance of the quantity of people in the operating room as a source of increased bacterial counts. Members of the surgical team who have direct contact with the sterile operating field have been linked to unusual outbreaks. Anesthesia personnel also may play a role in postsurgical infections. Although not directly involved in the operative field, they perform a variety of procedures leading up to the operation.

25.3 Patient's Individual Risk Factors

A critical component of preventing postoperative infection is assessing a patient's individual risk factors. While the significance of some risk factors remains controversial, a high body mass index (BMI), diabetes mellitus, malnutrition, preoperative anemia, cardiovascular disease, and immunosuppressive drugs are well documented as factors increasing infection risk [9, 28, 29]. In 2013, investigators at the Kaiser Permanente Orange County Department of Orthopedic Surgery reported the risk factors associated with SSIs, after analyzing over 56,000 knees [30]. After fully adjusting their model, they reported a patient with a BMI of over 35 was 1.47 times more likely to develop deep SSI, patients were 1.28 times more likely to develop an infection if they had diabetes mellitus and 3.23 times more likely to develop an infection if they had been previously diagnosed with posttraumatic arthritis. Other risk factors such as the male sex put patients at a hazard ratio of 1.89, and an American Society of Anesthesiologists (ASA) score of over 3 made a patient 1.65 times more likely to develop an infection. If a patient is noted to have multiple risk factors, proper counseling and measures should be taken to decrease their risk and increase their compliance with future instructions. To best prevent infection and minimize risk, preventative strategies should span across the preoperative, intraoperative, and postoperative stages [9]. For example, in the case of patients at increased risk of infection, the type of antibiotic and duration of the antibiotic prophylaxis must also be carefully evaluated [31, 32].

25.4 Properties of a Prophylactic Antibiotic

Bacteriostatic antibiotics limit the growth of bacteria predominantly by interrupting bacterial protein production or by inhibiting precursors in folic acid synthesis and DNA replication. These bacteriostatic agents inhibit the growth and reproduction of bacteria without killing them. Bactericidal antibiotics kill the bacteria. The beta-lactams accomplish this by inhibiting cell wall synthesis and inducing cytolysis [33]. Most of the prophylactic antibiotics used in orthopedic surgery are categorized as bactericidal. These include the penicillins, the cephalosporins, vancomycin, and the aminoglycosides. Clindamycin, a lincosamide, is considered bacteriostatic. High concentrations of most bacteriostatic agents can be bactericidal, whereas low concentrations of bactericidal agents can be only bacteriostatic [34].

The most important consideration in choosing an antibiotic for prophylaxis is its spectrum of action. While the chosen antibiotic may not cover the entire spectrum of organisms that may be encountered, it must be active against the bacteria that commonly cause postoperative infection. Other factors to consider include the pharmacokinetics and pharmacodynamics of the drug. Specifically, the agent must have a half-life that covers the decisive interval (the first 2 h after incision or contamination with therapeutic tissue concentrations from the time of incision to wound closure). Failure to maintain tissue concentrations of the drug above the minimum inhibitory concentration increases the risk of wound infection [35]. Repeat doses of antibiotics may be necessary if the procedure is long, if multiple transfusions are needed, or if the antibiotic is cleared rapidly. The final consideration should be the cost associated with the use of the antibiotic, which should include the costs of drug monitoring, administration, repeat doses, adverse effects, and failure of prophylaxis (e.g., wound infection sequelae).

25.5 Antibiotic Selection and Dosage in Primary TKA

Systemic antibiotics are known to reduce the risk of perioperative and/or postoperative infection [11, 36, 37]. However, some previous studies had reported that systemic antibiotics may not prevent all postoperative infections [7, 38, 39]. Furthermore, conventional systemic dosages may not provide adequate tissue concentrations against more resistant organisms, such as coagulase-negative staphylococci. According to the Surgical Care Improvement Project (SCIP) Advisory Committee, part of a US initiative to reduce surgical morbidity and mortality by 25% by 2010, and the American Academy of Orthopaedic Surgeons (AAOS), the preferred antimicrobials for patients undergoing total hip or knee arthroplasty are the cephalosporins, in particular cefazolin and cefuroxime [10, 15, 40, 41]. The cephalosporins have been the antibiotics of choice for both the prophylaxis and the treatment of orthopedic infections for at least three decades. Cefazolin has been extensively studied and its favorable activity against gram-positive organisms and its effectiveness against most clinically important aerobic gram-negative bacilli and nonbacteroid anaerobes have contributed to its widespread acceptance. In addition, cephalosporins have excellent distribution profiles in bone, synovium, muscle, and hematomas [42]. Studies have documented that minimum bactericidal concentrations for most non-methicillin-resistant Staphylococcus aureus organisms are achieved rapidly in these tissues [43].

Cefazolin is often dosed at 1 g for patients who weigh <80 kg or 2 g for patients who weigh >80 kg. In patients weighing >120 kg, a 3-g dose can be considered [44, 45] (Table 25.1). Cefuroxime is dosed at 1.5 g. It is recommended that, for extended operative times, cefazolin be readministered every 2–5 h; cefuroxime, every 3–4 h [11] (Table 25.1). Both of these cephalosporins are safe and have an effective spectrum of action against the most commonly encountered organisms, specifically gram-positive bacteria and 40% of gram-negative bacteria.

Anaphylactic reactions to cephalosporins are rare events, but they do occur and thus have led to the recommendation against their use in patients with known anaphylaxis to other beta-lactam antibiotics. Some of the more common reactions include skin rash (a rate of 1–5%), eosinophilia (3–10%), diarrhea (1–10%), and pseudomembranous colitis (<1%) [42].

Clindamycin and vancomycin are currently the preferred alternative antibiotics for people with an established allergy to a beta-lactam or with a contraindication to its use and at institutions with high rates of methicillin-resistant Staphylococcus aureus infection. Clindamycin has good bioavailability, and at 30 min after infusion has been shown to exceed the minimum inhibitory concentration for Staphylococcus

Table 25.1 Antibiotic dosage for routine prophylaxis in primary TKA

Antibiotic	Dosage	Time before surgery/tourniquet	Redosing schedule (h)
Cefazolin	1 g (<80 kg body weight) 2 g (60–120 kg body weight) 3 g (>120 kg body weight)	Within 30–40 min	2–5
Cefuroxime	1.5 g	Within 30–40 min	3–4
Clindamycin	900 mg	Within 30–40 min	3–6
Vancomycin	15 mg/kg (weight-based)	Within 60–90 min	6–12
Daptomycin	6 mg/kg (weight-based)	Within 30–60 min	24

aureus in both animal and human cortical bone samples [11]. The recommended dose of clindamycin is 600–900 mg and for extended operative time, every 3–6 h (Table 25.1). The most severe adverse effect of clindamycin is *C. difficile*-associated diarrhea (the most frequent cause of pseudomembranous colitis). Other side effects include the development of a rash, abdominal pain, cramps, and in high doses a metallic taste in the mouth.

Although clindamycin is effective against many MRSA species, vancomycin is a bactericidal agent that provides coverage against a greater percentage of MRSA species, making it a better choice to cover MRSA. Vancomycin is a large tricyclic glycopeptide molecule that has historically been the first line of treatment for *methicillin-resistant Staphylococcus aureus* infections [46]. The bactericidal action of vancomycin is a result of the inhibition of bacterial cell wall synthesis through the disruption of peptidoglycan biosynthesis. It is active against most gram-positive organisms including *Staphylococcus aureus*, *Staphylococcus epidermidis* (including heterogeneous methicillin-resistant strains), *streptococci*, *enterococci*, and *Clostridium*. Vancomycin lacks activity against *gram-negative bacteria*, fungi, or *mycobacteria*. Similar to cefazolin, vancomycin reaches high concentrations in bone, synovial tissue, and muscle within minutes after administration [47, 48].

Adverse reactions to vancomycin such as infusion-related pruritus and erythema can occur. Red man syndrome, a pruritic, erythematous rash on the upper trunk and face that is occasionally accompanied by hypotension, is associated with its rapid infusion and histamine release in approximately 5–13% of people [49]. This has led to the recommendation that vancomycin be administered slowly, at a rate of 1 g over 60 min. The recommended dose, which is based on body mass, is 10–15 mg/kg, up to a limit of 1 g, in patients with normal renal function [15]. When vancomycin is used for prophylaxis, its infusion should begin 1–2 h before initiation of the operation (compared with within 1 h for cefazolin) to ensure that the entire dose is administered and adequate concentrations reach the tissues prior to the surgical incision [50]. For extended operative times, repeat administration is recommended in 6–12 h [11] (Table 25.1).

Nephrotoxicity and ototoxicity occur in <1% of patients, with nephrotoxicity being associated with concomitant aminoglycoside use. Other complications include hypersensitivity rash, reversible neutropenia, and drug fever. Daptomycin should be considered as an alternative for people with known anaphylactic or severe reactions to vancomycin [15] (Table 25.1).

Patient-specific factors should be considered with respect to vancomycin dosage. One report found that 69% of patients receiving vancomycin at the standard 1-g dose were being underdosed based on their actual weight [51, 52]. This suggests that, given the high rates of obesity in arthroplasty patients, a weight-based dose of 15 mg/kg should be used.

With regard to the selection and effectiveness of antibiotic prophylaxis, the clinician must consider whether the organism identified on cultures at SSI presentation was within the spectrum of the original prophylaxis administered at the time of the primary surgery. A recent study of 163 patients with PJI demonstrated that, in 63% of patients, the infections were caused by a bacterium that was resistant to the original prophylaxis. MRSA was isolated from 26% of patients with cultures positive for infection [53].

Over the past decade, hospitals and emergency rooms have seen a changing pattern of infections caused by *Staphylococcus*. Usually resistant strains of *Staphylococcus* were reported in hospital settings and high-risk patient populations, such as intravenous drug users and people with chronic indwelling catheters. Recent articles have described an alarming upward trend in the prevalence of community-acquired methicillin-resistant *Staphylococcus aureus* strains in low-risk patients. One report from a large urban hospital in Chicago showed that the prevalence of community-acquired *methicillin-resistant Staphylococcus aureus* skin and soft-tissue infections increased 6.84-fold: from 24.0 cases per 100,000 people in 2000 to 164.2 cases per 100,000 people in 2005 [54]. Additional studies from large county institutions in Dallas and Atlanta have demonstrated similar trends of increasing prevalence of community-acquired *methicillin-resistant Staphylococcus aureus*, with the conclusion being that this is now the predominant organism in skin and soft-tissue infections [55].

Given the varying levels of antibiotic-resistant organisms present at institutions, it is important to customize antibiotics based on local trends. The use of a local and up-to-date antibiogram and consultation with an infectious disease specialist can help clinicians estimate the prevalence of antibiotic-resistant organisms, aiding selection of effective prophylactic agents. Given the increasing prevalence of MRSA, we must specifically address whether every arthroplasty patient should routinely receive vancomycin, either as a single medication or as a supplemental antibiotic. Current guidelines suggest that vancomycin is a reasonable choice of antibiotic for patients with a beta-lactam allergy, those known to be colonized with MRSA, and those at high risk of developing a MRSA infection (e.g., patients in regions with a high prevalence of MRSA, institutionalized patients, healthcare workers) [14, 45]. The 2013 Proceedings of the International Consensus on Periprosthetic Joint Infection broadly support the routine use of vancomycin in patients who

are known MRSA carriers, those with a known anaphylactic allergy to penicillin, or those at high risk of MRSA infection [40]. Additionally, the routine use of dual antibiotics is generally not supported [56].

Sewick et al. [38] compared dual prophylaxis with cefazolin and vancomycin versus cefazolin alone. In their retrospective analysis of 1828 primary THAs and TKAs, with 1-year follow-up, the authors found that the rates of infection with cefazolin and vancomycin versus cefazolin alone did not significantly differ (1.1% and 1.4%, respectively; $P = 0.636$). The prevalence of MRSA infections was significantly lower in the dual antibiotic group than in the cefazolin group (0.02% and 0.08%, respectively; $P < 0.05$). However, these infections were very rare in the cohort; therefore, the number needed to treat to prevent one MRSA infection was very high [43]. Tyllianakis et al. [57], in a prospective randomized study comparing cefuroxime to two antistaphylococcal agents (fusidic acid and vancomycin), for prophylaxis in total hip arthroplasty (THA) and total knee arthroplasty (TKA), investigated the incidence of SSI in an institute, where methicillin-resistant *Staphylococcus aureus* (MRSA) and methicillin-resistant *Staphylococcus epidermidis* (MRSE) prevalence exceeds 25% of orthopedic infections. Four hundred thirty-five patients, who were included in the study, were followed up for a mean time of 3.8 (2–5) years. The authors found that the use of alternative antibiotic agents (including vancomycin) was no better than cefuroxime alone in preventing SSIs. Wyles et al. [58], investigating 29,695 arthroplasties (22,705 patients) performed from 2004 to 2017 at the Mayo Clinic, in order to characterize antibiotic choices for perioperative TKA and THA prophylaxis, assess antibiotic allergy testing efficacy, and determine rates of prosthetic joint infection (PJI) based on perioperative antibiotic regimen, found that PJI rates were significantly higher when non-cefazolin antibiotics were used for perioperative TKA and THA prophylaxis. Given the low rate of true penicillin allergy positivity, and the readily modifiable risk factor that antibiotic choice provides, they also emphasized the role of perioperative testing and clearance for all patients presenting with penicillin and cephalosporin allergies.

Currently, the evidence to support the use of vancomycin for routine prophylaxis is controversial. Up to date, the American Academy of Orthopaedic Surgeons (AAOS) generally recommended vancomycin for patients with beta-lactam allergy, those with a known MRSA colonization, or those in institutions with a high prevalence of MRSA [59]. Moreover in a separate information statement, "The Use of Prophylactic Antibiotics in Orthopaedic Medicine and the Emergence of Vancomycin-Resistant Bacteria," AAOS stated: "Vancomycin may be appropriate as a prophylactic antimicrobial for patients undergoing joint replacement at institutions that have identified a significant prevalence (e.g., >10–20%) of *methicillin-resistant S. aureus* (MRSA) and *S. epidermidis* among orthopedic patients" [60]. However based on the abovementioned papers that show no clear superiority of vancomycin compared to cephalosporins in reducing postoperative SSI rates after primary TKA, non-consensus actually exists on its routine prophylactic use also in institutions with a high prevalence of MRSA. Moreover, Song et al. [61], investigating the outcome of cefazolin prophylaxis in 1323 TKAs performed in a hospital with a high endemic rate of MRSA infection, found that antimicrobial prophylaxis using only cefazolin can maintain low SSI rates if other adequate infection management measures, such as the use of an appropriate antiseptic agent for surgical scrub and skin preparation, HEPA filter, laminar air flow, and traffic control, are employed, even where there is a high prevalence of MRSA infection.

The unwillingness to use vancomycin as a routine prophylactic agent can be referred to the limited number of antibiotics available to treat *methicillin-resistant Staphylococcus aureus* as well as when antimicrobial profiles did not support its use. In addition, the fear of promoting possible vancomycin-resistant strains of staphylococci and the emergence of vancomycin-resistant enterococci caused physicians to be appropriately cautious about its use. The use of oral vancomycin to treat pseudomembranous colitis contributed to the emergence of vancomycin-resistant enterococci [46]. The first staphylococci with reduced susceptibility to vancomycin were reported in Japan in 1997 [62].

These staphylococci, labeled "*vancomycin-intermediate Staphylococcus aureus*," did not possess the resistance genes but had a reduced susceptibility to vancomycin. Since then, other strains with reduced susceptibility (heteroresistant vancomycin-intermediate *Staphylococcus aureus*) as well as resistant strains (vancomycin-resistant *Staphylococcus aureus*) have been identified but occur infrequently [63]. To help combat these resistant strains, new antibiotics that greatly expand the pharmacologic arsenal have been introduced. These newer antibiotics include linezolid, quinupristin/dalfopristin, daptomycin, and tigecycline. Whether a single preoperative parenteral dose of vancomycin is associated with increased vancomycin resistance or decreased vancomycin susceptibility has not been demonstrated. Conversely, prolonged exposure to antibiotics has been identified as a risk factor for promoting bacterial resistance [64].

Meehan et al. [15], in order to decrease all the risks related to the use of vancomycin as routine antibiotic prophylaxis in primary TKA, suggested to add a single preoperative dose of vancomycin along with the cefazolin to provide prophylaxis against these resistant organisms and the other common bacterial causes of infection in institutions with a high prevalence of MRSA infection.

25.6 Intraosseus Regional Prophylaxis

For antibiotic prophylaxis to be effective, the concentration of antibiotic in the tissues must exceed the minimum inhibitory concentration (MIC) of organisms that commonly cause infection for the period between skin incision and wound closure. *CoNS*, one of the most common causes of infection post-TKA, have relatively high MICs against cephalosporins. Conventional systemic dosing of prophylactic cephalosporins may therefore lead to inadequate tissue concentrations against these organisms [65]. Vancomycin has been proposed as an alternative [66]; however, it requires a prolonged administration time, can cause systemic toxicity, and risks promoting further antibiotic resistance. Recently, the attention of the research has been focused on low-dose prophylactic antibiotic through intraosseous regional administration (IORA). This route of drug administration may diminish all the previous issues and in primary TKA achieves higher tissue concentrations than systemic administration by limiting distribution of the drug to the targeted limb [67].

IORA involves intraosseous injection of antibiotics through a specific cannula (Vidacare, San Antonio, TX, USA; FDA-approved) inserted into the proximal tibial bone after tourniquet inflation and before skin incision. Even in adults, intraosseous injection is equivalent to IV administration and is reliably successful in primary TKA, reaching concentrations 6–10 times higher than systemic administration [68–71]. In an animal model of TKA, IORA was also shown to provide more effective prophylaxis against PJI [72].

This approach seems to be very effective in case of obesity. Obesity is an important risk factor for PJI after TKA [73, 74], a devastating complication for the patient [2] and the healthcare system [67]. In a meta-analysis of 83,001 patients, obesity was associated with an odds ratio of 2.2 for superficial infections and 2.4 for deep infections [75]. Furthermore, registry data show a 7% increase in risk per unit of body mass index (BMI) above a threshold of 35 [76]. A number of potential mechanisms are implicated. Obese patients have disrupted microcirculation and macrocirculation [73, 77], decreased wound healing [73, 77], and impaired immune function [73, 78]. Surgically, they are associated with greater difficulty [79] and longer surgical time [80], prolonging exposure to microorganisms. The higher risk of PJI has led some authors to suggest refusing TKA in patients above a certain BMI threshold [81].

In the nonobese TKA population, IORA of prophylactic antibiotics provides tissue concentrations 5–8 times higher than systemic administration in TKA [70]. However, the physiology in the obese patient unpredictably alters pharmacokinetics for different drugs [82]. For vancomycin, there is a higher volume of distribution and a shorter elimination half-life in the morbidly obese to nonobese individuals [83]. Thus, vancomycin requires total body weight-based dosing to achieve ideal target steady-state concentrations when given systemically [84]. The importance of higher dose of vancomycin is emphasized with bony infections as it displays poor bone penetration in animal models [85]. Chin et al. [86] in a randomized study comparing standard body weight-adjusted vancomycin prophylaxis versus low-dose vancomycin IORA in two groups of 11 obese patients found a statistically significant higher antibiotic concentration in bones of IORA patients.

Based on these assumptions an increased use of this approach should be considered providing higher tissue concentration of antibiotic prophylaxis than systemic administration. Moreover, IORA optimizes time of antibiotic administration and reduces the risk of systemic adverse effects, while providing high tissue antibiotic concentrations during TKA.

25.7 Timing and Duration of Action in Primary TKA

To be effective as an antimicrobial prophylaxis, the serum and tissue drug levels must be greater than the minimum inhibitory concentrations (MICs) for the target organisms for the period between skin incision and wound closure. Therefore, the goal should be to infuse antibiotics within adequate interval before incision or tourniquet inflation (whichever comes first). This allows an optimal antibiotic concentration at the surgical site when the procedure begins [14]. SSI risk increases incrementally with a longer interval between infusion and incision. Administration of antibiotics within 30 min before the incision was associated with a trend toward a lower risk of infection (1.6%) than administration 31–60 min (2.4%) before incision (odds ratio 1.74; 95% confidence interval, 0.98–3.04) [87]. If administered too rapidly, vancomycin can cause a histamine release, resulting in hypotension and a skin reaction called red man syndrome; therefore, infusion of vancomycin should take place over a longer period of time than that for other antibiotics—60–120 min instead of the typical 30–60 min. Additionally, tissue penetration affects the varying infusion times for antibiotics. Cefazolin has a rapid tissue penetration into bone, synovium, and soft tissue [10]. Because slower tissue penetration vancomycin needs to be administered earlier. Moreover, while cefazolin viability is not affected by patient weight, vancomycin shows a substantial difference in trabecular bone concentrations with respect to patient weight with lower body mass index (BMI) achieving greater concentrations [88]. The only exception to these guidelines is in the setting of revision arthroplasty when preoperative cultures of aspiration are negative but there is a high index of suspicion for an infection. In these cases, prophylactic antibiotics should not be administered until deep intra-articular cultures are obtained. Once these cultures are obtained, then the antibiotics can be administered.

To maintain adequate serum concentrations, antibiotics should be redosed during longer surgeries (e.g., 4 h) and when there is increased blood loss (>2000 mL) and/or fluid resuscitation (>2000 mL) [89]. Finally, 24 h is considered the ideal duration for prophylactic antibiotic treatment. Many studies have failed to demonstrate any benefit associated with the use of antibiotics beyond 24 h in elective, clean surgical case [90–92]. In a study of the short-term use of antibiotic prophylaxis in patients undergoing THA and TKA procedures, Heydemann and Nelson [90] found no difference in infection rates between a 24-h and a 7-day dose of nafcillin or cefazolin. In a retrospective review of 1341 THA and TKA procedures, Williams and Gustilo [91] came to the same results in patients treated with either a 24-h or a 3-day course of cefazolin. The risks of excessive antimicrobial treatment, including toxicity and development of antibiotic-resistant organisms, have led to the recommendation for a 24-h course of antibiotics [53]. Limiting unnecessary antibiotic exposure can minimize adverse effects associated with overuse, such as *C. difficile* infection [93]. Hospital-associated *C. difficile* infections carry serious morbidity and result in extended hospital stays and increased costs of care [94].

25.8 Role of Screening for Methicillin-Resistant *Staphylococcus aureus* Carriers

There is increasing evidence that *S aureus* colonization is a risk factor for SSI. Patients undergoing orthopedic surgery are colonized with *S aureus* at rates similar to those of the general population and, in that undergoing total joint arthroplasty, nearly 20% are *S aureus* carriers [95–97]. In this scenario, prophylactic antimicrobials may be modified depending on the results of the screening test. Patients may be screened to determine whether they are colonized with drug-resistant bacteria. Nasal carriers have increased rates of skin colonization, which is important to note because the skin is directly exposed to the surgical field at incision. In those cases, attempts at eliminating these drug-resistant bacteria can be made. This approach has been used with success in The Netherlands and is thought to be a contributor to the fact that ≤1% of *Staphylococcus aureus* isolates are methicillin-resistant there. At 49 hospitals in The Netherlands reporting to the European Antimicrobial Resistance Surveillance System during the years 1999 through 2004, only 58 (0.78%) of 7420 cultures were positive for methicillin-resistant *Staphylococcus aureus* isolates [98].

A universal program of *S aureus* screening and decolonization before high-risk orthopedic procedures (e.g., TJA, spine fusion) has been developed [96]. Patients' nares are cultured 7–10 days before the procedure. All patients are then given a prescription for nasal mupirocin for decolonization. On the day of surgery, patients are asked if they complied with the protocol. For those who report compliance, the cultures are checked and, if they test positive for MRSA, they receive vancomycin prophylaxis within 30 min of the skin incision and the typical preoperative preparation for their surgery. Patients whose cultures are negative receive the typical cephalosporin prophylaxis before the incision. If patients did not comply with the protocol and their cultures are negative or positive for methicillin-sensitive *S aureus* only, they also receive the typical cephalosporin or clindamycin prophylactic antibiotics before the incision. Patients who did not comply and have nasal cultures positive for MRSA receive preoperative vancomycin prophylaxis, are decolonized with mupirocin after surgery, and placed on isolation precautions after surgery until the decolonization protocol is complete. After adoption of this universal screening and decolonization protocol, the overall MRSA burden for the hospital was shown to decrease, and the overall deep infection rate associated with TJA was reduced from 1.45 to 1.28% after initiation of the protocol [97, 99]. However, this difference was not statistically significant and, to reach adequate power, 57,604 patients would be needed in each group.

As an alternative to obtaining preoperative cultures, polymerase chain reaction (PCR)-based testing has emerged as an effective tool for detecting MRSA colonization [95, 97, 100]. The accuracy of PCR-based tests for detection of *S aureus* has been validated in the literature and has been found to be sensitive, specific, and cost-effective [78, 101].

There is increasing evidence that *S aureus* carrier screening and decolonization have the ability to decrease perioperative infection rates; these procedures can be highly cost-effective and may improve outcomes [102]. It should be noted that the decolonization is not permanent, and patients who are decolonized have a significant risk of being recolonized [103]. This means that patients decolonized for a procedure will need to be rescreened if they undergo a second procedure or if their surgery is postponed. Additional studies are needed to determine the ideal screening and decolonization protocol and whether it is the decolonization process itself, administration of vancomycin for MRSA-colonized patients, or a combination of the two that is driving the trend of reduced infection rates.

25.9 Local Antibiotic Prophylaxis

Polymethyl methacrylate (PMMA) bone cement is commonly used for fixation of TKA components and its primary function is to transfer load force from prosthesis to bone. Initial medical applications of PMMA were in dentistry beginning in 1940 and in orthopedic surgery with John Charnley's early work on THA between 1950 and 1960.

Bone cement has the capacity to release antibiotic molecules if any antibiotic is included in it, and these elution properties are improved as cement porosity is increased. In vitro studies have shown high local antibiotic concentration for many hours or few days after its use. Mixing antibiotics into bone cement allows for direct delivery of antibiotics to the implant and surgical site immediately following surgery. Buchholz et al. [104] were the first to report on the addition of aminoglycoside antibiotics to Palacos bone cement in a large series of exchange arthroplasties. The aminoglycosides are a class of antibiotics that can be used in a prophylactic fashion, being that they are administered locally rather than parenterally. They cause bacterial cell death by an intracellular mechanism, binding to a 30S subunit of the ribosome and thereby inhibiting protein synthesis. This practice is common and widely accepted in revision arthroplasty either in the creation of a spacer in the first stage of the procedure or as part of the cementing process in the replantation stage [105]. However, the use of antibiotic-loaded bone cement in primary TKA is controversial. Many authors have recommended the use of antibiotic-loaded bone cement (ALBC) in TKA for infection prophylaxis, but the evidence based on data from National Registries, randomized clinical trials and meta-analysis suggests a protective effect of ALBC against infection when used in hips, but not (or only mild) in knees. A possible explanation is that the quantity of locally delivered antibiotics after TKA is small.

There are some concerns about the routine use of ALBC in primary TKA as prophylaxis against infection. Firstly, there is a risk of hypersensitivity or toxicity even when the chance is highly improbable. Secondly, there is a reduction in the mechanical properties of the cement, but this can be probably neglected if the antibiotic is used in low doses, not more than 1 g per 40 g cement package. Another significant concern is the increased economic cost, which could be overlooked if there were enough savings in treating fewer prosthetic infections. Finally, there is also a risk of selection of antibiotic-resistant strains of bacteria and this could be the main concern. If used, the choice of the antibiotic mixed in ALBC should consider microbiological aspects (broad antimicrobial spectrum and low rate of resistant bacteria), physical and chemical aspects (thermal stability, high water solubility), pharmacological characteristics (low risk to allergic reactions or toxicity), and economic aspects (not too expensive). Currently, the most commonly used antibiotics in ALBC are gentamicin, tobramycin, and vancomycin.

Several properties of bone cement are important to consider when creating an antibiotic-cement mixture [106, 107]. First, PMMA polymerization is an exothermic reaction; therefore, antibiotics must be heat stable. Second, the antibiotic itself must be water soluble to allow diffusion into the surrounding tissues. It must have a bactericidal effect at the tissue concentration and be released gradually over an extended period of time. Furthermore, the antibiotic must result in minimal local inflammatory or allergic reaction. Finally, composition of different bone cements differs and so the chance for release of antibiotics is not the same.

The mechanical and chemical stability of a variety of antibiotic-cement combinations has been studied. During the polymerization reaction of bone cement, there is an increase in temperature that causes the formation of air bubbles. Some of these bubbles escape from cement, but some others do not escape, causing some porosity in it. The final porosity of bone cement depends not only on the composition and method of manipulation, but also on the viscosity of the cement [108]. An increased cement porosity causes a decrease in the mechanical properties, but an increase in the capacity of the cement to release antibiotic molecules if any antibiotic is included in it. Historically, concerns about whether antibiotic loading decreases the strength of PMMA cement have been expressed. Lautenschlager et al. [109] showed that adding large doses of gentamicin (4.5 g per 40 g cement)

or liquid antibiotics caused a significant decrease in compressive strength to substandard levels. However, at the lower doses used for prophylaxis (2 g per 40 g cement), this change in strength is likely negligible [110, 111].

The initial release after exposure of ALBC to a fluid is mainly a surface phenomenon, while sustained release over the next days is a bulk diffusion phenomenon [108]. The elution of antibiotics from ALBC has been advocated to be effective for many days [43], but some other authors sustain that the process is sufficient for only few hours [112, 113]. Nevertheless, the hydrophobicity of the cement limits the antibiotic release at less than 10%, and most of this antibiotic is released during the first hours after surgery [108, 114, 115]. Three days after its use there is no effect of antibiotic in the ALBC in in vitro studies [114]. The elution can be improved by using liquid antibiotics instead of powder ones in the cement, but this choice creates a reduction in the compressive strength of the cement [116].

Aminoglycoside antibiotics (e.g., gentamicin, tobramycin) have favorable properties for this application [105]. Other antibiotics, including vancomycin, erythromycin, and colistin, have been used, as well.

Antibiotics contained in ALBC, though at low levels, are systemically absorbed and can potentially cause allergic reactions. Particular attention should be paid to an individual's antibiotic allergy history prior to implantation of any ALBC. The most frequently used antibiotics in ALBC are aminoglycosides (gentamicin and tobramycin), which very rarely cause allergic reactions. The possibility of an allergic reaction may become greater if other antibiotics such as cephalosporins are used [117].

There is an increasing concern in the emergence of drug-resistant organisms. No direct evidence links the development of bacterial resistance to the routine use of ALBC in primary arthroplasties and some authors do not believe that this risk is increased [118]. There is some evidence supporting the concern about antimicrobial resistance and the risk of selecting resistant mutans bacteria: in vitro studies show up to 8% of the antibiotic in ALBC is quickly released after surgery, and thereafter there is a low-dose release, that may not be effective at fighting infection, but can cause antibiotic microbial resistance. Prolonged exposure to antibiotic at a dose concentration below the inhibitory one allows the development of mutational resistance in bacteria [108, 112]. Josefsson et al. [119] found that 88% of the infected patients who had received gentamicin-loaded cement in primary arthroplasty showed at least one gentamicin-resistant isolate. Aminoglycoside (gentamicin and tobramycin) resistance rate is higher if an antibiotic spacer is used in 2-stage revision arthroplasty [120], suggesting that the risk of selecting resistant mutans when using ALBC is real. In a large series of patients, Hansen et al. [121] found that the introduction of routine ALBC in TKA in a hospital did not cause any significant change in the infecting pathogen profile or any alarming increase in antibiotic resistance, but they recognized that the sample size of the infected cohort might not be big enough. Recently Wu et al. [122], analyzing the incidence of SSI and PJI in a group of 3152 patients who underwent TKA between 2009 and 2013, found that the incidence of SSI and deep-implant SSI was 1.52% and 0.79%, respectively. An optimal dose of systemic antibiotics adjusted by patients' body weight for prophylaxis and the use of ALBC were significant protective factors for SSI. Meanwhile, the use of ALBC also significantly decreased the risk of PJI ($P < 0.01$).

The United States Food and Drug Administration (FDA) has approved the use of premixed antibiotic bone cement (either gentamicin or tobramycin) for prophylaxis in a second-stage reimplantation following a previous infection at the site of an arthroplasty, but not as prophylaxis in routine primary arthroplasties. Outside the USA, the use of antibiotic cement for routine primary THA or TKA has been well studied. Large studies of data from the Scandinavian registry established the efficacy of antibiotic cement in THA [123, 124]. In a recent study of TKAs from the Canadian registry, Bohm et al. [125] analyzed a sample of 36,681 TKAs. In 45% of these procedures, antibiotic-loaded cement was used. No significant difference between the groups treated with

or without antibiotic-loaded cement was found with regard to 2-year revision rates for infection or any other cause. In a large, prospective, randomized controlled trial, Hinarejos et al. [126] examined the efficacy of antibiotic-loaded cement in reducing the incidence of infection following TKA. The authors randomized 2948 patients to TKA with standard cement or with erythromycin/colistin-containing cement. The authors reported comparable rates of deep infection in the two groups: a rate of 1.4% in the antibiotic group versus 1.35% in the standard cement group ($P = 0.96$). Similarly, Kleppel et al. [51] doing a systematic review did not found a statistically significant difference between ALBC and non-ALBC groups. Currently, no conclusive evidence exists regarding the efficacy of antibiotic-loaded cement in primary TKA.

Finally, the issue of cost is critical. The average cost of premixed antibiotic in PMMA is approximately $300 per bag [8]. Illingworth et al. [8] reported that the cost of premixed antibiotic-loaded bone cement for 100 procedures (two bags per procedure) would be about $60,000. This is similar to the cost of treating one prosthetic infection. Therefore, for routine antibiotic-loaded cement to be cost-effective, it would have to demonstrably prevent one infection for every 100 primary arthroplasty procedures. An absolute decrease in infection rate of 1% would be difficult to achieve in practice, given that the baseline infection rates are already low (1–2%). Gutowski et al. [127] performed a similar cost analysis for antibiotic-loaded bone cement used in TKA and found that there is likely a cost benefit with hand-mixed cement, with the average cost per infection prevented ranging from $2112 to $37,176. This is lower than the cost of a revision procedure. The cost of premixed cement for TKA was $112,606 per infection spared. From a merely economic point of view, the use of ALBC might only be justified in high-risk groups of patients such as those having rheumatoid arthritis [128], immunodepression, morbid obesity [129–131], and diabetes [129, 132, 133], or patients with previous history of infection or fracture in the knee, and those having long surgeries [78, 91, 113, 162], groups where a much higher infection rate than the average could be expected. Moreover, a recent study stated that the use of ALBC in primary TKA might not be justified even in the group of patients considered as high risk [134].

Currently, given the mixed results regarding its efficacy, no recommendation can be made regarding the routine use of antibiotic-loaded cement in primary arthroplasty. One common practice is to use it only in patients with a high risk of infection (e.g., patients with diabetes mellitus, morbid obesity, prior history of PJI). The 2013 Proceedings of the International Consensus on Periprosthetic Joint Infection echoes this recommendation, with 90% agreement on the statement that antibiotic-loaded PMMA should be used in elective arthroplasty in high-risk patients only [40].

25.10 Antibiotic Prophylaxis in Revision TKA

The use of a preoperative systemic antibiotic prophylaxis has been demonstrated to be effective in reducing the infection rate in primary TKA. However, no consensus exists on the efficacy of antibiotic prophylaxis in TKA revision surgery, mainly in case of PJI. To date there has not been any sort of systematic review of RCTs examining the effect of antibiotic prophylaxis solely on revision TKA. There have been systematic reviews and meta-analysis that have examined the effect of antibiotic prophylaxis on primary and revision TKA collectively, without separating them out [135, 136]. Several studies also recognize that the periprosthetic infection rate is 2–3 times higher in revision TKA than in primary TKA [137, 138]. Moreover, other studies have shown that patients are at a 9–13 times higher risk of infection in a revision TKA procedure than in a primary TKA [138, 139]. Further, the infection rates in revision TKA have also more than doubled from 1.4% in the 1991–1994 timeframe to 3.0% in the 2007–2010 timeframe [140]. Despite the statistically significant higher infection rates seen in revision TKA, surprisingly, the current strong consensus is that periop-

erative antibiotic prophylaxis should be the same for primary and uninfected revision TKA [121]. Moreover, preoperative antibiotics are sometimes withheld in patients undergoing revision arthroplasty, as there is concern that occult infection may be present and the administration of antibiotics might affect intraoperative culture results [16]. This would be important if true, as culture results are integral to the diagnosis of PJI and antibiotic sensitivities obtained from these cultures are critical for guiding subsequent antimicrobial therapy. However, recent papers [141, 142] show that preoperative antibiotics should not be withheld before revision TKA surgery because culture results were not affected by a single dose of prophylactic antibiotics.

As previously reported, the most common organisms for implant infection are *Staphylococcus aureus* (50–65%) and *Staphylococcus epidermis* (25–30%) [143, 144]. However, in revision surgery there is also a constant risk of hospital acquired bacterial infections that are resistant to the antibiotics commonly used prophylactically in arthroplasty surgery [59]. These nosocomial infections include *C. difficile* and methicillin-resistant *Staphylococcus aureus* (MRSA). This is especially important in revision procedures as patients undergoing these procedures have an increased risk of developing bacterial infections due to their more advanced age and length of hospital stay, compared to primary TKA procedures.

In the USA, over the 2006–2012 period there has been a tremendous increase (35%) of TKA revision surgery. This increase in revision procedures in excess of the increase in the number of primary TKA implants is likely due to the prevalence of over seven million people living with THA and TKAs [145]. A main reason for revision has been due to infection, with approximately 35% of large joint implants (THA/TKA) being revised for this reason [146–148].

Based on these assumptions, new prospective randomized studies will have to be carried out to evaluate if it is necessary to adopt a different antibiotic prophylaxis strategy in case of aseptic revision of TKA. In those cases, probably the surgeon should carefully consider the age of the patient, the risk factors, the associated diseases, the duration and the complexity of the surgery, in order to customize the choice of antibiotics to be used for prophylaxis.

In case of PJI, the approach is different and more studies are available. A PJI typically develops in one of three ways: through perioperative colonization of the implant, hematogenous seeding caused by a bacteremia, or spread from an infection of the surrounding tissue [149]. Moreover, PJI can be classified in three categories based on time of occurrence. Early infections occur within 3 months after surgery. Delayed PJIs appear 3–24 months after implantation and late PJIs after 24 months [67]. Usually early and hematogenous PJIs are classified as acute infections, which often have an acute onset and are caused by virulent microorganisms [67].

The recommended treatment of an acute PJI is drainage, antibiotics, irrigation, and retention of the prosthesis (DAIR) [67, 150]. DAIR, for hip and knee prostheses, has a success rate of approximately 70% [150–152]. In the empirical phase, intravenous antibiotics are started blind after surgery until the causative microorganisms are determined in microbiological cultures [153, 154]. The importance of tailored antibiotic treatment during the targeted phase is well known [155]. However, far less literature is available on which antibiotic to use in the empirical phase.

25.11 Local Antibiotic Prophylaxis in Revision TKA

Revision TJA, even when performed for aseptic reasons, is well known to be associated with significantly higher infection rates as compared to primary procedures. Consequently, many authors advocate for the routine prophylactic use of ABLC in these surgeries. This is supported by a prospective pseudorandomized study of 189 first-time aseptic revision knee arthroplasties, which found a markedly lower deep infection rate at a mean of 89 months in patients whose components were fixed with cement containing 1 g of vancomycin per 40 g bag of plain cement (zero) compared with those who received plain bone cement (7%) [156]. A review of aseptic revision

cases performed between 2001 and 2012 and tracked through the US Kaiser Permanente Joint Replacement Registry found that the use of ALBC was associated with 50% reduction in all-cause re-revision [157]. Registry data confirm the widespread adoption of routine ALBC use in revision surgery. The Australian Joint Replacement Registry reported that 9 of the top 10 types of bone cement used in revision TJA in 2015 were ALBC, representing between 93 and 99% of all cemented component revisions [33]. In this context, the routine use of ALBC in cemented aseptic revision TJA can be considered the standard of care, conferring benefits in terms of both reduced infection rates and all-cause re-revision.

Most commercial preparations of ALBC are limited to aminoglycosides (gentamicin or tobramycin), which have been shown to have favorable bactericidal activity profile against both methicillin-susceptible and methicillin-resistant staphylococci within the joint space. Aminoglycoside resistance in staphylococci is a known issue, however, and increased resistance has been demonstrated after the use of high-dose ALBC in septic revision joint surgery [120]. Thus, there may be a theoretical benefit in adding low-dose vancomycin to ALBC in aseptic revision cases in which the patient had previously received aminoglycoside cement and/or is being treated in an institution with high rates of aminoglycoside resistance. However, this must be balanced against the risk of consequent selection of vancomycin-resistant organisms. At present, given the effectiveness of aminoglycoside-ALBC in reducing infection rates and lack of evidence supporting routine addition of vancomycin to aminoglycoside-ALBC, it is recommended that this is reserved for treatment of active infection.

The optimal dose ALBC in aseptic revision TKA remains controversial. Commercial preparations of ALBC using a base with favorable elution properties contain as little as 0.5 g of antibiotic (e.g., Palacos R + G; Zimmer Biomet), and these appear to be sufficient to confer benefits in reducing the risk of re-revision. Conversely, for surgeon-prepared ALBC, doses of ≥2 g of powdered antibiotic per 40 g bag of cement seem to be well tolerated in terms of mechanical characteristics.

In case of delayed and late PJI, ALBC is routinely used in two-stage septic revision surgery, with the purpose to leverage ALBC as a local drug delivery mechanism. Although historically periprosthetic infections were treated with resection arthroplasty and placement of antibiotic laden cement beads, contemporary approaches rely on ALBC-containing spacers to maintain joint space and function, while facilitating local antibiotic delivery. A number of different cement spacer designs are used, with the most marked difference being between static and dynamic spacers. In the latter category, these can be further subdivided based on whether the cement is preset or mixed and molded in the operating room; the bearing surfaces (e.g., cement-on-bone, cement-on-cement, metal-on-poly); whether they are molded or hand formed; and whether they use specific commercial products (e.g., preformed spacers, commercial molds) or regular off-the-shelf arthroplasty components. Although pros and cons exist to each spacer option, there is no consistent benefit of one design over another in terms of effectiveness in eradicating infection when principles of two-stage revision arthroplasty, such as the concomitant use of systemic antibiotics, are otherwise adhered to [40]. However, one disadvantage of preformed spacers is an inability to tailor the antibiotic regimen to the infecting organism.

It is generally accepted that high doses of antibiotics should be used in ALBC at the time of first-stage revision, with the goal of prolonged elution of antibiotics into the joint space and achievement of effective antimicrobial concentrations within the joint space and over a sustained period. Because these spacers are by definition temporary, strategies for optimal elution can be pursued without major concern about the potential adverse effect of mechanical properties of cement. In general, greater amounts of antibiotic will increase elution rates and length of time that effective intra-articular concentrations will be maintained. No high-quality data exist comparing clinical effectiveness of different antibiotic concentrations [158]. However, a general consensus exists that low-dose ALBC preparations of 1 g antibiotic per 40 g bag are insufficient for therapeutic use, whereas doses >8 g per bag have been reported to adversely affect handling characteristics during spacer formation [159]. Effective infection control has been reported with doses as low as 1.2 g per bag, the most commonly reported doses in the literature ranging from 3.4 to 8.6 g of antibiotic per bag of cement [22]. Although isolated case reports of adverse events have been attributed to systemic antibiotic toxicity, these seem to be exceptionally rare and insufficient evidence exists to justify decreasing antibiotic concentrations.

Antibiotic elution rates are known to be the product of several factors that can be varied independent of the concentration of antibiotic used, including cement surface area and porosity. Several cement preparation strategies have been shown to increase the elution of antibiotics and should be used when forming spacers for first-stage revision procedures. These include high-speed hand-mixing (3+ cycles per second) under atmospheric pressure, adding powdered antibiotics after cement mixing is complete, not crushing antibiotic crystals, and not adding additional liquid monomer in an attempt to compensate for the increased volume of powder added [160–162]. It is worth noting that higher concentrations of powdered antibiotics increase cement porosity, further increasing their elution.

Selection of antibiotics for surgeon-mixed high-dose ALBC should be guided by the sensitivity profiles of the infecting organisms, while ensuring that they meet the prerequisite criteria for effective local activity (i.e., heat stable and water soluble). The most commonly used antibiotics include the aminoglycosides, such as gentamicin and tobramycin; vancomycin; and cephalosporins, such as cefazolin [22]. For susceptible organisms, the use of cefazolin either in place of or in combination with vancomycin may be advantageous because of its bactericidal activity and superior elution characteristics [163].

The use of at least two different classes of antibiotics is recommended. In vitro studies have demonstrated a synergistic effect of bi- and tri-antibiotic cement on elution rates, although evidence concerning a synergistic effect on bacterial growth is equivocal [163, 164]. However, inclusion of more than one class of antibiotic maximizes the likelihood of effective local antimicrobial activity.

Particular care should be taken with antibiotic selection for ALBC in patients who have failed previous spacer implantation because aminoglycoside-reported resistance rates for isolates from these patients were between 1.7 and 2.5 times those from patients with first-time periprosthetic infections [120].

At the time of component reimplantation similar to aseptic revision procedures, the use of cemented fixation after periprosthetic infections is routine for knees. Given the evidence supporting the benefits of ALBC in aseptic revision surgery, little controversy exists surrounding its use at the time of definitive component reimplantation after periprosthetic infection when cemented fixation is used. Available strategies for cemented fixation include using a commercially prepared low-dose ALBC or a custom-mixed ALBC prepared in the operating room.

Commercially available low-dose ALBC in the United States is FDA approved specifically (and only) for use in second-stage revision. Custom-mixed ALBC provides theoretical advantages by allowing for tailoring of antibiotics based on local resistance patterns and/or sensitivities of organisms isolated from the infected joint, while providing elution characteristics similar to commercially prepared cement [165]. However, little guidance is available from the literature in terms of outcomes with either approach.

If a custom-mixed ALBC is used, given the previously described evidence concerning antibiotic concentration and mechanical properties of cement, it would seem reasonable to limit concentrations to no more than 2 g per 40 g bag [120, 156]. Similarly, liquid antibiotics should be avoided [109]. Consideration should be given to using more than one antibiotic, given the synergistic effects and broader antimicrobial activity spectrum that can be achieved [163, 164]. To maximize mechanical characteristics, the antibiotics should be added to the cement powder first, followed by the addition of the monomer and vacuum mixing [161].

References

1. Kurtz S, Ong K, Lau E, Mowat F, Halpern M. Projections of primary and revision hip and knee arthroplasty in the United States from 2005 to 2030. J Bone Joint Surg Am. 2007;89(4):780–5.
2. Kurtz SM, Lau E, Watson H, Schmier JK, Parvizi J. Economic burden of periprosthetic joint infection in the United States. J Arthroplast. 2012;27(8 Suppl):61–5.
3. Bengtson S, Knutson K. The infected knee arthroplasty. A 6-year follow-up of 357 cases. Acta Orthop Scand. 1991;62:301–11.
4. Blom AW, Brown J, Taylor AH, Pattison G, Whitehouse S, Bannister GC. Infection after total knee arthroplasty. J Bone Joint Surg Br. 2004;86:688–91.
5. Nickinson R, Board T, Gambhir A, Porter M, Kay P. The microbiology of the infected knee arthroplasty. Int Orthop. 2010;34:505–10.
6. Phillips JE, Crane TP, Noy M, Elliott TSJ, Grimer RJ. The incidence of deep prosthetic infections in a specialist orthopaedic hospital: a 15-year prospective survey. J Bone Joint Surg Br. 2006;88:943–8.
7. World Health Organization. WHO guidelines for safe surgery: 2009: safe surgery saves lives. http://whqlibdoc.who.int/publications/2009/9789241598552_eng.pdf. Accessed 18 Nov 2010.
8. Illingworth KD, Mihalko WM, Parvizi J, Sculco T, McArthur B, el Bitar Y, Saleh KJ. How to minimize infection and thereby maximize patient outcomes in total joint arthroplasty: a multicenter approach. AAOS exhibit selection. J Bone Joint Surg Am. 2013;95(8):e50.
9. Papas PV, Congiusta D, Scuderi GR, Cushner FD. A modern approach to preventing prosthetic joint infections. J Knee Surg. 2018;31(7):610–7.
10. Prokuski L. Prophylactic antibiotics in orthopaedic surgery. J Am Acad Orthop Surg. 2008;16(5):283–93.
11. Fletcher N, Sofianos D, Berkes MB, Obremskey WT. Prevention of perioperative infection. J Bone Joint Surg Am. 2007;89:1605–18.
12. Davis N, Curry A, Gambhir AK, Panigrahi H, Walker CR, Wilkins EG, Worsley MA, Kay PR. Intraoperative bacterial contamination in operations for joint replacement. J Bone Joint Surg Br. 1999;81:886–9.
13. Page CP, Bohnen JM, Fletcher JR, McManus AT, Solomkin JS, Wittmann DH. Antimicrobial prophylaxis for surgical wounds. Guidelines for clinical care. Arch Surg. 1993;128:79–88.
14. Bratzler DW, Houck PM; Surgical Infection Prevention Guidelines Writers Workgroup; American Academy of Orthopaedic Surgeons; American Association of Critical Care Nurses; American Association of Nurse Anesthetists; American College of Surgeons; American College of Osteopathic Surgeons; American Geriatrics Society; American Society of Anesthesiologists; American

Society of Colon and Rectal Surgeons; American Society of Health-System Pharmacists; American Society of Peri Anesthesia Nurses; Ascension Health; Association of peri Operative Registered Nurses; Association for Professionals in Infection Control and Epidemiology; Infectious Diseases Society of America; Medical Letter; Premier; Society for Healthcare Epidemiology of America; Society of Thoracic Surgeons; Surgical Infection Society; Surgical Infection Prevention Guideline Writers Work Group. Antimicrobial prophylaxis for surgery: an advisory statement from the National Surgical Infection Prevention Project. Clin Infect Dis. 2004;38:1706–15.

15. Meehan J, Jamali AA, Nguyen H. Prophylactic antibiotics in hip and knee arthroplasty. J Bone Joint Surg Am. 2009;91(10):2480–90.

16. Mangram AJ, Horan TC, Pearson ML, Silver LC, Jarvis WR. Guideline for prevention of surgical site infection, 1999. Hospital Infection Control Practices Advisory Committee. Infect Control Hosp Epidemiol. 1999;20:250–78.

17. Burke JF. The effective period of preventive antibiotic action in experimental incisions and dermal lesions. Surgery. 1961;50:161–8.

18. Tachdjian MO, Compere EL. Postoperative wound infections in orthopedic surgery: evaluation of prophylactic antibiotics. J Int Coll Surg. 1957;28(6 Pt 1):797–805.

19. Aslam S, Darouiche RO. Prosthetic joint infections. Curr Infect Dis Rep. 2012;14(5):551–7.

20. Bernard L, Sadowski C, Monin D, Stern R, Wyssa B, Rohner P, Lew D, Hoffmeyer P. The value of bacterial culture during clean orthopedic surgery: a prospective study of 1,036 patients. Infect Control Hosp Epidemiol. 2004;25:512–4.

21. Osmon DR. Antimicrobial resistance: guidelines for the practicing orthopaedic surgeon. Instr Course Lect. 2002;51:527–37.

22. Costerton JW, Stewart PS, Greenberg EP. Bacterial biofilms: a common cause of persistent infections. Science. 1999;284:1318–22.

23. Zimmerli W, Moser C. Pathogenesis and treatment concepts of orthopaedic biofilm infections. FEMS Immunol Med Microbiol. 2012;65(2):158–68.

24. Lamagni T. Epidemiology and burden of prosthetic joint infections. J Antimicrob Chemother. 2014;69(Suppl 1):i5–i10.

25. Del Pozo JL, Patel R. Clinical practice: infection associated with prosthetic joints. N Engl J Med. 2009;361(8):787–94.

26. Hare R, Thomas CG. The transmission of Staphylococcus aureus. Br Med J. 1956;2:840–4.

27. Ritter MA. Operating room environment. Clin Orthop Relat Res. 1999;369:103–9.

28. Daines BK, Dennis DA, Amann S. Infection prevention in total knee arthroplasty. J Am Acad Orthop Surg. 2015;23(06):356–64.

29. Peersman G, Laskin R, Davis J, Peterson M. Infection in total knee replacement: a retrospective review of 6489 total knee replacements. Clin Orthop Relat Res. 2001;392:15–23.

30. Namba RS, Inacio MCS, Paxton EW. Risk factors associated with deep surgical site infections after primary total knee arthroplasty: an analysis of 56,216 knees. J Bone Joint Surg Am. 2013;95(09):775–82.

31. De Francesco CJ, Fu MC, Kahlenberg CA, Miller AO, Bostrom MP. Extended antibiotic prophylaxis may be linked to lower peri-prosthetic joint infection rates in high-risk patients: an evidence-based review. HSS J. 2019;15(3):297–301.

32. Inabathula A, Dilley JE, Ziemba-Davis M, Warth LC, Azzam KA, Ireland PH, Meneghini RM. Extended oral antibiotic prophylaxis in high-risk patients substantially reduces primary total hip and knee arthroplasty 90-day infection rate. J Bone Joint Surg Am. 2018;100(24):2103–9.

33. Australian Orthopaedic Association: National Joint Replacement Registry Supplemental report: cement in hip and knee arthroplasty, Adelaide, Australia. 2016. https://aoanjrr.sahmri.com/documents/10180/275107/Cement%20in%20Hip%20 and%20Knee%20Arthroplasty.

34. Mandell GL, Bennet JE, Dolin R, editors. Mandell, Douglas, and Bennett's principles and practice of infectious diseases, vol. 2. 6th ed. New York: Elsevier/Churchill Livingstone; 2005.

35. Forse RA, Karam B, MacLean LD, Christou NV. Antibiotic prophylaxis for surgery in morbidly obese patients. Surgery. 1989;106:750–7.

36. Holtom PD. Antibiotic prophylaxis: current recommendation. J Am Acad Orthop Surg. 2006;14:S98–S100.

37. Ridgeway S, Wilson J, Charlet A, Kafatos G, Pearson A, Coello R. Infection of the surgical site after arthroplasty of the hip. J Bone Joint Surg Br. 2005;87:844–50.

38. Sewick A, Makani A, Wu C, O'Donnell J, Baldwin KD, Lee GC. Does dual antibiotic prophylaxis better prevent surgical site infections in total joint arthroplasty? Clin Orthop Relat Res. 2012;470(10):2702–7.

39. Windsor RE, Bono JV. Infected total knee replacements. J Am Acad Orthop Surg. 1994;2:44–53.

40. Parvizi J, Gehrke T, Chen AF. Proceedings of the International Consensus on Periprosthetic joint infection. Bone Joint J. 2013;95-B(11):1450–2.

41. Rosenberger LH, Politano AD, Sawyer RG. The surgical care improvement project and prevention of post-operative infection, including surgical site infection. Surg Infect. 2011;12(3):163–8.

42. Neu HC. Cephalosporin antibiotics as applied in surgery of bones and joints. Clin Orthop Relat Res. 1984;190:50–64.

43. Schurman DJ, Hirshman HP, Kajiyama G, Moser K, Burton DS. Cefazolin concentrations in bone and synovial fluid. J Bone Joint Surg Am. 1978;60:359–62.

44. Brill MJ, Houwink AP, Schmidt S, Van Dongen EP, Hazebroek EJ, van Ramshorst B, Deneer VH, Mouton JW, Knibbe CA. Reduced subcutane-

ous tissue distribution of cefazolin in morbidly obese versus non-obese patients determined using clinical microdialysis. J Antimicrob Chemother. 2014;69(3):715–23.

45. Ho VP, Nicolau DP, Dakin GF, Pomp A, Rich BS, Towe CW, Barie PS. Cefazolin dosing for surgical prophylaxis in morbidly obese patients. Surg Infect (Larchmt). 2012;13(1):33–7.

46. Levine DP. Vancomycin: understanding its past and preserving its future. South Med J. 2008;101:284–91.

47. Eshkenazi AU, Garti A, Tamir L, Hendel D. Serum and synovial vancomycin concentrations following prophylactic administration in knee arthroplasty. Am J Knee Surg. 2001;14:221–3.

48. Graziani AL, Lawson LA, Gibson GA, Steinberg MA, MacGregor RR. Vancomycin concentrations in infected and noninfected human bone. Antimicrob Agents Chemother. 1988;32:1320–2.

49. Sivagnanam S, Deleu D. Red man syndrome. Crit Care. 2003;7:119–20.

50. McNamara DR, Steckelberg JM. Vancomycin. J Am Acad Orthop Surg. 2005;13:89–92.

51. Kheir MM, Tan TL, Azboy I, Tan DD, Parvizi J. Vancomycin prophylaxis for total joint arthroplasty: incorrectly dosed and has a higher rate of periprosthetic infection than cefazolin. Clin Orthop Relat Res. 2017;475(7):1767–74.

52. Liu C, Kakis A, Nichols A, Ries MD, Vail TP, Bozic KJ. Targeted use of vancomycin as perioperative prophylaxis reduces periprosthetic joint infection in revision TKA. Clin Orthop Relat Res. 2014;472(1):227–31.

53. Peel TN, Cheng AC, Buising KL, Choong PF. Microbiological aetiology, epidemiology, and clinical profile of prosthetic joint infections: are current antibiotic prophylaxis guidelines effective? Antimicrob Agents Chemother. 2012;56(5):2386–91.

54. Hota B, Ellenbogen C, Hayden MK, Aroutcheva A, Rice TW, Weinstein RA. Community-associated methicillin-resistant Staphylococcus aureus skin and soft tissue infections at a public hospital: do public housing and incarceration amplify transmission? Arch Intern Med. 2007;167:1026–33.

55. Fridkin SK, Hageman JC, Morrison M, Sanza LT, Como-Sabetti K, Jernigan JA, Harriman K, Harrison LH, Lynfield R, Farley MM. Active bacterial core surveillance program of the emerging infections program network. Methicillin-resistant Staphylococcus aureus disease in three communities. N Engl J Med. 2005;352:1436–44.

56. Parvizi J, Pawasarat IM, Azzam KA, Joshi A, Hansen EN, Bozic KJ. Periprosthetic joint infection: the economic impact of methicillin-resistant infections. J Arthroplast. 2010;25(Suppl 6):103–7.

57. Tyllianakis ME, Karageorgos AC, Marangos MN, Saridis AG, Lambiris EE. Antibiotic prophylaxis in primary hip and knee arthroplasty: comparison between cefuroxime and two specific antistaphylococcal agents. J Arthroplast. 2010;25(7):1078–82.

58. Wyles CC, Hevesi M, Osmon DR, Park MA, Habermann EB, Lewallen DG, Berry DJ, Sierra RJ. 2019 John Charnley Award: increased risk of prosthetic joint infection following primary total knee and hip arthroplasty with the use of alternative antibiotics to cefazolin: the value of allergy testing for antibiotic prophylaxis. Bone Joint J. 2019;101-B(6_Suppl_B):9–15.

59. American Academy of Orthopaedic Surgeons. Recommendations for the use of intravenous antibiotic prophylaxis in primary total joint arthroplasty. 2004. http://www.aaos.org/about/papers/advistmt/1027.asp.

60. American Academy of Orthopaedic Surgeons. The use of prophylactic antibiotics in orthopaedic medicine and the emergence of vancomycin-resistant bacteria. 1998. Revised 2002. http://www.aaos.org/about/papers/advistmt/1016.asp.

61. Song KH, Kang YM, Sin HY, Yoon SW, Seo HK, Kwon S, Shin MJ, Chang CB, Kim TK, Kim HB. Outcome of cefazolin prophylaxis for total knee arthroplasty at an institution with high prevalence of methicillin-resistant Staphylococcus aureus infection. Int J Infect Dis. 2011;15(12):e867–70.

62. Centers for Disease Control and Prevention (CDC). Reduced susceptibility of Staphylococcus aureus to vancomycin—Japan, 1996. MMWR Morb Mortal Wkly Rep. 1997;46:624–6.

63. Centers for Disease Control and Prevention (CDC). Staphylococcus aureus resistant to vancomycin—United States, 2002. MMWR Morb Mortal Wkly Rep. 2002;51:565–7.

64. Eggimann P, Pittet D. Infection control in the ICU. Chest. 2001;120:2059–93.

65. Yamada K, Matsumoto K, Tokimura F, Okazaki H, Tanaka S. Are bone and serum cefazolin concentrations adequate for antimicrobial prophylaxis? Clin Orthop Relat Res. 2011;469(12):3486–94.

66. Smith EB, Wynne R, Joshi A, Liu H, Good RP. Is it time to include vancomycin for routine perioperative antibiotic prophylaxis in total joint arthroplasty patients? J Arthroplast. 2012;27:55–60.

67. Zimmerli W, Trampuz A, Ochsner PE. Prosthetic-joint infections. N Engl J Med. 2004;351(16):1645–54.

68. Angthong C, Krajubngern P, Tiyapongpattana W, Pongcharoen B, Pinsornsak P, Tammachote N, Kittisupaluck W. Intraosseous concentration and inhibitory effect of different intravenous cefazolin doses used in preoperative prophylaxis of total knee arthroplasty. J Orthop Traumatol. 2015;16(4):331–4.

69. Young SW, Zhang M, Freeman JT, Vince KG, Coleman B. Higher cefazolin concentrations with intraosseous regional prophylaxis in TKA. Clin Orthop Relat Res. 2013;471(1):244–9.

70. Young SW, Zhang M, Freeman JT, Mutu-Grigg J, Pavlou P, Moore GA. The Mark Coventry Award: higher tissue concentrations of vancomycin with low dose intraosseous regional versus systemic prophylaxis in TKA: a randomized trial. Clin Orthop Relat Res. 2014;472:57–65.

71. Young SW, Zhang M, Moore GA, Pitto RP, Clarke HD, Spangehl MJ. The John N. Insall Award: higher tissue concentrations of vancomycin achieved with intraosseous regional prophylaxis in revision TKA: a randomized controlled trial. Clin Orthop Relat Res. 2018;476(1):66–74.

72. Young SW, Roberts T, Johnson S, Dalton JP, Coleman B, Wiles S. Regional intraosseous administration of prophylactic antibiotics is more effective than systemic administration in a mouse model of TKA. Clin Orthop Relat Res. 2015;473:3573–84.

73. de Heredia FP, Gómez-Martínez S, Marcos A. Obesity, inflammation and the immune system. Proc Nutr Soc. 2012;71(2):332–8.

74. Jung P, Morris AJ, Zhu M, Roberts SA, Frampton C, Young SW. BMI is a key risk factor for early periprosthetic joint infection following total hip and knee arthroplasty. N Z Med J. 2017;130(1461): 24–34.

75. Kerkhoffs GM, Servien E, Dunn W, Dahm D, Bramer JA, Haverkamp D. The influence of obesity on the complication rate and outcome of total knee arthroplasty: a meta-analysis and systematic literature review. J Bone Joint Surg Am. 2012;94(20):1839–44.

76. Wagner ER, Kamath AF, Fruth K, Harmsen WS, Berry DJ. Effect of body mass index on reoperation and complications after total knee arthroplasty. J Bone Joint Surg Am. 2016;98(24):2052–60.

77. Yosipovitch G, DeVore A, Dawn A. Obesity and the skin: skin physiology and skin manifestations of obesity. J Am Acad Dermatol. 2007;56(6):901–16.

78. Luteijn JM, Hubben GA, Pechlivanoglou P, Bonten MJ, Postma MJ. Diagnostic accuracy of culture-based and PCR-based detection tests for methicillin-resistant Staphylococcus aureus: a meta- analysis. Clin Microbiol Infect. 2011;17(2):146–54.

79. Lozano LM, Núñez M, Segur JM, Maculé F, Sastre S, Núñez E, Suso S. Relationship between knee anthropometry and surgical time in total knee arthroplasty in severely and morbidly obese patients: a new prognostic index of surgical difficulty. Obes Surg. 2008;18(9):1149–53.

80. Gadinsky NE, Manuel JB, Lyman S, Westrich GH. Increased operating room time in patients with obesity during primary total knee arthroplasty: conflicts for scheduling. J Arthroplasty. 2012;27(6):1171–6.

81. Naziri Q, Issa K, Malkani AL, Bonutti PM, Harwin SF, Mont MA. Bariatric orthopaedics: total knee arthroplasty in super-obese patients (BMI > 50 kg/m2). Survivorship and complications. Clin Orthop Relat Res. 2013;471(11):3523–30.

82. Hanley MJ, Abernethy DR, Greenblatt DJ. Effect of obesity on the pharmacokinetics of drugs in humans. Clin Pharmacokinet. 2010;49(2):71–87.

83. Polso AK, Lassiter JL, Nagel JL. Impact of hospital guideline for weight-based antimicrobial dosing in morbidly obese adults and comprehensive literature review. J Clin Pharm Ther. 2014;39(6): 584–608.

84. Bauer LA, Black DJ, Lill JS. Vancomycin dosing in morbidly obese patients. Eur J Clin Pharmacol. 1998;54(8):621–5.

85. Darley ES, MacGowan AP. Antibiotic treatment of gram-positive bone and joint infections. J Antimicrob Chemother. 2004;53(6):928–35.

86. Chin SJ, Moore GA, Zhang M, Clarke HD, Spangehl MJ, Young SW. The AAHKS Clinical Research Award: intraosseous regional prophylaxis provides higher tissue concentrations in high BMI patients in total knee arthroplasty: a randomized trial. J Arthroplast. 2018;33(7S):S13–8.

87. Steinberg JP, Braun BI, Hellinger WC, Kusek L, Bozikis MR, Bush AJ, Dellinger EP, Burke JP, Simmons B, Kritchevsky SB. Trial to Reduce Antimicrobial Prophylaxis Errors (TRAPE) Study Group: timing of antimicrobial prophylaxis and the risk of surgical site infections: results from the trial to reduce antimicrobial prophylaxis errors. Ann Surg. 2009;250(1):10–6.

88. Sharareh B, Sutherland C, Pourmand D, Molina N, Nicolau DP, Schwarzkopf R. Effect of body weight on cefazolin and vancomycin trabecular bone concentrations in patients undergoing total joint arthroplasty. Surg Infect. 2016;17(1):1–7.

89. Bosco JA, Bookman J, Slover J, Edusei E, Levine B. Principles of antibiotic prophylaxis in total joint arthroplasty: current concepts. J Am Acad Orthop Surg. 2015;23(8):e27–35.

90. Heydemann JS, Nelson CL. Short-term preventive antibiotics. Clin Orthop Relat Res. 1986;205:184–7.

91. Williams DN, Gustilo RB. The use of preventive antibiotics in orthopaedic surgery. Clin Orthop Relat Res. 1984;190:83–8.

92. Wymenga AB, Hekster YA, Theeuwes A, Muytjens HL, van Horn JR, Slooff TJ. Antibiotic use after cefuroxime prophylaxis in hip and knee joint replacement. Clin Pharmacol Ther. 1991;50(2):215–20.

93. Tokarski AT, Karam JA, Zmistowski B, Deirmengian CA, Deirmengian GK. Clostridium difficile is common in patients with postoperative diarrhea after hip and knee arthroplasty. J Arthroplast. 2014;29:1110–3.

94. Campbell R, Dean B, Nathanson B, Haidar T, Strauss M, Thomas S. Length of stay and hospital costs among high-risk patients with hospital-origin Clostridium difficile-associated diarrhea. J Med Econ. 2013;16(3):440–8.

95. Bode LG, Kluytmans JA, Wertheim HF, Bogaers D, Vandenbroucke-Grauls CM, Roosendaal R, Troelstra A, Box AT, Voss A, van der Tweel I, van Belkum A, Verbrugh HA, Vos MC. Preventing surgical-site infections in nasal carriers of Staphylococcus aureus. N Engl J Med. 2010;362(1):9–17.

96. Hadley S, Immerman I, Hutzler L, Slover J, Bosco J. Staphylococcus aureus decolonization protocol decreases surgical site infections for total joint replacement. Arthritis. 2010;2010:924518.

97. Kim DH, Spencer M, Davidson SM, Li L, Shaw JD, Gulczynski D, Hunter DJ, Martha JF, Miley GB,

Parazin SJ, Dejoie P, Richmond JC. Institutional prescreening for detection and eradication of methicillin-resistant Staphylococcus aureus in patients undergoing elective orthopaedic surgery. J Bone Joint Surg Am. 2010;92(9):1820–6.

98. European Antimicrobial Resistance Surveillance System (EARSS). Annual report 2004. Bilthoven: RIVM; 2005.

99. Ramos N, Skeete F, Haas JP, Hutzler L, Slover J, Phillips M, Bosco J. Surgical site infection prevention initiative: patient attitude and compliance. Bull NYU Hosp Jt Dis. 2011;69(4):312–5.

100. Hacek DM, RobbWJ PSM, Kudrna JC, Stamos VP, Peterson LR. Staphylococcus aureus nasal decolonization in joint replacement surgery reduces infection. Clin Orthop Relat Res. 2008;466(6):1349–55.

101. Shrestha NK, Shermock KM, Gordon SM, Tuohy MJ, Wilson DA, Cwynar RE, Banbury MK, Longworth DL, Isada CM, Mawhorter SD, Procop GW. Predictive value and cost-effectiveness analysis of a rapid polymerase chain reaction for preoperative detection of nasal carriage of Staphylococcus aureus. Infect Control Hosp Epidemiol. 2003;24(5):327–33.

102. Slover J, Haas JP, Quirno M, Phillips MS, Bosco JA III. Cost-effectiveness of a Staphylococcus aureus screening and decolonization program for high-risk orthopedic patients. J Arthroplast. 2011;26(3):360–5.

103. Immerman I, Ramos NL, Katz GM, Hutzler LH, Phillips MS, Bosco JA III. The persistence of Staphylococcus aureus decolonization after mupirocin and topical chlorhexidine: implications for patients requiring multiple or delayed procedures. J Arthroplast. 2012;27(6):870–6.

104. Buchholz HW, Elson RA, Engelbrecht E, Lodenkämper H, Rottger J, Siegel A. Management of deep infection of total hip replacement. J Bone Joint Surg Br. 1981;63:342–53.

105. Joseph TN, Chen AL, Di Cesare PE. Use of antibiotic-impregnated cement in total joint arthroplasty. J Am Acad Orthop Surg. 2003;11(1):38–47.

106. Arora M, Chan EK, Gupta S, Diwan AD. Polymethylmethacrylate bone cements and additives: a review of the literature. World J Orthop. 2013;4(2):67–74.

107. Jiranek WA, Hanssen AD, Greenwald AS. Antibiotic-loaded bone cement for infection prophylaxis in total joint replacement. J Bone Joint Surg Am. 2006;88(11):2487–500.

108. van de Belt H, Neut D, Schenk W, van Horn JR, van Der Mei HC, Busscher HJ. Staphylococcus aureus biofilm formation on different gentamicin-loaded polymethylmethacrylate bone cements. Biomaterials. 2001;22:1607–11.

109. Lautenschlager EP, Jacobs JJ, Marshall GW, Meyer PR Jr. Mechanical properties of bone cements containing large doses of antibiotic powders. J Biomed Mater Res. 1976;10(6):929–38.

110. Bourne RB. Prophylactic use of antibiotic bone cement: an emerging standard. In the affirmative. J Arthroplasty. 2004;19(4 Suppl 1):69–72.

111. Hanssen AD. Prophylactic use of antibiotic bone cement: an emerging standard. In opposition. J Arthroplasty. 2004;19(4 Suppl 1):73–7.

112. Hendriks JG, Neut D, van Horn JR, van der Mei HC, Busscher HJ. Bacterial survival in the interfacial gap in gentamicin-loaded acrylic bone cements. J Bone Joint Surg Br. 2005;87:272–6.

113. Klekamp J, Dawson JM, Haas DW, DeBoer D, Christie M. The use of vancomycin and tobramycin in acrylic bone cement: biomechanical effects and elution kinetics for use in joint arthroplasty. J Arthroplast. 1999;14:339–46.

114. Dunne NJ, Hill J, McAfee P, Kirkpatrick R, Patrick S, Tunney M. Incorporation of large amounts of gentamicin sulphate into acrylic bone cement: effect on handling and mechanical properties, antibiotic release, and biofilm formation. Proc Inst Mech Eng H. 2008;222:355–65.

115. Powles JW, Spencer RF, Lovering AM. Gentamicin release from old cement during revision hip arthroplasty. J Bone Joint Surg Br. 1998;80:607–10.

116. Chang YH, Tai CL, Hsu HY, Hsieh PH, Lee MS, Ueng SW. Liquid antibiotics in bone cement: an effective way to improve the efficiency of antibiotic release in antibiotic loaded bone cement. Bone Joint Res. 2014;3:246–51.

117. Cummins JS, Tomek IM, Kantor SR, Furnes O, Engesaeter LB, Finlayson SR. Cost-effectiveness of antibiotic-impregnated bone cement used in primary total hip arthroplasty. J Bone Joint Surg Am. 2009;91:634–41.

118. Dunbar MJ. Antibiotic bone cements: their use in routine primary total joint arthroplasty is justified. Orthopedics. 2009;32.

119. Josefsson G, Kolmert L. Prophylaxis with systematic antibiotics versus gentamicin bone cement in total hip arthroplasty. A ten-year survey of 1,688 hips. Clin Orthop Relat Res. 1993;(292):210–4.

120. Corona PS, Espinal L, Rodríguez-Pardo D, Pigrau C, Larrosa N, Flores X. Antibiotic susceptibility in gram-positive chronic joint arthroplasty infections: increased aminoglycoside resistance rate in patients with prior aminoglycoside-impregnated cement spacer use. J Arthroplast. 2014;29:1617–21.

121. Hansen EN, Adeli B, Kenyon R, Parvizi J. Routine use of antibiotic laden bone cement for primary total knee arthroplasty: impact on infecting microbial patterns and resistance profiles. J Arthroplast. 2014;29:1123–7.

122. Wu CT, Chen IL, Wang JW, Ko JY, Wang CJ, Lee CH. Surgical site infection after Total knee arthroplasty: risk factors in patients with timely administration of systemic prophylactic antibiotics. J Arthroplast. 2016;31(7):1568–73.

123. Engesaeter LB, Lie SA, Espehaug B, Furnes O, Vollset SE, Havelin LI. Antibiotic prophylaxis in total hip arthroplasty: effects of antibiotic prophylaxis systemically and in bone cement on the revision rate of 22,170 primary hip replacements

followed 0-14 years in the Norwegian Arthroplasty Register. Acta Orthop Scand. 2003;74(6):644–51.

124. Espehaug B, Engesaeter LB, Vollset SE, Havelin LI, Langeland N. Antibiotic prophylaxis in total hip arthroplasty: review of 10,905 primary cemented total hip replacements reported to the Norwegian arthroplasty register, 1987 to 1995. J Bone Joint Surg Br. 1997;79(4):590–5.

125. Bohm E, Zhu N, Gu J, de Guia N, Linton C, Anderson T, Paton D, Dunbar M. Does adding antibiotics to cement reduce the need for early revision in total knee arthroplasty? Clin Orthop Relat Res. 2014;472(1):162–8.

126. Hinarejos P, Guirro P, Leal J, et al. The use of erythromycin and colistin-loaded cement in total knee arthroplasty does not reduce the incidence of infection: a prospective randomized study in 3000 knees. J Bone Joint Surg Am. 2013;95(9):769–74.

127. Gutowski CJ, Zmistowski BM, Clyde CT, Parvizi J. The economics of using prophylactic antibiotic-loaded bone cement in total knee replacement. Bone Joint J. 2014;96-B(1):65–9.

128. Liu HT, Chiu FY, Chen CM, Chen TH. The combination of systemic antibiotics and antibiotics impregnated cement in primary total knee arthroplasty in patients of rheumatoid arthritis-evaluation of 60 knees. J Chin Med Assoc. 2003;66:533–6.

129. Dowsey MM, Choong PF. Obese diabetic patients are at substantial risk for deep infection after primary TKA. Clin Orthop Relat Res. 2009;467:1577–81.

130. Malinzak RA, Ritter MA, Berend ME, Meding JB, Olberding EM, Davis KE. Morbidly obese, diabetic, younger, and unilateral joint arthroplasty patients have elevated total joint arthroplasty infection rates. J Arthroplast. 2009;24:84–8.

131. Pulido L, Ghanem E, Joshi A, Purtill JJ, Parvizi J. Periprosthetic joint infection: the incidence, timing, and predisposing factors. Clin Orthop Relat Res. 2008;466:1710–5.

132. Jämsen E, Nevalainen P, Kalliovalkama J, Moilanen T. Preoperative hyperglycemia predicts infected total knee replacement. Eur J Intern Med. 2010;21:196–201.

133. Mraovic B, Suh D, Jacovides C, Parvizi J. Perioperative hyperglycemia and postoperative infection after lower limb arthroplasty. J Diabetes Sci Technol. 2011;5:412–8.

134. Qadir R, Sidhu S, Ochsner JL, Meyer MS, Chimento GF. Risk stratified usage of antibiotic-loaded bone cement for primary total knee arthroplasty: short term infection outcomes with a standardized cement protocol. J Arthroplast. 2014;29:1622–4.

135. Albuhairan B, Hind D, Hutchinson A. Antibiotic prophylaxis for wound infections in total joint arthroplasty: a systematic review. J Bone Joint Surg. 2008;90-B(7):915–9.

136. Glenny AM, Song F. Antimicrobial prophylaxis in total hip replacement: a systematic review. Health Technol Assess. 1999;3(21):1–57.

137. Mortazavi SMJ, Schwartzenberger J, Austin MS, Purtill JJ, Parvizi J. Revision total knee arthroplasty infection: incidence and predictors. Clin Orthop Relat Res. 2010;468:2052–9.

138. Mortazavi SMJ, Molligan J, Austin MS, Purtill JJ, Hozack WJ, Parvizi J. Failure following revision total knee arthroplasty: infection is the major cause. Int Orthop. 2011;35:1157–64.

139. Ong KL, Lau E, Suggs J, Kurtz SM, Manley MT. Risk of subsequent revision after primary and revision total joint arthroplasty. Clin Orthop Relat Res. 2010;468(11):3070–6.

140. Slover J, Zuckerman JD. Increasing use of total knee replacement and revision surgery (2012). J Am Med Assoc. 2012;308(12):1266–8.

141. Burnett RS, Aggarwal A, Givens SA, McClure JT, Morgan PM, Barrack RL. Prophylactic antibiotics do not affect cultures in the treatment of an infected TKA: a prospective trial. Clin Orthop Relat Res. 2010;468(1):127–34.

142. Tetreault MW, Wetters NG, Aggarwal V, Mont M, Parvizi J, Della Valle CJ. The Chitranjan Ranawat Award: should prophylactic antibiotics be withheld before revision surgery to obtain appropriate cultures? Clin Orthop Relat Res. 2014;472(1):52–6.

143. American Society of Health-System Pharmacists. ASHP therapeutic guidelines on antimicrobial prophylaxis in surgery. Am J Health Syst Pharm. 1999;56:1839–88.

144. Mulcahy H. Chew current concepts in knee replacement: complications. Am J Roentgenol. 2014;202:W76–86.

145. Kremers HM, Larson DR, Crowson CS, Kremers WK, Washington RE, Steiner CA, Jiranek WA, Berry DJ. Prevalence of total hip and knee replacement in the United States. J Bone Joint Surg Am. 2015;97:1386–97.

146. Sierra RJ, Cooney WP, Pagnano MW, Trousdale RT, Rand JA. Reoperations after 3200 revision TKAs: rates, etiology, and lessons learned. Clin Orthop Relat Res. 2004;425:200–6.

147. Voigt J, Mosier M, Darouiche R. Systematic review and meta-analysis of randomized controlled trials of antibiotics and antiseptics for preventing infection in people receiving primary total hip and knee prostheses. Antimicrob Agents Chemother. 2015;59(11):6696–707.

148. Voigt J, Mosier M, Darouiche R. Antibiotics and antiseptics for preventing infection in people receiving revision total hip and knee prostheses: a systematic review of randomized controlled trials. BMC Infect Dis. 2016;749:1–9.

149. Widmer AF. New developments in diagnosis and treatment of infection in orthopedic implants. Clin Infect Dis. 2001;33(s2):S94–106.

150. de Vries L, van der Weegen W, Neve WC, Das H, Ridwan BU, Steens J. The effectiveness of debridement, antibiotics and irrigation for periprosthetic joint infections after primary hip and knee arthroplasty. A 15 years retrospective study

in two community hospitals in the Netherlands. J Bone Joint Infect. 2016;1:20–4.

151. Kuiper JWP, Willink RT, Moojen DJF, van den Bekerom MP, Colen S. Treatment of acute periprosthetic infections with prosthesis retention: review of current concepts. World J Orthop. 2014;5(5):667.

152. Vahedi H, Aali-Rezaie A, Shahi A, Conway JD. Irrigation, débridement, and implant retention for recurrence of periprosthetic joint infection following two-stage revision Total knee arthroplasty: a matched cohort study. J Arthroplast. 2019;34(8):1772–5.

153. Moran E, Masters S, Berendt AR, McLardy-Smith P, Byren I, Atkins BL. Guiding empirical antibiotic therapy in orthopaedics: the microbiology of prosthetic joint infection managed by debridement, irrigation and prosthesis retention. J Infect. 2007;55(1):1–7.

154. Sousa R, Pereira A, Massada M, Vieira Da Silva M, Lemos R, Costa E, Castro J. Empirical antibiotic therapy in prosthetic joint infections. Acta Orthop Belg. 2010;76(2):254–9.

155. Argenson JN, Arndt M, Babis G, Battenberg A, Budhiparama N, Catani F, Chen F, de Beaubien B, Ebied A, Esposito S, Ferry C, Flores H, Giorgini A, Hansen E, Hernugrahanto KD, Hyonmin C, Kim TK, Koh IJ, Komnos G, Lausmann C, Loloi J, Lora-Tamayo J, Lumban-Gaol I, Mahyudin F, Mancheno-Losa M, Marculescu C, Marei S, Martin KE, Meshram P, Paprosky WG, Poultsides L, Saxena A, Schwechter E, Shah J, Shohat N, Sierra RJ, Soriano A, Stefánsdóttir A, Suleiman LI, Taylor A, Triantafyllopoulos GK, Utomo DN, Warren D, Whiteside L, Wouthuyzen-Bakker M, Yombi J, Zmistowski B. Hip and knee section, treatment, debridement and retention of implant: proceedings of International Consensus on Orthopedic Infections. J Arthroplast. 2019;34(2S):S399–419.

156. Chiu FY, Lin CF. Antibiotic-impregnated cement in revision total knee arthroplasty. A prospective cohort study of one hundred and eighty-three knees. J Bone Joint Surg Am. 2009;91(3):628–33.

157. Bini SA, Chan PH, Inacio MC, Paxton EW, Khatod M. Antibiotic cement was associated with half the risk of re-revision in 1,154 aseptic revision total knee arthroplasties. Acta Orthop. 2016;87:55–9.

158. Iarikov D, Demian H, Rubin D, Alexander J, Nambiar S. Choice and doses of antibacterial agents for cement spacers in treatment of prosthetic joint infections: review of published studies. Clin Infect Dis. 2012;55:1474–80.

159. Hsieh PH, Chen LH, Chen CH, Lee MS, Yang WE, Shih CH. Two-stage revision hip arthroplasty for infection with a custommade, antibiotic-loaded, cement prosthesis as an interim spacer. J Trauma. 2004;56:1247–52.

160. Amin TJ, Lamping JW, Hendricks KJ, McIff TE. Increasing the elution of vancomycin from high-dose antibiotic-loaded bone cement: a novel preparation technique. J Bone Joint Surg Am. 2012;94:1946–51.

161. Miller R, McLaren A, Leon C, McLemore R. Mixing method affects elution and strength of high-dose ALBC: a pilot study. Clin Orthop Relat Res. 2012;470:2677–83.

162. Pithankuakul K, Samranvedhya W, Visutipol B, Rojviroj S. The effects of different mixing speeds on the elution and strength of high-dose antibiotic-loaded bone cement created with the hand-mixed technique. J Arthroplast. 2015;30:858–63.

163. Paz E, Sanz-Ruiz P, Abenojar J, Vaquero-Martin J, Forriol F, Del Real JC. Evaluation of elution and mechanical properties of high-dose antibiotic-loaded bone cement: comparative "in vitro" study of the influence of vancomycin and cefazolin. J Arthroplast. 2015;30:1423–9.

164. Duey RE, Chong AC, McQueen DA, Womack JL, Song Z, Steinberger TA, Wooley PH. Mechanical properties and elution characteristics of polymethylmethacrylate bone cement impregnated with antibiotics for various surface area and volume constructs. Iowa Orthop J. 2012;32:104–15.

165. McLaren AC, Nugent M, Economopoulos K, Kaul H, Vernon BL, McLemore R. Hand-mixed and premixed antibiotic-loaded bone cement have similar homogeneity. Clin Orthop Relat Res. 2009;467:1693–8.

Preoperative Management: Staphylococcus aureus Decolonisation

T. W. Hamilton, A. Alvand, and A. J. Price

26.1 Introduction

Prosthetic joint infection is a catastrophic and an under-recognised complication of knee replacement. Infection can be acute or chronic and represents the most common indication for revision surgery in the first 2 years following implantation [1]. In the UK, the overall revision rate for infection following primary knee replacement, both total and unicompartmental, is 0.92 (95%CI 0.90–0.95) revisions per 1000 prosthesis years with lower revision rates for unicompartmental including patellofemoral replacement as compared to total knee replacement [1]. Management of prosthetic joint infection (PJI) comes at a significant cost to both the patient and healthcare system and despite a better understanding of PJI, and the risk factors for it, the incidence is increasing, in part through improved diagnosis [2, 3].

Reducing the incidence of PJI requires a multifaceted, multi-disciplinary, approach. Prior to surgery, risk factors for PJI need to be screened for, with modifiable risk factors optimised. Once risk factors for PJI have been optimised, then a patient may be booked for surgery and pre-, intra- and post-operative infection prevention packages implemented to further minimise the risk of this devastating complication. Medical optimisation of the patient prior to surgery has been covered in the last chapter. This chapter will focus on preoperative screening and decolonisation of *S. aureus* prior to knee replacement. It will cover the epidemiology of *S. aureus* colonisation, incidence of invasive infection in colonised and non-colonised individuals, methods of decolonisation and the outcomes of decolonisation prior to surgery. Finally, we will review the current international guidelines on decolonisation and outline our local approach.

26.2 Epidemiology of Staphylococcus aureus Colonisation

Colonisation with *S. aureus* is common and can be persistent or intermittent [4]. Around 20% of the population are persistently colonised with relatively high, yet typically asymptomatic, bacterial loads, whilst many more individuals are intermittently colonised, typically with lower bacterial loads [5]. The Danish Twin Study has identified that in the older adults genetics exhibits only a modest influence on risk of persistent nasal *S. aureus* colonisation, whereas male gender, non-smoking status, chronic skin condition, and living

T. W. Hamilton · A. Alvand · A. J. Price (✉)
Nuffield Orthopaedic Centre, OUH NHS Trust, Oxford, UK

Nuffield Department of Orthopaedics Rheumatology and Musculoskeletal Science, Univeristy of Oxford, Oxford, UK
e-mail: thomas.hamilton@ndorms.ox.ac.uk;
abtin.alvand@ndorms.ox.ac.uk;
andrew.price@ndorms.ox.ac.uk

© ISAKOS 2022
U. G. Longo et al. (eds.), *Infection in Knee Replacement*,
https://doi.org/10.1007/978-3-030-81553-0_26

or working on a farm are associated with an increased risk [6, 7].

The primary site for *S. aureus* colonisation is the anterior nares, and colonisation at this location is predictive for colonisation at extra-nasal sites including the skin, throat, perineum, vagina and gastrointestinal tract [4]. Of those colonised at any site with *S. aureus* around 50% are colonised in the anterior nares thus to assess for colonisation status in addition to the anterior nares swabbing of extra-nasal sites should also be considered [4].

Nasal colonisation with *S. aureus* has been reported in around a quarter of patients undergoing joint arthroplasty [8, 9]. Whilst the majority or these are methicillin-sensitive *S. aureus* (MSSA) between 1 and 4% are methicillin-resistant *S. aureus* (MRSA) [8, 9]. Whilst there is some evidence that the overall prevalence of colonisation with *S. aureus* is decreasing over time, it has been reported that there has been a relative increase in the prevalence of MRSA nasal carriage [10].

26.3 Incidence of Invasive Infection in Colonised and Non-colonised Individuals

Persistent colonisation with *S. aureus* is associated with an increased risk of invasive infection compared to that seen in non-colonised individuals [4]. This is particularly true in individuals with regular healthcare contact and in those patients with indwelling devices, such as orthopaedic surgical patients, where a 3- to 11-fold increase in risk has been reported [11]. In hospitalised non-surgical, non-bacteraemic, patients with known *S. aureus* nasal colonisation, it has been reported that the risk of developing a *S. aureus* bacteraemia is three times higher (RR 3.0, 95%CI 2.0–4.7) than non-colonised individuals [12]. In colonised individuals who develop a bacteraemia genotyping has demonstrated that around 80% the isolates from the blood are clonally identical to those from the anterior nares [13, 14]. Data indicate that, compared to MSSA, the risk of invasive infection with MRSA colonisation is substantially higher; however, it is unclear

whether this increased risk is related to the relative virulence of the organism or whether this is due to the fact that those colonised with MRSA represent patients with greater medical comorbidity, broader antibiotic exposure and with longer hospital stays [14–16].

S. aureus is one of the most commonly isolated organisms in prosthetic joint infection and nasal carriage of *S. aureus* has been reported to be one of the most important risk factors for developing surgical site infection with *S. aureus* with surgical site infections noted to be higher in colonised as compared to non-colonised individuals [8, 17]. Based on these observations and work in other areas of healthcare decolonisation of patients colonised with *S. aureus*, both MSSA and MRSA, presents a potential opportunity to reduce the burden of surgical site infection following joint replacement.

26.4 Methods of Decolonisation

Decolonisation can be targeted at both nasal and extra-nasal sites and may be delivered selectively to patients that are known to be colonised with either MSSA or MRSA (or those at high risk of colonisation), or may be delivered universally to all patients undergoing joint replacement.

Nasal decolonisation has traditionally been performed using Mupirocin 2% ointment applied topically two to three times a day for 5 days to the inner surface of each nostril. Mupirocin is a topical antibacterial agent active against *S. aureus*, including MRSA. It is also active against other *Staphylococci*, *Streptococci* and gram-negative organisms such as *E. coli* and *H. influenzae*. Recently however, Mupirocin resistant *S. aureus* has reported to be increasing with the prevalence of Mupirocin resistant MSSA reported to be around 8% and Mupirocin resistant MRSA 14% [18]. Based on this, in combination with the need for multiple days treatment, which risks noncompliance, other methods of decolonisation have been trialled, including photo-disinfection as well as a single topical nasal treatment with either povidone iodine or chlorhexidine gluconate with promising results [19–23].

Extra-nasal decolonisation can be performed by skin washing prior to surgery which is intended to reduce the bacterial load and intuitively should involve the whole body such that, in addition to the surgical site, known extra-nasal colonisation sites are targeted. Skin washing can be performed using an antibacterial or antiseptic soap, povidone iodine or chlorhexidine gluconate. There remains uncertainty as to the effectiveness of preoperative skin washing, the optimal time to start cleaning and optimum agent to use [24–27]. In the UK, where skin washing is performed, chlorhexidine gluconate is probably the most common agent used as it has activity against many pathogens including MRSA.

Whilst decolonisation is successful in the majority of patients, it has been reported that up to twenty percent remain colonised with *S. aureus* despite treatment [28, 29]. The reasons for this remain unclear and whether this represents failure of treatment, potentially due to Mupirocin resistance, or non-compliance is uncertain. As such the optimal decolonisation regime remains unclear and whether to re-assess patients for colonisation following treatment remains controversial and further research is needed to clarify these areas [18, 19].

26.5 Outcomes of Decolonisation Prior to Surgery

The effect of *S. aureus* decolonisation on the risk of surgical site infection following hip and knee replacement has been the subject of several studies (Table 26.1). A recent meta-analysis found that *S. aureus* decolonisation significantly reduced the risk of overall surgical site infection (both superficial and deep infections, Odds Ratio 0.43 95%CI 0.31–0.59) as well as both superficial (Odds Ratio 0.43 95%CI 0.25–0.73) and deep prosthetic joint infections (Odds Ratio 0.40 95%CI 0.21–0.77) following hip and knee replacement surgery [40]. Whilst these results indicate that screening and decolonisation of *S. aureus* is associated with a reduction in prosthetic joint infection, it is important to acknowledge that these results represent the outcomes

seen in predominantly retrospective and non-randomised studies and as such does not take into account other improvements in practice that have been implemented to reduce prosthetic joint infection.

26.6 Current Guidelines

World Health Organisation

- *Nasal Decontamination.*
  - Does not specify about universal screening and decolonisation.
  - Topical Mupirocin for decolonisation of MRSA and/or MSSA colonised patients.
- *Skin Decontamination.*
  - Shower or bathe the night prior to surgery.
  - Consider cleansing with chlorhexidine gluconate body wash.

International Consensus Meeting

- *Nasal Decontamination.*
  - No definitive recommendation on screening and decolonisation.
  - No consensus for decolonisation method for colonised patients.
- *Skin Decontamination.*
  - Whole-body skin cleansing with chlorhexidine gluconate.
  - Start at least the night prior to surgery.

National Institute for Clinical Excellence

- *Nasal Decontamination.*
  - Consider topical Mupirocin where S. aureus is a likely cause of a surgical site infection.
- *Skin Decontamination.*
  - Shower or bathe the night prior to or day of surgery using soap.
  - Consider cleansing with chlorhexidine gluconate body wash.

Our institution has adopted a universal decolonisation policy. Our local practice is that all patients undergo nasal swab to assess for MRSA

Table 26.1 Incidence of surgical site infection before and after implementation of a decolonisation programme for *S. aureus* in patients undergoing hip and knee replacement

			Incidence surgical site infection	
Study	Screening	Intervention	Intervention	Control
Rao 2011 [27]	Nasal swab	N: Mupirocin 5d S: CHG 5d	1.32% (17/1285)	2.70% (20/741)
Sankar 2005 [30]	Nasal and extra-nasal swabs	N: Mupirocin/povidone iodine/triclosan	0% (0/231)	0.61% (1/164)
Hacek 2008 [31]	Nasal swab	N: Mupirocin 5d S: Nil	1.21% (11/912)	2.60% (14/583)
Hadley 2010 [32]	Nasal swab	N: Mupirocin 5d S: CHG 5d	1.28% (21/1644)	1.45% (6/414)
Kim 2010 [8]	Nasal swab	N: Mupirocin 5d S: CHG 5d	0.19% (13/7019)	0.45% (24/5293)
Gottschalk 2014 [33]	Nasal swab	N: Mupirocin 7d S: CHG 1d	1.9% (2/108)	12.9% (9/70)
Baratz 2015 [29]	Nasal swab	N: Mupirocin 5d S: CHG 5d	0.79% (27/3434)	1.07% (33/3080)
McDonald 2015 [34]	Nasal swab	N: Mupirocin 5d S: CHG 5d	0.66% (2/305)	1.8% (11/596)
Sporer 2016 [35]	Nasal swab	N: Mupirocin 5d S: CHG 5d	0.34% (33/9690)	1.11% (16/1443)
Hofmann 2017 [36]	No screening	N: Mupirocin 2d S: Nil	0.74% (4/538)	2.02% (10/496)
Stanbough 2017 [37]	No screening	N: Mupirocin 5d S: CHG 5d	0.22% (5/2205)	0.76% (15/1981)
Jeans 2018 [38]	Nasal & extra-nasal swabs	N: Mupirocin 5d S: Octenisan 5d	1.41% (131/9318)	1.92% (69/3593)
Pelfort 2019 [39]	Nasal swab	N: Mupirocin 5d S: CHG 5d	1.24% (5/403)	4.25% (17/400)

CHG chlorhexidine gluconate, *N* nasal, *S* skin

colonisation 2 weeks before surgery followed by, in all patients, independent of *Staphylococcus* colonisation (both MSSA and MRSA), decolonisation treatment. The rationale for assessing for MRSA colonisation is that contact precautions are taken with all inpatients with a history of MRSA colonisation with these patients nursed in a side room and placed last on the surgical list.

Staphylococcus decolonisation treatment consists of a topical nasal chlorhexidine with neomycin cream (Naseptin, Alliance Pharmaceuticals Limited) together with a chlorhexidine skin wash. The protocol differs based on whether patients are MRSA colonised or not. In MRSA colonised patients, the topical nasal chlorhexidine with neomycin cream is applied three times daily for 5 days prior to surgery and the chlorhexidine wash (HiBiScrub 4%, Molnlycke Health Care Ltd) is used for a similar duration twice a day. In patients with an allergy to either chlorhex-

idine or neomycin or who have a peanut or soya allergy, Mupirocin (Bactroban 2% cream, GlaxoSmithKline UK Ltd) is used. In patients having an allergy to the chlorhexidine wash, Octenisan antimicrobial wash (Schulke) is used. In patients not MRSA colonised, independent of known MSSA colonisation, topical nasal chlorhexidine with neomycin cream is applied three times daily for 1 day prior to surgery and the chlorhexidine wash (HiBiScrub 4%, Molnlycke Health Care Ltd) is used the night before and on the morning of surgery only. Patients are not routinely swabbed to confirm decolonisation.

Our centre is part of the Quality Improvement in Surgical Teams (QIST) Collaborative model. This ongoing cluster-randomised trial led by Northumbria Healthcare NHS Foundation Trust, in partnership with the British Orthopaedic Association hopes to improve the evidence for screening for and decolonisation of *S. aureus* with the results informing practice in the UK and worldwide [41].

References

1. National Joint Registry for Endlgnad, Wales, Northern Ireland and the Isle of Man 16th annual report; 2019.
2. Kurtz SM, et al. Economic burden of periprosthetic joint infection in the United States. J Arthroplast. 2012;27(8 Suppl):61–5.e1.
3. Lenguerrand E, et al. Description of the rates, trends and surgical burden associated with revision for prosthetic joint infection following primary and revision knee replacements in England and Wales: an analysis of the National Joint Registry for England, Wales, Northern Ireland and the Isle of Man. BMJ Open. 2017;7(7):e014056.
4. Brown AF, et al. Staphylococcus aureus colonization: modulation of host immune response and impact on human vaccine design. Front Immunol. 2014;4:507.
5. Kluytmans J, van Belkum A, Verbrugh H. Nasal carriage of Staphylococcus aureus: epidemiology, underlying mechanisms, and associated risks. Clin Microbiol Rev. 1997;10(3):505–20.
6. Andersen PS, et al. Influence of host genetics and environment on nasal carriage of staphylococcus aureus in Danish middle-aged and elderly twins. J Infect Dis. 2012;206(8):1178–84.
7. Andersen PS, et al. Risk factors for Staphylococcus aureus nasal colonization in Danish middle-aged and elderly twins. Eur J Clin Microbiol Infect Dis. 2013;32(10):1321–6.
8. Kim DH, et al. Institutional prescreening for detection and eradication of methicillin-resistant Staphylococcus aureus in patients undergoing elective orthopaedic surgery. J Bone Joint Surg Am. 2010;92(9):1820–6.
9. Sousa RJ, et al. Preoperative Staphylococcus aureus screening/decolonization protocol before Total joint arthroplasty-results of a small prospective randomized trial. J Arthroplast. 2016;31(1):234–9.
10. Gorwitz RJ, et al. Changes in the prevalence of nasal colonization with Staphylococcus aureus in the United States, 2001-2004. J Infect Dis. 2008;197(9):1226–34.
11. Sakr A, et al. Staphylococcus aureus nasal colonization: an update on mechanisms, epidemiology, risk factors, and subsequent infections. Front Microbiol. 2018;9:2419.
12. Wertheim HF, et al. Risk and outcome of nosocomial Staphylococcus aureus bacteraemia in nasal carriers versus non-carriers. Lancet. 2004;364(9435):703–5.
13. von Eiff C, et al. Nasal carriage as a source of Staphylococcus aureus bacteremia. Study Group. N Engl J Med. 2001;344(1):11–6.
14. Stenehjem E, et al. Longitudinal evaluation of clinical and colonization methicillin-resistant Staphylococcus aureus isolates among veterans. Infect Control Hosp Epidemiol. 2015;36(5):587–9.
15. Stenehjem E, Stafford C, Rimland D. Reduction of methicillin-resistant Staphylococcus aureus infection among veterans in Atlanta. Infect Control Hosp Epidemiol. 2013;34(1):62–8.
16. Goyal N, Aggarwal V, Parvizi J. Methicillin-resistant Staphylococcus aureus screening in total joint arthroplasty: a worthwhile endeavor. J Knee Surg. 2012;25(1):37–43.
17. Kalmeijer MD, et al. Nasal carriage of Staphylococcus aureus is a major risk factor for surgical-site infections in orthopedic surgery. Infect Control Hosp Epidemiol. 2000;21(5):319–23.
18. Dadashi M, et al. Mupirocin resistance in Staphylococcus aureus: a systematic review and meta-analysis. J Glob Antimicrob Resist. 2020;20:238–47.
19. Ramos N, et al. Surgical site infection prevention initiative - patient attitude and compliance. Bull NYU Hosp Jt Dis. 2011;69(4):312–5.
20. Anderson MJ, et al. Efficacy of skin and nasal povidone-iodine preparation against mupirocin-resistant methicillin-resistant Staphylococcus aureus and S. aureus within the anterior nares. Antimicrob Agents Chemother. 2015;59(5):2765–73.
21. Torres EG, et al. Is preoperative nasal povidone-iodine as efficient and cost-effective as standard methicillin-resistant Staphylococcus aureus screening protocol in total joint arthroplasty? J Arthroplast. 2016;31(1):215–8.
22. Phillips M, et al. Preventing surgical site infections: a randomized, open-label trial of nasal mupirocin ointment and nasal povidone-iodine solution. Infect Control Hosp Epidemiol. 2014;35(7):826–32.
23. Bryce E, et al. Nasal photodisinfection and chlorhexidine wipes decrease surgical site infections: a historical control study and propensity analysis. J Hosp Infect. 2014;88(2):89–95.
24. Webster J, Osborne S. Preoperative bathing or showering with skin antiseptics to prevent surgical site infection. Cochrane Database Syst Rev. 2015;2:CD004985.
25. Kapadia BH, Elmallah RK, Mont MA. A randomized, clinical trial of preadmission chlorhexidine skin preparation for lower extremity total joint arthroplasty. J Arthroplasty. 2016;31(12):2856–61.
26. Colling K, et al. Pre-operative antiseptic shower and bath policy decreases the rate of S. aureus and methicillin-resistant S. aureus surgical site infections in patients undergoing joint arthroplasty. Surg Infect. 2015;16(2):124–32.
27. Rao N, et al. Preoperative screening/decolonization for Staphylococcus aureus to prevent orthopedic surgical site infection: prospective cohort study with 2-year follow-up. J Arthroplast. 2011;26(8):1501–7.
28. Moroski NM, Woolwine S, Schwarzkopf R. Is preoperative staphylococcal decolonization efficient in total joint arthroplasty. J Arthroplast. 2015;30(3):444–6.
29. Baratz MD, et al. Twenty percent of patients may remain colonized with methicillin-resistant Staphylococcus aureus despite a decolonization pro-

tocol in patients undergoing elective total joint arthroplasty. Clin Orthop Relat Res. 2015;473(7):2283–90.

30. Sankar B, Hopgood P, Bell KM. The role of MRSA screening in joint-replacement surgery. Int Orthop. 2005;29(3):160–3.

31. Hacek DM, et al. Staphylococcus aureus nasal decolonization in joint replacement surgery reduces infection. Clin Orthop Relat Res. 2008;466(6):1349–55.

32. Hadley S, et al. Staphylococcus aureus decolonization protocol decreases surgical site infections for total joint replacement. Arthritis. 2010;2010:924518.

33. Gottschalk MB, et al. Decreased infection rates following total joint arthroplasty in a large county run teaching hospital: a single surgeon's experience and possible solution. J Arthroplast. 2014;29(8):1610–6.

34. McDonald LT, et al. Winning the war on surgical site infection: evidence-based preoperative interventions for total joint arthroplasty. AORN J. 2015;102:182. e1–182.e11.

35. Sporer SM, Rogers T, Abella L. Methicillin-resistant and methicillin-sensitive Staphylococcus aureus screening and decolonization to reduce surgical site infection in elective total joint arthroplasty. J Arthroplast. 2016;31(9 Suppl):144–7.

36. Hofmann KJ, et al. Triple prophylaxis for the prevention of surgical site infections in total joint arthroplasty. Curr Orthop Pract. 2017;28(1):66–9.

37. Stambough JB, et al. Decreased hospital costs and surgical site infection incidence with a universal decolonization protocol in primary total joint arthroplasty. J Arthroplast. 2017;32(3):728–34.

38. Jeans E, et al. Methicillin sensitive staphylococcus aureus screening and decolonisation in elective hip and knee arthroplasty. J Infect. 2018;77(5):405–9.

39. Pelfort X, et al. Reduction of periprosthetic Staphylococcus aureus infection by preoperative screening and decolonization of nasal carriers undergoing total knee arthroplasty. Acta Orthop Traumatol Turc. 2019;53(6):426–31.

40. Zhu X, et al. Can nasal Staphylococcus aureus screening and decolonization prior to elective total joint arthroplasty reduce surgical site and prosthesis-related infections? A systematic review and meta-analysis. J Orthop Surg Res. 2020;15(1):60.

41. No authors listed. QIST: Anaemia & MSSA Collaborative. https://qist.org.uk/ Accessed 9 Oct 2020.

Intraoperative Prevention Strategies to Prevent Infection

Christopher Vertullo

C. Vertullo (✉)
Knee Research Australia,
Gold Coast, QLD, Australia

27.1 Introduction

In modern knee replacement, surgical site infection (SSI) is now the most common reason for revision despite it being a largely avoidable complication, hence the infection prevention chapters of this book are probably the most pertinent [1]. This chapter deals with an important part of the optimisation of surgery outcomes, intraoperative management, and as such most of the principles discussed apply to all aspects of clean elective orthopaedic surgery.

The burden of infection in total knee replacement is devastating for the patient as it occurs usually in the early expected implant survivorship, with younger patients most at risk. As a result, SSI rates are increasingly being used as a quality indicator and comparison benchmark within and across healthcare facilities [2]. A multimodal methodology is compulsory in PJI prevention, and a meticulous approach is important with each component.

For this narrative review, it is assumed the patient will arrive in the operating theatre complex with any immune-compromise reversed, nutrition and body mass index optimised, normothermic, non-anaemic, decolonised and/or screened preoperatively for colonisation with potential skin pathogens such as resistant and sensitive Staph aureus and other Staph species, with optimal blood sugars if the patient is a diabetic and cessation of tobacco products well prior. The details of preoperative optimisation will have been dealt with in preceding chapters.

One on the difficulties in making recommendations around infection prevention best-practice is the quality of the data and the strength of recommendations based around that data. The GRADE categories [3] (Grading of Recommendations Assessment, Development and Evaluation) allow clinicians to grade the quality or certainty of evidence and hence the strength of recommendations. The World Health Organisation's Global Guidelines for the Prevention of Surgical Site Infection uses the GRADE system to guide surgeons as to optimal technique to prevent SSI and is recommended reading; however, many of the recommendations are not arthroplasty specific.

27.2 Antibiotic Prophylaxis

The timing and type of preoperative antibiotics deserves very careful consideration to achieve adequate plasma levels of an appropriate prophylactic antibiotic for the typical local infecting organisms, typically an intravenous first-generation cephalosporin unless the patient is MRSA colonised, prior to the incision being

© ISAKOS 2022
U. G. Longo et al. (eds.), *Infection in Knee Replacement*,
https://doi.org/10.1007/978-3-030-81553-0_27

made and as part of a pre-surgical checklist to avoid errors of omission [4]. Prophylaxis with cefazolin has the lowest risk of later infection compared to alternative antibiotics such as vancomycin with a lower risk of adverse events, hence true allergy screening is recommended [5].

Optimal timing of surgical antibiotic prophylaxis remains uncertain; however, strong evidence suggest administration after incision or tourniquet application increases risk of SSI, as does inadequate levels at the time of surgical closure [2].

Hence, timing should be prior to the incision being made, with reference to the half-life of the chosen antibiotic. If the interval since the initial antibiotic dose is greater than 4 h, further dosing during the procedure is appropriate. For primary TKR, second dosing would be unusual. Underdosing, particularly with vancomycin and in obese individuals is common. Readers are encouraged to review the previous chapter on optimal antibiotic prophylaxis.

The role of intraosseous antibiotics under tourniquet for primary and revision TKR has promising preclinical data [5–7], with 5–20 times plasma levels achieved compared to IV prophylaxis, but routine use in primary TKR remains uncertain [8]. In meta-analysis, no evidence exists that extended course of prophylaxis reduces infection risk [9, 10]; however, the overall GRADE of evidence of the available literature is low (high risk of bias, high risk of publication bias and low precision).

27.3 The Operating Room

A carefully monitored, robust quality assured process following clearly defined national and international standards is required to maintain the Operating Room (OR) infection prevention measures for appropriate environmental cleaning and waste disposal. The entire operating room must be cleaned daily [11], starting from the least soiled and moving to the most soiled areas, using techniques that prevent mists or aerosol creation. After each procedure, soiled and high touch areas require cleaning and disinfecting. Instrument decontamination, cleaning, disinfection and sterilisation must be stan-dardised to national and international standards [12]. A team approach between surgeons and nurses is vital to ensure that all equipment is visibly clean and sterile prior to commencing, especially loan equipment, and that the operating field is sterile and clearly defined. Theatre traffic must be reduced as much as possible to minimise aerosol creation. The long-standing recommendations against the use of laminar flow remains, with no evidence in 12 observational trials of it being of no benefit with greater cost [13]; however, this data has been criticised for the biases inherent in observation registry data [14].

27.4 Hand Preparation

Hand preparation should be undertaken by either hand-scrubbing with antimicrobial aqueous soap or hand-rubbing with alcohol-based hand rub complying with international standards, after an initial hand clean-up with soap prior to entering the OR [15]. Low GRADE evidence suggests alcohol-based hand-rubbing may be superior to antimicrobial aqueous hand-scrubbing, while aqueous chlorhexidine may be superior to iodine aqueous solutions if scrubbing [2].

27.5 Gloves

In a recent meta-analysis, evidence supporting reduced SSI with multiple glove changing remained weak [16], hence authors recommended gloves should be changed after draping, hourly, with any visible penetration and before handling implants [16].

27.6 Surgical Site Preparation

Prior to entering the OR, the surgical site should have been washed with either plain soap, chlorhexidine gluconate soap or chlorhexidine gluconate impregnated cloths, prior to the surgery [17]. It remains unclear of the optimal washing period pre-surgery; however, consensus currently suggests 3 days.

Moderate evidence suggest best-practice site preparation involves never shaving the skin as it increases the infection risk, keeping clipping to the minimum required and only using as a single use device outside the operating theatre [18]. The optimum timing of hair clipping prior to the surgery remains uncertain.

The WHO strongly recommends alcohol-based chlorhexidine gluconate preparation should be utilised with less risk of SSI when compared to alcohol-based povidone-iodine and aqueous solutions with alcoholic and aqueous povidone-iodine having similar SSI rates for all surgical cases based on meta-analysis [2]. The recent cluster-randomised ACAISA trial compared chlorhexidine alcohol versus iodine alcohol for surgical site skin preparation in an elective arthroplasty, finding results contrary to the WHO, with no difference for the primary outcome measure of SSI, but lower prosthetic joint infections. The differences may be attributable the ACASIA being arthroplasty specific. At this stage, it is recommended that prep solutions all contain 70% alcohol and either povidone-iodine or chlorhexidine until more data is available. It is important to recognise that alcoholic preparations are flammable and preparation technique should avoid saturated drapes and or pooling. A recent trial by Morrison et al. [19] suggested a repeated alcoholic iodine preparation just prior to iodine-impregnated incision drape application had a lower SSI than a single preparation; however, it should be recognised that a higher risk of intraoperative fire can occur with this technique [20]. There is no evidence that film-forming cyanoacrylate sealants such as InteguSeal reduce infection rates [21].

27.7 Intra-Articular Dilute Povidone-Iodine Lavage

The benefit of a dilute 500 ml, 0.35% povidone-iodine lavage for 3 min prior to closure in primary arthroplasty has mixed results with observational evidence [22–24], overall suggesting no benefit. In revision total knee arthroplasty, a recent randomised clinical trial [25] of 478 patients undergoing aseptic revision TKA and THA had a lower infection rate with the dilute betadine lavage. The WHO recommends dilute povidone-iodine lavage for clean wounds [2].

27.8 Drapes and Gowns

Sterile impermeable reusable or single use drapes and gowns should be used, with no difference in SSI rates between the two [2, 26]. Conversely, despite theoretical claims of locking in dermal bacteria, plastic adhesive drapes do not reduce the risk of SSI [27] and may cause patient harm through allergy and skin damage. No evidence exists regarding changing gowns or drapes intraoperatively.

27.9 Perioperative Hyperoxygenation

The benefits of 80% fraction of inspired oxygen intraoperatively and post-operatively remain controversial. The WHO strongly recommends perioperative hyperoxygenation to those undergoing general anaesthesia with endotracheal intubation [2]; however, other recent meta-analysis question this recommendation, stating possibly increased mortality with no decrease in SSI [28]. No arthroplasty literature exists in this area.

27.10 Normothermia and Normovolemia Maintenance

Anaesthesia impairs patients' abilities to maintain body temperature, and heat loss is increased due to cool intravenous fluids and irrigation fluids. The WHO recommends active perioperative patient warming based on moderate evidence of reduced SSI in non-arthroplasty literature [2]. While many methods exist for active warming [29], forced air warming may be counterproductive due to aerosol creation.

With the use of tranexamic acid, significant hypovolemia in primary TKR would be atypical; however, in revision surgery normovolaemia needs to be maintained as some evidence in the non-arthroplasty literature suggests lower SSI with a goal directed-fluid therapy [2].

27.11 Dressings, Drains, Sutures and Closure

A variety of antimicrobial sutures are currently available, with the most closely studied being Triclosan (5-chloro-2-(2,4-dichlorophenoxy) phenol), a broad-spectrum bactericidal agent used in a variety of applications including household soaps, which at a higher concentration is bactericidal, and at lower concentration is bacteriostatic [2]. The benefits of Triclosan sutures in arthroplasty remain uncertain, with the WHO recommending their use for all types of surgery; however, two recent clinical trials both failed to show a reduced risk of SSI [30, 31] with them. No data supports changing instruments for closure [2]. While the evidence is fragile, staples have a higher risk of superficial SSI [32, 33] than suture closure.

A recent Cochrane review suggested negative pressure wound therapy reduced the risk of SSI by approximately 33% with moderate evidence [34]; however, its routine use in knee arthroplasty remains uncertain compared to situations with questionable skin integrity. In recent Cochrane review [35], there was no evidence supporting the use of advanced dressing such as hydrocolloid, hydroactive, silver-containing (metallic or ionic) and polyhexamethylene biguanide (PHMB) dressings compared to standard dry absorbant dressings.

The role of surgical drains increasing SSI risk remains uncertain, with some authors finding increased risk [36] with their use, and other describing decreased risk [37]. If drains are used, no evidence supports lower SSI risk with early removal of the drain [2].

27.12 Surgical Hoods and Body Exhaust Suits

When surgical hoods are discussed, it is important to recognise between the two different systems that are available, the original cumbersome negative pressure body exhaust suits (BES) intro-duced by Charnley, and later, the more portable positive pressure surgical helmet systems (SHS) [38]. BES that are characterised by bulky aspiration tubing and a negative intra-suit pressure, have clinical evidence in meta-analysis supporting their ability to reduce deep infection compared to standard surgical gowns [38].

SHS have been described as a "personal protection device", are typically characterised by a fan on a helmet with a positive pressure within the suit, blowing air across the surgeon's face and neck. In contrast to the BES, SHS have not been shown to reduce SSI [38] or wound contamination [39, 40] when compared to standard surgical gowns and in registry studies may increase rates [41]. While taping the gown glove interface does not alter contamination rate [40], authors have suggested using SHS solely as personal protective equipment and wearing a balaclava underneath to reduce bacterial load from the wearer's face and neck [39].

27.13 Prosthesis Design and Antibiotic-Loaded Bone Cement

Despite some controversy around the benefits of antibiotic-loaded bone cement [42], a recent meta-analysis of nine randomised clinical trials using Cochrane methodology and prosthetic joint infection as the primary outcome measure suggested that it did reduce the risk of SSI in TKR [43]. The optimum antibiotics and dosing remain uncertain, with the two most common antibiotics utilised being vancomycin and aminoglycosides such as tobramycin and gentamycin. It should be noted that many randomised clinical trials in this area are underpowered to adequately investigate the primary outcome measure of prosthetic joint infection and observational studies and registry analysis are at risk of selection bias, where high risk patients receive antibiotic-loaded bone cement at higher rates than low risk patients. Future arthroplasty registry imbedded cluster-randomised trials would be a low-cost solution to providing more robust data in this area.

Recently, the interaction of prosthesis design and infection risk has been investigated in registry studies, with up to 100% greater revision for infection risk with posterior stabilised TKR compared to cruciate retaining and over 25% higher for non-cross linked polyethylene [1, 44]. As observational registry studies are at a risk of confounder bias, registry imbedded cluster-randomised trials would be beneficial.

27.14 Blood Management

The interaction of chemoprophylaxis with infection risk remains uncertain and is a complex area with competing risks of mortality and morbidity. Readers are encouraged to refer to the chapter dealing with thromboprophylaxis and haematoma. Some forms of chemoprophylaxis, particularly rivaroxaban [45], have been reported to increase infection rate in smaller observation studies; however, larger registry studies have not shown higher infection risk with direct oral anticoagulants when compared to aspirin [46]. Tranexamic acid has been reported to reduced infection risk [47, 48] in observational studies.

27.15 Post-operative Care

General principles of appropriate wound care are important to follow. Additionally, evidence suggests that post-operative recovery in either specialist elective surgery hospitals or "ring-fenced" elective areas within a non-elective hospital reduces infection risk [49].

References

1. Vertullo CJ, de Steiger RN, Lewis PL, Lorimer M, Peng Y, Graves SE. The effect of prosthetic design and polyethylene type on the risk of revision for infection in total knee replacement: an analysis of 336,997 prostheses from the Australian Orthopaedic Association National Joint Replacement Registry. J Bone Joit Surg. 2018;100(23):2033–40.
2. World Health Organization. Global guidelines for the prevention of surgical site infection; 2016.
3. Guyatt GH, Oxman AD, Vist GE, Kunz R, Falck-Ytter Y, Alonso-Coello P, et al. GRADE: an emerging consensus on rating quality of evidence and strength of recommendations. BMJ. 2008;336(7650):924–6.
4. WHO Surgical Safety Checklist [Internet]. https://www.who.int/patientsafety/safesurgery/checklist/en/.
5. Wyles CC, Hevesi M, Osmon DR, Park MA, Habermann EB, Lewallen DG, et al. John Charnley Award: increased risk of prosthetic joint infection following primary total knee and hip arthroplasty with the use of alternative antibiotics to cefazolin: the value of allergy testing for antibiotic prophylaxis. Bone Joint J. 2019;101-B(6_Suppl_B):9–15.
6. Young SW, Zhang M, Moore GA, Pitto RP, Clarke HD, Spangehl MJ. The John N. Insall Award: higher tissue concentrations of vancomycin achieved with intraosseous regional prophylaxis in revision TKA: a randomized controlled trial. Clin Orthop. 2017;476(1):9.
7. Symonds T, Parkinson B, Hazratwala K, McEwen P, Wilkinson M, Grant A. Use of regional administration of prophylactic antibiotics in total knee arthroplasty: administration of prophylactic antibiotics. ANZ J Surg. 2018;88(9):848–53.
8. Batty LM, Lanting B. Contemporary strategies to prevent infection in hip and knee arthroplasty. Curr Rev Musculoskelet Med. 2020;13(4):400–8.
9. Ryan SP, Kildow BJ, Tan TL, Parvizi J, Bolognesi MP, Seyler TM. Is there a difference in infection risk between single and multiple doses of prophylactic antibiotics? A meta-analysis. Clin Orthop. 2019;477(7):1577–90.
10. Siddiqi A, Forte SA, Docter S, Bryant D, Sheth NP, Chen AF. Perioperative antibiotic prophylaxis in total joint arthroplasty: a systematic review and meta-analysis. J Bone Joint Surg. 2019;101(9):828–42.
11. Dancer SJ. Controlling hospital-acquired infection: focus on the role of the environment and new technologies for decontamination. Clin Microbiol Rev. 2014;27(4):665–90.
12. ISO/TC 198: sterilization of health care products [Internet]. https://www.iso.org/committee/54576.html.
13. Bischoff P, Kubilay NZ, Allegranzi B, Egger M, Gastmeier P. Effect of laminar airflow ventilation on surgical site infections: a systematic review and meta-analysis. Lancet Infect Dis. 2017;17(5):553–61.
14. Jutte PC, Traversari RA, Walenkamp GH. Laminar flow: the better choice in orthopaedic implants. Lancet Infect Dis. 2017 Jul;17(7):695–6.
15. Tanner J, Swarbrook S, Stuart J. Surgical hand antisepsis to reduce surgical site infection. In: The Cochrane Collaboration, editor. Cochrane Database of Systematic Reviews [Internet]. Chichester: Wiley; 2008 [cited 2020 Jul 21]. p. CD004288.pub2. http://doi.wiley.com/10.1002/14651858.CD004288.pub2.
16. Kim K, Zhu M, Munro JT, Young SW. Glove change to reduce the risk of surgical site infection or prosthetic joint infection in arthroplasty surgeries: a systematic review. ANZ J Surg. 2019;89(9):1009–15.

17. Institute for Healthcare Improvement. How-to guide: prevent surgical site infection for hip and knee arthroplasty [Internet]. http://www.ihi.org/resources/Pages/Tools/HowtoGuidePreventSSIforHipKneeArthroplasty.aspx.

18. Tanner J, Norrie P, Melen K. Preoperative hair removal to reduce surgical site infection. Cochrane Wounds Group, editor. Cochrane Database Syst Rev [Internet]. 2011 [cited 2020 Jul 20]. http://doi.wiley.com/10.1002/14651858.CD004122.pub4.

19. Morrison TN, Chen AF, Taneja M, Küçükdurmaz F, Rothman RH, Parvizi J. Single vs repeat surgical skin preparations for reducing surgical site infection after total joint arthroplasty: a prospective, randomized, double-blinded study. J Arthroplasty. 2016;31(6):1289–94.

20. Kezze I, Zoremba N, Rossaint R, Rieg A, Coburn M, Schälte G. Risks and prevention of surgical fires: a systematic review. Anaesthesist. 2018;67(6):426–47.

21. Dohmen PM. Impact of antimicrobial skin sealants on surgical site infections. Surg Infect. 2014;15(4):368–71.

22. Brown NM, Cipriano CA, Moric M, Sporer SM, Della Valle CJ. Dilute betadine lavage before closure for the prevention of acute postoperative deep periprosthetic joint infection. J Arthroplast. 2012;27(1):27–30.

23. Hernandez NM, Hart A, Taunton MJ, Osmon DR, Mabry TM, Abdel MP, et al. Use of povidone-iodine irrigation prior to wound closure in primary total hip and knee arthroplasty: an analysis of 11,738 cases. J Bone Joint Surg. 2019;101(13):1144–50.

24. Kim C-H, Kim H, Lee SJ, Yoon JY, Moon J-K, Lee S, et al. The effect of povidone-iodine lavage in preventing infection after total hip and knee arthroplasties: systematic review and meta-analysis. J Arthroplasty. 2020;35:2267–73.

25. Calkins TE, Culvern C, Nam D, Gerlinger TL, Levine BR, Sporer SM, et al. Dilute betadine lavage reduces the risk of acute postoperative periprosthetic joint infection in aseptic revision total knee and hip arthroplasty: a randomized controlled trial. J Arthroplasty. 2020;35(2):538–543.e1.

26. Rutala WA, Weber DJ. A review of single-use and reusable gowns and drapes in health care. Infect Control Hosp Epidemiol. 2001;22(4):248–57.

27. Webster J, Alghamdi A. Use of plastic adhesive drapes during surgery for preventing surgical site infection. Cochrane Wounds Group, editor. Cochrane Database Syst Rev [Internet]. 2015 [cited 2020 Jul 27]. http://doi.wiley.com/10.1002/14651858.CD006353.pub4.

28. Wetterslev J, Meyhoff CS, Jørgensen LN, Gluud C, Lindschou J, Rasmussen LS. The effects of high perioperative inspiratory oxygen fraction for adult surgical patients. Cochrane Anaesthesia Group, editor. Cochrane Database Syst Rev [Internet]. 2015 [cited 2020 Jul 21]. http://doi.wiley.com/10.1002/14651858.CD008884.pub2.

29. Warttig S, Alderson P, Campbell G, Smith AF. Interventions for treating inadvertent postoperative hypothermia. Cochrane Anaesthesia, Critical and Emergency Care Group, editor. Cochrane Database Syst Rev [Internet]. 2014 [cited 2020 Jul 27]. https://doi.org/10.1002/14651858.CD009892.pub2.

30. Sprowson AP, Jensen C, Parsons N, Partington P, Emmerson K, Carluke I, et al. The effect of triclosan-coated sutures on the rate of surgical site infection after hip and knee arthroplasty: a double-blind randomized controlled trial of 2546 patients. Bone Joint J. 2018;100-B(3):296–302.

31. Sukeik M, George D, Gabr A, Kallala R, Wilson P, Haddad FS. Randomised controlled trial of triclosan coated *vs* uncoated sutures in primary hip and knee arthroplasty. World J Orthop. 2019;10(7):268–77.

32. Krishnan RJ, Crawford EJ, Syed I, Kim P, Rampersaud YR, Martin J. Is the risk of infection lower with sutures than with Staples for skin closure after orthopaedic surgery? A meta-analysis of randomized trials. Clin Orthop. 2019;477(5):922–37.

33. Smith TO, Sexton D, Mann C, Donell S. Sutures versus staples for skin closure in orthopaedic surgery: meta-analysis. BMJ. 2010;340(mar16 1):c1199.

34. Norman G, Goh EL, Dumville JC, Shi C, Liu Z, Chiverton L, et al. Negative pressure wound therapy for surgical wounds healing by primary closure. Cochrane Wounds Group, editor. Cochrane Database Syst Rev [Internet]. 2020 15 [cited 2020 Jul 31]. http://doi.wiley.com/10.1002/14651858.CD009261.pub6.

35. Dumville JC, Gray TA, Walter CJ, Sharp CA, Page T, Macefield R, et al. Dressings for the prevention of surgical site infection. Cochrane Wounds Group, editor. Cochrane Database Syst Rev [Internet]. 2016 [cited 2020 Jul 31]. http://doi.wiley.com/10.1002/14651858.CD003091.pub4.

36. Minnema B, Vearncombe M, Augustin A, Gollish J, Simor AE. Risk factors for surgical-site infection following primary total knee arthroplasty. Infect Control Hosp Epidemiol. 2004;25(6):477–80.

37. Kong L, Cao J, Zhang Y, Ding W, Shen Y. Risk factors for periprosthetic joint infection following primary total hip or knee arthroplasty: a meta-analysis: risk factors for PJI following TJA. Int Wound J. 2017 Jun;14(3):529–36.

38. Young SW, Zhu M, Shirley OC, Wu Q, Spangehl MJ. Do "surgical helmet systems" or "body exhaust suits" affect contamination and deep infection rates in arthroplasty? A systematic review. J Arthroplasty. 2016;31(1):225–33.

39. Vijaysegaran P, Knibbs LD, Morawska L, Crawford RW. Surgical space suits increase particle and microbiological emission rates in a simulated surgical environment. J Arthroplast. 2018;33(5):1524–9.

40. Shirley OC, Bayan A, Zhu M, Dalton JP, Wiles S, Young SW. Do surgical helmet systems affect intraoperative wound contamination? A randomised controlled trial. Arch Orthop Trauma Surg. 2017;137(11):1565–9.

41. Hooper GJ, Rothwell AG, Frampton C, Wyatt MC. Does THE use of laminar flow and space

suits reduce early deep infection after total hip and knee replacement?: the ten-year results of the New Zealand Joint Registry. J Bone Joint Surg Br. 2011;93-B(1):85–90.

42. Fillingham Y, Greenwald AS, Greiner J, Oshkukov S, Parsa A, Porteous A, et al. Hip and knee section, prevention, local antimicrobials: proceedings of international consensus on orthopedic infections. J Arthroplast. 2019;34(2):S289–92.

43. Sebastian S, Liu Y, Christensen R, Raina DB, Tägil M, Lidgren L. Antibiotic containing bone cement in prevention of hip and knee prosthetic joint infections: a systematic review and meta-analysis. J Orthop Transl. 2020;23:53–60.

44. Vertullo CJ, Lewis PL, Peng Y, Graves SE, de Steiger RN. The effect of alternative bearing surfaces on the risk of revision due to infection in minimally stabilized Total knee replacement: an analysis of 326,603 prostheses from the Australian Orthopaedic Association National Joint Replacement Registry. J Bone Joit Surg. 2018;100(2):115–23.

45. Brimmo O, Glenn M, Klika AK, Murray TG, Molloy RM, Higuera CA. Rivaroxaban use for thrombosis

prophylaxis is associated with early periprosthetic joint infection. J Arthroplast. 2016;31(6):1295–8.

46. Matharu GS, Garriga C, Whitehouse MR, Rangan A, Judge A. Is aspirin as effective as the newer direct oral anticoagulants for venous thromboembolism prophylaxis after total hip and knee arthroplasty? An analysis from the National Joint Registry for England, Wales, Northern Ireland, and the Isle of Man. J Arthroplast. 2020;35:2631.

47. Yazdi H, Klement MR, Hammad M, Inoue D, Xu C, Goswami K, et al. Tranexamic acid is associated with reduced Periprosthetic joint infection after primary total joint arthroplasty. J Arthroplast. 2020;35(3):840–4.

48. Drain NP, Gobao VC, Bertolini DM, Smith C, Shah NB, Rothenberger SD, et al. Administration of tranexamic acid improves long-term outcomes in total knee arthroplasty. J Arthroplast. 2020;35(6):S201–6.

49. Biant LC, Teare EL, Williams WW, Tuite JD. Eradication of methicillin resistant *Staphylococcus aureus* by "ring fencing" of elective orthopaedic beds. BMJ. 2004;329(7458):149–51.

Dental Procedures After Joint Replacement

Kohei Nishitani and Shuichi Matsuda

28.1 Introduction

Prosthetic joint infection (PJI) is one of the most devastating problems following arthroplasty, and thus, orthopedic surgeons want to avoid it at all costs. Many orthopedic surgeons may consider that dental procedures may cause bacteremia, which is managed with antibiotics. Thus, antibiotics are better to be used during dental procedures in patients who have joint prostheses. In this chapter, we first describe the relationship between dental procedures and bacteremia. Next, we describe whether the dental procedure is a risk factor of PJI and whether antibiotic prophylaxis effectively inhibits PJI. We then provide an overview of the recent guidelines for dental procedures and prophylaxis for patients with a joint prosthesis. Finally, we discuss how this issue can be managed in practical setting.

28.2 Dental Procedure and Bacteremia

The oral cavity is one of the most common bacterial sites in the human body. The human oral microbiome comprises more than 2000 bacterial taxa, including a large number of pathogens involved in the periodontal, respiratory, cardiovascular, and systemic diseases [1]. These bacteria can enter the bloodstream by dental procedures. Surprisingly, even daily oral care activities such as brushing and flossing as well as clinical procedures, such as scaling, planing, and oral surgical procedures may cause temporary bacteremia. For patients with healthy oral conditions, brushing is usually safe without causing bacteremia [2]. However, in patients with oral problems such as periodontitis, brushing is associated with an incidence of bacteremia in about 10 and 20% of patients [3–5], and after scaling and planing, in 13–75% of patients [3, 4, 6, 7]. More aggressive procedures, such as root-canal procedures and tooth extraction, cause bacteremia with a higher probability of 30–80% [8–11]. As many reports describe, non-invasive and invasive dental procedures have a risk of bacteremia, especially in patients who have poor oral conditions.

Antibiotics and topical antimicrobial prophylaxis effectively reduce the bacteremia caused by dental procedures. For example, Lockhart et al. randomized 290 patients into toothbrushing, single-tooth extraction with amoxicillin prophylaxis, or single-tooth extraction with identical placebo groups [10], and showed that the cumulative incidence of bacteria was 23%, 33%, and 60% for tooth brushing, extraction-oral amoxicillin, and extraction-placebo groups, respectively (P < 0.0001). Dios PD et al. randomized 220

K. Nishitani · S. Matsuda (✉)
Department of Orthopaedic Surgery, Graduate School of Medicine, Kyoto University, Kyoto, Japan
e-mail: nkohei@kuhp.kyoto-u.ac.jp;
smat522@kuhp.kyoto-u.ac.jp

© ISAKOS 2022
U. G. Longo et al. (eds.), *Infection in Knee Replacement*,
https://doi.org/10.1007/978-3-030-81553-0_28

patients for dental extraction into four groups: a control group, an oral amoxicillin group, an oral clindamycin group, and an oral moxifloxacin group, and venous blood samples were collected from each patient at baseline, and various time points after dental extractions [12]. Results indicate the effectiveness of amoxicillin and moxifloxacin, showing 96%, 46%, 85%, and 57% bacteremia incidence rates at 30 s, and 20%, 4%, 22%, and 7% bacteremia incidence rates at 1 h, in control, amoxicillin, clindamycin, and moxifloxacin groups, respectively. Simple tooth extraction resulted in the second-highest median incidence of bacteremia and the highest median prevalence of bacteremia for all procedures, and the effectiveness of antibiotic prophylaxis has also been reported in numerous literature [13].

28.3 Dental Procedure and Prosthetic Joint Infection

There are many reports of PJI associated with dental procedures. It has been estimated that 6–13% of PJI cases are due to oral flora [14]. In the current review by Slullitel et al., nine studies focused on PJI diagnosis after dental procedures, in which total infections associated with a dental procedure ranged from 0 to 15.9% [15]. For example, Barbari et al. reported 35/339 (10.3%) PJI-related dental work [16]. Their report included organisms of potential oral or dental origin, such as *beta-hemolytic* (n = 13) and Viridans group *streptococci* (n = 11), *Peptostreptococcus* (n = 5), *Streptococcus*-like organisms (n = 2), *Abiotrophia/Granulicatella* species (n = 2), *Gemella* species (n = 1) and *Actinomyces* species (n = 1). In other reports, Uçkay et al. reported 3/71 (4.2%) dental works that were related to PJI caused by *Streptococcus oralis* (n = 1), *Streptococcus milleri* (n = 1), *Staphylococcus aureus* (n = 1) [17], and LaPorte et al. reported 3/52 (5.8%) PJI caused by *Streptococcus viridans* (n = 2), and *Peptostreptococcus* (n = 1) [18]. In recent years, there have been several case reports that show PJI in dental flora due to dental procedures [19–22]. Although many studies show the relationship

between organisms in dental flora and hematogenous PJI, a case-control study by Skaar et al. found no association between dental procedures and PJI [23]. In their report, 42 cases of PJI and 126 matched controls without PJI were analyzed. They reported that control participants were more likely to have undergone invasive dental procedures than case participants, although this result was not significant (hazard ratio = 0.78 [95% confidence interval [CI], 0.18–3.39]; odds ratio [OR] = 0.56 [95% CI, 0.18–1.74]). In a population-based cohort study using the Taiwan National Health Insurance Research Database, a dental cohort comprised of 57,066 patients who received dental treatment was compared with a 1:1 matched nondental cohort [24]. In their report, PJI occurred in 328 patients (0.57%) in the dental cohort and 348 patients (0.61%) in the nondental cohort, with no between-cohort difference in the 1-year cumulative incidence (0.6% in both, P = 0.3).

Although literatures describe that dental procedures cause bacteremia, and there are many reports of PJI by dental flora, there is much controversy regarding routine prophylaxis in patients with a history of joint replacement undergoing dental procedures. In a study of 1000 patients with 1112 joint replacements, the patients were advised not to take prophylactic antibiotics before any dental or surgical procedures. In this population, 284 infections developed in various organs, including the oral cavity, but none of these patients developed hematogenous infections [25]. In a case-control study by Berbari et al., 339 patients with total hip or knee infection and 339 controls undergoing total hip or knee replacement without infection during the same period were compared. Dental procedures are distinguished as high-risk (dental hygiene, mouth surgery, periodontal treatment, dental extraction, and therapy for dental abscess) and low-risk (restorative dentistry, dental filing, endodontic treatment, and fluoride treatment) dental procedures. As a result, they reported no increased risk of prosthetic hip or knee infection for patients who were undergoing high-risk (adjusted OR, 0.8; 95% CI, 0.4–1.6) or low-risk dental procedures (adjusted OR, 0.6; 95% CI, 0.4–1.1). Additionally, antibiotic prophylaxis in high-risk (adjusted OR, 0.9; 95% CI, 0.5–1.6) or low-risk (adjusted OR, 1.2; 95% CI, 0.7–2.2) dental procedures did not decrease the risk of subsequent total hip or knee infection [16]. In a population-based cohort study using the Taiwan National Health Insurance Research Database, the dental cohort was further distinguished as an antibiotic (n = 6513) and nonantibiotic subcohorts (n = 6513) [24]. PJI occurred in 13 patients (0.2%) in the antibiotic subcohort and in 12 patients (0.18%) in the nonantibiotic subcohorts (P = 0.8). Multivariate-adjusted analyses confirmed that there were no association between PJI incidence and prophylactic antibiotics (adjusted hazard ratio, 1.03; 95% CI: 0.47–2.27).

The time after arthroplasty may be a confounder for the risk of dental procedures. In an animal study, bacteremia caused hematogenous infection in a rabbit cemented stainless-steel implant in the early period; however, the rabbit became resistant to infection 3 weeks postoperatively [26]. In clinical studies, the timing after arthroplasty was related to hematogenous infection, which was higher during the first 2 years after arthroplasty [27]. A possible explanation for this might be that active local inflammation and osseointegration activity around components may lead to a higher blood flow to the prosthetic joint and the potential for organism seeding onto the implant surface [14, 15]. The number of bacteria in the blood flow also affected PJI. Zimmerli et al. found that a 10^2 *Staphylococcus aureus* colony forming unit (CFU) inoculum injected into the region of the foreign material was required to induce infection in >95% of guinea pigs. Another report found that 10^4–10^6 CFU intravenous *Staphylococcus aureus* injections were required to cause endocarditis in rabbit [28, 29]. Although the dose-effect of the inoculation was evident in animal models, the magnitude of bacteremia required to cause clinically significant bacterial disease in humans is unknown.

28.4 Current Guidelines for Dental Procedures for Patients with Total Joint Prosthesis

Professional guidelines have provided evidence-based approaches regarding the relationship between oral procedures and PJI and antibiotic prophylaxis effectiveness. In the current guidelines published within the last 10 years, the American Academy of Orthopaedic Surgeons (AAOS) and the American Dental Association (ADA) released a new guideline in 2012. In this guideline, a vigorous literature review provides an overview of the evidence to explain the proposed association between dental procedures and orthopedic implant infection (Fig. 28.1) [13]. The guideline shows strong evidence between oral procedure and the occurrence of bacteremia, and moderate evidence strength between oral organisms and PJI. However, no evidence has described that oral procedures cause PJI via bacteremia.

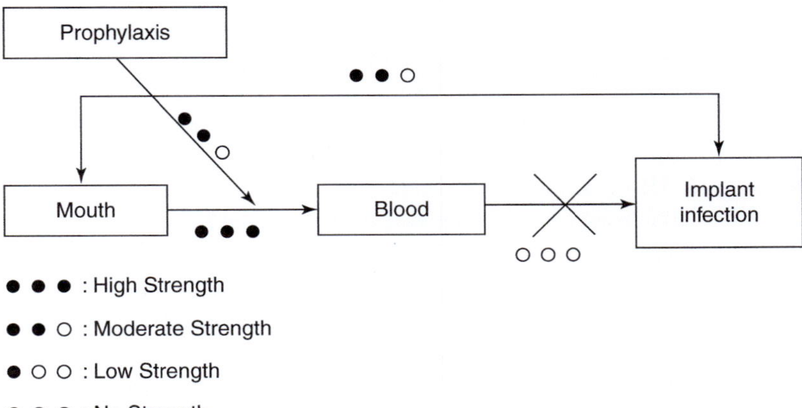

Fig. 28.1 The strength of evidences among oral bacteria, bacteremia, and PJI. (From ADA and AAOS guideline in 2012 [13] with modification)

With this accumulation of evidence, this guideline provided three recommendations [13]: (1) The practitioner might consider discontinuing the practice of routinely prescribing prophylactic antibiotics for patients with hip and knee prosthetic joint implants undergoing dental procedures (Grade of Recommendation: Limited); (2) We are unable to recommend for or against the use of topical oral antimicrobials in patients with prosthetic joint implants or other orthopedic implants undergoing dental procedures (Grade of Recommendation: Inconclusive); (3) In the absence of reliable evidence linking poor oral health to prosthetic joint infection, it is the opinion of the workgroup that patients with prosthetic joint implants or other orthopedic implants maintain appropriate oral hygiene (Grade of Recommendation: Consensus). The 2014 ADA guidelines followed the AAOS and ADA 2012 guidelines. They conclude that evidence fails to demonstrate an association between dental procedures and PJI or any effectiveness for antibiotic prophylaxis, with a recommendation that in general, for patients with prosthetic joint implants, prophylactic antibiotics are not recommended prior to dental procedures to prevent PJI [30]. Although the two abovementioned guidelines did not recommend routinely using antibiotics for dental procedures, they also described that treatment decisions should be made in light of all circumstances presented by the patient. Treatments and procedures applicable to individual patient rely on mutual communication between patient, physician, dentist, and other healthcare practitioners [13]. This suggests that orthopedic surgeons, dentists, and patients should consider individual risk to decide the use of antibiotics for dental procedures.

In guidelines from an orthopedic surgeon's viewpoint, the first International Consensus Meeting (ICM) on Periprosthetic Joint Infection had some consensus statement on dental procedures for patients with PJI [31]. For the question "Should a patient with total joint arthroplasty (TJA) be given routine dental antibiotic prophylaxis?", the Consensus states "The use of dental antibiotic prophylaxis in patients with TJA should be individualized based on patient risk factors and the complexity of the dental procedure to be performed." with a strong consensus (agree rate: 81%). Although there is no consensus that antibiotic prophylaxis before dental work can reduce PJI, most PJIs occur within the first 2 years postoperatively [18, 32]. Thus, this guideline concludes that using antibiotic prophylaxis for dental procedures after TJA to decrease the risk of bacteremia following dental procedures is justifiable to decrease the risk of sustaining a PJI within the first 2 years postoperatively [31]. However, in the second ICM consensus statement, for the question "What is the role of prophylactic antibiotics for invasive procedures (dental, gastrointestinal, urologic, etc.) in the presence of an arthroplasty to prevent subsequent PJI?", the recommendation stated that there is no role for routine prophylactic antibiotic administration prior to dental procedures (Level of Evidence: Limited, Weak Consensus) [33]. In the second ICM consensus statement, they also recommend that nonurgent invasive dental procedures, if possible, be delayed until the osseointegration of uncemented components is complete [33].

28.5 Practical Usage of Antibiotics for Patients with Prosthesis

Antibiotic prophylaxis against dental procedures should be addressed on a patient-by-patient basis, considering individual risk factors and the risk of the dental procedure. Who would be effectively protected by antibiotics before the dental procedure? Patients who were considered to be given antibiotics in the past guideline are likely to benefit most from antibiotics. In the advisory statement of ADA and AAOS in 2009 and first ICM consensus statement, high-risk patients included immunocompromised patients, patients with inflammatory arthropathy such as rheumatoid arthritis and systemic lupus erythematosus, immunosuppressed patients; patients with *Human Immunodeficiency Virus*, patients with previous joint infection, hemophilia, malnourishment, type 1 diabetes, or malignancy, and patients with mega prosthesis [34–38]. The following factors are determined by a dental care provider: high gingival score and gingival index, high plaque score and plaque index, gum probing depth, and periodontitis [5, 39, 40]. Although the guidelines did not list any special situations, clinicians may consider antibiotic prophylaxis despite the lack of scientific evidence. To help clinicians make decisions regarding antibiotic prophylaxis for dental procedures, AAOS and ADA developed a tool for the appropriate use criteria (AUC) of antibiotics usage to assist orthopedic surgeons and dentists to aid their patients [41]. Clinicians can utilize the aforementioned AUC for the "Management of Patients with Orthopaedic Implants Undergoing Dental Procedures (2016)" in the ORTHO GUIDELINES website (http://www.orthoguidelines.org/go/auc/). By choosing an appropriate indication profile for planned dental procedure, immunocompromised status, diabetic glycemic control, history of periprosthetic or deep PJI that required an operation, and timing since joint replacement procedure, the clinicians can obtain recommendations if antibiotic prophylaxis is "rarely appropriate," "maybe appropriate," or is "appropriate."

If prophylaxis was performed, what kind of antibiotics were suitable for the prophylaxis of dental procedures to reduce the risk of PJI? Because there is no evidence for the prophylaxis of PJI after dental procedures, antibiotics that effectively reduce bacteremia after dental procedures would be the clue for drug selection. The advisory statement of ADA and AAOS in 2003 provides the suggested antibiotic prophylaxis regimens, classified by patient type [42]. The suggested regimen is as follows: for patients who are not allergic to penicillin, 2 g of oral cephalexin, cephradine, or amoxicillin 1 h prior to the dental procedure; for patients not allergic to penicillin and unable to take oral medications, 1 g of cefazolin or 2 g of ampicillin intramuscularly or intravenously 1 h prior to the dental procedure; for patients allergic to penicillin, 600 mg of clindamycin orally 1 h prior to the dental procedure; and for patients allergic to penicillin and unable to take oral medications, 600 mg of clindamycin intravenously 1 h prior to the dental procedure. No second doses are recommended for any of these dosing regimens. The first ICM consensus also referred to several antibiotics to reduce the burden of bacteria released during dental procedures [31], with 2 g of amoxicillin, recommended to be administered a maximum of 1 h prior to the procedure [10, 12, 43, 44]. In the current concept review in 2014, Young et al. reported a relative decrease in bacteremia was decreased by antibiotics at 5 min postoperatively [14]. They also found a favorable bacterial reduction in oral amoxicillin (OR, 0.135; 95% CI, 0.097–0.187) and oral clindamycin (OR, 0.407; 95% CI, 0.223–0.725) vs. no antibiotic control.

Finally, physicians must be aware that the administration of antibiotics to individuals is not without its problems and may result in drug-related adverse effects such as swelling or itching, *C. difficile* colitis, and even more severe adverse effects such as anaphylaxis. The potential to cause the emergence of drug-resistant organisms is also considered. Young et al. provided an interesting analysis of the risk and benefit of antibiotic usage for dental procedures [14]. In their analyses, using 6–13% of PJI cases as being due to oral flora in approximately 140,000 PJIs out of 7,000,000 people with prosthetic joints, 8400 to 18,200 PJIs were secondary to oral bacteremia, and amoxicillin administered before the dental procedure may decrease PJI to 1746 and 3784 cases, respectively. Given a 2% antibiotic-related side effect incidence rate, if all 7,000,000 people with prosthetic joints had antibiotics, 140,000 side effects might have occurred. In their comment, 37–80 patients (140,000/[1746–3784]) would experience an adverse antibiotic effect for every PJI. The seriousness of PJI and antibiotic-related side effects cannot be the same. Therefore, this may be a somewhat radical calculation, but it is agreeable that the risk of abusing antibiotics cannot be overlooked. Therefore, carefully evaluating the patient-by-patient risk-benefit for antibiotic administration is mandatory for the dentist and orthopedic surgeon.

28.6 Conclusions

In conclusion, dental procedures cause bacteremia, and antibiotic prophylaxis reduces it. However, there is limited evidence that shows dental procedures are associated with PJI or antibiotic prophylaxis before dental procedures reduce PJI. Thus, recent guidelines do not recommend the routine use of antibiotics for dental procedures. Hence, it is important for physicians and dentists to consider the individual patient risk and procedural risk to decide whether to use antibiotics before dental procedures, considering the side effects and potential drug resistance. The risk and benefit analysis of using antibiotics is better shared by the patient, dentist, and orthopedic surgeon.

References

1. Warinner C, Rodrigues JFM, Vyas R, Trachsel C, Shved N, Grossmann J, et al. Pathogens and host immunity in the ancient human oral cavity. Nat Genet. 2014;46:336–44.
2. Hartzell JD, Torres D, Kim P, Wortmann G. Incidence of bacteremia after routine tooth brushing. Am J Med Sci. 2005;329:178–80.
3. Kinane DF, Riggio MP, Walker KF, MacKenzie D, Shearer B. Bacteraemia following periodontal procedures. J Clin Periodontol. 2005;32:708–13.
4. Forner L, Larsen T, Kilian M, Holmstrup P. Incidence of bacteremia after chewing, tooth brushing and scaling in individuals with periodontal inflammation. J Clin Periodontol. 2006;33:401–7.
5. Lockhart PB, Brennan MT, Thornhill M, Michalowicz BS, Noll J, Bahrani-Mougeot FK, et al. Poor oral hygiene as a risk factor for infective endocarditis-related bacteremia. J Am Dent Assoc. 2009;140:1238–44.
6. Lafaurie GI, Mayorga-Fayad I, Torres MF, Castillo DM, Aya MR, Barón A, et al. Periodontopathic microorganisms in peripheric blood after scaling and root planing. J Clin Periodontol. 2007;34:873–9.
7. Zhang W, Daly CG, Mitchell D, Curtis B. Incidence and magnitude of bacteraemia caused by flossing and by scaling and root planing. J Clin Periodontol. 2013;40:41–52.
8. Wahlmann U, Al-Nawas B, Jütte M, Wagner W. Clinical and microbiological efficacy of single dose cefuroxime prophylaxis for dental surgical procedures. Int J Antimicrob Agents. 1999;12:253–6.
9. Savarrio L, Mackenzie D, Riggio M, Saunders WP, Bagg J. Detection of bacteraemias during non-surgical root canal treatment. J Dent. 2005;33:293–303.
10. Lockhart PB, Brennan MT, Sasser HC, Fox PC, Paster BJ, Bahrani-Mougeot FK. Bacteremia associated with toothbrushing and dental extraction. Circulation. 2008;117:3118–25.
11. Barbosa M, Carmona IT, Amaral B, Limeres J, Álvarez M, Cerqueira C, et al. General anesthesia increases the risk of bacteremia following dental extractions. Oral Surg Oral Med Oral Pathol Oral Radiol Endod. 2010;110:706–12.
12. Diz Dios P, Tomás Carmona I, Limeres Posse J, Medina Henríquez J, Fernández Feijoo J, Álvarez FM. Comparative efficacies of amoxicillin, clindamycin, and moxifloxacin in prevention of bacteremia following dental extractions. Antimicrob Agents Chemother. 2006;50:2996–3002.
13. American Academy of Orthopaedic Surgeons & American Dental Association. Prevention of orthopaedic implant infection in patients undergoing dental procedures. http://www.orthoguidelines.org/topic?id=1002. Accessed 12 Oct 20120.
14. Young H, Hirsh J, Hammerberg EM, Price CS. Dental disease and periprosthetic joint infection. J Bone Joint Surg Am. 2014;96:162–8.
15. Slullitel PA, Oñativia JI, Piuzzi NS, Higuera-Rueda C, Parvizi J, Buttaro MA. Is there a role for antibiotic prophylaxis prior to dental procedures in patients with total joint arthroplasty? A systematic review of the literature. J Bone Joint Infect. 2020;5:7–15.
16. Berbari EF, Osmon DR, Carr A, Hanssen AD, Baddour LM, Greene D, et al. Dental procedures as risk factors for prosthetic hip or knee infection: a hospital-based prospective case-control study. Clin Infect Dis. 2010;50:8–16.
17. UCkay I, Lübbeke A, Emonet S, Tovmirzaeva L, Stern R, Ferry T, et al. Low incidence of haematogenous seeding to total hip and knee prostheses in patients with remote infections. J Infect. 2009;59:337–45.
18. Laporte DM, Waldman BJ, Mont MA, Hungerford DS. Infections associated with dental procedures in total hip arthroplasty. J Bone Joint Surg Br. 1999;81:56–9.
19. Al-Himdani S, Woodnutt D. Group C streptococcal septic arthritis of a prosthetic hip joint following dental treatment. BMJ Case Rep. 2015;2015:bcr2015211203.
20. Klein R, Dababneh AS, Palraj BRV. Streptococcus gordonii prosthetic joint infection in the setting of vigorous dental flossing. BMJ Case Reports. 2015;2015:bcr2015211203.
21. Quénard F, Seng P, Lagier J-C, Fenollar F, Stein A. Prosthetic joint infection caused by Granulicatella adiacens: a case series and review of literature. BMC Musculoskelet Disord. 2017;18:276–5.
22. Olson LB, Turner DJ, Cox GM, Hostler CJ. Streptococcus salivarius prosthetic joint infection following dental cleaning despite antibiotic prophylaxis. Case Rep Infect Dis. 2019;2019:8109280.
23. Skaar DD, O'Connor H, Hodges JS, Michalowicz BS. Dental procedures and subsequent prosthetic joint infections: findings from the Medicare current beneficiary survey. J Am Dent Assoc. 2011;142:1343–51.
24. Kao F-C, Hsu Y-C, Chen W-H, Lin J-N, Lo Y-Y, Tu Y-K. Prosthetic joint infection following invasive dental procedures and antibiotic prophylaxis in patients with hip or knee arthroplasty. Infect Control Hosp Epidemiol. 2017;38:154–61.
25. Ainscow DA, Denham RA. The risk of haematogenous infection in total joint replacements. J Bone Joint Surg Br. 1984;66:580–2.

26. Southwood RT, Rice JL, McDonald PJ, Hakendorf PH, Rozenbilds MA. Infection in experimental arthroplasties. Clin Orthop Relat Res. 1987;(224):33–6.

27. Deacon JM, Pagliaro AJ, Zelicof SB, Horowitz HW. Prophylactic use of antibiotics for procedures after total joint replacement. J Bone Joint Surg Am. 1996;78:1755–70.

28. Perlman BB, Freedman LR. Experimental endocarditis. II. Staphylococcal infection of the aortic valve following placement of a polyethylene catheter in the left side of the heart. Yale J Biol Med. 1971;44:206–13.

29. Perlman BB, Freedman LR. Experimental endocarditis. 3. Natural history of catheter induced staphylococcal endocarditis following catheter removal. Yale J Biol Med. 1971;44:214–24.

30. Sollecito TP, Abt E, Lockhart PB, Truelove E, Paumier TM, Tracy SL, Tampi M, Beltrán-Aguilar ED, Frantsve-Hawley J. The use of prophylactic antibiotics prior to dental procedures in patients with prosthetic joints: evidence-based clinical practice guideline for dental practitioners--a report of the American Dental Association Council on Scientific Affairs. J Am Dent Assoc. 2015;146:11–8.

31. Proceedings of the International Consensus meeting on periprosthetic joint infection. https://www.efort.org/wp-content/uploads/2013/10/Philadelphia_Consensus.pdf. Accessed 12 Oct 20120.

32. Kurtz SM, Ong KL, Lau E, Bozic KJ, Berry D, Parvizi J. Prosthetic joint infection risk after TKA in the medicare population. Clin Orthop Relat Res. 2010;468:52–6.

33. Arnold WV, Bari AK, Buttaro M, Huang R, Mirez JP, Neira I, et al. General assembly, prevention, postoperative factors: proceedings of International Consensus on Orthopaedic Infections. J Arthroplast. 2019;34:S169–74.

34. Jacobson JJ, Millard HD, Plezia R, Blankenship JR. Dental treatment and late prosthetic joint infections. Oral Surg Oral Med Oral Pathol. 1986;61:413–7.

35. Murray RP, Bourne MH, Fitzgerald RH. Metachronous infections in patients who have had more than one total joint arthroplasty. J Bone Joint Surg Am. 1991;73:1469–74.

36. Jacobson JJ, Patel B, Asher G, Woolliscroft JO, Schaberg D. Oral staphylococcus in older subjects with rheumatoid arthritis. J Am Geriatr Soc. 1997;45:590–3.

37. Berbari EF, Hanssen AD, Duffy MC, Steckelberg JM, Ilstrup DM, Harmsen WS, et al. Risk factors for prosthetic joint infection: case-control study. Clin Infect Dis. 1998;27:1247–54.

38. Nadlacan LM, Hirst P. Infected total knee replacement following a dental procedure in a severe haemophiliac. Knee. 2001;8:159–61.

39. Bhanji S, Williams B, Sheller B, Elwood T, Mancl L. Transient bacteremia induced by toothbrushing a comparison of the Sonicare toothbrush with a conventional toothbrush. Pediatr Dent. 2002;24:295–9.

40. Forner L, Nielsen CH, Bendtzen K, Larsen T, Holmstrup P. Increased plasma levels of IL-6 in bacteremic periodontis patients after scaling. J Clin Periodontol. 2006;33:724–9.

41. American Dental Association–Appointed Members of the Expert Writing and Voting Panels Contributing to the Development of American Academy of Orthopaedic Surgeons Appropriate Use Criteria. American Dental Association guidance for utilizing appropriate use criteria in the management of the care of patients with orthopaedic implants undergoing dental procedures. J Am Dent Dent Assoc. 2017;148:57–9.

42. American Dental Association, American Academy of Orthopaedic Surgeons. Antibiotic prophylaxis for dental patients with total joint replacements. Am Dent Assoc. 2003;134:895–9.

43. Roberts GJ, Radford P, Holt R. Prophylaxis of dental bacteraemia with oral amoxycillin in children. Br Dent J. 1987;162:179–82.

44. Vergis EN, Demas PN, Vaccarello SJ, Yu VL. Topical antibiotic prophylaxis for bacteremia after dental extractions. Oral Surg Oral Med Oral Pathol Oral Radiol Endod. 2001;91:162–5.

Hematoma and Thromboprophylaxis

Shinichiro Nakamura

29.1 Hematoma

Postoperative hematoma can be a reason for surgical site infection (SSI). The use of closed drainage has been advocated because there is less infection, postoperative pain, and swelling as well as better healing of the soft tissues and quicker mobilization of the extremities [1–3]. Kim et al. conducted a prospective study of 69 patients who had a primary simultaneous bilateral total knee arthroplasty (TKA) to assess the effect of postoperative suction drainage on infection and would healing. The knees that had no drains had a higher incidence of drainage from the wound, had soaked dressings requiring dressing reinforcements, and had more ecchymosis and erythema around the wound. Although the incidence of infection in the two groups is not statistically different, the development of infection in two knees in which drains were not used suggests that suction drainage may reduce deep infection [1].

Recently conflicting results have been reported, and an increasing number of studies have demonstrated no benefit to the use of closed drainage [4–6]. Li et al. conducted a prospective randomized, controlled trial in 100 patients to compare the postoperative use of wound drains with the use of no drains in patients who underwent unilateral primary TKA. The group treated without a drain needed comparatively less blood transfused. Differences in wound infection, incidence of deep vein thrombosis, and range of motion were not statistically significant [4].

Several systemic review and meta-analysis studies to assess the benefit and drawback of closed drainage were published [7, 8]. Si et al. reported that no significant differences in infection rate or blood loss were found between the closed drainage and nondrainage TKAs, and there was also no significant difference in hematoma formation, deep venous thrombosis, postoperative VAS score, or range of motion between the two groups [7]. Zhang et al. also reported no significant difference in total blood loss, hemoglobin drop, superficial wound infection, prosthetic joint infection, formation of deep vein thrombosis, duration of hospital stay, and range of movement [8].

The incidence of postoperative hematoma is decreasing with the use of local infiltration of anesthesia and tranexamic acid. The usage of a closed drainage in TKA will decrease in the future.

S. Nakamura (✉)
Department of Orthopedic Surgery, Kyoto University, Graduate School of Medicine, Kyoto, Japan
e-mail: shnk@kuhp.kyoto-u.ac.jp

© ISAKOS 2022
U. G. Longo et al. (eds.), *Infection in Knee Replacement*,
https://doi.org/10.1007/978-3-030-81553-0_29

29.2 Timing of Drain Removal

Closed suction drainage of wounds has been well established as a principle of management following joint arthroplasty, although the efficacy of this practice has been questioned recently. Drinkwater et al. conducted a prospective clinical trial, in which surgeons were asked to randomly allocate the time that the drains were left in situ after surgery [9]. The likelihood of bacterial colonization increased while wound drainage decreased with time. The proportion of drains contaminated after 24 h was significantly higher. The authors suggested that the optimal time to remove drains is 24 h after total joint arthroplasty. As fast-track program has been implemented in TKA, whether drainage tube could be removed early, and the ideal timing for removal after fast-track primary TKA has been a new topic. Zhang et al. evaluated the safety and feasibility of early removal of drainage tube in a prospective cohort study. A wound drainage tube was indwelled for 6, 12, and 18 h. There was no statistically significant difference in the volume of total and hidden blood loss among three groups, but as the time of drainage prolonged, total volume of drainage and dominant blood loss increased gradually. Early removal of wound drainage tube could drain the hematocele and reduce the risk of infection, and it doesn't increase the sense of pain, inflammatory reaction, limb swelling, and total blood loss. It's safe and feasible to remove the drainage tube within 6–12 h after fast-track primary TKA [10].

There is no direct evidence to suggest that the use of surgical drains leads to an increase in the rate of subsequent SSI. The recommended time to remove drains is within 24 h because of higher contamination. The use of surgical drains leads to a higher volume of blood loss and an increased need for allogenic blood transfusion, which may indirectly increase the rate of SSI.

29.3 Tranexamic Acid (TXA)

Tranexamic acid (TXA) is an antifibrinolytic agent, which has become an integral component in postoperative blood management in orthopedic surgery [11, 12]. The published literature on TXA has dramatically expanded over the past several years. In a meta-analysis study, topical, intravenous (IV), and oral TXA formulations were all superior to placebo in terms of decreasing blood loss and risk of transfusion, and strong evidence supports the efficacy of TXA to decrease blood loss and the risk of transfusion after primary TKA [11]. Relatively large reductions in the mean difference of blood loss between 225 and 331 mL were observed in favor of TXA treatments compared with placebo.

Preoperative anemia is associated with development of subsequent postoperative periprosthetic infection, medical complication, and mortality [13, 14]. Greenky et al. defined anemia as hemoglobin 12 g/dL in women and hemoglobin 13 g/dL in men. An allogenic transfusion was received in 44% of anemic patients, compared with only 13.4% of nonanemic patients. Postoperative periprosthetic infection occurred more frequently in anemic patients at an incidence of 4.3% in anemic patients compared with 2% in nonanemic patients. Allogeneic blood transfusions are also associated with infection and reoperation [15, 16]. Newman et al. showed that the rate of reoperations for suspected infection was higher among patients with perioperative allogeneic exposure (1.67%) as compared with all others (0.72%, $p = 0.014$) [16]. Friedman et al. investigated the types of postoperative infection including lower or upper respiratory tract and lung infection, bone and joint infection, wound inflammation or infection, urinary tract infection, and other infections. The rates of any infection, lower or upper respiratory tract and lung infection, and wound inflammation or infection were significantly increased in patients receiving allogeneic blood transfusion [15].

The direct effect of TXA on SSI has been unclear so far. Lacko aimed to analyze the effect of intravenous administration of TXA on reducing the risk of revision for acute and delayed periprosthetic joint infection. Cumulative revision rate of TKA was significantly lower in the TXA group (0.13% vs. 1.08%, $p = 0.043$). The use of TXA was shown as the significant protective factor [odds ratio (OR): 0.109; 95% confidence interval (CI): 0.0128–0.929; p = 0.043] [17]. Further research should be conducted to examine whether TXA is effective for SSI. The administration of TXA potentially reduces the incidence of SSI by reducing postoperative anemia and the need for allogenic blood transfusion.

29.4 Thromboprophylaxis

29.4.1 Prevention of Venous Thromboembolism (VTE)

VTE is a serious complication following major orthopedic surgery. Several guidelines are suggested to reduce postoperative pulmonary embolism and deep vein thrombosis. The American Academy of Orthopaedic Surgeons (AAOS) guidelines on preventing venous thromboembolic disease in patients undergoing elective hip and knee arthroplasty, suggests the use of pharmacologic agents and/or mechanical compressive devices for the prevention of venous thromboembolism in patients undergoing elective hip or knee arthroplasty, and who are not at elevated risk beyond that of the surgery itself for venous thromboembolism or bleeding. In the absence of reliable evidence, it is the opinion of this work group that patients undergoing elective hip or knee arthroplasty, and who have also had a previous venous thromboembolism, receive pharmacologic prophylaxis and mechanical compressive devices [18].

In antithrombotic therapy and prevention of thrombosis, 9th ed: American College of Chest Physicians (ACCP) Evidence-Based Clinical Practice Guidelines, strategies for thromboprophylaxis after major orthopedic surgery are included. In patients undergoing TKA, use of one of the following is recommended for a minimum of 10–14 days rather than no antithrombotic prophylaxis: low-molecular-weight heparin (LMWH), fondaparinux, apixaban, dabigatran, rivaroxaban, low-dose unfractionated heparin (LDUH), adjusted-dose vitamin K antagonist (VKA), aspirin (all Grade 1B), or an intermittent pneumatic compression device (IPCD) (Grade 1C) [19].

The incidence of VTE after total hip arthroplasty (THA) or TKA is reduced by the use of thromboprophylaxis. However, current evidence is unclear about which prophylactic strategy (or strategies) is/are optimal or suboptimal. Therefore, it is unable to recommend for or against specific prophylactics in these patients. In the absence of reliable evidence about how long to employ these prophylactic strategies, patients and physicians discuss the duration of prophylaxis.

29.5 Complication of Bleeding

The incidence of VTE after THA or TKA is reduced due to thromboprophylaxis. However, these medications have a number of limitations that impede their use, including increased bleeding risk. The potential for bleeding secondary to prophylaxis has been associated with prolonged recovery, infections, wound failure, and readmission. Therefore, the risk vs. benefit is a primary consideration when a provider chooses VTE prophylaxis in these patients.

Concerning bleeding, Lindquist et al. compared postoperative bleeding rates in patients receiving aspirin to patients who received enoxaparin or rivaroxaban after undergoing elective total joint arthroplasty [20]. Those who received aspirin or enoxaparin were less likely to experience any bleeding compared to those patients who received rivaroxaban ($P < 0.05$). There was also a lower rate of major bleeding in these groups. Suen et al. conducted systematic review of the surgical site bleeding complications of thromboprophylactic agents. LMWH increased the risk of surgical site bleeding compared with control, warfarin, and dabigatran and trended toward an increased risk compared with apixaban. The risk of surgical site bleeding was similar with LMWH and rivaroxaban [21].

29.6 Complication of Wound Complication

Wound-related complications following arthroplasty can cause restricted joint movement, reoperation, infection, and revision arthroplasty. Jameson evaluated the surgically relevant complications of using either rivaroxaban or an LMWH as thromboprophylaxis, based on prospectively collected national data. The rivaroxaban group had a higher wound complication rate and a lower deep venous thrombosis rate; there were no differences in symptomatic pulmonary embolism or all-cause mortality [22]. Bloch et al. reported the impact of dabigatran on wound leakage. The use of dabigatran led to a significant increase in postoperative wound leakage (20% with dabigatran, 5% with a multimodal regimen; $p < 0.001$), which also resulted in an increased duration of hospital stay [23].

Garfinkel et al. conducted a retrospective review of a prospectively collected total joint arthroplasty registry to examine whether the choice of aspirin vs. factor Xa inhibitors for VTE prophylaxis is associated with differences in the rates of bleeding and wound complications in the early postoperative period. Six of 32 patients (18.7%) in the Xa inhibitor group had a postoperative bleeding/wound complication (4 delayed healing/blistering, 1 hematoma/excessive ecchymosis, and 1 readmission for cellulitis). There were no bleeding/wound complications in the aspirin group ($P < 0.03$). Factor Xa inhibitors were associated with a higher incidence of bleeding/wound complications in comparison with aspirin [24]. The choice of VTE prophylaxis should be based on the perceived risks of bleeding and wound complications compared to the risks of VTE in each patient.

29.7 Infection After Thromboprophylaxis

TKA is a relatively safe procedure, with <1% of these procedures complicated postoperatively by periprosthetic joint infection [25, 26]. Managing and/or eliminating risk factors that predispose a patient to periprosthetic joint infection is critically important. The use of certain agents to prevent deep vein thrombosis after arthroplasty has been linked to an increased risk of adverse effects including wound drainage and infection.

Chahal et al. measured the return to theatre rate for any cause related to wound complications in patients undergoing total hip replacement and total knee replacement and compared these rates between patients on oral rivaroxaban 10 mg OD and subcutaneous enoxaparin 40 mg OD. In this retrospective cohort study, it was found that patients who received rivaroxaban were more than twice as likely to return to theatre for wound complications compared to patients receiving enoxaparin. Although not statistically significant, this increase is in line with previous studies. Infection rates increased from 0.9 to 1.9% after the introduction of rivaroxaban and microbiologically confirmed superficial infections rose from 1.3 to 3.1% after rivaroxaban was introduced. These rises were not statistically significant [27].

Brimmo et al. compared the early deep postoperative surgical site infection and subsequent reoperation rates in THA and TKA patients treated with either oral rivaroxaban or any other form of chemical thromboprophylaxis [28]. Patients were divided into two groups: the study group received rivaroxaban, whereas the control group received another form of chemical thromboprophylaxis for at least 2 weeks postoperative. There were no significant differences between groups regarding demographics, risk factors, or illness severity scores. Incidence of early deep SSI in the rivaroxaban group was higher than in the control group (2.5% vs. 0.2%; $P < 0.015$). The use of rivaroxaban for thromboprophylaxis led to a significantly increased incidence of deep SSI in a continuous series of patients.

Aspirin is a widely used antiplatelet drug. It prevents platelet aggregation by inhibiting the production of thromboxane A2 by activated platelets [29]. AAOS has endorsed aspirin for VTE prevention after total joint arthroplasty (TJA) [30]. In 2012, ACCP evidence-based clinical practice guidelines (9th edition), for the first time, acknowledged the usage of aspirin for prophylaxis of pulmonary embolism (PE) after TJA (Grade IB recommendation) [19].

Raphael et al. compared the (1) overall frequency of symptomatic PE, (2) risk of symptomatic PE after propensity matching that adjusted for potentially confounding variables, and (3) other complications and length of stay before and after propensity matching in patients undergoing

TJA at our institution who received either aspirin or warfarin prophylaxis. The overall symptomatic PE rate was lower ($p < 0.001$) in patients receiving aspirin (0.14%) than in the patients receiving warfarin (1.07%). This difference did not change after matching. The aspirin group also had significantly fewer symptomatic DVTs and wound-related problems and shorter hospital stays, which did not change after matching [31].

Huang et al. compare the rates of periprosthetic joint infection (PJI) at our institution in patients receiving aspirin compared with warfarin for VTE prophylaxis following TJA. Incidence of PJI was significantly lower at 0.4% (8 of 1456 patients) in patients receiving aspirin as VTE prophylaxis compared to 1.5% (24 of 1700 patients) in patients receiving warfarin ($P < 0.001$). Rate of postoperative PE was also lower in the aspirin group at 0.1% (1 of 1456 patients) compared to 0.3% (5 of 1700 patients) in the warfarin group ($P < 0.001$). Multivariate analysis identified warfarin prophylaxis compared to aspirin as an independent risk factor for PJI following TJA ($P = 0.018$). Patients receiving aspirin prophylaxis have fewer wound-related complications following primary TJA, which theoretically explains its added benefits in reducing the incidence of SSI. The use of aspirin compared to warfarin for VTE prophylaxis provides adequate protection against postoperative VTE while reducing the risk of SSI following TJA [32].

In a majority of studies evaluating VTE prophylaxis in patients undergoing TJA, aspirin appears to result in a lower risk of SSI than anticoagulants (vitamin K antagonists, heparin-based products, factor Xa inhibitors, and direct thrombin inhibitors).

References

1. Kim YH, Cho SH, Kim RS. Drainage versus nondrainage in simultaneous bilateral total knee arthroplasties. Clin Orthop Relat Res. 1998;347:188–93.
2. Omonbude D, El Masry MA, O'Connor PJ, Grainger AJ, Allgar VL, Calder SJ. Measurement of joint effusion and haematoma formation by ultrasound in assessing the effectiveness of drains after total knee replacement: a prospective randomised study. J Bone Joint Surg Br. 2010;92(1):51–5. https://doi.org/10.1302/0301-620X.92B1.22121.
3. Ovadia D, Luger E, Bickels J, Menachem A, Dekel S. Efficacy of closed wound drainage after total joint arthroplasty. A prospective randomized study. J Arthroplast. 1997;12(3):317–21. https://doi.org/10.1016/s0883-5403(97)90029-2.
4. Li C, Nijat A, Askar M. No clear advantage to use of wound drains after unilateral total knee arthroplasty: a prospective randomized, controlled trial. J Arthroplast. 2011;26(4):519–22. https://doi.org/10.1016/j.arth.2010.05.031.
5. Niskanen RO, Korkala OL, Haapala J, Kuokkanen HO, Kaukonen JP, Salo SA. Drainage is of no use in primary uncomplicated cemented hip and knee arthroplasty for osteoarthritis: a prospective randomized study. J Arthroplast. 2000;15(5):567–9. https://doi.org/10.1054/arth.2000.6616.
6. Ritter MA, Keating EM, Faris PM. Closed wound drainage in total hip or total knee replacement. A prospective, randomized study. J Bone Joint Surg Am. 1994;76(1):35–8. https://doi.org/10.2106/00004623-199401000-00005.
7. Si HB, Yang TM, Zeng Y, Shen B. No clear benefit or drawback to the use of closed drainage after primary total knee arthroplasty: a systematic review and meta-analysis. BMC Musculoskelet Disord. 2016;17:183. https://doi.org/10.1186/s12891-016-1039-2.
8. Zhang Q, Liu L, Sun W, Gao F, Zhang Q, Cheng L, Li Z. Are closed suction drains necessary for primary total knee arthroplasty?: A systematic review and meta-analysis. Medicine (Baltimore). 2018;97(30):e11290. https://doi.org/10.1097/MD.0000000000011290.
9. Drinkwater CJ, Neil MJ. Optimal timing of wound drain removal following total joint arthroplasty. J Arthroplast. 1995;10(2):185–9. https://doi.org/10.1016/s0883-5403(05)80125-1.
10. Zhang S, Xu B, Huang Q, Yao H, Xie J, Pei F. Erratum: early removal of drainage tube after fast-track primary total knee arthroplasty. J Knee Surg. 2017;30(6):e1. https://doi.org/10.1055/s-0037-1599280.
11. Fillingham YA, Ramkumar DB, Jevsevar DS, Yates AJ, Shores P, Mullen K, Bini SA, Clarke HD, Schemitsch E, Johnson RL, Memtsoudis SG, Sayeed SA, Sah AP, Della Valle CJ. The efficacy of tranexamic acid in total knee arthroplasty: a network meta-analysis. J Arthroplast. 2018;33(10):3090–3098.e3091. https://doi.org/10.1016/j.arth.2018.04.043.
12. Tsukada S, Wakui M. Combined intravenous and intra-articular tranexamic acid in simultaneous bilateral total knee arthroplasty without tourniquet use. J Bone Joint Surg Open Access. 2017;2(2):e0002. https://doi.org/10.2106/JBJS.OA.17.00002.
13. Greenky M, Gandhi K, Pulido L, Restrepo C, Parvizi J. Preoperative anemia in total joint arthroplasty: is it associated with periprosthetic joint infection? Clin Orthop Relat Res. 2012;470(10):2695–701. https://doi.org/10.1007/s11999-012-2435-z.
14. Viola J, Gomez MM, Restrepo C, Maltenfort MG, Parvizi J. Preoperative anemia increases postopera-

tive complications and mortality following total joint arthroplasty. J Arthroplast. 2015;30(5):846–8. https://doi.org/10.1016/j.arth.2014.12.026.

15. Friedman R, Homering M, Holberg G, Berkowitz SD. Allogeneic blood transfusions and postoperative infections after total hip or knee arthroplasty. J Bone Joint Surg Am. 2014;96(4):272–8. https://doi.org/10.2106/JBJS.L.01268.

16. Newman ET, Watters TS, Lewis JS, Jennings JM, Wellman SS, Attarian DE, Grant SA, Green CL, Vail TP, Bolognesi MP. Impact of perioperative allogeneic and autologous blood transfusion on acute wound infection following total knee and total hip arthroplasty. J Bone Joint Surg Am. 2014;96(4):279–84. https://doi.org/10.2106/JBJS.L.01041.

17. Lacko M, Jarcuska P, Schreierova D, Lackova A, Gharaibeh A. Tranexamic acid decreases the risk of revision for acute and delayed periprosthetic joint infection after total knee replacement. Joint Dis Relat Surg. 2020;31(1):8–13. https://doi.org/10.5606/ehc.2020.72061.

18. Mont MA, Jacobs JJ, Boggio LN, Bozic KJ, Della Valle CJ, Goodman SB, Lewis CG, Yates AJ Jr, Watters WC III, Turkelson CM, Wies JL, Donnelly P, Patel N, Sluka P, Aaos. Preventing venous thromboembolic disease in patients undergoing elective hip and knee arthroplasty. J Am Acad Orthop Surg. 2011;19(12):768–76. https://doi.org/10.5435/00124635-201112000-00007.

19. Falck-Ytter Y, Francis CW, Johanson NA, Curley C, Dahl OE, Schulman S, Ortel TL, Pauker SG, Colwell CW Jr. Prevention of VTE in orthopedic surgery patients: antithrombotic therapy and prevention of thrombosis, 9th ed: American College of Chest Physicians evidence-based clinical practice guidelines. Chest. 2012;141(2 Suppl):e278S–325S. https://doi.org/10.1378/chest.11-2404.

20. Lindquist DE, Stewart DW, Brewster A, Waldroup C, Odle BL, Burchette JE, El-Bazouni H. Comparison of postoperative bleeding in total hip and knee arthroplasty patients receiving rivaroxaban, enoxaparin, or aspirin for thromboprophylaxis. Clin Appl Thromb Hemost. 2018;24(8):1315–21. https://doi.org/10.1177/1076029618772337.

21. Suen K, Westh RN, Churilov L, Hardidge AJ. Low-molecular-weight heparin and the relative risk of surgical site bleeding complications: results of a systematic review and meta-analysis of randomized controlled trials of venous thromboprophylaxis in patients after total joint arthroplasty. J Arthroplast. 2017;32(9):2911–2919.e2916. https://doi.org/10.1016/j.arth.2017.04.010.

22. Jameson SS, Rymaszewska M, Hui AC, James P, Serrano-Pedraza I, Muller SD. Wound complications following rivaroxaban administration: a multicenter comparison with low-molecular-weight heparins for thromboprophylaxis in lower limb arthroplasty. J Bone Joint Surg Am. 2012;94(17):1554–8. https://doi.org/10.2106/JBJS.K.00521.

23. Bloch BV, Patel V, Best AJ. Thromboprophylaxis with dabigatran leads to an increased incidence of wound leakage and an increased length of stay after total joint replacement. Bone Joint J. 2014;96-B(1):122–6. https://doi.org/10.1302/0301-620X.96B1.31569.

24. Garfinkel JH, Gladnick BP, Roland N, Romness DW. Increased incidence of bleeding and wound complications with factor-Xa inhibitors after total joint arthroplasty. J Arthroplast. 2018;33(2):533–6. https://doi.org/10.1016/j.arth.2017.08.039.

25. Lidgren L, Knutson K, Stefansdottir A. Infection and arthritis. Infection of prosthetic joints. Best Pract Res Clin Rheumatol. 2003;17(2):209–18. https://doi.org/10.1016/s1521-6942(03)00002-0.

26. Phillips JE, Crane TP, Noy M, Elliott TS, Grimer RJ. The incidence of deep prosthetic infections in a specialist orthopaedic hospital: a 15-year prospective survey. J Bone Joint Surg Br. 2006;88(7):943–8. https://doi.org/10.1302/0301-620X.88B7.17150.

27. Chahal GS, Saithna A, Brewster M, Gilbody J, Lever S, Khan WS, Foguet P. A comparison of complications requiring return to theatre in hip and knee arthroplasty patients taking enoxaparin versus rivaroxaban for thromboprophylaxis. Ortop Traumatol Rehabil. 2013;15(2):125–9. https://doi.org/10.5604/15093492.1045953.

28. Brimmo O, Glenn M, Klika AK, Murray TG, Molloy RM, Higuera CA. Rivaroxaban use for thrombosis prophylaxis is associated with early periprosthetic joint infection. J Arthroplast. 2016;31(6):1295–8. https://doi.org/10.1016/j.arth.2015.12.027.

29. Catella-Lawson F, Reilly MP, Kapoor SC, Cucchiara AJ, DeMarco S, Tournier B, Vyas SN, FitzGerald GA. Cyclooxygenase inhibitors and the antiplatelet effects of aspirin. N Engl J Med. 2001;345(25):1809–17. https://doi.org/10.1056/NEJMoa003199.

30. Johanson NA, Lachiewicz PF, Lieberman JR, Lotke PA, Parvizi J, Pellegrini V, Stringer TA, Tornetta P 3rd, Haralson RH III, Watters WC 3rd. Prevention of symptomatic pulmonary embolism in patients undergoing total hip or knee arthroplasty. J Am Acad Orthop Surg. 2009;17(3):183–96. https://doi.org/10.5435/00124635-200903000-00007.

31. Raphael IJ, Tischler EH, Huang R, Rothman RH, Hozack WJ, Parvizi J. Aspirin: an alternative for pulmonary embolism prophylaxis after arthroplasty? Clin Orthop Relat Res. 2014;472(2):482–8. https://doi.org/10.1007/s11999-013-3135-z.

32. Huang R, Buckley PS, Scott B, Parvizi J, Purtill JJ. Administration of aspirin as a prophylaxis agent against venous thromboembolism results in lower incidence of periprosthetic joint infection. J Arthroplast. 2015;30(9 Suppl):39–41. https://doi.org/10.1016/j.arth.2015.07.001.

Daniel Pérez-Prieto

30.1 Introduction

Polymethyl methacrylate (PMMA) or bone cement has been used since the late 1940s [1]. The first available reports are about its use for fracture fixation and even bone substitution in femoral and humeral head fractures [2, 3]. The mechanical properties of PMMA and the versatility it offers in terms of shape conformation as well as for substitution and fixation favored its introduction in the field of orthopedics. In 1964, John Charnley published the first study on cemented prosthesis. It is the one currently in use, albeit with some slight differences [4]. Then again, in subsequent decades some reports on its disadvantages like an allergic reaction, cardiac arrest, pulmonary embolism, among others, were also published [5–8].

The use of PMMA in orthopedic infections was first proposed by Buchholz in 1970. However, it was difficult to convince the orthopedic community that antibiotics could elute from a stony material such as PMMA [9–11]. Nevertheless, he continued with the use of antibiotic-loaded bone cement (ALBC) for the treatment of prosthetic infections and published promising results in 1981 [12]. Buchholz pioneered one-stage exchange by using ALBC with two purposes, for fixation for a permanent implant and infection treatment in prosthetic joint infections (PJI).

The use of ALBC became popular and new indications such as prophylaxis were started in this decade [13]. Therefore, the purpose is not only for fixation of a permanent implant but also infection prophylaxis.

All the previously cited studies were about hip prosthesis. Ten years later, in 1983, John Insall described a new technique to treat PJI. It was denominated the two-stage exchange for knee PJI [14]. Although an ALBC spacer was not used in the interval, Borden and Wilde introduced the use of an ALBC spacer for the interim in TKA two-stage exchange a few years later [15, 16]. In this case, ALBC was used for void filling and space maintenance with a temporary implant along with infection treatment. In that decade, reports on one-stage exchange for TKA infections using ALBC were also published by groups distinct from the Buchhold group. However, the aims were the same, infection treatment and prosthesis fixation [17].

30.2 Characteristics

PMMA is a resistant plastic also known as acrylic. It has multiple uses such as headlights in vehicles, photo frames, tablecloths, and other household items like lamps. In medicine, it is

D. Pérez-Prieto (✉)
Universitat Autònoma de Barcelona, Hospital del Mar, ICATME-Hospital Universitari Dexeus, Board of Trustees Pro-Implant Foundation, Barcelona, Spain

© ISAKOS 2022
U. G. Longo et al. (eds.), *Infection in Knee Replacement*,
https://doi.org/10.1007/978-3-030-81553-0_30

used in the making of diagnostic tools, but its main use is as bone cement for dentist, orthopedic surgeons, and neurosurgeons.

The mechanical properties of bone cement are considerable, and it is rigid at room temperature. In contrast, it has low impact resistance and is sensitive to heat [18].

The composition of commercial acrylic bone cement differs in some modifications. It also comes with the addition of co-polymers of PMMA and some different co-monomers in the liquid. Bone cement powder predominantly contains PMMA in powder form that also carries radiopacifiers like barium sulfate or zirconium dioxide. In the case of ALBC, the antibiotic is usually incorporated into the powder phase [18].

The modifications of each brand make for the differences in mechanical properties as well as in the hydrophilic characteristics of the bone cement. The latter are crucial in ALBC as the elution of most antibiotics depends on how hydrophilic the cement is. The liberation of the antibiotic from the ALBC also depends on the porosity of the cement mantle and the total surface of the cement as the antibiotic only elutes from the outer surface, which can absorb fluid and then release it together with the antibiotics [19].

It is true that the characteristics of the powdered polymer and the liquid monomer influence antibiotic release, as stated before, but the opposite is also true. The addition of antibiotics affects its mechanical characteristics. Liquid antibiotics cause greater loss of compressive strength than powder preparations [20]. It has been found that the addition of antibiotics amounting to up to 10% of the weight of the PMMA barely affects mechanical strength [21, 22]. Other properties that can affect its mechanical characteristics are fatigue limit, fracture toughness, and the polymerization rate, which may differ between brands [22, 23].

30.3 Clinical Uses of the ALBC in the Knee Surgery

As previously stated, ALBC was first used for hip prosthesis but soon became popular among knee surgeons and its use spread worldwide. In fact, contrary to hip prosthesis, total knee arthroplasty (TKA) is rarely uncemented nowadays. According to the Nordic registries, up to 90% of TKA are cemented [24].

Although the use of ALBC around the knee can be very different (osteomyelitis treatment, Masquelet technique, open fracture dead space management, etc.), this chapter will focus only the use of ALBC in the prosthetic field.

ALBC can be employed in cases of primary TKA in which the aim will be fixation and infection prevention. In cases of TKA revision, the surgeon can also use ALBC for fixation and infection prevention when dealing with aseptic revisions. It can also be used for fixation and infection treatment in cases of one-stage septic revision and two-stage septic revision with a short interval. In all those instances, the cement will be permanently left in the patient. Finally, ALBC can be utilized for dead space management and infection treatment, which is the case of temporary spacers in the first stage of two-stage septic revisions [25, 26].

30.4 ALBC in Primary TKA

The prevention of PJI is a major concern among orthopedic surgeons. One of the most important measures to reduce the risk of infection is intravenous antibiotic prophylaxis. It has shown an 81% reduction in the relative risk [27]. The rationale for the combination of both local and systemic prophylaxis is based on multiple factors. Among them, there is a broadening of the antimicrobial spectrum, an improved antimicrobials synergistic effect, pharmacokinetics optimization and its action as a local antimicrobial barrier [28].

Cephalosporins are the most frequent antibiotic prophylaxis used in orthopedic surgery and aminoglycosides are the predominant ones in ALBC. While the first group covers most Gram-positive bacteria, the second is effective against Gram-negative that may not be susceptible to first-generation cephalosporins [26]. Moreover, the synergistic effect of beta-lactams and aminoglycosides has been well-known for decades [29, 30].

From the pharmacokinetic point of view, ALBC provides a high local concentration of antibiotic. That is something that is difficult to achieve when antibiotics are given intravenously. In that sense, Hendricks et al. found that the concentrations of gentamicin inside the gap between the bone and the prosthesis within the 2 h after surgery were about 1000 times higher than the minimal inhibitory concentration (MIC) for staphylococci [31]. This concentration may effectively decontaminate the prosthesis-related interfacial gap of any accidental contamination during surgery. Therefore, ALBC would act as a local barrier for accidental contamination.

For all the previously stated reasons, ALBC for PJI prevention in primary prosthesis is widely used in northern Europe. However, its use is not yet approved for that purpose in the United States. It is only approved for prophylaxis in revision cases in the USA [28, 32].

For local prophylaxis with ALBC, there is good evidence supporting its use for cemented hip arthroplasties [33–35]. In the case of TKA, the results from different studies are heterogeneous. Hinarejos et al., in one of the largest prospective randomized TRIAL with ALBC, found no differences between the ALBC and the plain cement group in terms of the infection rate [36]. On the other hand, Chiu did find a reduction of infection when cement loaded with cefuroxime was employed [37]. Additionally, data from arthroplasty registries seem to suggest that ALBC might reduce PJI after TKA [38, 39]. Aminoglycosides are the group of antibiotics most used in ALBC in the Finland, England, and Wales. They are the countries of origin of those studies. On the other hand, colistin, which has a limited spectrum against Gram-negative bacteria, and erythromycin, a bacteriostatic and with high rates of resistance to staphylococci were used in the study done by Hinarejos et al. [36, 38, 40]. This may be the reason for the different results obtained as the latter combination is not the optimal one.

In any case, what it is clear is that for fixation of a primary TKA along with prophylaxis, a low dose of antibiotic is advocated for to avoid mechanical property weakening. Aminoglycosides are the best antimicrobials to add (0.5 g of gentamicin per 40 g of PMMA or 1 g of tobramycin per 40 g of PMMA).

30.5 ALBC in Revision TKA

The reasons for TKA revision are varied. Nevertheless, the most important one that must be ruled out before surgery is infection. This is clear as the approach is completely different and not diagnosing PJI can make curing the infection more difficult in the long run. The big challenge in PJI is low-grade chronic infections as most of them are only accompanied by pain [41]. No other sign or symptom is seen in most of PJI caused by coagulase-negative staphylococci or *cutibacterium* spp. Therefore, it is crucial to use a pro-active and thorough diagnostic protocol to identify them and prevent unsuspected intraoperative positive cultures [42, 43]. In that sense, the criteria proposed by Zimmerli has been found to be more reliable in identifying PJI, specially low-grade infections [41, 43, 44].

Once PJI has been ruled out, aseptic revision is performed. In this case, ALBC has been clearly found to be superior to bone cement without antibiotics [45–48]. In that sense, the use of ALBC can be considered the gold standard for care in TKA revision [46]. There are several theories to explain these results. The most accepted is that some of those supposed aseptic revisions were actually low-grade infections that were not identified as previously stated [43, 49]. Some other reasons might be that the bone and soft tissues are of poor quality and less vascularized than in primary cases and therefore more prone to infection [50]. Moreover, the surgical duration of a revision is normally superior to a primary surgery and the blood loss is usually greater, which are factors that have been related to increased risk of infection [50–52].

As mentioned, ALBC in revision cases can be used for infection prevention in aseptic revisions. It is also used for infection prevention in second-stage reimplantation when there is a long interval between procedures in a two-stage exchange. In this case, infection has been cured after TKA removal and debridement and the interval with the knee spacer and systemic antibiotic treatment [25, 44, 53, 54]. In both cases, ALBC is used for prosthesis fixation and therefore its mechanical properties must be preserved.

To do so, a precise mixing technique that respects the prescribed mixing time and is done in vacuum is mandatory. Moreover, antibiotics must not exceed 10% of the weight of the PMMA to prevent weakening of the cement and the subsequent loss of strength [26]. The use of ALBC with a combination of two antibiotics is generally recommended in revision cases because of the synergistic effect and the broad spectrum of the combination. Moreover, studies seem to suggest there is better performance than with ALBC with gentamicin alone and it can also prevent resistant bacteria selection [34, 55].

In both aseptic revisions and the second stage of the two-stage septic revisions, a commercially available ALBC with two antibiotics is recommended for the previously stated reasons.

When dealing with one-stage exchange PJI revision, in which infection has not yet been cured, ALBC is used for the treatment of the infection as well as prosthesis fixation. The local activity of antibiotics along with prosthesis exchange, surgical debridement, and systemic antibiotics are used to cure infection [54, 56, 57]. The identification of the microorganism and its antibiotic susceptibility are crucial if this approach is used [57, 58]. Ideally, the microorganism is identified preoperatively, and the bone cement is loaded with antibiotics that are active against that microorganism. However, preoperative bacterial isolation is sometimes not possible. For those cases, a two-stage exchange with a short interval of approximately 2 weeks has been proposed [53, 59]. By doing so, the bacteria can be identified by means of intraoperative tissue cultures and prosthesis sonication. To do the implantation of the prosthesis in such a short interval, the bacteria must be susceptible to antibiofilm antibiotics [53, 60]. This interim and bacteria identification will also allow for the identification of the best ALBC antibiotic combination. It is important to mention that not all antibiotic combinations are commercially available. Therefore, an "off-label" hand-made mixing technique must be used in most of the cases [26]. Antibiotic mixing according to bacterial isolation can be seen in Table 30.1 [26, 58].

30.6 ALBC for Knee Spacers

Knee spacers are used in the two-stage septic revision technique. They can be either static or dynamic, self-made or preformed. Their differences are not the issue of the present chapter. Since they are used temporarily, high antibiotic doses can be used to treat infection regardless of the impact it can have on the mechanical properties [61]. It has been proven that antibiotic elution for the commonly used interim times is enough to eradicate infection [62]. Large amounts of antibiotic have been found when the spacer is analyzed after removal [63, 64]. However, it is worth knowing that if the spacer is left in place for a longer period (usually longer that 6–8 weeks), it may behave like a foreign body and biofilm may attach itself since antibiotic elution decreases [62, 65]. When using a self-made spacer, antibiotics for ALBC can be tailored to the preoperative cultures (when available) and the desired amount can be increased to even more than 10% of the weight of the PMMA [26, 61]. In addition, the mixing technique can be modified to obtain a "bad quality" cement. This means doing it without a vacuum to increase the number of bubbles which will explode afterwards eluting the antibiotics. Elution from the spacer also depends on the surface. A simple technique, making indentations with a scalpel, can increase the elution [66]. The legal issues around the off-label use of this mixing technique and manual addition of antibiotics mentioned in the previous point are less important here since the spacer is only a temporary device for a short period of time. The antibiotic combination in accordance with the microbiological results can be seen in Table 30.1 [26, 58].

30.7 Antibiotics for Bone Cement

Not all antibiotics are suitable for mixing with bone cement. The optimal characteristics of the antibiotics to be mixed with PMMA can be seen in Table 30.2 [61, 67].

Liquid antibiotics have a significant damaging effect on the mechanical properties of the bone cement, especially the compressive strength [68]. Some antibiotics, like rifampin, can impair

Table 30.1 Local antimicrobials in bone cement (PMMA) (additionally to systemic antimicrobial treatment)

Situation	Antimicrobial (AM)	Fixation cement (prophylactic dose: per 40 g PMMA cement) Black: industrially admixed AM Blue: manually admixed AM	Spacer cement (therapeutic dose: per 40 g PMMA cement)
Standard situation • Susceptible or unknown pathogen(s)	Gentamicin + Clindamycin	1 g 1 g	1 g 1 g (+2 g vancomycin)
Special situations • *Staphylococcus* spp. (oxacillin-/methicillin-resistant) or *Enterococcus* spp.	Gentamicin + Vancomycin *or* Daptomycin	0.5 g 2 g –	0.5 g 2 g (+2 g[a]) 2 g
• Vancomycin-resistant enterococci (VRE)	Gentamicin + Linezolid *or* Daptomycin *or* Fosfomycin-sodium[b]	0.5 g 1 g 2 g 1 g	0.5–1 g 2 g 3 g 2 g
• Resistant gram-negative pathogens (e.g., *E. coli, Klebsiella, Enterobacter, Pseudomonas* spp.)	Gentamicin [+] Colistin[c] *or* Fosfomycin-sodium[b] *or* Meropenem *or* Ciprofloxacin	0.5 g 2 g (=60 Mio E) 1 g 2 g 2 g	0.5–1 g 4 g (=120 Mio E) 2 g 3 g[d] 3 g
• Yeasts (*Candida* spp.) or molds (e.g., *Aspergillus* spp.)	Gentamicin [+] Amphotericin B liposomal (Ambisome®) *or* Voriconazole	0.5 g 0.1 g[e] 0.2 g	0.5–1 g 0.2 g[a,e] 0.4 g[d]

General considerations:
- When additional antimicrobials are admixed, industrially impregnated cements are preferred over plain cements (better mechanical properties and elution due to synergistic release)
- Antimicrobial susceptibility testing results are applicable for systemic antimicrobial application and might not be valid for local antimicrobial application due to high local concentrations and synergistic activity
- Side effects and interactions of local antimicrobials are rare. However, serum concentrations of vancomycin and gentamicin should be monitored in patients with kidney insufficiency and/or intravenous application
- Only use sterile antimicrobials in powder form. Liquid antimicrobials are not recommended due to inhomogeneous distribution in PMMA. Antibiotics that interfere with polymerization process (rifampin or metronidazole) or which are thermolabile or sensitive to oxidation (e.g., some beta lactams) should not be used
- Data on mechanical stability are not available for combinations of more than two antimicrobials. If possible, the total amount of antimicrobials should not exceed 10% of the PMMA powder weight (=4 g per 40 g)
- Recommendations are based on studies with PALACOS®/COPAL® PMMA cements and literature data. Elution data depend on the PMMA cement basis used
- Do not use vacuum mixing for preparation of spacer cement (higher porosity → better antimicrobial elution)

[a]These AM concentrations do not fulfill the mechanical ISO requirements for fixation cement
[b]Fosfomycin-sodium is preferred over fosfomycin-calcium due to better mechanical properties of PMMA
[c]Available as colistin-sodium or colistin-sulfate (equal efficacy)
[d]Improved efficacy and antimicrobial release in combination with gentamicin 1 g and clindamycin 1 g
[e]Literature is still controversial regarding minimal effective concentrations

cement polymerization and therefore hamper the curing process. The thermal stability of the antibiotic is also crucial as the exothermal reaction of the cement curing process may impair antibiotics like cloxacillin. Nevertheless, in vitro studies about the mechanical properties of ALBC are not always similar to in vivo results [69]. The brand of antibiotic added even has a different impact on the mechanical strength of the ALBC [22]. What is clear is that the more antibiotic added, the more impairment of the mechanical characteristics.

As a general rule, low antibiotic doses (<2.5% PMMA weight) are used for PJI prevention. For fixation of revision cases (either septic or aseptic), medium doses of up to 7% of the weight of the PMMA are recommended (<10% in any case). For spacer purpose in PJI treatment, 10% or more is usually used [28].

Table 30.2 Ideal properties of antibiotics to be used in antibiotic-loaded bone cement

- Availability in powder form
- Wide antibacterial spectrum
- Bactericidal at low concentrations
- Elution from PMMA in high concentrations for prolonged periods
- Thermal stability
- Low or no risk of allergy or delayed hypersensitivity
- Low influence on the mechanical properties of the cement
- Low serum protein binding

30.8 Types and Combination

Aminoglycosides are the most frequently used antibiotics worldwide. Gentamicin and tobramycin are mostly used for PJI prophylaxis (alone) and in combination for revision [67]. Commercially available bone cements loaded with two antibiotics are limited. The combination of gentamicin with clindamycin is recommended for aseptic revisions or PJI caused by anaerobes (*cutibacterium* spp.). The combination of gentamicin with vancomycin is recommended for septic revisions secondary to staphylococci (especially when dealing with MRSA) [26].

When it comes to self-made hand mixing in the operating theater, one must keep in mind that the cement characteristics on the brand's label are being modified and therefore an off-label use is being done. In that sense, there are studies that show that mechanical strength and antibiotic elution are worsened when the antibiotic is added manually [70, 71]. However, there are PJI cases that cannot be treated with the commercially available ALBC, for instance fungi PJI. For those cases, Table 30.1 summarizes the optimal antibiotic combination for PMMA.

30.9 Resistances

The selection of resistant bacteria is always a possibility when an antibiotic is used. Some factors that can favor this phenomenon are inadequate doses with a threshold under the MIC for the microorganism and a short antibiotic concentration time above the MIC. In that sense, ALBC provides high elution of antibiotics that are clearly above the MIC of the bacteria causing PJI in the first hours [19]. However, the major concern is whether the ALBC can provide an antibiotic concentration over the MIC for a long period, specially in cases of coagulase-negative staphylococci. There has been a shift towards higher MICs in those cases in the recent years. These assumptions are particularly important in the case of ALBC with gentamicin used for PJI treatment in which a higher rate of gentamicin-resistant staphylococci has been found in the recent years [19, 72]. When aminoglycosides are used alone for prevention, resistance selection is not a concern since the high amount of local antibiotics are enough to eradicate intraoperative contamination that is caused by a small inoculum of bacteria.

In the cases of PJI, the combination of two or more antibiotics is crucial for the synergistic effect, to improve antibiotic elution and to broaden the treatment spectrum. The same explanation is true for primary cases in high-risk patients [34, 73, 74].

30.10 ALBC Costs

One of the major concerns with the use of ALBC is the added cost that it implies. In revision cases, there is no doubt relative to the use of ALBC. However, the issue of cost arises in primary cases when ALBC is used as a prophylactic measure. Most of the cost-effective studies on ALBC come from the USA. Therefore, there are some peculiarities. The diagnostic criteria for PJI proposed by American societies of infectious diseases and orthopedics is different from the one proposed by the European society. Furthermore, the costs for PJI treatment and ALBC are clearly different. Moreover, since the PJI rate in primary TKA is quite low, it would be difficult to take any preventive measure to reduce this low rate even further.

In that sense, Sanz-Ruiz studied those variations and found ALBC to be cost-effective when the PJI rate is 4% or greater [75].

References

1. Vishnevetskaya RI. [Use of polymethyl metacrylate for osteosynthesis and arthroplasty]. Gosp Delo. 1947;(4):42–7.
2. Leibson ND. [Polymethylmethacrylate in skull defects]. Vopr Neirokhir. 1948;12(1):11–20.
3. Cottalorda J. Aubrespy null. [Arthroplasty with acrylic head in traumatism of the shoulder]. Mars Chir. 1951;3(4):455–60.
4. Charnley J. The bonding of prostheses to bone by cement. J Bone Joint Surg Br. 1964;46:518–29.
5. Powell JN, McGrath PJ, Lahiri SK, Hill P. Cardiac arrest associated with bone cement. Br Med J. 1970;3(5718):326.
6. Ratliff AH, Clement JA. Pulmonary embolism and bone cement. Br Med J. 1971;2(5760):532.
7. Kepes ER, Undersood PS, Becsey L. Intraoperative death associated with acrylic bone cement. Report of two cases. JAMA. 1972;222(5):576–7.
8. Fisher AA. Paresthesia on the fingers accompanying dermatitis due to methylmethacrylate bone cement. Contact Dermatitis. 1979;5(1):56–7.
9. Wahlig H, Buchholz HW. [Experimental and clinical studies on the release of gentamicin from bone cement]. Chir Z Alle Geb Oper Medizen. 1972;43(10):441–5.
10. Buchholz HW. Modification of the Charnley artificial hip joint. Clin Orthop. 1970;72:69–78.
11. Charnley J. The future of total hip replacement. Hip. 1982:198–210.
12. Buchholz HW, Elson RA, Engelbrecht E, Lodenkämper H, Röttger J, Siegel A. Management of deep infection of total hip replacement. J Bone Joint Surg Br. 1981;63-B(3):342–53.
13. Wannske M, Tscherne H. [Results of prophylactic use of Refobacin-Palacos in implantation of endoprostheses of the hip joint in Hannover]. Aktuelle Probl Chir Orthop. 1979;(12):201–5.
14. Insall JN, Thompson FM, Brause BD. Two-stage reimplantation for the salvage of infected total knee arthroplasty. J Bone Joint Surg Am. 1983;65(8):1087–98.
15. Borden LS, Gearen PF. Infected total knee arthroplasty. A protocol for management. J Arthroplast. 1987;2(1):27–36.
16. Wilde AH, Ruth JT. Two-stage reimplantation in infected total knee arthroplasty. Clin Orthop. 1988;236:23–35.
17. Freeman MA, Sudlow RA, Casewell MW, Radcliff SS. The management of infected total knee replacements. J Bone Joint Surg Br. 1985;67(5):764–8.
18. Ginebra M-P, Montufar EB. 9 - Cements as bone repair materials. In: Pawelec KM, Planell JA, editors. Bone repair biomaterials. 2nd ed. [Internet]. Woodhead Publishing; 2019 [cited 2020 Jun 14]. p. 233–71. (Woodhead Publishing Series in Biomaterials). http://www.sciencedirect.com/science/article/pii/B9780081024515000093.
19. Berberich C, Sanz-Ruiz P. Risk assessment of antibiotic resistance development by antibiotic-loaded bone cements: is it a clinical concern? EFORT Open Rev. 2019;4(10):576–84.
20. Armstrong MS, Spencer RF, Cunningham JL, Gheduzzi S, Miles AW, Learmonth ID. Mechanical characteristics of antibiotic-laden bone cement. Acta Orthop Scand. 2002;73(6):688–90.
21. Paz E, Sanz-Ruiz P, Abenojar J, Vaquero-Martín J, Forriol F, Del Real JC. Evaluation of elution and mechanical properties of high-dose antibiotic-loaded bone cement: comparative "in vitro" study of the influence of vancomycin and cefazolin. J Arthroplast. 2015;30(8):1423–9.
22. Lee S-H, Tai C-L, Chen S-Y, Chang C-H, Chang Y-H, Hsieh P-H. Elution and mechanical strength of vancomycin-loaded bone cement: in vitro study of the influence of brand combination. PLoS One. 2016;11(11):e0166545.
23. Lewis G. Not all approved antibiotic-loaded PMMA bone cement brands are the same: ranking using the utility materials selection concept. J Mater Sci Mater Med. 2015;26(1):5388.
24. Niemeläinen MJ, Mäkelä KT, Robertsson O, W-Dahl A, Furnes O, Fenstad AM, et al. The effect of fixation type on the survivorship of contemporary total knee arthroplasty in patients younger than 65 years of age: a register-based study of 115,177 knees in the Nordic Arthroplasty Register Association (NARA) 2000-2016. Acta Orthop. 2020;91(2):184–90.
25. Zimmerli W, Trampuz A, Ochsner PE. Prosthetic-joint infections. N Engl J Med. 2004;351(16):1645–54.
26. Kühn K-D, Renz N, Trampuz A. [Local antibiotic therapy]. Unfallchirurg. 2017;120(7):561–72.
27. AlBuhairan B, Hind D, Hutchinson A. Antibiotic prophylaxis for wound infections in total joint arthroplasty: a systematic review. J Bone Joint Surg Br. 2008;90(7):915–9.
28. Kühn K-D, editor. Management of periprosthetic joint infection: a global perspective on diagnosis, treatment options, prevention strategies and their economic impact [Internet]. Berlin: Springer; 2018 [cited 2020 Jun 14]. https://www.springer.com/gp/book/9783662544686.
29. Zinner SH, Klastersky J, Gaya H, Bernard C, Ryff JC. In vitro and in vivo studies of three antibiotic combinations against gram-negative bacteria and Staphylococcus aureus. Antimicrob Agents Chemother. 1981;20(4):463–9.
30. Watanakunakorn C. In vitro activity of ceftriaxone alone and in combination with gentamicin, tobramycin, and amikacin against Pseudomonas aeruginosa. Antimicrob Agents Chemother. 1983;24(2):305–6.
31. Hendriks JGE, Neut D, van Horn JR, van der Mei HC, Busscher HJ. The release of gentamicin from acrylic bone cements in a simulated prosthesis-related interfacial gap. J Biomed Mater Res B Appl Biomater. 2003;64(1):1–5.
32. Carpenter W, Hamilton DH, Luthringer T, Buchalter D, Schwarzkopf R. The evolution of cement fixa-

tion in total knee arthroplasty. Surg Technol Int. 2019;35:355–62.

33. Engesaeter LB, Lie SA, Espehaug B, Furnes O, Vollset SE, Havelin LI. Antibiotic prophylaxis in total hip arthroplasty: effects of antibiotic prophylaxis systemically and in bone cement on the revision rate of 22,170 primary hip replacements followed 0-14 years in the Norwegian Arthroplasty Register. Acta Orthop Scand. 2003;74(6):644–51.

34. Sprowson AP, Jensen C, Chambers S, Parsons NR, Aradhyula NM, Carluke I, et al. The use of high-dose dual-impregnated antibiotic-laden cement with hemiarthroplasty for the treatment of a fracture of the hip: the fractured hip infection trial. Bone Joint J. 2016;98-B(11):1534–41.

35. Colas S, Collin C, Piriou P, Zureik M. Association between total hip replacement characteristics and 3-year prosthetic survivorship: a population-based study. JAMA Surg. 2015;150(10):979–88.

36. Hinarejos P, Guirro P, Leal J, Montserrat F, Pelfort X, Sorli ML, et al. The use of erythromycin and colistin-loaded cement in total knee arthroplasty does not reduce the incidence of infection: a prospective randomized study in 3000 knees. J Bone Joint Surg Am. 2013;95(9):769–74.

37. Chiu F-Y, Chen C-M, Lin C-FJ, Lo W-H. Cefuroxime-impregnated cement in primary total knee arthroplasty: a prospective, randomized study of three hundred and forty knees. J Bone Joint Surg Am. 2002;84(5):759–62.

38. Jameson SS, Asaad A, Diament M, Kasim A, Bigirumurame T, Baker P, et al. Antibiotic-loaded bone cement is associated with a lower risk of revision following primary cemented total knee arthroplasty: an analysis of 731,214 cases using National Joint Registry data. Bone Joint J. 2019;101-B(11):1331–47.

39. Jämsen E, Furnes O, Engesaeter LB, Konttinen YT, Odgaard A, Stefánsdóttir A, et al. Prevention of deep infection in joint replacement surgery. Acta Orthop. 2010;81(6):660–6.

40. Jämsen E, Huhtala H, Puolakka T, Moilanen T. Risk factors for infection after knee arthroplasty. A register-based analysis of 43,149 cases. J Bone Joint Surg Am. 2009;91(1):38–47.

41. Pérez-Prieto D, Portillo ME, Puig-Verdié L, Alier A, Martínez S, Sorlí L, et al. C-reactive protein may misdiagnose prosthetic joint infections, particularly chronic and low-grade infections. Int Orthop. 2017;41(7):1315–9.

42. Jacobs AME, Bénard M, Meis JF, van Hellemondt G, Goosen JHM. The unsuspected prosthetic joint infection : incidence and consequences of positive intra-operative cultures in presumed aseptic knee and hip revisions. Bone Joint J. 2017;99-B(11):1482–9.

43. Renz N, Yermak K, Perka C, Trampuz A. Alpha defensin lateral flow test for diagnosis of periprosthetic joint infection: not a screening but a confirmatory test. J Bone Joint Surg Am. 2018;100(9): 742–50.

44. Zimmerli W. Clinical presentation and treatment of orthopaedic implant-associated infection. J Intern Med. 2014;276(2):111–9.

45. Chiu F-Y, Lin C-FJ. Antibiotic-impregnated cement in revision total knee arthroplasty. A prospective cohort study of one hundred and eighty-three knees. J Bone Joint Surg Am. 2009;91(3):628–33.

46. Gandhi R, Backstein D, Zywiel MG. Antibiotic-laden bone cement in primary and revision hip and knee arthroplasty. J Am Acad Orthop Surg. 2018;26(20):727–34.

47. Bini SA, Chan PH, Inacio MCS, Paxton EW, Khatod M. Antibiotic cement was associated with half the risk of re-revision in 1,154 aseptic revision total knee arthroplasties. Acta Orthop. 2016;87(1):55–9.

48. Kleppel D, Stirton J, Liu J, Ebraheim NA. Antibiotic bone cement's effect on infection rates in primary and revision total knee arthroplasties. World J Orthop. 2017;8(12):946–55.

49. Renz N, Mudrovcic S, Perka C, Trampuz A. Orthopedic implant-associated infections caused by Cutibacterium spp. - a remaining diagnostic challenge. PLoS One. 2018;13(8):e0202639.

50. Badawy M, Espehaug B, Fenstad AM, Indrekvam K, Dale H, Havelin LI, et al. Patient and surgical factors affecting procedure duration and revision risk due to deep infection in primary total knee arthroplasty. BMC Musculoskelet Disord. 2017;18(1):544.

51. Nikolaus OB, McLendon PB, Hanssen AD, Mabry TM, Berbari EF, Sierra RJ. Factors associated with 20-year cumulative risk of infection after aseptic index revision total knee arthroplasty. J Arthroplast. 2016;31(4):872–7.

52. Rhee C, Lethbridge L, Richardson G, Dunbar M. Risk factors for infection, revision, death, blood transfusion and longer hospital stay 3 months and 1 year after primary total hip or knee arthroplasty. Can J Surg. 2018;61(3):165–76.

53. Winkler T, Stuhlert MGW, Lieb E, Müller M, von Roth P, Preininger B, et al. Outcome of short versus long interval in two-stage exchange for periprosthetic joint infection: a prospective cohort study. Arch Orthop Trauma Surg. 2019;139(3):295–303.

54. Renner L, Perka C, Trampuz A, Renz N. [Treatment of periprosthetic infections]. Chir Z Alle Geb Oper Medizen. 2016;87(10):831–8.

55. Mohamed NS, Wilkie WA, Remily EA, Nace J, Delanois RE, Browne JA. Antibiotic choice: the synergistic effect of single vs dual antibiotics. J Arthroplast. 2020;35(3S):S19–23.

56. Kendoff D, Gehrke T. Surgical management of periprosthetic joint infection: one-stage exchange. J Knee Surg. 2014;27(4):273–8.

57. Friesecke C, Wodtke J. [Periprosthetic knee infection. One-stage exchange]. Orthopade. 2006;35(9):937–8, 940–5.

58. Izakovicova P, Borens O, Trampuz A. Periprosthetic joint infection: current concepts and outlook. EFORT Open Rev. 2019;4(7):482–94.

59. Tomislav M, Antea B, Josko J, Luka S, Darinka V. Functional recovery after two-stage short-interval revision of chronic periprosthetic knee joint infection. Int Orthop. 2020.

60. Karczewski D, Winkler T, Renz N, Trampuz A, Lieb E, Perka C, et al. A standardized interdisciplinary algorithm for the treatment of prosthetic joint infections. Bone Joint J. 2019;101-B(2):132–9.

61. Anagnostakos K. Therapeutic use of antibiotic-loaded bone cement in the treatment of hip and knee joint infections. J Bone Joint Infect. 2017;2(1):29–37.

62. Anagnostakos K, Meyer C. Antibiotic elution from hip and knee acrylic bone cement spacers: a systematic review. Biomed Res Int. 2017;2017:4657874.

63. Kummer A, Tafin UF, Borens O. Effect of sonication on the elution of antibiotics from polymethyl methacrylate (PMMA). J Bone Joint Infect. 2017;2(4):208–12.

64. Mariaux S, Furustrand Tafin U, Borens O. Diagnosis of persistent infection in prosthetic two-stage exchange: evaluation of the effect of sonication on antibiotic release from bone cement spacers. J Bone Joint Infect. 2018;3(1):37–42.

65. Sorlí L, Puig L, Torres-Claramunt R, González A, Alier A, Knobel H, et al. The relationship between microbiology results in the second of a two-stage exchange procedure using cement spacers and the outcome after revision total joint replacement for infection: the use of sonication to aid bacteriological analysis. J Bone Joint Surg Br. 2012;94(2):249–53.

66. Salih S, Paskins A, Nichol T, Smith T, Hamer A. The cement spacer with multiple indentations: increasing antibiotic elution using a cement spacer "teabag". Bone Joint J. 2015;97-B(11):1519–24.

67. Hinarejos P, Guirro P, Puig-Verdie L, Torres-Claramunt R, Leal-Blanquet J, Sanchez-Soler J, et al. Use of antibiotic-loaded cement in total knee arthroplasty. World J Orthop. 2015;6(11):877–85.

68. Hsieh P-H, Tai C-L, Lee P-C, Chang Y-H. Liquid gentamicin and vancomycin in bone cement: a potentially more cost-effective regimen. J Arthroplast. 2009;24(1):125–30.

69. Sanz-Ruiz P, Paz E, Abenojar J, Carlos del Real J, Vaquero J, Forriol F. Effects of vancomycin, cefazolin and test conditions on the wear behavior of bone cement. J Arthroplast. 2014;29(1):16–22.

70. Neut D, van de Belt H, van Horn JR, van der Mei HC, Busscher HJ. The effect of mixing on gentamicin release from polymethylmethacrylate bone cements. Acta Orthop Scand. 2003;74(6):670–6.

71. DeLuise M, Scott CP. Addition of hand-blended generic tobramycin in bone cement: effect on mechanical strength. Orthopedics. 2004;27(12):1289–91.

72. Corona PS, Espinal L, Rodríguez-Pardo D, Pigrau C, Larrosa N, Flores X. Antibiotic susceptibility in gram-positive chronic joint arthroplasty infections: increased aminoglycoside resistance rate in patients with prior aminoglycoside-impregnated cement spacer use. J Arthroplast. 2014;29(8):1617–21.

73. Stefánsdóttir A, Johansson D, Knutson K, Lidgren L, Robertsson O. Microbiology of the infected knee arthroplasty: report from the Swedish Knee Arthroplasty Register on 426 surgically revised cases. Scand J Infect Dis. 2009;41(11–12):831–40.

74. Corró S, Vicente M, Rodríguez-Pardo D, Pigrau C, Lung M, Corona PS. Vancomycin-gentamicin prefabricated spacers in 2-stage revision arthroplasty for chronic hip and knee periprosthetic joint infection: insights into reimplantation microbiology and outcomes. J Arthroplast. 2020;35(1):247–54.

75. Sanz-Ruiz P, Matas-Diez JA, Sanchez-Somolinos M, Villanueva-Martinez M, Vaquero-Martín J. Is the commercial antibiotic-loaded bone cement useful in prophylaxis and cost saving after knee and hip joint arthroplasty? The Transatlantic Paradox. J Arthroplasty. 2017;32(4):1095–9.

31

Mark Roussot, Justin Chang, Warran Wignadasan, and Sam Oussedik

31.1 Introduction

Delayed or inadequate treatment of septic arthritis can rapidly result in irreversible joint destruction, systemic sepsis, and even death as it has a mortality rate of 9–11% [1]. This rate is considerably higher in elderly patients, the presence of multifocal disease, significant co-morbidity and treatment failure [2, 3].

A previous history of native joint infection presents unique challenges with risk of prosthetic joint infection (PJI) that is difficult to quantify [4–7]. While total knee arthroplasty (TKA) can provide a durable solution with excellent functional results, it is imperative that the treatment strategy is patient specific, well planned, and performed with attention to detail in order to avoid potentially devastating and costly sequelae [8].

In this chapter we will briefly discuss the key aspects of the pathogenesis, explore the role of TKA in the context of previous knee infection, provide a synopsis of the evidence and experience for TKA and the treatment strategies utilized, and recommend a strategy for the evaluation and management of patients with post-infection arthropathy for whom knee arthroplasty is considered.

The focus will predominantly be on bacterial and mycobacterial knee infections.

31.2 Pathogenesis

The incidence of septic arthritis is bimodal, predominantly affecting young children and older adults. The spectrum of knee infections that may result in debilitating arthropathy includes intra-articular infections, with or without osteomyelitis, and can arise from a variety of systemic, local or iatrogenic causes, as highlighted in Table 31.1.

The most common pathogen is *S. aureus*, with *Staphylococcus epidermidis* and *Streptococci* less commonly implicated [1]. Other organisms are also associated with certain population groups, such as group A

M. Roussot · S. Oussedik (✉)
Department of Trauma and Orthopaedics, University College London Hospitals, London, UK
e-mail: mark.roussot@nhs.net

J. Chang
Department of Trauma and Orthopaedics, University College London Hospitals, London, UK

Humber River Hospital, Toronto, ON, Canada
e-mail: justin.chang@mail.utoronto.ca

W. Wignadasan
Department of Trauma and Orthopaedics, University College London Hospitals, London, UK

Chelsea and Westminster Hospital, London, UK
e-mail: w.wignadasan@nhs.net

© ISAKOS 2022
U. G. Longo et al. (eds.), *Infection in Knee Replacement*,
https://doi.org/10.1007/978-3-030-81553-0_31

Table 31.1 Summary of causes of prior knee infection

Origin of infection	Proportion (%)		
	Seo et al. [9] (N = 62)	Lee et al. [10] (N = 20)	Jerry et al. [11] (N = 65)
Post-operative	50	35	49
Hematogenous	35	50	26
IA injection	10	0	25
Miscellaneous	5	15	17

Streptococcus and *Enterobacter* in children, *Salmonella* in patients with sickle-cell disease, methicillin-resistant *S. aureus* (MRSA) in intravenous drug users (IVDUs), mycobacterial and fungal infections in the context of immunocompromise [1, 12]. Although these associations may guide initial empiric therapy, pathogen identification is an important aspect of managing the initial infection as well as the potential long-term sequelae. A multi-disciplinary approach to these cases should be adopted. The increasing prevalence of drug-resistant organisms such as MRSA and methicillin-resistant coagulase negative staphylococcus (MRCNS) add to the complexity of treatment and necessitate input from a specialist in microbiology or infectious diseases. Figure 31.1 represents the individual and pooled proportion of organisms identified in patients undergoing TKA with a history of prior septic arthritis for the 3 largest published series [9, 11, 13]. This highlights the diversity of primary bacterial knee infections encountered prior to arthroplasty and demonstrates the groups of bacteria that show a tendency to persist or cause prosthetic joint infection, which are maybe different to those identified initially.

Staph aureus virulence factors have a significant role in the promotion of joint destruction in septic arthritis [14], and the presence of Panton-Valentine leucocidin (PVL) has been associated with a higher incidence of fulminant infections, complications and treatment resistance [15].

Tuberculosis (TB) remains a significant cause of morbidity with an estimated worldwide prevalence greater than ten million [16]. Extra-

pulmonary musculoskeletal disease is reported in 1–3% of those cases and the knee joint is the most frequent musculoskeletal site after the spine and hip [17, 18].

31.3 Patterns of Arthropathy

Patient age influences the pattern of arthropathy that develops. In young children, reduced range of motion, growth disturbance and malalignment are the most frequently encountered sequelae [19], that may be followed by subsequent attempts at correction of deformity, leg length discrepancy and flexion contractures. Older adults may have significant comorbidities such as inflammatory arthropathy, diabetes, renal disease or pre-existent osteoarthritis [1].

Gächter described a classification system of arthroscopic findings of septic arthritis (Table 31.2) and demonstrated that more advanced stages (III and IV) are associated with multiple surgical procedures and treatment failure, and subsequent authors have correlated these stages with delayed treatment and adverse clinical outcomes [20–22].

In the case of TB infection, the radiographic appearance of the knee on presentation as described by Kerri and Martini (Table 31.3) is predictive of outcome, whereby the atrophic or arthritic types showing joint space narrowing and/or gross anatomic disorganisation are more likely to result in deformity, stiffness or even ankylosis [24, 25].

Primary TKA has been performed with a history of fungal infection, such as *Sporothrix schenckii* and *Candida Albicans*, but this is rare, and mostly limited to case reports [26, 27].

31.4 The Role of Arthroplasty in the Context of Previous Knee Infection

Historically, the presence or history of infection has been a contraindication to arthroplasty, and advanced, debilitating joint destruction in this context has been managed with resection arthroplasty or arthrodesis if surgery is contemplated [28]. While these can control infection and relieve pain [29], they lead to a marked reduction in function [30]. With increasing experience in the management of prosthetic joint infections, the understanding of biofilm and virulence factors, and a team approach, arthroplasty has become a viable option.

At present, the literature reporting on knee arthroplasty following septic arthritis is sparse and limited to case reports and case series. Sixteen studies have been identified reporting on >5 cases of knee arthroplasty for arthritis follow-

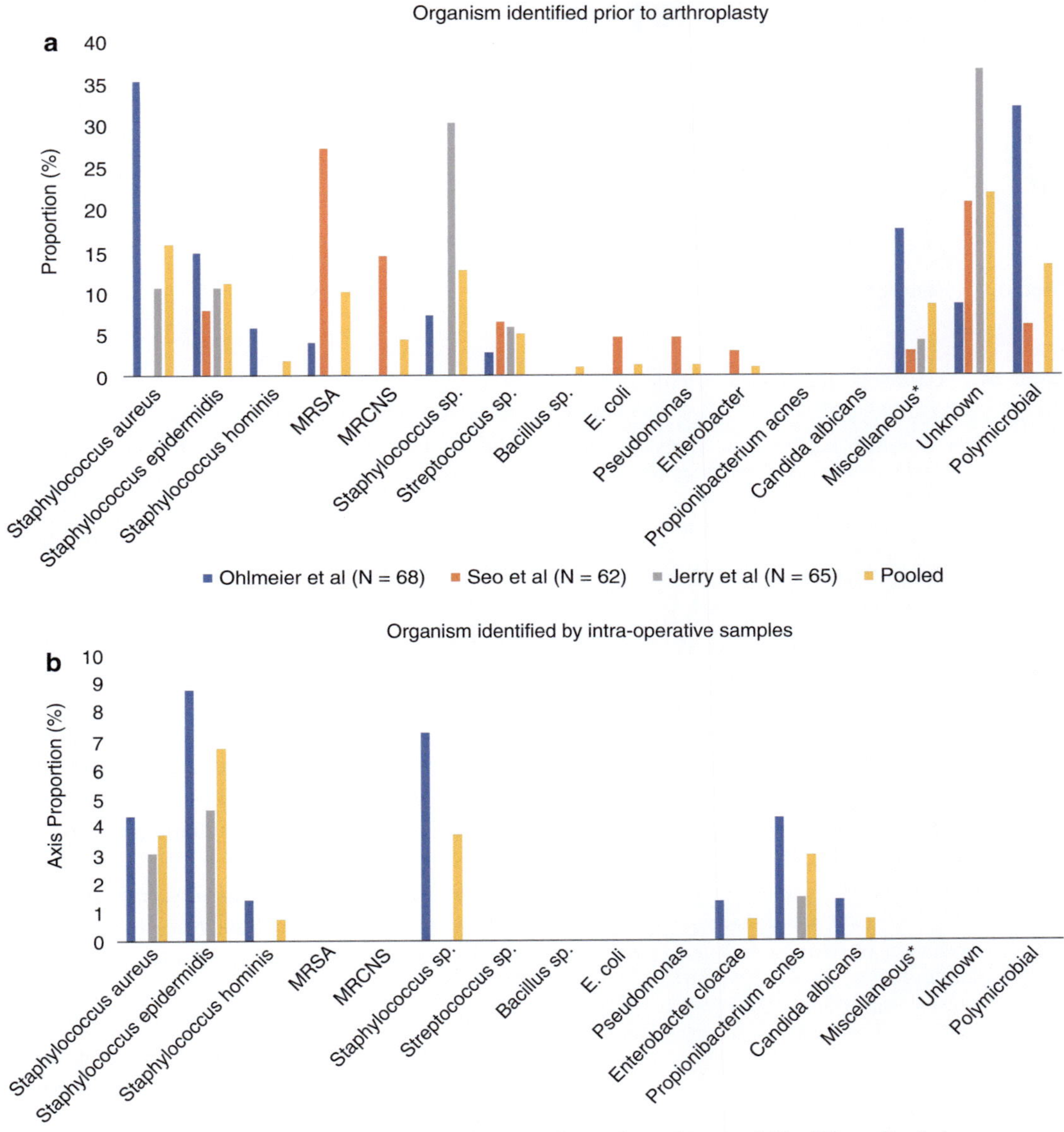

Fig. 31.1 Individual and pooled proportions of pathogens identified in patients undergoing TKA from Ohlmeier et al., Seo et al., and Jerry et al. MRCNS, methicillin-resistant coagulase negative Staphylococci; MRSA, methicillin-resistant *S. aureus*

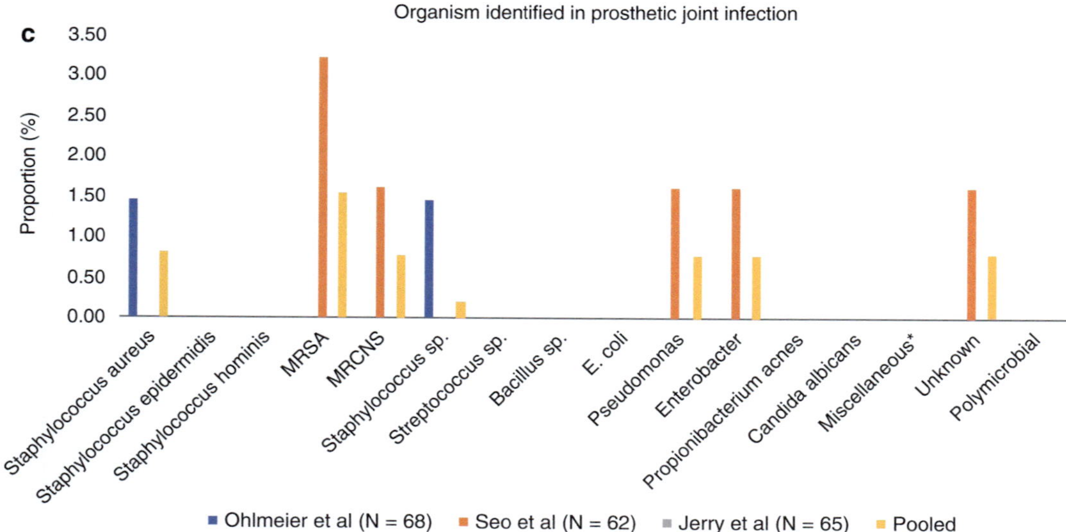

Fig. 31.1 (continued)

Table 31.2 Gächter grading of septic arthritis [23]

Stage	Criteria
I	Opacity of fluid, redness of the synovial membrane, possible petechial bleeding, no radiological alterations
II	Severe inflammation, fibrinous deposition, pus, no radiological alterations
III	Thickening of the synovial membrane, compartment formation ("sponge-like" arthroscopic view, especially in the suprapatellar pouch), no radiological alterations
IV	Aggressive pannus with infiltration of the cartilage, possibly undermining the cartilage, radiological signs of subchondral osteolysis, possible osseous erosions and cysts

Table 31.3 Kerri and Martini radiographic classification of tuberculosis of the knee [25]

Stage	Criteria
1	No bone lesions. Localised osteoporosis
2	One or more erosions (or cavities) in the bone. Discrete diminution of the joint space
3	Involvement and destruction of the whole joint without gross anatomical disorganisation
4	Gross anatomical disorganisation

ing bacterial or tuberculous infection of the native knee, summarised in Tables 31.4 and 31.5. Prior to the report of 68 patients by Ohlmeier et al. in 2019 [13], the largest published series of TKA following knee infection was published in 1988 and included 65 patients (65 knees) [11]. Some authors have taken almost a decade to accumulate less than 20 cases [31, 32].

Pooling of data and comparison of results is challenging because of the marked heterogeneity in terms of age of onset of infection (childhood vs. adult), type of infection (joint with or without osteomyelitis), type of procedure performed (single- vs. 2-stage), time interval between index infection and arthroplasty, interval between stages, the pathogen, and the antimicrobial strategy. Nonetheless, these studies provide valuable insight into the unique challenges in this context.

There are two broad clinical scenarios related to knee infection in which the role of knee arthroplasty has been practised and studied:

1. The treatment of post-infective arthropathy.
2. The management of active or evolving knee infection that is resistant to standard medical and surgical treatment.

The latter stems from our evolving experience from the treatment of PJI, where many of the management principles have been extensively studied.

Table 31.4 Summary of studies reporting on arthroplasty following bacterial infection of the knee

| Study | N | | Years since infection | Follow-up in years | Antimicrobials | | Persistent or re-infection rate | | Outcome measures | | |
Author Journal Year	Patients (knees)	Type of infection	Mean (range)	Mean (range)	Drug (duration)	Staging	%	Other complications	Survivorship	Knee scores	ROM
Ohlmeier et al. J Arthroplasty 2020	68 (68)	Bacterial	9.6 (0–63)	5 (1–9)	2 g vancomycin De-escalated to beta-lactam after 10.5 days (1–30) or culture specific ALBC (per 40 g) 2 g vancomycin + 1 g gentamicin ± 2 g meropenem Or 1 g clindamycin + 1 g gentamycin ± 2 g vancomycin	Single	2.9%	Arthrofibrosis (1.5%) Aseptic loosening (1.5%) Wound healing (2.9%) Haematoma (2.9%) Nerve palsy (1.5%) Non-surgical (15%)	97.1% at 5 years	OKS last FU 34.6 (8–48) KSS Last FU 14.9 (4–20)	
Xu et al. BMC MD 2019	(19)	Bacterial	4.9 ± 3.8 months between stages	4.7 (2.2–10.8)	IV antibiotics ≥6 weeks after 1st stage and 5 days after 2nd stage ACCS (per 40 g) 4–6 g vancomycin + 2–4 g meropenem 2nd stage 1 g vancomycin per 40 g cement for implant	2-stage	16%	Not reported	Survivorship 1-year 94.7% 2-year 89.5%	NR	NR

(continued)

Table 31.4 (continued)

Study	N		Years since infection	Follow-up in years	Antimicrobials		Persistent or re-infection rate			Outcome measures		
Author Journal Year	Patients (knees)	Type of infection	Mean (range)	Mean (range)	Drug (duration)	Staging	%	Other complications	Survivorship	Knee scores	ROM
Seo et al. J Arthroplasty 2014	62 (62)	Bacterial	4.3 (0.3–22)	6.1 (2–10.4)	ALBC 500 mg erythromycin + 240 mg colistin per 40 g cement for implant	Single	9.7%	Wound healing problems (6.5%) MUA (4.8%) Superficial wound infection (1.6%)		UCLA Pre-op 3.3 (2–5) Last FU 6.8 (5–9) KSS Pre-op 58 (36–74) Last FU 86 (58–96) WOMAC Pre-op 76.9 (68–86) Last FU 34.5 (20–48)	ROM Pre-op 99° (50–140) Last FU 125° (90–140)

Shaikh et al CORR 2014	1st stage 15 2nd stage 13	Bacterial (10) Fungal (2) TB (1)	Interval between 1st and 2nd stage 4 months (2–29 months)	4 (2–7)	IV ABs minimum 2 weeks post 1st stage, based on pre-operative and intra-operative cultures Anti-tuberculous medication (12 m post TKA) ACCS (per 40 g) 4 g Vancomycin + 2 g Streptomycin ±400 mg Amphotericin B for fungal infections 2nd stage 1 g Vancomycin per 40 g cement for implant	2-stage	0%	NR		KSS Pre-op 41 (26–73) Last FU 85 (46–93) WOMAC Pre-op 51 (40–65) Last FU 18 (11–31) VAS for pain Pre-op 66 (50–75) Last FU 18 (0–40)	ROM Pre-op 103° (60–155) Last FU 115° (75–150)
Chen et al. Orthopaedics 2013	22	Any	Not reported	NR	NR	Single	NR	NR	NR	NR	NR

(continued)

Table 31.4 (continued)

Study	N		Years since infection	Follow-up in years	Antimicrobials		Persistent or re-infection rate		Outcome measures		
Author Journal Year	Patients (knees)	Type of infection	Mean (range)	Mean (range)	Drug (duration)	Staging	%	Other complications	Survivorship	Knee scores	ROM
Bauer et al. Orthop Traumatol Surg Res 2010	31	Bacterial	Resolved: 5 years (2–18) Evolutive: for failed treatment of infection 2nd stage After mean 6w (4w–6m) when CRP stable for 2 weeks	5 (2–13)	Single stage: according to initial infection, continued until culture results 2-stage Dual antibiotic therapy for 93 days (45–180 days) Cement spacer without antibiotics	Single stage for 14 knees (Resolved septic arthritis) 2-stage for 17 knees (Evolutive septic arthritis)	7% (single stage) 12% (2-stage)	Not reported		KSS (single) Post-op 91 (75–100) KSS (2-stage) 83 (65–100)	

Bae et al. JBJS Br 2005	32 (32) 20 ankylosed 12 partially ankylosed	Bacterial (14) TB (18)	18.2 (1–51)	10 (5–13)	IV cephalosporin immediately after tourniquet deflation, continued for 2 weeks 1 g cephalosporin per 40 g bone cement Anti-tuberculous medication for 6 months	Single	3.1%	Flexion contractures (22%) Superficial infection (3%) Fracture (3%) Transient peroneal nerve palsy (3%)		HSS Knee score Pre-op 60 (26–87) for ankylosed knees 52 (29–66) for partially ankylosed knees Post-op 85 (64–94) for ankylosed knees 87 (69–97) for partially ankylosed knees	Mean post-op improvement in ROM 66° Post-op ROM 75° (30–115) for completely ankylosed knees Post-op ROM 99° (60–130 for partially ankylosed knees
Nazarian et al. J Arthoplasty 2003	14 (14)	Bacterial	2.1 (3 weeks to 7.8 years)	4.5 (2–7)	IV cefazolin, converted to oral cephalexin Or based on cultures vancomycin 1 g + tobramycin 2.4 g per 40 g cement	2-staged with ACCS, 6-week interval	0%	Patella subluxation (5%) Haematoma (5%) DVT (5%) Wound healing problem (5%)		Pre-op KSS 46 Last FU KSS 89	ROM >110° in 50% No flexion contractures >5°

(continued)

Table 31.4 (continued)

Study Author Journal Year	N Patients (knees)	Type of infection	Years since infection Mean (range)	Follow-up in years Mean (range)	Antimicrobials Drug (duration)	Staging	Persistent or re-infection rate %	Other complications	Outcome measures Survivorship	Knee scores	ROM
Lee et al. CORR 2002	19 (20)	Bacterial	23.3 (1–66)	5 (2–11)	Use of systemic antibiotics not reported 1 g Vancomycin or 1.2 g tobramycin per 40 g cement	Single (18) 2-staged (2) with ACCS and 6-week interval	5%	MUA (15%) Marginal skin necrosis (10%) Revision for aseptic loosening (5%) Haematoma (5%) Superficial wound infection (5%)		KSS Pre-op 39 (7–58) Last FU 91 (78–99)	ROM Pre-op 9 (0–40) to 86 (45–100) Post-op 1 (range 0–7) to 100 (85–110)
Jerry et al. CORR 1988	65 (65)	Bacterial	17.6 (1–65)	6.1 (2–15)	Semisynthetic penicillin or cephalosporin for 48–72 h ALBC not used	Single stage (65)	7.7% overall 15% for bone and joint infection 4% for joint infection	Superficial infection (8%) Haematoma (6%) Fracture (5%) Extensor mechanism disruption (3%)		HSS knee score improved from 54 pre-op to 80 at last FU	ROM pre-op 6° (±9) to 90° (±23) pre-op, 4 (±10) to 87° (±32) post-op

ACCS antibiotic-containing cement spacer, *ALBC* antibiotic-loaded bone cement, *DVT* deep vein thrombosis, *FU* follow-up, *HSS* Hospital For Special Surgery, *KSS* Knee Society Score, *MUA* manipulation under anaesthesia, *OKS* Oxford Knee Score, *ROM* range of motion, *UCLH* University of California, Los Angeles

Table 31.5 Summary of studies reporting on arthroplasty following mycobacterial infections of the knee

Study	N	Years since infection	Follow-up in years		Antimicrobials Pre-TKA	Antimicrobials Post-TKA	Persistent or re-infection rate		Outcome measures	
Author Journal Year	Patients (knees)	Mean (range)	Mean (range)	Staging	Drug (duration)	Drug (duration)	%	Other complications	Knee score	ROM
Zeng et al. Int Orthop 2016	9 (9)	8.7 (3–25)	4.4 (2–7)	Single (5) 2-stage (4)	Isoniazid Rifampicin Ethambutol Pyrazinamide (≥3 months)	Cefazolin 48 h Isoniazid Rifampicin Ethambutol Pyrazinamide (12 months)	0%	Nil	HSS Pre-op 44 (30–60) Last FU 82.7 (64–92)	Pre-op 56° (10–90) Last FU 94° (80–110)
Habaxi et al. Eur Rev Med Pharmacol Sci 2014	10 (10)	Active TB	1.2 (0.5–2.3)	Single	Isoniazid Rifampicin Ethambutol Pyrazinamide (2–4 weeks pre-op) Topical Streptomycin during TKA	Not reported	10% (1)	Nil	HSS Pre-op 25 ± 2 Last FU 87 ± 5	Pre-op Not reported Last FU 95° ± 5°
Öztürkmen et al. KSSTA 2013	12	Active TB 4 ± 1.5 months post diagnosis	6.1 ± 1.8	2-stage	1st stage: ACCS 2.4 g tobramycin + 2 g vancomycin per 40 g bone cement Interval: Rifampicin, isoniazid, pyrazinamide, ethambutol	After 2nd stage: Isoniazid Rifampicin Ethambutol Pyrazinamide (2 months) Isoniazid Rifampicin (min 10 months)	0%	NR	NR	NR

(continued)

Table 31.5 (continued)

Study	N	Years since infection	Follow-up in years		Antimicrobials Pre-TKA	Antimicrobials Post-TKA	Persistent or re-infection rate		Outcome measures	
Author Journal Year	Patients (knees)	Mean (range)	Mean (range)	Staging	Drug (duration)	Drug (duration)	%	Other complications	Knee score	ROM
Su et al. CORR 1996	15 (16)	2.1 (0.2–6)	6.3 (3.4–11)	Single	2–20 months (8) No treatment (8), undiagnosed TB	Isoniazid Rifampicin Ethambutol Pyrazinamide Minimum 12 months	31% (5) overall 50% (4/8) without pre-operative anti-TB drugs 12.5% (1/8) with pre-operative anti-TB drugs	Resection arthroplasty (6%) Revision for mechanical failure (6%) Periprosthetic fracture (6%)	KSS Pre-op 30.5 Last FU 83 KSS Function Pre-op 36 Last FU 74	NR
Kim JBJS Am 1988	19 (22)	1 (0.25–5)	2.7 (2–4)	Single (21) 2-stage (1)	Isoniazid Rifampicin Ethambutol Pyridoxine Streptomycin 3 months (6 pts) 11–47 months (8 pts) No treatment (5 pts)	Isoniazid Rifampicin Ethambutol Pyridoxine Streptomycin All 5 drugs: 2 months isoniazid. rifampicin. ethambutol. and pyridoxine: 16 months	16% (3)	NR	NR	NR
Eskola et al. JBJS Br 1988	6 (6)	35 (4–66)	6.3 (3–10)	Single	Rifampicin Isoniazid (2–3 weeks) (3 patients) No TB Rx (3 pts) Flucloxacillin (6 patients)	3 weeks Rifampicin Isoniazid (3 patients) 5 days Flucloxacillin (6 patients)	17% (1)—did not receive pre-op anti-TB Rx	Nil	HK Knee Score Pre-op 43 (25–60) Last FU 80 (45–100)	Pre-op 80 (20–110) Last FU flexion 67 (30–100)

FU follow-up, *HSS* Hospital For Special Surgery, *KSS* Knee Society Score, *OKS* Oxford Knee Score, *ROM* range of motion, *TB* tuberculosis, *UCLH* University of California, Los Angeles

31.5 Challenges and Controversies in Evaluation and Management

31.5.1 Incomplete History

Patients with knee arthrosis may present several years after the original knee infection, and a detailed history of the original pathogen, sensitivities and treatment may be incomplete. Indeed, the interval between the infection and arthroplasty is as long as six decades in some reports [10, 11, 13]. The pre-operative evaluation, therefore, requires great attention to the history, clinical examination, and special investigations (inflammatory markers, imaging and tissue biopsies).

31.5.2 Comorbidities

Comorbidities such as diabetes, chronic renal disease and rheumatoid arthritis are not uncommon in adults with infection-related arthropathy. This adds complexity to perioperative management and may increase the risk associated with arthroplasty [10, 11, 33].

31.5.3 Joint Versus Bone and Joint Infection

The presence or a history of osteomyelitis have been shown to have a higher risk of PJI in comparison to isolated intra-articular infection of the knee, and has been proposed as a contraindication to arthroplasty [11]. However, the application of a 2-stage approach with radical debridement and cement spacer at the first stage has been the proposed method of mitigating this risk [10, 31–34].

31.5.4 Anatomical Challenges

Soft tissue scarring, decreased blood supply, difficult exposure and increased operative time have been reported as surgical challenges [11]. This is especially pronounced in cases of complete or partial ankylosis, for which more extensile approach, capsular release and bony resection may be required to achieve adequate range of motion (ROM) [30]. Childhood infections may be associated with growth disturbances, malalignment and leg length discrepancy, which not only require careful pre-operative planning and implant selection, but may also require consideration of an extra-articular deformity correction.

31.5.5 Timing of Arthroplasty

Perhaps the most controversial challenge is to determine the appropriate timing of arthroplasty, for which there is more speculation than consensus.

Kim et al. [35] recommended an infection-free interval of at least 10 years prior to considering arthroplasty for the hip, based on their series of 170 total hip arthroplasty (THAs) for sequelae of childhood hip infections. In all but 1 patient (2 hips), the infection-free interval was >10 years. With a mean follow-up of 9.8 years, the only PJI in this cohort was documented in the patient with an infection-free interval of 7 years, although revision for aseptic loosening and osteolysis occurred in approximately 17% of patients.

Other authors have reported good outcomes with shorter intervals. Bauer et al. regarded patients with a minimum of 2 years free from infection as "resolved" or "quiescent", for whom they performed single-stage TKA, and the patients who failed medical and surgical management of infection were treated with debridement, synovectomy and 2-stage TKA [34].

Two of the largest series reported by Seo et al. [9] (62 knees) and Ohlmeier et al. [13] (68 knees) described an infection-free interval of at least 2 years and 1 year respectively, showing a PJI rate of 9.7% and 2.9%, respectively.

The International Consensus on Orthopaedic Infections guidelines recommend, "in the absence of concrete evidence", that arthroplasty is delayed "at least until completion of antibiotic treatment and resolution of clinical signs of infection but no earlier than 3 months from the inciting event" [7]. Although there are no single accurate markers of resolution of infection, as demonstrated in a recent meta-analysis [36], the use of multiple tools is advocated.

Ohlmeier et al. defined resolution of infection as:

1. Absence of clinical signs and symptoms for acute infection or local inflammation.
2. No signs of active infection on plain radiographs.
3. Normal serum inflammatory markers (ESR, CRP, total leucocyte count).
4. 14-day culture negative results during routine microbiological analysis of synovial fluid taken pre-operatively
5. Minimum 1-year follow-up.

Validating the most accurate combination of metrics may be an area for future research.

31.5.6 Single Versus Staged Approach

Arthroplasty in the context of resolved or quiescent infection has been performed as a single or staged procedure. In patients with evolving active infection, a 2-staged approach is advocated, which essentially comprises of an aggressive debridement, antibiotic spacer, prolonged antibiotic therapy and then reconstruction once infection has resolved. These are different clinical scenarios, and only 2 studies of bacterial [10, 34] and 2 studies of tuberculous [37, 38] knee infections have reported on the use of both approaches. Either approach requires an experienced team and specialist microbiological support. The outcomes for these strategies are discussed in the next section.

31.5.7 Single-Stage Technique

A standard medial parapatellar approach with due respect to previous skin incisions is usually sufficient. Radical debridement, including a total synovectomy, and antibiotic-loaded bone cement (ALBC) for the definitive implants is generally recommended prior to implantation, with multiple samples for culture and histology [9, 13].

31.5.8 Two-Staged Technique

Based on the experience from the staged management of PJI, this approach involves debridement of infected tissue, including any sinuses, synovectomy and debridement of affected bone [33, 39]. It is essential to do this patiently and thoroughly. Deep cultures are taken, and copious irrigation is performed. Some authors advocate the use of intra-operative frozen section [9, 10, 32, 33], although the value in this context is debated [40]. Various solutions have been utilised, including saline, antiseptic solution and antibiotic-containing solution, without clear evidence favouring any particular recipe [39].

The distal femoral and proximal tibial bone cuts can then be made. Here, the choice of instrumentation requires consideration. Extramedullary referencing and navigation may avoid the potential for dissemination of microbials into the canal that may occur with intra-medullary referencing. Although both, extra- [33] and intra-medullary [31] referencing techniques, have been utilised.

To manage dead space, deliver antibiotics and prevent contractures, an antibiotic-containing cement spacer (ACCS) is introduced. This can be made with commercially available moulds or manufactured intra-operatively using a cement mould of trial implants [31, 41]. An articulating spacer promotes maintenance of ROM and improved function during the interval, and is preferred to a static spacer in the absence of soft tissue loss, gross instability or orthoplastic soft tissue reconstruction [39].

Perioperative antibiotic cover is followed by culture-specific antibiotics, which are continued for a minimum of 6 weeks, and ceased when clinical evaluation and inflammatory markers suggest resolution of infection [33, 34]. The second stage is planned after a 2-week antibiotic holiday to facilitate intra-operative evaluation and further cultures—if the infection persists, then the first stage should be repeated [33, 34].

Patella resurfacing appears to be selective [30], routine [9, 33] or not performed, usually in the case of poor bone stock or compromised extensor mechanism [30].

31.5.9 Type, Duration and Mode of Delivery of Antibiotics

Although there is substantial variability in the antimicrobial protocols described (as indicated in Tables 31.4 and 31.5), it is important to adhere to the following principles.

Multimodal antibiotic delivery that is culture specific and based on the advice of a specialist microbiologist is recommended [13, 39]. Perioperative parenteral antibiotics may be given after deep cultures are taken and continued until clinical examination and inflammatory markers indicate resolution of infection. This usually takes at least 6 weeks, although oral equivalents with good bioavailability may be a suitable alternative.

The choice of antimicrobials for an ACCS is governed by cultures, and requires water soluble, heat stable agents, preferably in crystalline form (improved biomechanical strength of cement) [42] to be added to the polymethylmethacrolate (PMMA) powder at the time of cement mixing [39]. Since the load tolerance and endurance of the spacer does not need to match that of the cement used for definitive implants, up to 20% of the mass of the spacer can be composed of antibiotics [39]. Whether this is interpreted as 8 g per 40 g cement powder (48 g in total) or 10 g per 40 g cement powder (50 g in total) shall be left to the reader. The potential to cause adverse systemic sequelae, such as nephrotoxicity, may limit the amount of antibiotic added. Although this is rare [43], it may be more relevant in patients with renal or hepatic dysfunction.

Using 2 (or more) antibiotic agents in the ACCS is common practice and is supported by evidence for the synergistic antimicrobial effect (e.g., gentamicin or tobramycin combined with vancomycin), but the mechanisms for this and optimal combinations are not well understood [42].

Examples of regimens utilised for ACCS per 40 g bone cement include:

- 4–6 g vancomycin + 2–4 g meropenem [32]
- 4 g vancomycin + 2 g streptomycin ± 400 mg amphotericin B for fungal infections [31]

Examples of ALBC regimens utilised for definitive implant per 40 g bone cement include:

- 2 g vancomycin + 1 g gentamicin ± 2 g meropenem or 1 g clindamycin + 1 g gentamycin ± 2 g vancomycin [13]
- 500 mg erythromycin + 240 mg colistin per 40 g cement for implant.

TB is not regarded as a biofilm producing organism, but the capacity to form granulomas and survive intra-cellularly mandates wide surgical debridement and prolonged antimicrobial therapy. Although the regimens utilised vary widely, some important principles should be highlighted.

Prevention of mycobacterial as well as bacterial infection is required during arthroplasty. ACCS containing 2.4 g tobramycin +2 g vancomycin per 40 g bone cement [44] has been used, although there is little (if any) antimycobacterial activity with these agents *(refs)*. Topical streptomycin, a second line antimycobacterial agent, has been used during definitive implantation [45].

The optimum duration of oral antimycobacterial chemotherapy is not known, but all studies reporting on TKA with a history of TB infection recommend a period of antimycobacterials preoperatively, ranging from 2 weeks to 47 months [37, 45, 46]. This is supported by case series that have reported higher rates of post-TKA reactivation of TB infection in patients that did not receive pre-operative antimycobacterials in comparison to patients that did [28, 46, 47]. Post-operative regimens are typically 12–18 months, and longer if the clinical examination and inflammatory markers suggest ongoing TB activity [37, 38, 44, 47]. Generally 4 drugs are used initially, namely isoniazid, rifampicin, ethambutol and pyrazinamide, with 1 study adding streptomycin as well [37]. While some authors recommend continuing isoniazid and rifampicin after the initial 2-month period [37, 44], others have recommended 4 drugs for the entire duration of therapy [38, 47].

No studies report on regimes for drug-resistant or multidrug-resistant TB. Treatment in this instance would be individualised and guided by specialist microbiological or infectious diseases recommendations.

A diagrammatic representation of the principles of the authors' preferred approach to arthroplasty following septic arthritis is summarised in Fig. 31.2.

31.6 Outcomes

Currently, there is no universally accepted, evidence-based definition of success for arthroplasty following septic arthritis [48]. Authors have used rates of recurrent infection, revision rates, range of motion and patient reported outcome measures (PROMs) as outcome measures, and/or based definitions of success on those used for the management of prosthetic joint infections [32]. Indeed, the definition of success may be specific for the individual and, therefore, the patients' perspective of their outcome is an essential element [48].

The International Consensus on Orthopaedic Infections [7] attempted to pool data from 9 studies to quantify the PJI rate for hip or knee arthroplasty following bacterial or mycobacterial septic arthritis. Overall, the PJI rate for 1300 total hip and knee arthroplasties was reported as approximately 6% (95% CI 4.24 to 7.94), with lower rates for childhood infection (2.18%, 95% CI 1.16 to 3.70) compared to adult onset (8.25%, 95% CI 6.48 to 10.55). TKA appears to have a slightly higher overall rate of PJI following bacterial or mycobacterial septic arthritis (8.26%, 95% CI 5.30 to 12.15), in comparison to total hip arthroplasty (5.2%, 95% CI 3.50 to 7.21).

Older age, high pre-operative CRP and drug-resistant organism were identified as risk factors for failure of 2-stage arthroplasty [32].

In their series of 65 TKAs, Jerry et al. [11] reported a PJI rate of 4% for patients with prior septic arthritis and 15% for patients with prior bone and joint infection and subsequently recommended avoiding TKA for patients where infection involved bone. Other authors have utilised a 2-stage approach for such cases.

The PJI rate varies from 2.9% to 9.7% [9, 13] for single -tage and 0% to 16% [31, 32] for 2-stage approaches, but the indications for each approach vary between studies and likely represent increasing complexity of the case and/or concomitant risk factors such as rheumatoid arthritis and immunosuppressive therapy as highlighted by Bauer et al. [34] and Lee et al. [10]. These are the only studies that have used both single- and two-staged approaches in their series. Bauer et al. reported 7% (1 case) PJI infection rate for single stage performed for "quiescent infections" and 12% (1 case) for 2-stage TKA performed for "evolutive infected joints". The only PJI in the series by Lee et al. occurred in a patient undergoing 2-staged arthroplasty.

The largest series by Ohlmeier et al. [13] reported PJI free survivorship (Kaplan–Meier analysis) of 97.1% at a mean of 5 years (range 1–9, SD ±2.5 years). Of the 68 knees, 4 underwent re-operations (5.9%), 2 of which were revision for PJI (2.9%), 1 revision for aseptic loosening (1.5%), and 1 open arthrolysis for arthrofibrosis (1.5%). Complications were recorded in 15 patients (22%), including wound healing (2 patients, 2.9%), post-operative hematoma requiring an arthrocentesis (2 patients, 2.9%), and a temporary nerve palsy (1 patient, 1.5%). The remaining 10 patients experienced non-surgical complications such as pneumonia or electrolyte imbalance.

Most studies also report on PROMs, such as Knee Society Score (KSS), Oxford Knee Score (OKS), Western Ontario and McMaster University Index (WOMAC) and Hospital for Special Surgery (HSS), as well as ROM, Tables 31.4 and 31.5. Commonly, significant improvement in PROMs and ROM is reported between pre-operative and last follow-up measurements and highlights benefit in pain and function that

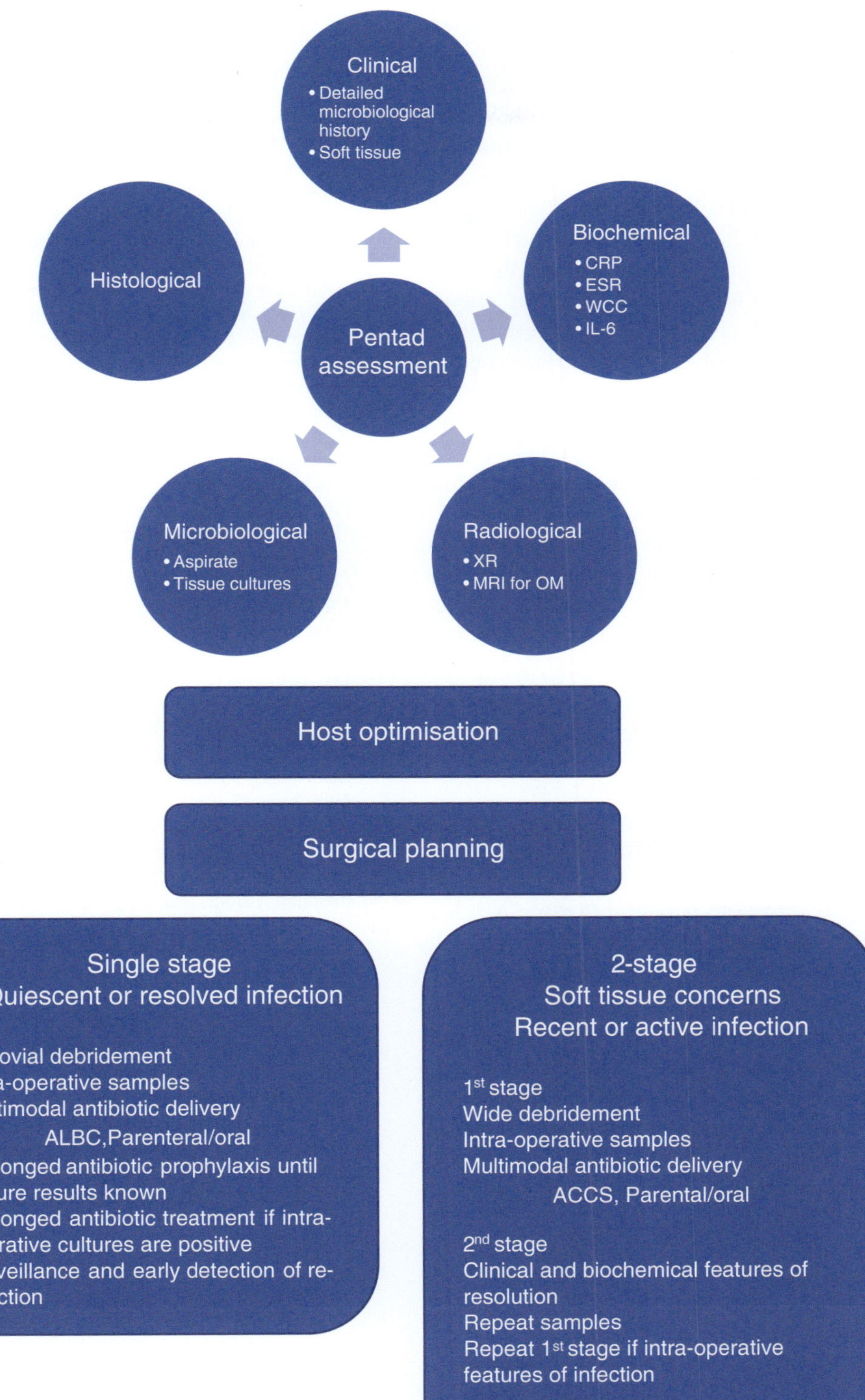

Fig. 31.2 Diagrammatic representation of authors' preferred approach

patients with infection-related knee arthrosis gain from reconstruction.

Reported results for TKA in the context of previous TB-related knee infections have similar variability between studies and approaches with PJI rates that range from 0 to 31%. However, the total number of patients (knees) being 71 (75) between 6 studies, challenges drawing clear conclusions. Despite the previous, it must be noted that low rates of reactivation and good clinical outcomes even in the treatment of active or recently diagnosed TB have been reported where antimycobacterial treatment is initiated prior to PJI in addition to prolonged post-operative therapy [37, 46, 47], and thorough surgical debridement is performed [44]. Additionally, reactivation of TB with a TKA in situ can be successfully treated with antimycobaterial therapy alone in many cases. Improvements in PROMs and ROM also support the notion that patients benefit greatly from reconstruction when indicated [28].

31.7 Conclusion

Successful eradication of native knee infection may require the excision of articular cartilage and subchondral bone. Alternatively, chronic or virulent acute infections may lead to extensive chondrolysis. Although arthroplasty has historically been viewed as being contraindicated in such situations, it is increasingly being used as an alternative to arthrodesis to improve patient functional outcomes. Although technically demanding and carrying greater risk, successful outcomes can be achieved by adherence to a thorough algorithm, emphasising the importance of contributions from a multi-disciplinary team.

References

1. Mathews CJ, Weston VC, Jones A, Field M, Coakley G. Bacterial septic arthritis in adults. Lancet. 2010;375(9717):846–55.
2. Maneiro JR, Souto A, Cervantes EC, Mera A, Carmona L, Gomez-Reino JJ. Predictors of treatment failure and mortality in native septic arthritis. Clin Rheumatol. 2015;34(11):1961–7.
3. Coakley G, Mathews C, Field M, Jones A, Kingsley G, Walker D, et al. BSR & BHPR, BOA, RCGP and BSAC guidelines for management of the hot swollen joint in adults. Rheumatology (Oxford). 2006;45(8):1039–41.
4. Lenguerrand E, Whitehouse MR, Beswick AD, Kunutsor SK, Foguet P, Porter M, et al. Risk factors associated with revision for prosthetic joint infection following knee replacement: an observational cohort study from England and Wales. Lancet Infect Dis. 2019;19(6):589–600.
5. Alamanda VK, Springer BD. The prevention of infection. Bone Joint J. 2019;101-B(1_Supple_A):3–9.
6. Marmor S, Kerroumi Y. Patient-specific risk factors for infection in arthroplasty procedure. Orthop Traumatol Surg Res. 2016;102(1):S113–S9.
7. Aalirezaie A, Arumugam SS, Austin M, Bozinovski Z, Cichos KH, Fillingham Y, et al. Hip and knee section, prevention, risk mitigation: proceedings of international consensus on orthopedic infections. J Arthroplasty. 2019;34(2s):S271–s8.
8. Haddad FS. Even the winners are losers. Bone Joint J. 2017;99-B(5):561–2.
9. Seo JG, Moon YW, Park SH, Han KY, Kim SM. Primary total knee arthroplasty in infection sequelae about the native knee. J Arthroplasty. 2014;29(12):2271–5.
10. Lee G-C, Pagnano MW, Hanssen AD. Total knee arthroplasty after prior bone or joint sepsis about the knee. Clin Orthop Relat Res. 2002;404:226–31.
11. Jerry JG, Rand JA, Ilstrup D. Old sepsis prior to total knee arthroplasty. Clin Orthop Relat Res. 1988;236:135–40.
12. Kang SN, Sanghera T, Mangwani J, Paterson JM, Ramachandran M. The management of septic arthritis in children: systematic review of the English language literature. J Bone Joint Surg Br. 2009;91(9):1127–33.
13. Ohlmeier M, Delgado G, Calderon CA, Hartwig C-H, Gehrke T, Citak M. Are patients with a history of septic arthritis undergoing total knee arthroplasty at higher risk for revision surgery? A single-center study. J Arthroplasty. 2020;35(7):1857–61.
14. Abdelnour A, Arvidson S, Bremell T, Rydén C, Tarkowski A. The accessory gene regulator (agr) controls Staphylococcus aureus virulence in a murine arthritis model. Infect Immun. 1993;61(9):3879–85.
15. Swaminathan A, Massasso D, Gotis-Graham I, Gosbell I. Fulminant methicillin-sensitive Staphylococcus aureus infection in a healthy adolescent, highlighting 'Panton-valentine leucocidin syndrome'. Intern Med J. 2006;36(11):744–7.
16. Global tuberculosis report 2018. France: World Health Organization; 2018.
17. Sanghvi DA, Iyer VR, Deshmukh T, Hoskote SS. MRI features of tuberculosis of the knee. Skeletal Radiol. 2009;38(3):267.
18. Dunn R, Ben HM. Spinal tuberculosis: review of current management. Bone Joint J. 2018;100(4):425–31.
19. Agarwal A, Aggarwal AN. Bone and joint infections in children: septic arthritis. Indian J Pediatr. 2016;83(8):825–33.

20. Kirpalani PA, In Y, Choi N, Koh H, Kim J, Han CW. Two-stage total knee arthroplasty for non-salvageable septic arthritis in diabetes mellitus patients. Acta Orthop Belg. 2005;71(3):315–20.

21. Yanmış I, Ozkan H, Koca K, Kılınçoğlu V, Bek D, Tunay S. The relation between the arthroscopic findings and functional outcomes in patients with septic arthritis of the knee joint, treated with arthroscopic debridement and irrigation. Acta Orthop Traumatol Turc. 2011;45(2):94–9.

22. Balabaud L, Gaudias J, Boeri C, Jenny J-Y, Kehr P. Results of treatment of septic knee arthritis: a retrospective series of 40 cases. Knee Surg Sports Traumatol Arthrosc. 2007;15(4):387–92.

23. Stutz G, Kuster MS, Kleinstück F, Gächter A. Arthroscopic management of septic arthritis: stages of infection and results. Knee Surg Sports Traumatol Arthrosc. 2000;8(5):270–4.

24. Hoffman EB, Allin J, Campbell JA, Leisegang FM. Tuberculosis of the knee. Clin Orthop Relat Res. 2002;398:100–6.

25. Kerri O, Martini M. Tuberculosis of the knee. Int Orthop. 1985;9(3):153–7.

26. Koëter S, Jackson R. Successful total knee arthroplasty in the presence of sporotrichal arthritis. Knee. 2006;13(3):236–7.

27. DeHart DJ. Use of itraconazole for treatment of sporotrichosis involving a knee prosthesis. Clin Infect Dis. 1995;21(2):450.

28. Sultan AA, Mahmood B, Samuel LT, George J, Faour M, Pelt CE, et al. Patients with a history of treated septic arthritis are at high risk of periprosthetic joint infection after total joint arthroplasty. Clin Orthop Relat Res. 2019;477(7):1605–12.

29. Lim HC, Bae JH, Hur CR, Oh JK, Han SH. Arthrodesis of the knee using cannulated screws. J Bone Joint Surg Br. 2009;91-B(2):180–4.

30. Bae D, Yoon K, Kim H, Song S. Total knee arthroplasty in stiff knees after previous infection. J Bone Joint Surg Br. 2005;87(3):333–6.

31. Shaikh AA, Ha C-W, Park Y-G, Park Y-B. Two-stage approach to primary TKA in infected arthritic knees using intraoperatively molded articulating cement spacers. Clin Orthop Relat Res. 2014;472(7):2201–7.

32. Xu C, Kuo FC, Kheir M, Li X, Chai W, Chen JY. Outcomes and predictors of treatment failure following two-stage total joint arthroplasty with articulating spacers for evolutive septic arthritis. BMC Musculoskelet Disord. 2019;20(1):272.

33. Nazarian DG, de Jesus D, McGuigan F, Booth RE Jr. A two-stage approach to primary knee arthroplasty in the infected arthritic knee. J Arthroplasty. 2003;18:16–21.

34. Bauer T, Lacoste S, Lhotellier L, Mamoudy P, Lortat-Jacob A, Hardy P. Arthroplasty following a septic arthritis history: a 53 cases series. Orthop Traumatol Surg Res. 2010;96(8):840–3.

35. Kim Y-H, Oh S-H, Kim J-S. Total hip arthroplasty in adult patients who had childhood infection of the hip. J Bone Joint Surg Am. 2003;85(2):198–204.

36. Lee YS, Fernando N, Koo KH, Kim HJ, Vahedi H, Chen AF. What markers best guide the timing of reimplantation in two-stage exchange arthroplasty for PJI? A systematic review and meta-analysis. Clin Orthop Relat Res. 2018;476(10):1972–83.

37. Kim YH. Total knee arthroplasty for tuberculous arthritis. J Bone Joint Surg Am. 1988;70(9):1322–30.

38. Zeng M, Xie J, Wang L, Hu Y. Total knee arthroplasty in advanced tuberculous arthritis of the knee. Int Orthop. 2016;40(7):1433–9.

39. Gehrke T, Alijanipour P, Parvizi J. The management of an infected total knee arthroplasty. Bone Joint J. 2015;97-b(10 Suppl A):20–9.

40. Tsaras G, Maduka-Ezeh A, Inwards CY, Mabry T, Erwin PJ, Murad MH, et al. Utility of intraoperative frozen section histopathology in the diagnosis of periprosthetic joint infection: a systematic review and meta-analysis. J Bone Joint Surg Am. 2012;94(18):1700–11.

41. Ha C-W. A technique for intraoperative construction of antibiotic spacers. Clin Orthop Relat Res. 2006;445:204–9.

42. Anagnostakos K, Meyer C. Antibiotic elution from hip and knee acrylic bone cement spacers: a systematic review. Biomed Res Int. 2017;2017:4657874.

43. Frommelt L. Principles of systemic antimicrobial therapy in foreign material associated infection in bone tissue, with special focus on periprosthetic infection. Injury. 2006;37(2):S87–94.

44. Oztürkmen Y, Uzümcügil O, Karamehmetoğlu M, Leblebici C, Caniklioğlu M. Total knee arthroplasty for the management of joint destruction in tuberculous arthritis. Knee Surg Sports Traumatol Arthrosc. 2014;22(5):1076–83.

45. Habaxi KK, Wang L, Miao XG, Alimasi WQ, Zhao XB, Su JG, et al. Total knee arthroplasty treatment of active tuberculosis of the knee: a review of 10 cases. Eur Rev Med Pharmacol Sci. 2014;18(23):3587–92.

46. Eskola A, Santavirta S, Konttinen YT, Tallroth K, Lindholm ST. Arthroplasty for old tuberculosis of the knee. J Bone Joint Surg Br. 1988;70(5):767–9.

47. Su JY, Huang TL, Lin SY. Total knee arthroplasty in tuberculous arthritis. Clin Orthop Relat Res. 1996;323:181–7.

48. Haddad FS, Oussedik S, Meek RMD, Konan S, Stockley I, Gant V. Orthopaedic infection: is consensus the answer? Bone Joint J. 2018;100-B(11):1405–6.

The Place of Antibiotic-Loaded Cement in TKA Infection

Francois Kelberine, Malek Meherzi,
and Jean Philippe Vivona

32.1 Introduction

Rate of infection after knee arthroplasty is depending on publications from 1–5% to 6% after TKA revision [1–5]. Primary TKA procedures are 2–3 times less susceptible to infection than TKA revisions [6, 7].

It has been reported in previous chapters.

After surgery, the inner bony tissue interacts with the biomaterial and forms a very thin biofilm as immune reaction toward the material [8]. If microorganisms reach the surface, they can adhere to it. Its persistence due to inflammation increases susceptibility to infection. And bacteria can themselves enhance the development of the biofilm. Surface roughness is of importance and cement is prone to bacteria adhesion [9, 10].

Conversely, the use of cement as a carrier for topical delivery for antibiotics has been initially described by Buchholz and Englebrecht using gentaline in Palacos resin [11]. It dramatically developed during last three decades in orthopedic field.

It is hypothesized that antibiotic-loaded cement (ABLC) help to treat local infections and will result in lower infection rates during primary and/or revision TKA surgery.

32.1.1 Bacteriology

Most prosthetic joint infections (PJI) involve gram-positive organisms (*Staphylococcus aureus*, *Staphylococcus epidermidis*, or group B streptococcus) or gram-negative bacteria.

Chiu reported that those organisms identified through culture in revision infections are more virulent and less sensitive to antibiotics than those found in primary TKA infections [12].

To be suitable for use in bone cement antibiotics might be bactericidal for these bacteria with minimal risks of side effect especially allergy. It must be water-soluble and thermally stable during exothermic polymerization [13]. Consequently, the most commonly used antibiotics for ABLC (including spacers) reported in the literature are gentamicin, tobramycin, vancomycin, and cephalosporins.

Elution of antibiotic from cement used for spacers allows the local delivery of antibiotics toward the infected bone and soft tissue at high concentrations, much higher than can be achieved by intravenous or oral routes late 4 months locally after implantation [14–16]. It has been shown that at least 3.6 g of antibiotic per 40 g of acrylic cement is desirable for effective elution kinetics and sustained therapeutic levels of antibiotic [17].

F. Kelberine (✉) · J. P. Vivona
Pôle Aixois de Chirurgie Articulaire et Sportive
(PACAS), Bastide d'Axium, 31 avenue de Lattre de
Tassigny, Aix en Provence, France
e-mail: fkelberine@pacas.fr

M. Meherzi
Centre Hospitalier de Bagnols sur Ceze,
Bagnols sur Ceze, France

© ISAKOS 2022
U. G. Longo et al. (eds.), *Infection in Knee Replacement*,
https://doi.org/10.1007/978-3-030-81553-0_32

Doses as high as 6 to 8 g of antibiotic per 40 g cement, when ABLC is used in the form of beads or spacers, have been shown to be safe clinically [18].

32.1.2 Mechanics

Mixing antibiotic to cement allows elution of antibiotic but modifies mechanical properties. Compressive and tensile strengths of ABLC decrease with the quantity of antibiotic powder (maximum 2 g/40 g of cement). Using liquid or powder forms change ratio elution: liquid is more detrimental to mechanical properties [19]. Polymerization forms bubbles depending on cement and temperature: some escape from cement, others are sealled in. Antibiotic is released from the surface of the cement and from cracks and voids within the cement.

Gradual diffusion of antibiotics into surrounding tissues over time depends on cement porosity. This is related to the type of antibiotic, the composition of cement (viscosity) and preparation (e.g., vacuum mixing devices minimize porosity).

So, the mechanical and elution properties of commercially available premixed ABLC products seem superior to those of hand-mixed preparations [10, 20–22] but controversial [23].

At last, the potential risk of selection of antibiotic-resistant strains of bacteria was not confirmed [24].

32.1.3 Place of ABLC in the Spectrum of Prosthetic Joint Infection (PJI)

After TKA, deep PJI occur in an early to moderate time period after the operation, while none of the studies reported chronic deep infection to be the most common type of infection [13].

ABLC are useful in early PJI (local beads) and in late chronic PJI in one step or two steps (spacers) revision.

They are used too to prevent infection in primary TKA and revision of aseptic TKA.

32.2 ALBC in Primary TKA

To prevent infection in primary TKA is controversial using an ABLC depends on cultural practices. It is largely used in the UK, Nordic countries, and Australia.

Initially proposed in 2004 by Bourne [25] or Hanssen [26] to mimic Nordic registries which was effective to decrease the rate of PJI after total hip arthroplasty.

At the knee level, Jameson reporting 731,214 cases from the UK registry note less revision (aseptic or PJI) in comparison with plain cement at 10 years [27]; Jamsen with the finish registry about 43,149 primary TKA as well [28].

But the other publications support the conclusion that ALBC could not prevent deep infection after primary TKA.

The results at 2 years follow-up after index surgery is a good threshold for analysis concerning infection as is linked to end of infection risk and mechanical changes for cement [29].

Bohm found no difference regarding the revision rate for infection nor any other cause (comorbidities included) [30].

Namba about 22,889 cases found no difference in the rate of deep infection between TKA with plain cement and those with ABLC, but a nonsignificant trend of higher proportion of aseptic loosening for the second group without risk factors [31].

Gandhi reached the same conclusion for 1625 TKA from a monocentric study [32].

A prospective randomized study by Hinarejos compared the rates of deep infection of ALBC versus plain cement for 2948 cases [33]. The use of erythromycin and colistin ALBC did not lead to a decrease in the rate of infection after primary TKA when systemic prophylactic antibiotics were used.

This is in accordance with other authors [34, 35], the result of the Australian Orthopædic Association registry and two recent meta-analysis from Schiavone-Pani or Kleppel [13, 36, 37].

If some report did not found risk factors in large series [31, 38], numerous authors recommend the use of ABLC in patient at higher risk of infection: diabetic, immunocompromised, morbidly obese, patients with previous history of fracture, contamination and/or infection of the knee [9, 10, 12, 29].

Lee includes thyroid, heart, or lung diseases [39].

Paucity of randomized clinical trials and the literature are not sufficient to confirm the reduction of the risk of infection with the use of ALBC in primary TKA.

It leads us to recommend with caution the use of ALBC only in high-risk patients.

In addition, culture from fluid or tissue at revision TKA can alter reliability of result when ABLC has been used at index surgery [40].

In primary TKA, the potential economic impact using ALBC is not valid [41, 42].

32.3 ALBC in Aseptic Revision of TKA

The occurrence of periprosthetic infection is 2 to 3 times higher in revision TKA than in primary THA/TKA [7].

The risk of infection following aseptic resurgery decreases by 6% at 89 months when using a vanco manually mixed ABLC [12]. In this level 1 prospective randomized study including 183 cases, local antibiotic delivery is very effective against infection with no infection in the ABLC group.

A retrospective study about 1154 re-TKA presents a high risk of failure (10%) and ABLC decreases by 50% the risk of all cause of re-revision [1].

The Kleppel's meta-analysis [13] reported two studies: at 62.5 months follow-up, the secondary infection rate is significantly lower with ALBC.

So the use of ALBC is clearly recommended in case of revision of TKA without sepsis. The effect of release of antibiotic is mainly at initial postoperative period [13].

Commercial gentamicin or tobramycin-LBC provide sufficient concentrations to be bactericidal even against methicillin-resistant organisms. The use of vancomycin should be considered in revisions following primary TKA in which gentamicin or tobramycin-loaded bone cement had been used because of the risk of gentamicin resistance [10].

32.4 Place of ABLC in Resurgery for PJI

32.4.1 Surgery in One Step

It concerns especially the early infection after primary TKA.

DAIR before 4 weeks can be effective in acute PJI. The procedure includes debridement, multiple bacteriological harvesting, change of PE. It is modified by addition of antibiotic (vancomycin) impregnated cement beads [8].

Small comparative studies [43–45] in combination with parenteral IV antibiotherapy can get 78% of healing in early cases. But with a higher risk of septic recurrence if the cement at index surgery was plain which is frequently the case [28].

32.4.2 Surgery in Two Steps

In case of late infection, the modified DAIR presents a high failure rate.

The treatment is first to implant a massive spacer to achieve high intra-articular concentrations of antibiotics while preserving joint space.

The final goal is to insert a new TKA once the infection has been healed.

The first step is to remove implants, *cement*, and debride the tissue. At this stage, the debridement is more important than the type of spacer or the additional antibiotic amount. Once the joint is cleaned, a spacer can be inserted.

The spacer is an ABLC which can be premolded by companies or molded peroperatively [46, 47].

Local antibiotic delivery via cement mixtures has been shown to achieve high local concentrations of antibiotic able to effectively treat the local bacterial burden [47].

But few premixed cements are available with a limited dose of antibiotic (1–2 g/40 g of cement). It needs to add antibiotic powder to reach high doses of antibiotics up to 8 g/40 mg.

The choice of antibiotic depends on individualized microbiological aspect (virulence of germ) and is often based on multiple preoperative punctures.

Surgeon creates his own antibiotic cement mixture peroperatively, producing a variable final product [47]. He can also ask manufacturer to prepare a personalized spacer [48].

Vancomycin may be added to ABLC which already includes gentamicin or tobramycin [10]. Other antibiotic can be added in specific cases (e.g., *ceftazidime for Pseudomonas aeruginosa*) [49]. Cephalosporins are not effective against methicillin-resistant organisms.

The local treatment is always combined with parenteral antibiotherapy.

Spacer induces a very low risk of nephrotoxicity due to systemic absorption up to 8 weeks [50–53]. Some cases have been reported [53–56] to justify monitoring when inserted especially in patients with bad renal function.

Mechanically, high antibiotics dose does not influence the properties of cement as the spacer is used temporarily. However, virulence of the infection and delay to resurgery can influence quality of bone and soft tissue [46].

It can be static or mobile. Mobile is supposed to get a better post op mobility after re-implantation [57]. Described initially by Scott, Chang use former TKA (autoclaved peroperatively after explantation with high dose of ABLC) as a spacer before to change it later [43, 58].

Nozdo [47] compared 140 different mobile spacers (prefabricated, two separate cement spacers molded by surgeon, tibial spacer, and femoral autoclaved implant) without difference between them.

Struelens reported fractures, dislocations, and knee subluxation with mobile spacers [59].

Finally, the mobile spacers did not confirm their efficacy neither in terms of mobility [60] nor in mid-term functions [46, 61].

The second and final step is to remove the spacer once the infection is healed and to reimplant a new arthroplasty with medium dose ALBC.

32.5 Guidelines

Use of ALBC is recommended:

1. As prophylaxy (low dose of antibiotic)
   (a) in primary TKA for high-risk patients only
   (b) in TKA aseptic revision
2. As treatment in PJI (high dose of antibiotic)
   (a) beads with modified DAIR in early infection
   (b) spacer for re-TKA in two steps.

References

1. Bini S, Chan P, Inacio M, Paxton E, Khatod M. Antibiotic cement was associated with half the risk of re-revision in 1154 aseptic revision total knee arthroplasties. Acta Orthop. 2015;87:55–9.
2. Bistolfi F, Albanese C, Vernè E, Miola M. PMMA-based bone cements and the problem of joint arthroplasty infections: status and new perspectives. Materials. 2019;12:4002.
3. Blom AW, Brown J, Taylor AH, Pattison G, Whitehouse S, Bannister GC. Infection after total knee arthroplasty. J Bone Joint Surg Br. 2004;86:688–91.
4. Kurtz SM, Ong KL, Lau E, Bozic KJ, Berry D, Parvizi J. Prosthetic joint infection risk after TKA in the medicare population. Clin Orthop Relat Res. 2010;468:52–6.
5. Zimmerli W, Trampuz A, Ochsner PE. Prosthetic-joint infections. N Engl J Med. 2004;351:1645–54.
6. Peersman G, Laskin R, Davis J, Peterson M. Infection in total knee replacement: a retrospective review of 6489 total knee replacements. Clin Orthop Relat Res. 2001;392:15–23.
7. Voigt J, Mosier M, Darouiche R. Antibiotics and antiseptics for preventing infection in people receiving revision total hip and knee prostheses: a systematic review of randomized controlled trials. BMC Infect Dis. 2016;16:749.
8. Van Vugt TAG, Arts JJ, Geurts JAP. Antibiotic-loaded polymethylmethacrylate beads and spacers in treatment of orthopedic infections and the role of biofilm formation. Front Microbiol. 2019;10:1626.
9. Bistolfi A, Massazza G, Verné E, Massè A, Deledda D, Ferraris S. Antibiotic-loaded cement in orthopedic surgery: a review. ISRN Orthop. 2011;2011:290851.
10. Jiranek W, Hanssen A, Greenwald A. Antibiotic-loaded bone cement for infection prophylaxis in total joint replacement. J Bone Jt Surg. 2006;88:2487–500.
11. Buchholz HW, Engelbrecht H. Depot effects of various antibiotics mixed with Palacos resins. Chirurg. 1970;41:511–5.
12. Chiu F, Lin C. Antibiotic-impregnated cement in revision total knee arthroplasty. J Bone Jt Surg Am Vol. 2009;91:628–33.
13. Kleppel D, Stirton J, Liu J, Ebraheim N. Antibiotic bone cement's effect on infection rates in primary and revision total knee arthroplasties. World J Orthop. 2017;8:946–55.
14. Mifsud M, McNally M. Local delivery of antimicrobials in the treatment of bone infections. Orthop Trauma. 2019;33:160–5.
15. Mutimer J, Gillespie G, Lovering AM, Porteus AJ. Measurements of in vivo intra-articular gen-

tamicin levels from antibiotic loaded articulating spacers in revision total knee replacement. Knee. 2009;16:39–41.

16. Vrabec G, Stevenson W, Elguizaoui S, Kirsch M, Pinkowski J. What is the intraarticular concentration of tobramycin using low-dose tobramycin bone cement in TKA: an in vivo analysis? Clin Orthop Relat Res. 2016;474:2441–7.

17. Penner MJ, Masri BA, Duncan CP. Elution characteristics of vancomycin and tobramycin combined in acrylic bone-cement. J Arthroplasty. 1996;11:939–44.

18. Springer BD, Lee GC, Osmon D, Haidukewych GJ, Hanssen AD, Jacofsky DJ. Systemic safety of high-dose antibiotic-loaded cement spacers after resection of an infected total knee arthroplasty. Clin Orthop Relat Res. 2004;427:47–51.

19. Seldes R, Winiarsky R, Jordan L, Baldini T, Brause B, Zodda F. Liquid gentamicin in bone cement. J Bone Jt Surg. 2005;87:268–72.

20. Brock HS, Moodie PG, Hendricks KJ, McIff TE. Compression strength and porosity of single-antibiotic cement vacuum-mixed with vancomycin. J Arthroplasty. 2010;25:990–7.

21. DeLuise M, Scott CP. Addition of hand-blended generic tobramycin in bone cement: effect on mechanical strength. Orthopedics. 2004;27:1289–91.

22. Mau H, Schelling K, Heisel C. Comparison of various vacuum mixing systems and bone cements as regards reliability, porosity and bending strength. Acta Orthop Scand. 2004;75:160–72.

23. Postak PD, Greenwald AS. Assuring cement fixation: all mixing systems are NOT the same. Proc Am Acad Orthop Surg. 2003;4:656.

24. Hansen E, Adeli B, Kenyon R, Parvizi J. Routine use of antibiotic laden bone cement for primary total knee arthroplasty: impact on infecting microbial patterns and resistance profiles. J Arthroplasty. 2014;29:1123–7.

25. Bourne R. Prophylactic use of antibiotic bone cement. J Arthroplasty. 2004;19:69–72.

26. Hanssen AD. Prophylactic use of antibiotic bone cement: an emerging standard in opposition. J Arthroplasty. 2004;19:73.

27. Jameson S, Asaad A, Diament M, Kasim A, Bigirumurame T, Baker P. Antibiotic-loaded bone cement is associated with a lower risk of revision following primary cemented total knee arthroplasty. Bone Joint J Br. 2019;101:1331–47.

28. Jämsen E, Huhtala H, Puolakka T, Moilanen T. Risk factors for infection after knee arthroplasty. A register-based analysis of 43,149 cases. J Bone Joint Surg Am. 2009;91:38–47.

29. Hinarejos P. Use of antibiotic-loaded cement in total knee arthroplasty. World J Orthop. 2015;6:877.

30. Bohm E, Zhu N, Gu J, de Guia N, Linton C, Anderson T. Does adding antibiotics to cement reduce the need for early revision in total knee arthroplasty? Clin Orthop Relat Res. 2013;472:162–8.

31. Namba R, Chen Y, Paxton E, Slipchenko T, Fithian D. Outcomes of routine use of antibiotic-loaded cement in primary total knee arthroplasty. J Arthroplasty. 2009;24:44–7.

32. Gandhi R, Razak F, Pathy R, Davey J, Syed K, Mahomed N. Antibiotic bone cement and the incidence of deep infection after total knee arthroplasty. J Arthroplasty. 2009;24:1015–8.

33. Hinarejos P, Guirro P, Leal J, Montserrat F, Pelfort X, Sorli M. The use of erythromycin and Colistin-loaded cement in total knee arthroplasty. Does not reduce the incidence of infection. J Bone Jt Surg. 2013;95:769–74.

34. Havelin LI, Espehaug B, Vollset SE, Engesaeter LB. The effect of the type of cement on early revision of Charnley total hip prostheses: a review of eight thousand five hundred and seventy nine primary arthroplasties from the Norwegian Arthroplasty Register. J Bone Joint Surg Am. 1995;77:1543–50.

35. Wang H, Qiu G, Lin J, Jin J, Qian W, Weng X. Antibiotic bone cement cannot reduce deep infection after primary total knee arthroplasty. Orthopedics. 2015;38:462–6.

36. Australian Orthopaedic Association. https://aoanjrr. dmac.adelaide.edu.au/documents/10180/172288/ Cement-in-Hip&Knee-Arthroplasty. Accessed 27 May 2015.

37. Schiavone Panni A, Corona K, Giulianelli M, Mazzitelli G, Del Regno C, Vasso M. Antibiotic-loaded bone cement reduces risk of infections in primary total knee arthroplasty? A systematic review. Knee Surg Sports Traumatol Arthrosc. 2016;24:3168–74.

38. Qadir R, Sidhu S, Ochsner J, Meyer M, Chimento G. Risk stratified usage of antibiotic-loaded bone cement for primary total knee arthroplasty: short term infection outcomes with a standardized cement protocol. J Arthroplasty. 2014;29:1622–4.

39. Lee Q, Mak W, Wong Y. Risk factors for periprosthetic joint infection in total knee arthroplasty. J Orthop Surg. 2015;23:282–6.

40. Fletcher MD, Spencer RF, Langkamer VG, Lovering AM. Gentamicin concentrations in diagnostic aspirates from 25 patients with hip and knee arthroplasties. Acta Orthop Scand. 2004;75:173–6.

41. Sanz-Ruiz P, Matas-Diez J, Sanchez-Somolinos M, Villanueva-Martinez M, Vaquero-Martín J. Is the commercial antibiotic-loaded bone cement useful in prophylaxis and cost saving after knee and hip joint arthroplasty? The transatlantic paradox. J Arthroplasty. 2017;32:1095–9.

42. Yayac M, Rondon AJ, Tan TL, Levy H, Parvizi J, Courtney PM. The economics of antibiotic cement in total knee arthroplasty: added cost with no reduction in infection rates. J Arthroplasty. 2019;34:2096–101.

43. Chang M, Lee S, Kang S, Hwang K, Park H, Lee K. A retrospective comparative study of infection control rate and clinical outcome between open debridement using antibiotic-impregnated cement beads and a two-stage revision in acute periprosthetic knee joint infection. Medicine. 2020;99:e18891.

44. Estes CS, Beauchamp CP, Clarke HD, et al. A two-stage retention debridement protocol for acute peri-

prosthetic joint infections. Clin Orthop Relat Res. 2010;468:2029–38.

45. Sherrell JC, Fehring TK, Odum S, et al. The Chitranjan Ranawat award: fate of two-stage reimplantation after failed irrigation and debridement for periprosthetic knee infection. Clin Orthop Relat Res. 2011;469:18–25.

46. Lachiewicz P, Wellman S, Peterson J. Antibiotic cement spacers for infected total knee arthroplasties. J Am Acad Orthop Surg. 2020;28:180–8.

47. Nodzo S, Boyle K, Spiro S, Nocon A, Miller A, Westrich G. Success rates, characteristics, and costs of articulating antibiotic spacers for total knee periprosthetic joint infection. Knee. 2017;24:1175–81.

48. Corona P, Barro V, Mendez M, Cáceres E, Flores X. Industrially prefabricated cement spacers: do vancomycin and gentamicin-impregnated spacers offer any advantage? Clin Orthop Relat Res. 2013;472:923–32.

49. Drexler M, Dwyer T, Kuzyk P, Kosashvilli Y, Abolghasemian M, Regev G. The results of two-stage revision TKA using ceftazidime–vancomycin-impregnated cement articulating spacers in Tsukayama type II periprosthetic joint infections. Knee Surg Sports Traumatol Arthrosc. 2015;24:3122–30.

50. Aeng ES, Shalansky KF, Lau TT, Zalunardo N, Li G, Bowie WR. Acute kidney injury with tobramycin-impregnated bone cement spacers in prosthetic joint infections. Ann Pharmacother. 2015;49:1207–13.

51. Edelstein A, Okroj K, Rogers T, Della Valle C, Sporer S. Systemic absorption of antibiotics from antibiotic-loaded cement spacers for the treatment of periprosthetic joint infection. J Arthroplasty. 2018;33:835–9.

52. Meng TJ, Koethe JR, Jenkins CA, Wright PW, Shinar AA, Miller GG. Acute kidney injury after placement of an antibiotic-impregnated cement spacer during revision total knee arthroplasty. J Arthroplasty. 2012;27:1221–7.

53. Van Raaij TM, Visser LE, Vulto AG, Verhaar JA. Acute renal failure after local gentamicin treatment in an infected total knee arthroplasty. J Arthroplasty. 2002;17:948–50.

54. Curtis JM, Sternhagen V, Batts D. Acute renal failure after placement of tobramycin-impregnated bone cement in an infected total knee arthroplasty. Pharmacotherapy. 2005;25:876–80.

55. Dovas S, Liakopoulos V, Papatheodorou L, Chronopoulou I, Papavasiliou V, Atmatzidis E, Giannopoulou M, Eleftheriadis T, Simopoulou T, Karachalios T, Stefanidis I. Acute renal failure after antibiotic-impregnated bone cement treatment of an infected total knee arthroplasty. Clin Nephrol. 2008;69:207–12.

56. Patrick BN, Rivey MP, Allington DR. Acute renal failure associated with vancomycin- and tobramycin-laden cement in total hip arthroplasty. Ann Pharmacother. 2006;40:2037–42.

57. Pitto R, Spika I. Antibiotic-loaded bone cement spacers in two-stage management of infected total knee arthroplasty. Int Orthop. 2004;28:129–33.

58. Scott IR, Stockley I, Getty CJ. Exchange arthroplasty for infected knee replacements. A new two-stage method. J Bone Joint Surg Br. 1993;75:28–31.

59. Struelens B, Claes S, Bellemans J. Spacer-related problems in two-stage revision knee arthroplasty. Acta Orthop Belg. 2013;79:422–6.

60. Guild GN III, Wu B, Scuderi GR. Articulating vs static antibiotic impregnated spacers in revision total knee arthroplasty for sepsis. A systematic review. J Arthroplasty. 2014;29:558–63.

61. Voleti PB, Baldwin KD, Lee GC. Use of static or articulating spacers for infection following total knee arthroplasty: a systematic literature review. J Bone Joint Surg Am. 2013;95:1594–9.

Operating Room Methods to Reduce Infection in Total Knee Arthroplasty

Alexander J. Nedopil and Stephen M. Howell

33.1 Introduction

This chapter presents the current evidence-based measures to maintain a clean environment in the operating room, including the most recent guidelines, with the goal to minimize surgical site infections (SSI) after total knee arthroplasty (TKA).

SSI is one of the most common postoperative adverse events with associated patient morbidity and healthcare costs. Hospital-acquired infections (HAIs) are a leading cause of death in the United States, with an estimated 99,000 deaths occurring because of HAI [1]. Over 20% of HAIs are classified as SSI [2]. SSI is associated with increased length of stay, higher costs, and significant morbidity for the patient. In the era of cost control, reducing SSI is imperative for patient safety and optimal utilization of limited resources.

A. J. Nedopil
Department of Orthopaedic Surgery, König-Ludwig-Haus, University of Würzburg, Würzburg, Germany

Department of Orthopedic Surgery at Adventist Health/Lodi Memorial, Sacramento and Lodi, CA, USA

S. M. Howell (✉)
Biomedical Engineering Graduate Group, University of California, Davis, CA, USA

Department of Orthopedic Surgery at Adventist Health/Lodi Memorial, Sacramento and Lodi, CA, USA

Prevention efforts should target all surgical procedures, especially those in which the human and financial burden is most significant. In 2020, primary TKA will account for approximately 1.07 million arthroplasty procedures (primary and revision) performed in the United States, followed by approximately 500,000 total hip arthroplasties (THAs) [3]. Primary shoulder, elbow, and ankle arthroplasties are much less common. By 2030, prosthetic joint arthroplasties are projected to increase to 3.8 million procedures per year [4]. Infection is the most common indication for revision in TKA and the third most common in THA [5]. By 2030, the infection risk for TKA and THA is expected to increase from 2.2% to 6.8% and 6.5%, respectively [4, 6]. In addition, owing to increasing risk and the number of individuals undergoing prosthetic joint arthroplasty procedures, the total number of hip and knee prosthetic joint infections is projected to increase to 221,500 cases per year by 2030, at the cost of more than $1.62 billion [4, 6].

The operating room represents the patient's environment most vulnerable to infection as the patient's physical barrier is weakened, and auto-regulatory functions (e.g., control of body temperature) are disabled. Therefore, it is of paramount importance to reduce the patient's exposure to pathogens in the operating room. Surgical equipment, anesthesia, and operating room personnel impact the risk of SSI.

© ISAKOS 2022
U. G. Longo et al. (eds.), *Infection in Knee Replacement*,
https://doi.org/10.1007/978-3-030-81553-0_33

The following sections of the chapter will address in a systematic fashion how surgical equipment, anesthesia, and surgical personnel can reduce the risk of SSI in TKA.

33.2 Surgical Equipment Considerations

The term equipment is defined in this chapter as resources provided to the surgical staff to perform a TKA. This includes the operating room's airflow technology, body exhaust suits, adhesive drapes, and single-use instrumentation.

33.3 Operating Room Airflow Technology

In 1969 Sir John Charnley, a pioneer of THA, began to focus on preventing infection through air quality control [7]. He pioneered a purpose-built ultraclean laminar airflow (LAF) enclosure that functioned as a separate "room within a room." In combination with occlusive operating exhaust gowns, he reduced his periprosthetic joint infection rate from 9.5% to 0.5% [8]. As LAF gradually became a culturally accepted standard, further evidence supported its use [9]. This multi-center randomized controlled trial involved 8055 hip and knee replacements and compared LAF systems to conventional theaters and body exhaust suits to conventional clothing. Vertical LAF and body exhaust suits were associated with the lowest rate of PJI (0.1%) and the lowest bacterial air count (0.4 bacteria carrying particles per m^3). When prophylactic antibiotic agents were used with LAF, the rate of PJI reduced from 3.4% to 0.3%. This study provided strong evidence supporting LAF systems. Further evaluation of 3175 arthroplasties revealed a reduced PJI rate after THA (2.0% to 1.2%) but an increased PJI rate after TKA (1.9% to 3.9%) with horizontal LAF [10]. A sub-analysis of confounding factors such as age, diagnosis, comorbidity, surgeon experience, and duration of surgery could not explain this difference.

More recently, there has been an increasing body of registry-based evidence that disputes the clinical efficacy of LAF. An analysis of 41,212 THAs and 20,554 TKAs from the German nosocomial infection surveillance system determined that hospitals with LAF systems had similar PJI rates to hospitals with conventional ventilation [11]. An interrogation of 51,485 THAs and 36,826 TKAs from the New Zealand Joint Registry found a substantially higher rate of early revision for PJI when procedures were performed with LAF compared with a conventional theater (0.15% vs. 0.06%) [12]. A more recent analysis of 91,585 THAs from the same registry observed nearly a twofold risk of revision for PJI within 6 months with LAF compared with conventional ventilation [13]. Data from the UK National Joint Registry has also been used to analyze the effect of LAF. In comparative series of 4915 THAs and 5928 TKAs, there was no substantial difference between LAF and conventional ventilation in the rate of SSI (0.92% vs. 1.14%, respectively) or revision for infection (0.53% vs. 0.45%, respectively) [14]. A meta-analysis of 196,819 hip or knee replacements revealed a higher risk of SSI with LAF (relative risks of 1.71 and 1.36 for THA and TKA, respectively) compared with conventional ventilation. A more recent meta-analysis of 12 studies consisting of 330,146 THAs and 134,368 TKAs showed no substantial difference in PJI risk for LAF compared with conventional ventilation (odds ratio 1.29 and 1.08 for THA and TKA, respectively) [15]. Based on these studies, the World Health Organization has now advised against the use of LAF to reduce the risk of SSI for patients undergoing arthroplasty surgery [16]. More recently, an International Consensus Meeting on PJI has also agreed that LAF is unnecessary for elective joint arthroplasty surgery [17].

33.4 Body Exhaust Suits

Body exhaust suits are commonly used during arthroplasty procedures. However, their role in reducing SSI and PJI is controversial. While negative-pressure body exhaust suits led to less air contamination, less wound contamination, and fewer PJI, positive-pressure body exhaust suits or surgical helmet systems were not shown to reduce contamination or deep infection during arthroplasty [18]. A fundamental principle of negative-pressure exhaust suits uses aspiration tubing to create negative pressure inside the suit, which removes shed particles from the surgical field [19]. The application of negative-pressure body exhaust suits, combined with ultraclean operating rooms, has reduced the infection rate from 1.5% to 0.6% [9]. These results, published in 1982, have led to a widespread acceptance of negative-pressure body exhaust suits as a means of reducing SSIs and PJIs.

However, exhaust tubing is not practical during surgery [20]. Consequently, portable surgical helmet systems were introduced in the 1990s. The surgical helmet system creates a positive-pressure environment inside the gown by drawing air through the hood material, using the material as a filter, and blowing air across the surgeon's face and neck. In contrast to the negative-pressure body exhaust suits, the positive-pressure surgical helmet systems currently in use did not demonstrate a reduction in SSI or PJI and have been associated with a paradoxical increase in deep infection rates compared to standard sterile gowning [18, 21]. Despite being widely used, the current evidence does not support surgical helmet systems to reduce SSI or PJI [18].

33.5 Adhesive Drapes

Adhesive plastic drapes, either plain or saturated with an antimicrobial agent (mostly an iodophor), are used on the patient's skin after completing the surgical site preparation. The drape adheres to the skin, and the surgeon cuts through the skin and the drape itself [22]. Such a drape is theoretically believed to represent a mechanical and microbial barrier to reduce the microorganisms' migration from the skin to the operative site [23]. However, some reports have shown an increased recolonization of the skin following antiseptic preparation underneath adhesive drapes compared to no drapes [24].

A Cochrane review and its updates on the effect of adhesive drapes to reduce SSI concluded that there is no evidence that adhesive drapes reduce SSI [22]. No recommendation is available on using sterile disposable or reusable drapes and surgical gowns for SSI prevention.

Based on current evidence, the WHO suggests not to use adhesive drapes with or without antimicrobial properties to prevent SSI.

33.6 Single-Use Instruments

The introduction of single-use sterile prepackaged instrumentation is a strategy growing in interest to reduce cost, infection, and improve quality and efficiency. The risk of SSI could potentially be reduced through single-use instrumentation compared to traditional, reusable instruments. Reusable instrumentation could become contaminated following re-sterilization, before use in surgery, and may be associated with SSI [25–27]. No evidence is currently available demonstrating a reduction in SSI or PJI with single-use instruments. However, clinical data suggests a reduction in SSI as surgical field contamination is reduced when performing a TKA with single-use instruments in comparison to reusable instruments [28].

33.7 Anesthesia Considerations

Anesthesia staff has the means to modulate the risk of SSI and PJI in the operating room by administering either general or regional anesthesia, by controlling the patient's body temperature, tissue oxygenation, metabolism, and by maintaining a clean work environment to reduce contamination of the surgical field.

33.8 General Vs. Regional Anesthesia

Regional anesthesia in TKA is claimed to decrease the incidence of deep-vein thrombosis and pulmonary embolism and reduce intraoperative bleeding, the need for transfusion, and the length of hospital stay [29–31]. However, spinal and epidural anesthesia and analgesia may cause hypotension, motor blockade, urinary retention, and pruritus [32]. Despite refinements made to reduce such complications, there is still the potential for inadvertent dural puncture and neurological injury, making these techniques less acceptable [33].

The risk of SSI is slightly reduced with regional vs. general anesthesia in patients undergoing TKA [34, 35]. However, none of the current guidelines recommend either for or against a specific mode of anesthesia.

33.9 Maintaining Normothermia

The body normally maintains its temperature between 36 °C and 38 °C by balancing heat production and heat loss to maintain a state of normothermia [36, 37]. These functions are controlled by the thermoregulatory systems in the central nervous system [37]. The body loses heat through radiation, conduction, evaporation, and convection. In surgery, this may occur via the normal process of heat moving away from the body (radiation), contact with cool operating surfaces (conduction), respiration (evaporation), and exposure to the airflow through the operating room (convection). The central nervous system is disrupted under general and regional anesthesia, and the body's thermoregulatory systems are unable to function appropriately; thus, both hypothermia, a core temperature < 36 °C, and hyperthermia, a core temperature > 38 °C, may occur during surgical procedures [37].

Hypothermia can lead to greater susceptibility to infections [38]. This effect can be considerable; a decrease of 1.9 °C in core temperature triples the relative risk of surgical periprosthetic infection and increases the hospitalization duration by 20%. Hypothermia increases patients' susceptibility to perioperative wound infections by causing vasoconstriction and impaired immunity [39]. The presence of sufficient intraoperative hypothermia triggers thermoregulatory vasoconstriction, decreasing the partial pressure of oxygen in tissues, thus lowering resistance to infection [40, 41].

Although it is often assumed that hypothermia is a result of lengthy procedures, the greatest temperature drops may, in fact, occur before surgery and during induction of anesthesia [42]. The administration of inhaled gases (e.g., isoflurane, sevoflurane, or nitrous oxide), or the use of intravenous anesthetic induction agents (e.g., propofol or opioids), cause peripheral vasodilation and cause the transfer of core body heat to the periphery [43]. Once hypothermia occurs, it is difficult to correct efficiently [42]. The type of anesthesia, spinal vs. general, has no effect on thermoregulation in patients undergoing TKA [42]. The patient's body temperature before and during TKA can drop by 1.5 °C [42].

Maintaining normothermia during TKA is an important step for reducing the risk of SSI. The means of achieving this goal include the use of pre- and intraoperative warming devices and the administration of pre-warmed intravenous fluids [44]. However, the best warming device to ensure normothermia remains unknown. Concerns regarding the use of air warmer and the potential for contamination have been raised by a few authors, although this has not been proven [45, 46].

33.10 Perioperative Oxygenation

There is evidence that optimized blood flow to the surgical incision decreases SSI rates by avoiding hypothermia, hypoxia, and decreased perfusion [47]. This has also been demonstrated for tourniquet use [48, 49]. Because inadequate tissue oxygen tension impairs tissue repair and oxidative killing of surgical pathogens, supplemental oxygen is another important mechanism for SSI reduction [50]. The WHO recognizes the importance of sufficient oxygenation to the surgical incision and recommends 80% fractions of inspired oxygen concentration during surgery and in the postoperative recovery unit [51].

33.11 Glycemic Control

Between 8% and 22% of patients who undergo total joint replacement have diabetes, and about one-third have undiagnosed hyperglycemia [52, 53]. Diabetes, especially when uncontrolled, is a significant risk factor for SSI [54]. Even non-diabetic patients who develop hyperglycemia postoperatively have a significantly increased risk of SSI, with current recommendations that peri- and postoperative glucose levels are strictly monitored and maintained <180 mg/dL [55]. The identification of patients with diabetes or hyperglycemia and the implementation of strict perioperative glycemic control minimizes the risk of infection [56]. Maintaining a blood glucose level < 180 mg/dL might be important even after the patient is discharged. With the trend towards outpatient TKA, the glycemic control adds another task to the patient's daily routine of home recovery. Even non-diabetic patients, who are not familiar with blood sugar testing, should be trained with this task before discharge.

33.12 Maintaining a Clean Work Environment

The Society for Healthcare Epidemiology of America (SHEA) established guidelines for anesthesia personnel to maintain a clean work environment with the purpose to reduce SSI by microbial cross-transmission from the anesthesia work area in the intraoperative environment [57]: Hand hygiene ideally should be performed according to the WHO 5 Moments for Hand Hygiene. These 5 Moments of Hand Hygiene are:

1. before touching a patient,
2. before clean/aseptic procedures,
3. after body fluid exposure/risk,
4. after touching a patient,
5. after touching the patient's surroundings.

SHEA recommends that hand hygiene be performed at the minimum before aseptic tasks (e.g., inserting central venous catheters, inserting arterial catheters, drawing medications, spiking IV bags); after removing gloves; when hands are soiled or contaminated (e.g., oropharyngeal secretions); before touching the contents of the anesthesia cart; and when entering and exiting the OR (even after removing gloves). These recommendations could mean that anesthesia providers have to perform hand hygiene up to 54 times per hour [58]. The current failure to perform hand hygiene for all anesthesia providers is 82% [58]. To facilitate hand hygiene, SHEA recommends positioning alcohol-based hand rub dispensers at the entrances to the operating room and near anesthesia providers inside the operating room.

To further reduce the risk of contamination in the OR, anesthesia providers should wear double gloves during airway management and remove the outer gloves immediately after airway manipulation. As soon as possible, providers should remove the inner gloves and perform hand hygiene.

33.13 Surgical Personnel

This section addresses methods the surgical personnel can apply to reduce the risk of wound contamination, SSI, and PJI. Intraoperative methods applied by the surgical team to reduce these risks are discussed in a different chapter.

33.14 Operating Room Traffic

Operating room (OR) traffic flow is linked to increased contamination rates [59]. It is hypothesized that OR personnel are the major contributors to OR contamination because of bacterial shedding, mainly from the skin, with shedding rates as high as 10,000 bacteria per minute [60–62]. The bacterial load in the OR is directly associated with the number of members present, with a 34-fold increase in bacterial counts with five OR personnel compared with an empty room [63, 64]. Also, increased personnel traffic implies more door openings, which is associated with increased bacterial counts [65]. Any obstacle in the directional airflow path coupled with repeated door openings creates air turbulence that allows the mixing of filtered air with unclean air [10, 61, 66]. The average frequency of door openings during a primary arthroplasty is 0.65/min [67]. The most common OR personnel entering and leaving the OR are the circulating nurses and surgical equipment representatives. For almost 50% of the room entries, no identifiable purpose could be identified. Hence, most OR personnel traffic is extraneous and can be reduced. Ideally, the anticipated implants are in the OR prior to the start of the case, and the exchange of anesthesia and scrub technician personnel is limited.

References

1. Klevens RM, Edwards JR, Richards CL Jr, Horan TC, Gaynes RP, Pollock DA, et al. Estimating health care-associated infections and deaths in US hospitals, 2002. Public Health Rep. 2007;122(2):160–6.
2. De Lissovoy G, Fraeman K, Hutchins V, Murphy D, Song D, Vaughn BB. Surgical site infection: incidence and impact on hospital utilization and treatment costs. Am J Infect Control. 2009;37(5):387–97.
3. Singh JA, Yu S, Chen L, Cleveland JD. Rates of total joint replacement in the United States: future projections to 2020–2040 using the National Inpatient Sample. J Rheumatol. 2019;46(9):1134–40.
4. Kurtz S, Ong K, Lau E, Mowat F, Halpern M. Projections of primary and revision hip and knee arthroplasty in the United States from 2005 to 2030. J Bone Joint Surg Am. 2007;89(4):780–5.
5. Bozic KJ, Kurtz SM, Lau E, Ong K, Chiu V, Vail TP, et al. The epidemiology of revision total knee arthroplasty in the United States. Clin Orthop Relat Res. 2010;468(1):45–51.
6. Kurtz SM, Lau E, Watson H, Schmier JK, Parvizi J. Economic burden of periprosthetic joint infection in the United States. J Arthroplasty. 2012;27(8 Suppl):61–5e1.
7. Charnley J, Eftekhar N. Postoperative infection in total prosthetic replacement arthroplasty of the hip-joint. With special reference to the bacterial content of the air of the operating room. Br J Surg. 1969;56(9):641–9.
8. Charnley J. Postoperative infection after total hip replacement with special reference to air contamination in the operating room. Clin Orthop Relat Res. 1972;87:167–87.
9. Lidwell OM, Lowbury EJ, Whyte W, Blowers R, Stanley SJ, Lowe D. Effect of ultraclean air in operating rooms on deep sepsis in the joint after total hip or knee replacement: a randomised study. Br Med J (Clin Res Ed). 1982;285(6334):10–4.
10. Salvati EA, Robinson RP, Zeno SM, Koslin BL, Brause BD, Wilson PD. Infection-rates after 3175 total hip and total knee replacements performed with and without a horizontal unidirectional filtered air-flow system. J Bone Jt Surg Am Vol. 1982;64(4):525–35.
11. Breier AC, Brandt C, Sohr D, Geffers C, Gastmeier P. Laminar airflow ceiling size: no impact on infection rates following hip and knee prosthesis. Infect Control Hosp Epidemiol. 2011;32(11):1097–102.
12. Hooper G, Rothwell A, Frampton C, Wyatt M. Does the use of laminar flow and space suits reduce early deep infection after total hip and knee replacement? The ten-year results of the New Zealand joint registry. J Bone Jt Surg. 2011;93(1):85–90.
13. Smith JO, Frampton CMA, Hooper GJ, Young SW. The impact of patient and surgical factors on the rate of postoperative infection after total hip arthroplasty—a New Zealand joint registry study. J Arthroplasty. 2018;33(6):1884–90.
14. Singh S, Reddy S, Shrivastava R. Does laminar airflow make a difference to the infection rates for lower limb arthroplasty: a study using the National Joint Registry and local surgical site infection data for two hospitals with and without laminar airflow. Eur J Orthop Surg Traumatol. 2017;27(2):261–5.
15. Bischoff P, Kubilay NZ, Allegranzi B, Egger M, Gastmeier P. Effect of laminar airflow ventilation on surgical site infections: a systematic review and meta-analysis. Lancet Infect Dis. 2017;17(5):553–61.
16. Organization WH. Global guidelines for the prevention of surgical site infection. Geneva: World Health Organization; 2016.
17. Schwarz EM, Parvizi J, Gehrke T, Aiyer A, Battenberg A, Brown SA, et al. 2018 international consensus meeting on musculoskeletal infection: research priorities from the general assembly questions. J Orthop Res. 2019;37(5):997–1006.
18. Young SW, Zhu M, Shirley OC, Wu Q, Spangehl MJ. Do 'Surgical helmet Systems' or 'Body exhaust Suits' affect contamination and deep infection rates in arthroplasty? A systematic review. J Arthroplasty. 2016;31(1):225–33.
19. Aggarwal VK, Weintraub S, Klock J, Stachel A, Phillips M, Schwarzkopf R, et al. Frank Stinchfield award: a comparison of prosthetic joint infection rates between direct anterior and non-anterior approach total hip arthroplasty. Bone Jt J. 2019;101-B(6_Supple_B):2–8.
20. Malik MH, Handford E, Staniford E, Gambhir AK, Kay PR. Comfort assessment of personal protection systems during total joint arthroplasty using a novel multi-dimensional evaluation tool. Ann R Coll Surg Engl. 2006;88(5):465–9.
21. Hooper GJ, Rothwell AG, Frampton C, Wyatt MC. Does the use of laminar flow and space suits reduce early deep infection after total hip and knee replacement?: the ten-year results of the New Zealand joint registry. J Bone Joint Surg Br. 2011;93(1):85–90.

22. Webster J, Alghamdi A. Use of plastic adhesive drapes during surgery for preventing surgical site infection. Cochrane Database Syst Rev. 2015;2015(4):CD006353.

23. French M, Eitzen HE, Ritter MA. The plastic surgical adhesive drape: an evaluation of its efficacy as a microbial barrier. Ann Surg. 1976;184(1):46.

24. Falk-Brynhildsen K, Friberg O, Soderquist B, Nilsson UG. Bacterial colonization of the skin following aseptic preoperative preparation and impact of the use of plastic adhesive drapes. Biol Res Nurs. 2013;15(2):242–8.

25. Mobley KS, Jackson JB 3rd. A prospective analysis of clinical detection of defective wrapping by operating room staff. Am J Infect Control. 2018;46(7):837–9.

26. Dancer SJ, Stewart M, Coulombe C, Gregori A, Virdi M. Surgical site infections linked to contaminated surgical instruments. J Hosp Infect. 2012;81(4):231–8.

27. Waked WR, Simpson AK, Miller CP, Magit DP, Grauer JN. Sterilization wrap inspections do not adequately evaluate instrument sterility. Clin Orthop Relat Res. 2007;462(462):207–11.

28. Mont MA, Johnson AJ, Issa K, Pivec R, Blasser KE, McQueen D, et al. Single-use instrumentation, cutting blocks, and trials decrease contamination during total knee arthroplasty: a prospective comparison of navigated and nonnavigated cases. J Knee Surg. 2013;26(4):285–90.

29. Sharrock NE, Haas SB, Hargett MJ, Urquhart B, Insall JN, Scuderi G. Effects of epidural anesthesia on the incidence of deep-vein thrombosis after total knee arthroplasty. J Bone Joint Surg Am. 1991;73(4):502–6.

30. Nielsen PT, Jorgensen LN, Albrecht-Beste E, Leffers AM, Rasmussen LS. Lower thrombosis risk with epidural blockade in knee arthroplasty. Acta Orthop Scand. 1990;61(1):29–31.

31. Jorgensen LN, Rasmussen LS, Nielsen PT, Leffers A, Albrecht-Beste E. Antithrombotic efficacy of continuous extradural analgesia after knee replacement. Br J Anaesth. 1991;66(1):8–12.

32. Gedney JA, Liu EH. Side-effects of epidural infusions of opioid bupivacaine mixtures. Anaesthesia. 1998;53(12):1148–55.

33. Moraca RJ, Sheldon DG, Thirlby RC. The role of epidural anesthesia and analgesia in surgical practice. Ann Surg. 2003;238(5):663–73.

34. Pugely AJ, Martin CT, Gao YB, Mendoza-Lattes S, Callaghan JJ. Differences in short-term complications between spinal and general anesthesia for primary total knee arthroplasty. J Bone Jt Surg Am Vol. 2013;95a(3):193–9.

35. Park YB, Chae WS, Park SH, Yu JS, Lee SG, Yim SJ. Comparison of short-term complications of general and spinal anesthesia for primary unilateral total knee arthroplasty. Knee Surg Relat Res. 2017;29(2):96–103.

36. Ellis FP. The control of operating-suite temperatures. Br J Ind Med. 1963;20(4):284–7.

37. Sappenfield JW, Hong CM, Galvagno SM. Perioperative temperature measurement and management: moving beyond the surgical care improvement project. J Anesthesiol Clin Sci. 2013;2(1):8.

38. Leijtens B, Koeter M, Kremers K, Koeter S. High incidence of postoperative hypothermia in total knee and total hip arthroplasty: a prospective observational study. J Arthroplasty. 2013;28(6):895–8.

39. Kurz A, Sessler DI, Lenhardt R. Perioperative normothermia to reduce the incidence of surgical-wound infection and shorten hospitalization. Study of wound infection and temperature group. N Engl J Med. 1996;334(19):1209–15.

40. Sessler DI, McGuire J, Sessler AM. Perioperative thermal insulation. Anesthesiology. 1991;74(5):875–9.

41. Ozaki M, Sessler DI, Suzuki H, Ozaki K, Tsunoda C, Atarashi K. Nitrous-oxide decreases the threshold for vasoconstriction less-than sevoflurane or isoflurane. Anesth Analg. 1995;80(6):1212–6.

42. Simpson JB, Thomas VS, Ismaily SK, Muradov PI, Noble PC, Incavo SJ. Hypothermia in total joint arthroplasty: a wake-up call. J Arthroplasty. 2018;33(4):1012–8.

43. Sessler DI. Perioperative thermoregulation and heat balance. Lancet. 2016;387(10038):2655–64.

44. Putzu M, Casati A, Berti M, Pagliarini G, Fanelli G. Clinical complications, monitoring and management of perioperative mild hypothermia: anesthesiological features. Acta Biomed. 2007;78(3):163–9.

45. McGovern PD, Albrecht M, Belani KG, Nachtsheim C, Partington PF, Carluke I, et al. Forced-air warming and ultra-clean ventilation do not mix: an investigation of theatre ventilation, patient warming and joint replacement infection in orthopaedics. J Bone Joint Surg Br. 2011;93(11):1537–44.

46. Legg AJ, Cannon T, Hamer AJ. Do forced air patient-warming devices disrupt unidirectional downward airflow? J Bone Joint Surg Br. 2012;94(2):254–6.

47. Allen DB, Maguire JJ, Mahdavian M, Wicke C, Marcocci L, Scheuenstuhl H, et al. Wound hypoxia and acidosis limit neutrophil bacterial killing mechanisms. Arch Surg. 1997;132(9):991–6.

48. Zhang W, Li N, Chen SF, Tan Y, Al-Aidaros M, Chen LB. The effects of a tourniquet used in total knee arthroplasty: a meta-analysis. J Orthop Surg Res. 2014;9(1):13.

49. Blanco JF, Diaz A, Melchor FR, da Casa C, Pescador D. Risk factors for periprosthetic joint infection after total knee arthroplasty. Arch Orthop Trauma Surg. 2020;140(2):239–45.

50. Greif R, Akca O, Horn EP, Kurz A, Sessler DI, Outcomes RG. Supplemental perioperative oxygen to reduce the incidence of surgical-wound infection. N Engl J Med. 2000;342(3):161–7.

51. Parvizi J, Shohat N, Gehrke T. Prevention of periprosthetic joint infection: new guidelines. Bone Jt J. 2017;99-B(4 Supple B):3–10.

52. Stryker LS, Abdel MP, Morrey ME, Morrow MM, Kor DJ, Morrey BF. Elevated postoperative blood glucose

and preoperative hemoglobin A1C are associated with increased wound complications following total joint arthroplasty. J Bone Joint Surg Am. 2013;95(9):808–14, S1-2.

53. Capozzi JD, Lepkowsky ER, Callari MM, Jordan ET, Koenig JA, Sirounian GH. The prevalence of diabetes mellitus and routine hemoglobin A1c screening in elective Total joint arthroplasty patients. J Arthroplasty. 2017;32(1):304–8.

54. Marchant MH Jr, Viens NA, Cook C, Vail TP, Bolognesi MP. The impact of glycemic control and diabetes mellitus on perioperative outcomes after total joint arthroplasty. J Bone Jt Surg. 2009;91(7):1621–9.

55. Mraovic B, Suh D, Jacovides C, Parvizi J. Perioperative hyperglycemia and postoperative infection after lower limb arthroplasty. J Diabetes Sci Technol. 2011;5(2):412–8.

56. Thompson BM, Stearns JD, Apsey HA, Schlinkert RT, Cook CB. Perioperative management of patients with diabetes and hyperglycemia undergoing elective surgery. Curr Diab Rep. 2016;16(1):2.

57. Munoz-Price LS, Bowdle A, Johnston BL, Bearman G, Camins BC, Dellinger EP, et al. Infection prevention in the operating room anesthesia work area. Infect Control Hosp Epidemiol. 2018;40(1):1–17.

58. Biddle C, Shah J. Quantification of anesthesia providers' hand hygiene in a busy metropolitan operating room: what would Semmelweis think? Am J Infect Control. 2012;40(8):756–9.

59. Andersson AE, Bergh I, Karlsson J, Eriksson BI, Nilsson K. Traffic flow in the operating room: an explorative and descriptive study on air quality during orthopedic trauma implant surgery. Am J Infect Control. 2012;40(8):750–5.

60. Ritter MA. Surgical wound environment. Clin Orthop Relat Res. 1984;190:11–3.

61. Ritter MA. Operating room environment. Clin Orthop Relat Res. 1999;369(369):103–9.

62. Tumia N, Ashcroft GP. Convection warmers—a possible source of contamination in laminar airflow operating theatres? J Hosp Infect. 2002;52(3):171–4.

63. Ritter MA, Eitzen H, French M, Hart JB. The operating room environment as affected by people and the surgical face mask. Clin Orthop Relat Res. 1975;111:147–50.

64. Ayliffe GA. Role of the environment of the operating suite in surgical wound infection. Rev Infect Dis. 1991;13 Suppl 10(Supplement_10):S800–4.

65. Smith EB, Raphael IJ, Maltenfort MG, Honsawek S, Dolan K, Younkins EA. The effect of laminar air flow and door openings on operating room contamination. J Arthroplasty. 2013;28(9):1482–5.

66. Young RS, O'Regan DJ. Cardiac surgical theatre traffic: time for traffic calming measures? Interact Cardiovasc Thorac Surg. 2010;10(4):526–9.

67. Panahi P, Stroh M, Casper DS, Parvizi J, Austin MS. Operating room traffic is a major concern during total joint arthroplasty. Clin Orthop Relat Res. 2012;470(10):2690–4.

Tourniquet

34

Ahmed A. Magan, Babar Kayani, Sandeep Singh, and Fares S. Haddad

34.1 Introduction

34.1.1 Definition of Tourniquet

It is essentially an external device that applies pressure to a limb, causing constriction of blood flow, therefore creating better visualising of the surgical field and it reduces blood loss.

34.1.2 History of Tourniquet

The use of tourniquet dates back as far as the era of Alexandra The Great's military empire around the fourth century. It was not until 1718 when Jean-Louis Petit popularised its use in the field of surgery. As an anatomist as well as a surgeon, he made a respectable contribution to the advancement of Trauma and Orthopaedic surgery [1]. He made a screw device which by turning constricted the blood flow. Hence it was named tourniquet, which comes from the French word 'tourner = to turn'. Over the centuries, his design evolved resulting in the different types of tourniquets that are in use today.

34.1.3 Tourniquet Use in Total Knee Arthroplasty (TKA)

The use of tourniquet in surgery has helped surgeons for centuries in minimising the amount of blood loss. Over the last several decades, the use of tourniquet has become controversial in lower limb arthroplasty. There is no conclusive evidence in the published literature, whether tourniquet should be routinely used in TKA. In orthopaedics currently, there are three schools of thought with regard to tourniquet usage; (1) use it for the entire case, (2) use in part (for cementing), (3) do not use it all. This chapter will cover essential topics regarding tourniquet usage and will include the relevant literature as well as focusing on infections.

34.1.4 Indications and Contraindications of Tourniquet Use in Surgery

Generally, it is indicated for procedures in which there is a likelihood of high blood loss or in delicate surgery in which the relevant anatomy needs to be identified during the approach.

A. A. Magan (✉) · S. Singh · F. S. Haddad
Department of Trauma and Orthopaedic Surgery, University College London Hospitals, London, UK

The Princess Grace Hospital, and The NIHR Biomedical Research Centre at UCLH, London, UK
e-mail: fsh@fareshaddad.net

B. Kayani
Department of Trauma and Orthopaedic Surgery, University College Hospital, Fitzrovia, London, UK

© ISAKOS 2022
U. G. Longo et al. (eds.), *Infection in Knee Replacement*,
https://doi.org/10.1007/978-3-030-81553-0_34

The main contraindication to tourniquet use is in patients with significant peripheral vascular disease. There are other situations in which tourniquet use may not be advised such as in some open injuries, intramedullary nailing and diabetic foot disease [2].

34.1.5 What Is Normal Tourniquet Pressure?

There is no universally agreed value to inflate the tourniquet pressure to although the vast majority would support using the lowest tourniquet pressure for the shortest period time if one has to use it. Several factors can influence the value to inflate above the systolic pressure. Some authors advocate inflating tourniquets to 2.5 times above the pre-anaesthetic resting systolic blood pressure and increasing further by 50 mmHg for obese patients [2]. A randomised control trial (RCT) compared two groups using tourniquet during TKA. One group had higher tourniquet pressure of 350 mmHg (set as standard), and the group had a lower tourniquet pressure set to 100mmHG above the patients' systolic pressure. The study consisted of 26 patients undergoing bilateral TKAs. They found using the lower tourniquet pressure (100 mmHg above the systolic) was as acceptable in controlling bleeding as the higher pressure (350 mmHg) group. Also, the lower tourniquet pressure group had less pain and faster recovery [3].

34.2 Tourniquet Use in TKA: Does It Influence the Risk of Infection?

34.2.1 Pathophysiology of Tourniquet Ischaemia, Wound Healing and Tourniquet Time

Healthy wound healing is dependent on adequate local cellular oxygenation, which in turn will reduce the risk of delayed wound healing or

infections [4]. Johnson in 1993 described it well in their study on wound healing following TKA. It explained the resultant wound ischaemia following the TKA. The wound edge oxygenation varied in the early postoperative period, and type of incision used (midline, medial, curved medial) had an influence on it [5]. Once a tourniquet is applied, around 1% of the normal circulation is perfusing the limb [5]. Furthermore, the paper pointed out that exsanguinating the limb prior to applying the tourniquet favoured any potentially opportunistic microbes present for two reasons. Firstly, once a tourniquet is applied, it leads to reduced circulatory defensive cells to kill off any bacteria that may be present. Secondly, if the antibiotics are not administered on time, it may result in inadequate therapeutic levels within the tissue. Possibly a combination of these two factors may contribute to the development of superficial wound healing problems or worse a deep infection.

There is a difference in skin edge perfusion with knee going into flexion in the early periods following TKA [6]. The lateral wound edge appears to have lower oxygen concentration compared to the medial edge wound [5] although this can be resolved by providing the patients with extra oxygen [7]. A large RCT found giving supplementary oxygen to patients undergoing colorectal resection halved their wound infection rate [8]. Given some of these factors, one might ask why to use the tourniquet if one's aim is to try and mitigate any risks of infection?

Tourniquet usage can result in ischaemia-related events. Clarke et al. looked at 31 patients undergoing TKA and divided them into groups: no tourniquet and two other groups in which tourniquet was inflated 125 mmHg or 250 mmHg above the mean anaesthetic systolic pressure. In this small series, they found all the groups had an element of critical hypoxia and this was most significant in the higher tourniquet pressure group. Also, in this group the duration of hypoxia persisted longer when compared to lower tourniquet pressure and the no tourniquet group [9].

A meta-analysis on the use of pneumatic tourniquet in TKA looked at 3 studies out of 13

RCTs that mentioned infection in their analysis. There were in total 223 patients and the study stated infection rate was higher in the tourniquet group than the control group, with RR 5.37 (95% confident interval (CI) 0.99–29.6) and *P*-value of 0.05. [10] Although at a glance, their results may appear significant; however, it must be interpreted with caution due to the small number of studies. It is difficult with certainty whether operative time or tourniquet is contributing to the development of prosthetic joint infection (PJI). In the published literature, some surgeons use tourniquet time and operative time almost interchangeably. Increased operative time will subsequently lead to the application of tourniquet for a more extended period which as a result of the prolonged surgery elevates the risk of PJI. For example, in a case-control study Blanco et al. reviewed retrospectively 132 patients records who had TKA in which of all the cases used tourniquet. The authors included in the study 66 TKAs with PJI and 66 TKAs without PJI as control. They concluded, prolonged operative >90 min and tourniquet time >60 min were the most relevant risk factor for PJI [11]. Carefully analysing their findings, one can conclude they found the risk of PJI increased after 60 min of operating time, further increasing fivefold every 15 min after 90 min of operative time. Table 34.1 below shows a summary of relevant studies of tourniquet use in TKA and infections.

34.3 Tourniquet Use on the Rate of Blood Loss, Operative Time and Deep Vein Thrombosis (DVT)

There is no substitute for excellent haemostasis during exposure and wound closure. Blood loss continues after the closure of the wound and this can be more than the blood loss in surgery. A recent meta-analysis of 11 RCTs involving 541 knees looked at tourniquet use and blood loss in TKA. It concluded tourniquet use in TKA

reduced blood loss during surgery as well as calculated blood loss and operative time. However, there was no difference in postoperative total blood loss or the need for blood transfusion [15].

This study also confirmed previous findings that the risk of having the thromboembolic event was fivefold higher with the use of tourniquet compared to without a tourniquet [15, 16]. Furthermore another two meta-analyses commented on the incidence of DVT being higher with the use of tourniquet, with similar fivefold increase as the previous studies [10, 17].

34.3.1 Tourniquet use in TKA: Pain and Range of Movement (ROM)

Previously published studies including RCTs (Table 34.1) suggested the use of tourniquet in TKA resulted in an increase in pain in the immediate period after surgery and it also affected the ability to straight leg raise. On the other hand, Deering's et al. published an informative systematic review and a meta-analysis last year which included 14 studies and 8 of them discussed pain [18]. These 8 studies consisted of 440 TKA, (221 TG vs. 219 NTG) and analysis showed no clinically important difference between the two groups 5.23 ± 1.94 cm vs. 3.78 ± 1.61 cm; standardised [STD] mean difference 0.88 mm; 95% confidence interval [CI], 0.54–1.23; $p < 0.001$. The authors used the Visual Analogue Scale (VAS) 0 mm to 100 mm and defined 20 mm on the VAS score as the minimum clinically important difference (MCID). Danoff et al. observational study of 139 total hip arthroplasty (THA) and 161 TKA demonstrated the MCID for worsening pain to be 23.6 for THA and 29.1 for TKA [19].

Deerings et al. found no clinically significant difference between TG and TNG on the range of movement patients achieved post-surgery. In addition, their results demonstrated no difference in the length of hospital stay between the two groups.

Table 34.1 Summary of RCTs looking at the correlation between Tourniquet use in TKA and infections

Authors and year	LoE	Aim of the study	No. cases	TG	NTG	Conclusion	Comments
Liu et al. (2017) [12]	I	Prospective RCT assessing the benefits of the use of a tourniquet in on limb in patients undergoing simultaneous bilateral TKAs	52	25	27	Use of tourniquet may save operative time but could also lead to increased postoperative pain, swelling, delayed straight leg raise and wound complications	The only **1 infection (deep)** was in the TG
Vandenbussche et al. (2002) [13]	I	Prospective RCT looking at the effects of tourniquet use in TKA	80	40	40	There were no significant differences between the two groups in terms of operative time, complications and length of hospital stay. NT group had more blood loss, better ROM until day 5, less pain for the first 6 h post-op	**No wound infections**
Clarke et al. (2001) [9]	I	RCT looking whether thigh tourniquet influenced wound hypoxia and was the cause of delay	31	21	10	If a tourniquet is used, then it should be inflated at the lowest possible pressure to minimise wound complications	The only **1 infection (2 skin flaps)** was in the TG. There were 3 skin flaps (×2 TG and 1× NTG) with delayed wound healing
Abdel-Salam et al. (1995) [14]	I	Prospective RCT looking at the effects of a tourniquet on wound healing, pain and muscle function	80	40	40	The complication rate was lower in the group with NT, better initial recovery and less pain	Tourniquet group had 5 **wound infections** vs. no cases in the NTG

LoE level of evidence, *TKA* total knee arthroplasty, *NTG* no tourniquet group, *TG* tourniquet group

34.4 Conclusions

Tourniquet use in TKA may lead to an increase in some complications following surgery. These include the incidence of wound infections, tourniquet pain, thromboembolic events, neurovascular injury and stiffness. On the other hand, proponents of tourniquet use argue that there is less blood loss, a shorter operative time and no clinically significant difference in overall outcome compared to those who have TKA without a tourniquet.

The current published Level 1 studies do not conclusively support whether tourniquet should be used routinely or not—in particular concerning the incidence of infection. Infection is a serious complication with associated high morbidity and mortality. PJIs have worse 5-year survival rate than some cancers. It is known that prolonged surgery time is associated with infection and by virtue, some authors report prolonged tourniquet time leads to infection. Until we have adequately powered level 1 studies, the current status quo will continue. In our practice, we do not routinely use a tourniquet and neither do we support its use in TKA.

References

1. Markatos K, Androutsos G, Karamanou M, Tzagkarakis G, Kaseta M, Mavrogenis A. Jean-Louis petit (1674–1750): a pioneer anatomist and surgeon and his contribution to orthopaedic surgery and trauma surgery. Int Orthop. 2018;42(8):2003–7. https://doi.org/10.1007/s00264-018-3978-8.

2. Khan AL, Gray A. Tourniquet uses and precautions. Surgery. 2014;32:131–3. https://doi.org/10.1016/j.mpsur.2013.12.014.
3. Worland RL, Arredondo J, Angles F, Lopez-Jimenez F, Jessup DE. Thigh pain following tourniquet application in simultaneous bilateral total knee replacement arthroplasty. J Arthroplasty. 1997;12(8):848–52. https://doi.org/10.1016/S0883-5403(97)90153-4.
4. Hunt TK. The physiology of wound healing. Ann Emerg Med. 1988;17(12):1265–73. https://doi.org/10.1016/S0196-0644(88)80351-2.
5. Johnson DP. Infection after knee arthroplasty. Acta Orthop Scand. 1993;252:1–48. https://doi.org/10.3109/17453679309153926.
6. Johnson DP, Eastwood DM, Bader DL. Biomechanical factors in wound healing following knee arthroplasty. J Med Eng Technol. 1991;15(1):8–14. https://doi.org/10.3109/03091909109015442.
7. Vince KG. Wound closure: healing the collateral damage. J Bone Jt Surg Ser B. 2012;94(11 Suppl A):126–33. https://doi.org/10.1302/0301-620X.94B11.30792.
8. Greif R, Akça O, Horn EP, Kurz A, Sessler DI. Supplemental perioperative oxygen to reduce the incidence of surgical-wound infection. N Engl J Med. 2000;342(3):161–7. https://doi.org/10.1056/NEJM200001203420303.
9. Clarke MT, Longstaff L, Edwards D, Rushton N. Tourniquet-induced wound hypoxia after total knee replacement. J Bone Jt Surg Ser B. 2001;83(1):40–4. https://doi.org/10.1302/0301-620X.83B1.10795.
10. Yi S, Tan J, Chen C, Chen H, Huang W. The use of pneumatic tourniquet in total knee arthroplasty: a meta-analysis. Arch Orthop Trauma Surg. 2014;134(10):1469–76. https://doi.org/10.1007/s00402-014-2056-y.
11. Blanco JF, Díaz A, Melchor FR, da Casa C, Pescador D. Risk factors for periprosthetic joint infection after total knee arthroplasty. Arch Orthop Trauma Surg. 2020;140(2):239–45. https://doi.org/10.1007/s00402-019-03304-6.
12. Liu PL, Li DQ, Zhang YK, et al. Effects of unilateral tourniquet used in patients undergoing simultaneous bilateral total knee arthroplasty. Orthop Surg. 2017;9(2):180–5. https://doi.org/10.1111/os.12329.
13. Vandenbussche E, Duranthon LD, Couturier M, Pidhorz L, Augereau B. The effect of tourniquet use in total knee arthroplasty. Int Orthop. 2002;26(5):306–9. https://doi.org/10.1007/s00264-002-0360-6.
14. Abdel-Salam A, Eyres KS. Effects of tourniquet during total knee arthroplasty. A prospective randomised study. J Bone Jt Surg Ser B. 1995;77(2):250–3. https://doi.org/10.1302/0301-620x.77b2.7706340.
15. Cai DF, Fan QH, Zhong HH, Peng S, Song H. The effects of tourniquet use on blood loss in primary total knee arthroplasty for patients with osteoarthritis: a meta-analysis. J Orthop Surg Res. 2019;14(1):348. https://doi.org/10.1186/s13018-019-1422-4.
16. Parmet JL, Horrow JC, Berman AT, Miller F, Pharo G, Collins L. The incidence of large venous emboli during total knee arthroplasty without pneumatic tourniquet use. Anesth Analg. 1998;87(2):439–44. https://doi.org/10.1097/00000539-199808000-00039.
17. Zhang W, Li N, Chen S, Tan Y, Al-Aidaros M, Chen L. The effects of a tourniquet used in total knee arthroplasty: a meta-analysis. J Orthop Surg Res. 2014;9(1):13. https://doi.org/10.1186/1749-799X-9-13.
18. McCarthy Deering E, Hu SY, Abdulkarim A. Does tourniquet use in TKA increase postoperative pain? A systematic review and meta-analysis. Clin Orthop Relat Res. 2019;477(3):547–58. https://doi.org/10.1097/CORR.0000000000000572.
19. Danoff JR, Goel R, Sutton R, Maltenfort MG, Austin MS. How much pain is significant? Defining the minimal clinically important difference for the visual analog scale for pain after Total joint arthroplasty. J Arthroplasty. 2018;33(7S):S71–S75.e2. https://doi.org/10.1016/j.arth.2018.02.029.

Intraarticular Injection Prior to Joint Replacement and its Relationship to Prosthetic Joint Infection

Darshan S. Angadi, Claire Bolton,
Vikram Kandhari, and Myles R. J. Coolican

35.1 Introduction

The management of symptomatic osteoarthritis (OA) of the knee includes well-described treatment options such as oral analgesia, non-steroidal anti-inflammatory medications, braces and sleeves, physiotherapy particularly strengthening exercises, dietary/lifestyle changes, intraarticular (IA) injection of therapeutic substances and when these modalities have failed to adequately control symptoms, arthroplasty is appropriate [1–5].

IA injections of the knee are routinely performed both in the outpatient clinic and operating room setting [3]. It has been reported that approximately 30% to 50% of patients undergoing arthroplasty have had an IA injection in the ipsilateral knee during the year leading up to the surgical procedure [6, 7]. However, compared to other nonoperative treatment modalities intraarticular injection procedure is relatively more invasive. Hence several investigators have reported the risks and complications associated with this procedure [8, 9]. Local complications such as painful effusion [10], skin lesions [11], skin necrosis [12] and septic arthritis [13–15] have been described following intraarticular injection.

Progression of symptoms despite the nonoperative treatment options is an indication for arthroplasty in the form of either a unicompartmental or total knee replacement (TKR) [2]. Outcomes of TKR may be influenced by some of the initial interventions used in the management of knee OA [16–18]. In this context, some investigators have evaluated the influence of preoperative IA injections on subsequent joint replacement [19–21].

This chapter discusses the risk of deep prosthetic joint infection (PJI) in TKR emanating from the practice of preoperative IA injections used in the management of knee OA and addresses some of the key questions encountered by clinicians in the decision-making process.

These include:

1. What are the common types of therapeutic substances used in IA injections of knee for the management of knee OA?
2. Which are the patient/clinician/procedure related factors that may influence the risk of PJI in TKR following IA injection in the preoperative period?
3. What is the current evidence to guide the safe surgical management when TKR is indicated in a patient with knee OA and previous history of ipsilateral IA injection?

D. S. Angadi · C. Bolton · V. Kandhari
M. R. J. Coolican (✉)
Sydney Orthopaedic Research Institute, Level 1, The Gallery, Chatswood, NSW, Australia
e-mail: myles@mylescoolican.com.au

© ISAKOS 2022
U. G. Longo et al. (eds.), *Infection in Knee Replacement*,
https://doi.org/10.1007/978-3-030-81553-0_35

35.2 Types of Therapeutic Substances Used in Intraarticular Injection

35.2.1 Corticosteroids

Methylprednisolone or triamcinolone are the most commonly used corticosteroids for intraarticular injections. Corticosteroids are typically combined with local anaesthetic such as lidocaine or bupivacaine [22]. Glucocorticoids reduce the proinflammatory effects of arachidonic acid by acting directly on nuclear steroid receptors which alter the synthesis of mRNA and proteins leading to changes in T-cell and B-cell functions, decreases in the levels of cytokines and enzymes, and inhibition of phospholipase A2 [23]. Corticosteroids reduce inflammation by altering B- and T-cell function as well as stimulating hyaluronic acid synthesis [22].

More recent studies have demonstrated that such changes in the pericellular matrix in which the chondrocytes are situated and to which they are adapted can have significant effects on the chondrocytes in terms of gene expression with subsequent effect on the anabolic/catabolic homeostatic balance [24]. This alteration in normal chondrocyte function may tip the balance from an anabolic to catabolic state with subsequent degenerative change seen in osteoarthritis [25]. In summary, IA corticosteroids may be useful in treating synoviocyte-mediated inflammation, thereby providing some symptom relief but have a negative effect on chondrocyte function.

In their guidelines, the American Academy of Orthopaedic Surgeons (AAOS) noted that given the inconclusive evidence they were not able to recommend for or against the use of intraarticular corticosteroids to treat knee OA [26]. However, an intraarticular steroid injection remains the first step in management for many patients after initial presentation to a surgeon.

35.2.2 Hyaluronic Acid (HA)

Hyaluronic Acid (HA) is a complex high molecular weight polysaccharide that is an essential component of proteoglycans found in synovial fluid [27]. It has a molecular weight in normal synovial fluid ranging from 6500 to 10,900 kDa [28]. In the normal adult knee, HA concentration ranges from 2 to 4 mg per ml and has a half-life of 20 hours [29]. It increases the viscosity of IA fluid and entangles between collagen fibres to trap water, providing increased compressive strength to articular cartilage [22, 30]. HA decreases inflammation by reducing oxidative stress and inhibiting macrophage phagocytosis [31].

In comparison to normal knee joint, the half-life of intrasynovial HA is reduced (11 to 12 h) in degenerative conditions such as knee OA [32]. Furthermore, HA has been demonstrated to undergo depolymerisation with reduced molecular weight ranging from 2700 to 4500 kDa [28].

Exogenous HA injections are known by the marketing term "viscosupplementation" to describe a combination of the presumed dual effects of adding viscous material to the joint and supplementing the supply of hyaluronic acid. Currently, the commercially available HA preparations are typically administered in single-dose regimens, but most require three to five weekly injections [22, 33]. These products vary in their molecular weight, method of production, half-lives and cost [33]. They are produced either from harvested rooster combs or via bacterial fermentation in vitro [34]. Higher molecular weight HA (above 6000 kDa) is suggested to have greater clinical efficacy, but the current literature is inconclusive [31, 32, 35, 36].

It must be noted that the AAOS guidelines do not recommend the use of HA injections for knee OA [26, 37]. However, the Federal Drug Administration (FDA) in the United States has approved their use in the treatment of knee OA as a medical device as opposed to pharmaceutical agents [38]. Furthermore, their use is approved only in the select cohort of patients where knee OA symptoms have progressed despite simple oral analgesics or nonpharmacologic therapy [22, 38].

35.2.3 Biological/Novel Agents

Several biological and novel agents have been introduced in the recent years in the management of knee OA with variable outcomes [39–45]. These include:

35.2.3.1 Platelet-Rich Plasma (PRP)

The rationale for PRP injection in knee OA is the direct introduction and subsequent utilisation of platelet-derived growth factors stored in the alpha granules of platelets to stimulate the natural healing cascade with regeneration of tissue and mediation of the anti-inflammatory response [40, 44, 45].

Several commercial systems are available which enable PRP preparation from the patient's venous blood, which is centrifuged to separate the platelets from red and white blood cells [42, 45, 46]. Several investigators have evaluated the clinical effectiveness of PRP in the management of knee OA [46–48]. Recent evidence has suggested that IA administration of leukocyte poor PRP in patients with knee OA can result in significant improvement in Western Ontario and McMaster Universities Osteoarthritis Index (WOMAC) scores compared to HA or placebo [49–51]. However, other investigators have reported no significant improvement with PRP treatment [52, 53]. The current AAOS guidelines do not recommend for or against the use of PRP for knee OA [26].

35.2.3.2 Mesenchymal Stem Cells (MSC)

Mesenchymal stem cells (MSC) derived from bone marrow, adipose tissue and amnion have been described in the recent literature as biological modalities useful in the management of patients with knee OA [42, 43, 54, 55]. Whilst the literature regarding these treatment options is rapidly evolving, they are performed predominantly in specialist centres [55–57].

The mechanism(s) through which MSC work in knee OA remains an area of ongoing research [57, 58]. Some investigators have suggested that IA injections of MSC may act via a combination of direct differentiation into chondrocytes, expression of appropriate extracellular matrix (ECM) proteins, and secretion of growth factors and cytokines that suppress inflammatory cell activation and stimulate tissue repair [55–57].

35.2.3.3 Autologous Cell Free Preparations (ACS/APS)

Two common forms of autologous cell free preparations used in the management of knee OA include autologous conditioned serum (ACS) and autologous protein serum (APS) [39, 59]. Currently, several commercially available kits are utilised to prepare ACS/APS from whole-blood samples of patients [60–63]. The obtained blood sample is further conditioned by incubation with glass beads and centrifugation, leading to an increase in the production of IL-1Ra as well as multiple other cytokines and growth factors [63, 64]. Broadly, both ACS and APS are injectable solutions enriched in endogenous cytokines which may help to restore joint homeostasis preventing degenerative changes in cartilage and bone [39, 59].

35.3 Current Evidence

35.3.1 Literature Search and Databases

A literature search of all the available evidence was undertaken (March 2020) using the healthcare database website (http://www.library.nhs.uk/hdas). The databases searched were Medline, CINAHL, Embase and the Cochrane library. Medline, CINAHL and Embase search was performed using Boolean statements and the wildcard symbol (*). A review of the Cochrane database for relevant articles was performed. An adjunctive bibliography search was undertaken to identify additional relevant studies through review articles, Google scholar (https://scholar.google.co.uk/) and the grey literature database—OpenGrey [65].

35.3.2 Search Criteria

Corticosteroids: The search criteria included "knee* AND (replacement* OR arthroplasty*) AND (intraarticular* OR joint*) AND inject* AND (steroid* OR corticosteroid*)".

Viscosupplementation: The search criteria included "knee* AND (replacement* OR arthroplasty*) AND (intraarticular* OR joint*) AND inject* AND (hyaluronic acid* OR viscosupplement*)".

Biological/novel agents: The search criteria included "knee* AND (replacement* OR arthroplasty*) AND (intraarticular* OR joint*) AND inject* AND [(platelet rich plasma* OR mesenchymal stem cells* OR autologous conditioned serum* OR autologous protein solution*)]".

35.3.3 Search Results

A brief survey of studies in the current literature is presented in Tables 35.1, 35.2 and 35.3.

Interestingly, despite the considerable amount of literature available regarding the biological/novel agents used in the management of knee OA, the current comprehensive search did not identify any study addressing the topic of PJI risk in TKR following their use in the preoperative period.

35.4 Pathogenesis of PJI in TKR Following IA Injection

Whilst the precise mechanism whereby an IA injection leads to PJI following TKR is unknown, there are a number of theories. It has been suggested that some of the depot preparations of corticosteroids may not dissolve completely and can remain trapped within the soft tissue areas of cystic degeneration [21]. These remnants may be reactivated during surgery and lead to risk of wound complications or PJI [21]. Other investigators have reported that skin bacteria may be introduced at the time of IA injection given the significant variations in the skin preparation and the aseptic technique used [66–69]. This view is supported by investigators who used the "spent needle" culture method and noted that despite alcohol skin preparation 14% to 28% needle tips showed evidence of organisms [70]. These organisms may remain dormant and later be activated by the surgery.

There is consensus that PJI in TKR patients is the result of a multiple factors [71–74]. However, given the paucity of high quality studies coupled with the conflicting conclusions arrived by the different investigators, there remains a lack of detailed understanding regarding the aetiopathological mechanisms leading to PJI in TKR patients who have received an IA injection in the preoperative period [7, 75, 76].

35.4.1 Corticosteroids

As evident from Table 35.1, the published studies evaluating the potential risk of PJI in TKR following an IA corticosteroid injection are varied. Furthermore, their retrospective design limits the level evidence with majority being level III/IV studies. This has been highlighted by the systematic reviews and meta-analyses on the topic [7, 75, 76]. The overall reported rate in the literature of PJI in TKR is relatively low at approximately 1% [71, 77, 78]. Hence it has been suggested that the minimum number of patients required per cohort to demonstrate a 50% increase in infection rates following IA corticosteroid injection is 2000 [79]. All the studies except that by Richardson et al. [80] do not satisfy this criteria.

In an initial study on this topic, Papavasiliou and colleagues investigated the association between preoperative corticosteroid injection and increased risk of PJI in TKR [66]. This retrospective cohort study divided the 144 patients into two groups; one group had received IA corticosteroids prior to TKR and a control group who had not. The authors reported three PJI cases in the study group. The time from last injection to surgery for the three infected cases was 8, 10 and 11 months. However, the timing of injection for those patients who did not develop infection was not stated. In contrast to the injection group, no infections were documented in the control group who had not received steroids prior to TKR ($p < 0.025$). The authors concluded that preoperative IA corticosteroid injection given within the 11-month period prior to TKR significantly increased the risk of deep infection. This study

Table 35.1 Survey of studies evaluating risk of PJI in TKR following preoperative corticosteroid injection

Study	Study design	Number of patients/TKR	Steroid (type and dose)	Place of injection	Follow-up after TKR (months)	PJI	Time between injection and TKR (months)	Odds ratio (95% CI) and p-value
Richardson et al. (2019)	Retrospective cohort	16,656 patients 6653 5569 4434	NR	NR	6	3.25%	≤3 >3–6 >6–12	1.21 (1.04–1.40), $p = 0.01$ 1.07 (0.90–1.27), $p = 0.41$ 1.17 (0.98–1.40), $p = 0.08$
Kokubun et al. (2017)	Retrospective cohort	442 TKR	Methylprednisolone 80 mg or Triamcinolone 40 mg	NR	51.5	3.0%	≤3 ≤6	1.09 (0.52–2.23), $p = 0.80$ 1.47 (0.71–3.04), $p = 0.29$
Khanuja et al. (2016)	Retrospective cohort	302 patients	Triamcinolone 40 mg	Clinic: 302	42	2.0%	5	0.5[a] (0.12–1.98), $p = 0.5$
Desai et al. (2009)	Retrospective cohort	90 TKR	Methylprednisolone 40 mg	Clinic: 30 OR: 60	12	0	≤12	NR
Horne et al. (2008)	Retrospective case-control	40 cases 352 control	NR	Clinic: 40	NR	11/40[b]	16	1.38 (0.55–3.31), $p = $ NR
Joshy et al. (2006)	Retrospective cohort	32 TKR	NR	NR	NR	NR	46	NR
Papavasiliou et al. (2006)	Retrospective cohort	54 patients	Methylprednisolone 40 mg	Clinic: 54	NR	5.6%	9.6	NR

PJI prosthetic joint infection, *TKR* total knee replacement, *OR* operating room, *NR* not reported, *CI* confidence interval
[a]Relative risk of PJI due to corticosteroid injection
[b]Number of patients in each subgroup is not reported

Table 35.2 Survey of studies evaluating risk of PJI in TKR following preoperative viscosupplementation injection

Study	Study design	Number of patients/ TKR	HA (type and dose)	Place of injection	Follow-up after TKR (months)	PJI rate	Time between injection and TKR (months)	Odds ratio (95% CI) and p-value
Richardson et al. (2019)	Retrospective cohort	3249 patients 646 1113 1490	NR	NR	6	4.18%	$\leq$3 >3–6 >6–12	1.55(1.02–2.25), $p = 0.02$ 0.84(0.55–1.23), $p = 0.39$ 0.83(0.57–1.16), $p = 0.28$
Kokubun et al. (2017)	Retrospective cohort	442 TKR	Synvisc-One[a] Orthovisc[a] Gel-One[a]	NR	51.5	3.0%	$\leq$3 $\leq$6	1.09(0.52–2.23), $p = 0.80$ 1.47(0.71–3.04), $p = 0.29$

PJI prosthetic joint infection, *TKR* total knee replacement, *HA* hyaluronic acid, *NR* not reported, *CI* confidence interval

[a]Number of patients in each subgroup is not reported

collated data only from the hospital records and potentially could have missed those patients who received steroid injections from GPs and inadvertently including those patients in the control group introducing an obvious selection bias. Furthermore, the authors did not provide information regarding other patients who may have had IA corticosteroid injection closer to surgery than 8 months without developing infection.

Joshy et al. [81] performed a retrospective matched case-control study involving a group of 32 patients who had PJI following TKR comparing them with a similar number of TKR patients without infection. The authors reported that previous steroid injection was not a risk factor for PJI. However, the very small sample size renders this study significantly underpowered.

In 2008, Horne et al. conducted a similar retrospective matched case-control comparing 40 patients with PJI with 352 patients without PJI following TKR. Apart from reviewing hospital records, the authors assessed the number of IA corticosteroid injections performed in the community by the patient's GP and rheumatologists using questionnaires. Thus, the comparative groups were reduced to 28 (PJI) and 219 (without PJI). They reported that 32% patients in the control group and 39% in the study group had received a corticosteroid injection. The authors concluded that this was not significant ($p = 0.44$). This study has several inconsistencies on closer inspection. The study group was initially reported to include 29 patients in the methods but subsequently reported as only 28 patients in the results section. The follow-up period was limited to only 6 months post TKR. Furthermore, corticosteroid injection prior to TKA was identified via the questionnaire only, without attempts to screen orthopaedic, rheumatology or general practitioner (GP) records. Therefore, this study is potentially subject to significant recall bias.

Subsequently, Desai et al. [79] in 2009 reported the outcomes of 90 TKRs with preoperative history of corticosteroid injection and 1 year follow-up. Interestingly, 60 knees were injected in the operating room (OR) and the remainder were performed in the outpatient clinic. The authors compared the above patients with a cohort of 180 TKR from the same institution without a history of preoperative corticosteroid injection and reported no PJI in either group. Forty five knees in the study group received an injection within the 12 months prior to surgery. However, the authors did not state how close to

Table 35.3 Survey of studies investigating risk of PJI in TKR based on timing of preoperative intraarticular injection

Study	Study design	Number of patients/TKR	Therapeutic substance	Place of injection	Follow-up after TKR (months)	PJI (%)	Time between injection and TKR (months)	Odds ratio (95% CI) and p-value
Bedard et al. (2017)	Retrospective cohort	29,603 patients	NR	NR	6	4.6	1	1.29 (1.03–1.62), $p = 0.024$
		1804				4.4	2	1.23 (1.06–1.42), $p = 0.005$
		5031				4.4	3	1.23 (1.07–1.40), $p = 0.003$
		5659				4.6	4	1.28 (1.11–1.50), $p = 0.001$
		4197				4.6	5	1.30 (1.09–1.54), $p = 0.003$
		3259				5.2	6	1.46 (1.21–1.76), $p < 0.001$
		2444				3.8	7	1.06 (0.83–1.35), $p = 0.625$
		1839				3.5	8	0.96 (0.72–1.27), $p = 0.779$
		1477				4.4	9	1.23 (0.93–1.62), $p = 0.141$
		1257				3.4	10	0.95 (0.68–1.33), $p = 0.766$
		1053				3.4	11	0.95 (0.65–1.38), $p = 0.781$
		850				3.8	12	1.07 (0.73–1.56), $p = 0.741$
		733						
Cancienne et al. (2015)	Retrospective cohort	22,240 patients	NR	NR	6	3.41	≤3	1.5 (1.2–1.8), $p < 0.0001$
		5313				2.48	>3–6	1.1 (0.9–1.3), $p = 0.52$
		8919				2.24	>6–12	1.0 (0.8–1.2), $p = 0.66$
		8008						

PJI prosthetic joint infection, *TKR* total knee replacement, *NR* not reported, *CI* confidence interval the TKR procedure those injections were given and did not state the mean time between injection and TKR for the study group. It must be noted that the method of performing steroid injections in an operating room is not common. Hence, the findings of this study may not be applicable to all centres. Additionally, the authors did not investigate whether the patients in either group received corticosteroid injection in the community leading to a selection bias.

Khanuja and colleagues reported the outcomes of 302 patients who had received IA corticosteroid injection prior to undergoing TKR [21]. All the IA corticosteroid (triamcinolone 40 mg) injections were performed during office visits under aseptic precautions following skin preparation with alcoholic chlorhexidine solution. They compared the outcomes of the above group with a control group of patients matched for gender, age, body mass index (BMI) and American Society of Anaesthesiologists (ASA) status (1:1 matching). They observed that there was no significant difference between the two groups with respect to PJI (2%—injection cohort and 1%—non-injection cohort; risk ratio = 0.5, p = 0.5). Interestingly, the authors stated that whilst all patients in the non-injection control group were drawn based on records of a single institution, they were unable to rule out that this group may have included patients who received IA injection at other institutions.

In 2017, Kokubun et al. reported on the outcomes and complications of 442 TKRs with a mean follow-up of 51 months from a single surgeon series [82]. They reported that 13 patients (3%) had a PJI with 175 patients (40%) having received 4 or more injections whilst 267 patients (60%) patients had received 3 or fewer injections. The authors concluded that preoperative corticosteroid injections do not significantly influence the risk of PJI in subsequent TKR. The authors acknowledge the low numbers in their data and use the principle "a priori" power analysis using the above infection rate. Additionally, the details as to whether the injections were performed in hospital or community settings are missing. This study included both corticosteroid and hyaluronic acid injections. However, it must be noted that the authors do not report the number of patients

in each group, thereby limiting the interpretation of their results.

In their study, Richardson et al. used a large national database in the United States to identify 58,337 patients who had undergone primary TKR between 2007 to 2016 [80]. Using procedure codes, patients who had an IA injection in the 12 months leading up to TKR and underwent surgical procedures for PJI in the 6 months post TKR were reviewed. They had a cohort of 16,656 patients with history of IA corticosteroid injection in the preoperative period and further divided these patients based on the time between the IA injection and TKR (Table 35.1). There were 6653 (39.9%) patients who had had IA corticosteroid injection less than 3 months prior to their TKR with a PJI rate of 3.25% compared to 2.74% in patients without history of IA injection thereby representing a 19% increased risk. After controlling for age, sex and medical comorbidities, there was a significantly higher risk of PJI; the odds ratio was 1.21 (Table 35.1). The authors found that corticosteroid injections given more than 3 months prior to the TKR posed no added infection risk.

35.4.2 Hyaluronic Acid

Only two studies in the current literature have investigated the risk of PJI with TKR in patients receiving viscosupplementation treatment in the preoperative period [80, 82] (Table 35.2). Both studies are methodologically different with the data for the study by Richardson et al. [80] derived from large national database whilst the data for the study by Kokubun et al. [82] represents a single surgeon series.

The primary research question which Richardson and colleagues have investigated is the influence of time gap between viscosupplementation injections and TKR procedure and the associated risk of PJI. Of their total of 3249 patients, a cohort of 646 (19.9%) received HA injections less than 3 months before their TKR with a reported PJI rate of 4.18% compared to 2.74% in the non-injection group. This represented a 53% relatively higher risk of PJI (odds ratio, 1.55).

In their study, Kokubun et al. [82] investigated the influence of the number of injections along with time between viscosupplementation and TKR procedure on PJI. The authors reported an infection rate of 3% in their cohort. The authors concluded that viscosupplementation injections with hyaluronic acid including the timing or number of injections have no relationship with PJI in TKR. However, their data has patients who received IA injections of both corticosteroids and hyaluronic acid. Consequently, several limitations of this study become apparent including the lack of clarity regarding the number of patients who received viscosupplementation treatment and the time gap between the injections and TKR. Hence, the results from this study need to be interpreted carefully with due consideration to all the inherent limitations from a single surgeon series data set.

35.4.3 Biological/Novel Agents

Several studies have been published in the recent past describing the clinical outcomes of knee OA treatment with PRP [45, 46], MSC [43, 58], ACS [61, 83, 84] and APS [63, 85] amongst other biological/novel agents. However, there is no study in the published literature evaluating the risk of PJI in TKR following these treatment modalities. Nonetheless, it is useful to note that septic arthritis has been reported as either a complication of treatment or as an adverse event in the setting of experimental studies involving some of the aforementioned products [86, 87]. Theoretically, given the invasive nature of injections the potential for introduction of occult infection into the knee is present but due to the paucity of studies it is difficult to estimate the risk of PJI in TKR following IA injection with these products.

35.5 Timing of Injection

Two recent studies used information collated from large databases to investigate the influence of the time gap between IA injection in the ipsilateral knee and the risk of PJI in subsequent TKR [20, 88] (Table 35.3).

Cancienne et al. [88] investigated the outcomes of 22,240 patients with TKR and a history of IA injection in the preoperative period (upto 12 months). Their control group matched for age, gender, BMI, diabetes and smoking consisted of 13,650 TKR patients without a history of IA injection. They observed that in the subgroup of 5313 patients who received IA injection less than 3 months before TKR had a higher rate of PJI of 3.41% (odds ratio, 1.5; $p < 0.0001$). There was no significant difference in infection rates in patients who underwent TKA between 3–6 months or 6–12 months after ipsilateral knee injection compared to the control cohort.

In their 2017 retrospective cohort study, Bedard and colleagues [20] used the Humana Health Insurance database to obtain information on the outcomes of TKR patients. They identified 29,603 TKR patients who had had an IA injection in the ipsilateral knee at least 1 year before the TKR. The control group consisted of 54,081 TKR patients with no preoperative IA injection in the ipsilateral knee joint. Both groups were matched as per the Charlson comorbidity index [89]. In the group of TKR patients who had an ipsilateral injection in the preoperative period, they noted that the risk of PJI was higher compared to the control group (4.4% vs. 3.59%; odds ratio, 1.23; $p < 0.001$). Furthermore, the risk of a postoperative infection resulting in return to the operating room within 6 months after TKR was also higher for patients that received an IA injection before ipsilateral TKR than those that did not (1.49% vs. 1.04%; odds ratio, 1.4; $p < 0.001$).

Both the above studies concluded that IA injection prior to TKR was associated with not only a higher risk of PJI but in addition the risk was time-dependent.

35.6 Other Evidence and Guidelines

A review of literature pertaining to injections into the hip joint and subsequent arthroplasty has similar findings to the aforementioned studies [75, 90–93]. The working group which was part of International Consensus Meeting (ICM) noted that there was limited information in the current literature to recommend the ideal timing for elective total ankle arthroplasty (TAA) after corticosteroid injection for the symptomatic native ankle joint [94]. They recommended that at least 3 months pass after corticosteroid injection and prior to performing TAA [94].

35.7 Conclusions

There is paucity of robust studies evaluating the adverse risk of PJI from the IA injection in subsequent TKR. This has contributed to the lack of consensus on this vital aspect of management of patients with symptomatic knee OA. There is global consensus that PJI in TKR patients is multifactorial with a complex interplay of risk factors. Whilst some risk factors are non-modifiable, factors such as IA injections and timing of TKR represent modifiable factors.

There is a need to continue further research on this topic to develop our understanding albeit with a combination of clinical studies, observational studies based on large databases, systematic reviews and meta-analysis of the available evidence.

IA injections continue to be a part of the management of patients with knee symptomatic OA. Hence these patients need to be appropriately counselled regarding the benefits and potential adverse effects including the risk of PJI in subsequent TKR. A minimum interval of 3 months between IA injection and TKR would be a safe approach to adopt until further evidence emerges to guide the management.

References

1. Parker DA, Scholes C, Neri T. Non-operative treatment options for knee osteoarthritis: current concepts. J ISAKOS. 2018;3(5):274–81.
2. Weber KL, Jevsevar DS, McGrory BJ. AAOS clinical practice guideline: surgical management of osteoarthritis of the knee: evidence-based guideline. J Am Acad Orthop Surg. 2016;24(8):e94–6.
3. Levy DM, Petersen KA, Scalley Vaught M, Christian DR, Cole BJ. Injections for knee osteoarthritis: corticosteroids, viscosupplementation, platelet-rich plasma, and autologous stem cells. Arthroscopy. 2018;34(5):1730–43.
4. McAlindon TE, Bannuru RR, Sullivan MC, Arden NK, Berenbaum F, et al. OARSI guidelines for the non-surgical management of knee osteoarthritis. Osteoarthr Cartil. 2014;22(3):363–88.
5. Klasan A, Putnis SE, Yeo WW, Fritsch BA, Coolican MR, et al. Advanced age is not a barrier to total knee arthroplasty: a detailed analysis of outcomes and complications in an elderly cohort compared with average age total knee arthroplasty patients. J Arthroplasty. 2019;34(9):1938–45.
6. Bedard NA, Dowdle SB, Anthony CA, DeMik DE, McHugh MA, et al. The AAHKS clinical research award: what are the costs of knee osteoarthritis in the year prior to total knee arthroplasty? J Arthroplasty. 2017;32(9):S8–S10.e11.
7. Marsland D, Mumith A, Barlow IW. Systematic review: the safety of intra-articular corticosteroid injection prior to total knee arthroplasty. Knee. 2014;21(1):6–11.
8. Ong KL, Runa M, Xiao Z, Ngai W, Lau E et al. Severe acute localized reactions following intra-articular hyaluronic acid injections in knee osteoarthritis. Cartilage. 2020:1947603520905113.
9. Kompel AJ, Roemer FW, Murakami AM, Diaz LE, Crema MD, et al. Intra-articular corticosteroid injections in the hip and knee: perhaps not as safe as we thought? Radiology. 2019;293(3):656–63.
10. Puttick MP, Wade JP, Chalmers A, Connell DG, Rangno KK. Acute local reactions after intraarticular hylan for osteoarthritis of the knee. J Rheumatol. 1995;22(7):1311–4.
11. Kunugiza Y, Tani M, Tomita T, Yoshikawa H. Staphylococcal scalded skin syndrome after intra-articular injection of hyaluronic acid. Mod Rheumatol. 2011;21(3):316–9.
12. Kim WB, Alhusayen RO. Skin necrosis from intra-articular hyaluronic acid injection. J Cutan Med Surg. 2015;19(2):182–4.
13. Albert C, Brocq O, Gerard D, Roux C, Euller-Ziegler L. Septic knee arthritis after intra-articular hyaluronate injection: two case reports. Joint Bone Spine. 2006;73(2):205–7.
14. Shemesh S, Heller S, Salai M, Velkes S. Septic arthritis of the knee following intraarticular injections in elderly patients: report of six patients. IMAJ Israel Med Assoc J. 2011;13(12):757.
15. Mohamed M, Patel S, Plavnik K, Liu E, Casey K, et al. Retrospective analysis of septic arthritis caused by intra-articular viscosupplementation and steroid injections in a single outpatient center. J Clin Med Res. 2019;11(7):480–3.
16. Kim SC, Jin Y, Lee YC, Lii J, Franklin PD, et al. Association of preoperative opioid use with mortality and short-term safety outcomes after total knee replacement. JAMA Netw Open. 2019;2(7):e198061.
17. Huber EO, Roos EM, Meichtry A, de Bie RA, Bischoff-Ferrari HA. Effect of preoperative neuromuscular training (NEMEX-TJR) on functional outcome after total knee replacement: an assessor-blinded

randomized controlled trial. BMC Musculoskelet Disord. 2015;16:101.

18. Chesham RA, Shanmugam S. Does preoperative physiotherapy improve postoperative, patient-based outcomes in older adults who have undergone total knee arthroplasty? A systematic review. Physiother Theory Pract. 2017;33(1):9–30.

19. Amin NH, Omiyi D, Kuczynski B, Cushner FD, Scuderi GR. The risk of a deep infection associated with intraarticular injections before a total knee arthroplasty. J Arthroplasty. 2016;31(1):240–4.

20. Bedard NA, Pugely AJ, Elkins JM, Duchman KR, Westermann RW, et al. The John N. Insall Award: do intraarticular injections increase the risk of infection after TKA? Clin Orthop Relat Res. 2017;475(1):45–52.

21. Khanuja HS, Banerjee S, Sodhi GS, Mont MA. Do prior intra-articular corticosteroid injections or time of administration increase the risks of subsequent periprosthetic joint infections after total knee arthroplasty? J Long Term Eff Med Implants. 2016;26(3):191–7.

22. Levy DM, Petersen KA, Vaught MS, Christian DR, Cole BJ. Injections for knee osteoarthritis: corticosteroids, viscosupplementation, platelet-rich plasma, and autologous stem cells. Arthroscopy. 2018;34(5):1730–43.

23. Law TY, Nguyen C, Frank RM, Rosas S, McCormick F. Current concepts on the use of corticosteroid injections for knee osteoarthritis. Phys Sportsmed. 2015;43(3):269–73.

24. Hayman DM, Blumberg TJ, Scott CC, Athanasiou KA. The effects of isolation on chondrocyte gene expression. Tissue Eng. 2006;12(9):2573–81.

25. Resteghini P. Injection therapy in the management of osteoarthritis of the knee. PhD Thesis. University of Brighton; 2010.

26. Jevsevar DS, Brown GA, Jones DL, Matzkin EG, Manner PA, et al. The American Academy of Orthopaedic surgeons evidence-based guideline on: treatment of osteoarthritis of the knee. JBJS. 2013;95(20):1885–6.

27. Leighton R, Fitzpatrick J, Smith H, Crandall D, Flannery CR, et al. Systematic clinical evidence review of NASHA (Durolane hyaluronic acid) for the treatment of knee osteoarthritis. Open Access Rheumatol Res Rev. 2018;10:43–54.

28. Balazs EA, Watson D, Duff IF, Roseman S. Hyaluronic acid in synovial fluid. I Molecular parameters of hyaluronic acid in normal and arthritic human fluids. Arthritis Rheum. 1967;10(4):357–76.

29. Zhang W, Robertson J, Jones A, Dieppe P, Doherty M. The placebo effect and its determinants in osteoarthritis: meta-analysis of randomised controlled trials. Ann Rheum Dis. 2008;67(12):1716–23.

30. Neustadt DH. Long-term efficacy and safety of intra-articular sodium hyaluronate (Hyalgan\®) in patients with osteoarthritis of the knee. Clin Exp Rheumatol. 2003;21(3):307–12.

31. Waddell DD. Viscosupplementation with hyaluronans for osteoarthritis of the knee. Drugs Aging. 2007;24(8):629–42.

32. Hunter DJ. Viscosupplementation for osteoarthritis of the knee. N Engl J Med. 2015;372(11):1040–7.

33. Strauss EJ, Hart JA, Miller MD, Altman RD, Rosen JE. Hyaluronic acid viscosupplementation and osteoarthritis: current uses and future directions. Am J Sports Med. 2009;37(8):1636–44.

34. McArthur BA, Dy CJ, Fabricant PD, Della Valle AG. Long term safety, efficacy, and patient acceptability of hyaluronic acid injection in patients with painful osteoarthritis of the knee. Patient Prefer Adherence. 2012;6:905–10.

35. Maneiro E, De Andrés M, Fernandez-Sueiro J, Galdo F, Blanco F. The biological action of hyaluronan on human osteoartritic articular chondrocytes: the importance of molecular weight. Clin Exp Rheumatol. 2004;22(3):307–12.

36. Evaniew N, Simunovic N, Karlsson J. Cochrane in CORR®: viscosupplementation for the treatment of osteoarthritis of the knee. Clin Orthop Relat Res. 2014;472(7):2028–34.

37. Brown GA. AAOS clinical practice guideline: treatment of osteoarthritis of the knee: evidence-based guideline. J Am Acad Orthop Surg. 2013;21(9):577–9.

38. Watterson JR, Esdaile JM. Viscosupplementation: therapeutic mechanisms and clinical potential in osteoarthritis of the knee. J Am Acad Orthop Surg. 2000;8(5):277–84.

39. Angadi DS, Macdonald H, Atwal N. Autologous cell-free serum preparations in the management of knee osteoarthritis: what is the current clinical evidence? Knee Surg Relat Res. 2020;32(1):16.

40. Campbell KA, Saltzman BM, Mascarenhas R, Khair MM, Verma NN, et al. Does intra-articular platelet-rich plasma injection provide clinically superior outcomes compared with other therapies in the treatment of knee osteoarthritis? A systematic review of overlapping meta-analyses. Arthroscopy. 2015;31(11):2213–21.

41. Chahla J, Mandelbaum BR. Biological treatment for osteoarthritis of the knee: moving from bench to bedside—current practical concepts. Arthroscopy. 2018;34(5):1719–29.

42. Delanois RE, Etcheson JI, Sodhi N, Henn Iii RF, Gwam CU, et al. Biologic therapies for the treatment of knee osteoarthritis. J Arthroplasty. 2019;34(4):801–13.

43. Jorgensen C. SP0108 MSC based therapy for severe osteoarthritis of the knee: the Adipoa experience. London: BMJ Publishing Group; 2015.

44. Mascarenhas R, Saltzman BM, Fortier LA, Cole BJ. Role of platelet-rich plasma in articular cartilage injury and disease. J Knee Surg. 2015;28(01):003–10.

45. Southworth TM, Naveen NB, Tauro TM, Leong NL, Cole BJ. The use of platelet-rich plasma in symptomatic knee osteoarthritis. J Knee Surg. 2019;32(01):037–45.

46. Lai LP, Stitik TP, Foye PM, Georgy JS, Patibanda V, et al. Use of platelet-rich plasma in intra-articular knee injections for osteoarthritis: a systematic review. PM R. 2015;7(6):637–48.

47. Annaniemi JA, Pere J, Giordano S. Platelet-rich plasma versus hyaluronic acid injections for knee osteoarthritis: a propensity-score analysis. Scand J Surg. 2019;108(4):329–37.

48. Shirokova K, Noskov S, Shirokova L. Comparison of clinical efficacy of platelet-rich plasma and autologous conditioned serum treatment in patients with osteoarthritis of the knee. Osteoarthr Cartil. 2017;25:S438.

49. Riboh JC, Saltzman BM, Yanke AB, Fortier L, Cole BJ. Effect of leukocyte concentration on the efficacy of platelet-rich plasma in the treatment of knee osteoarthritis. Am J Sports Med. 2016;44(3):792–800.

50. Cerza F, Carnì S, Carcangiu A, Di Vavo I, Schiavilla V, et al. Comparison between hyaluronic acid and platelet-rich plasma, intra-articular infiltration in the treatment of Gonarthrosis. Am J Sports Med. 2012;40(12):2822–7.

51. Buendía-López D, Medina-Quirós M, Fernández-Villacañas Marín MÁ. Clinical and radiographic comparison of a single LP-PRP injection, a single hyaluronic acid injection and daily NSAID administration with a 52-week follow-up: a randomized controlled trial. J Orthop Traumatol. 2018;19(1):3–3.

52. Filardo G, Di Matteo B, Di Martino A, Merli ML, Cenacchi A, et al. Platelet-rich plasma intra-articular knee injections show no superiority versus visco-supplementation: a randomized controlled trial. Am J Sports Med. 2015;43(7):1575–82.

53. Cole BJ, Karas V, Hussey K, Merkow DB, Pilz K, et al. Hyaluronic acid versus platelet-rich plasma: a prospective, double-blind randomized controlled trial comparing clinical outcomes and effects on intra-articular biology for the treatment of knee osteoarthritis. Am J Sports Med. 2017;45(2):339–46.

54. Jiang Y, Iwata S, Yang C, Shirakawa K, Matsuoka T. Cartilage regeneration by autologous adipose-derived mesenchymal stem cells for the treatment of osteoarthritis. Cytotherapy. 2019;21(5, supplement):S83–4.

55. Orozco L, Munar A, Soler R, Alberca M, Soler F, et al. Treatment of knee osteoarthritis with autologous mesenchymal stem cells: a pilot study. Transplantation. 2013;95(12):1535–41.

56. Jo CH, Lee YG, Shin WH, Kim H, Chai JW, et al. Intra-articular injection of mesenchymal stem cells for the treatment of osteoarthritis of the knee: a proof-of-concept clinical trial. Stem Cells. 2014;32(5):1254–66.

57. Vega A, Martín-Ferrero MA, Del Canto F, Alberca M, García V, et al. Treatment of knee osteoarthritis with allogeneic bone marrow mesenchymal stem cells: a randomized controlled trial. Transplantation. 2015;99(8):1681–90.

58. Vangsness CT Jr, Jack Farr I, Boyd J, Dellaero DT, Mills CR, et al. Adult human mesenchymal stem cells delivered via intra-articular injection to the knee following partial medial meniscectomy: a randomized, double-blind, controlled study. JBJS. 2014;96(2):90–8.

59. Vitali M, Ometti M, Drossinos A, Pironti P, Santoleri L, et al. Autologous conditioned serum: clinical and functional results using a novel disease modifying agent for the management of knee osteoarthritis. J Drug Assess. 2020;9(1):43–51.

60. Baltzer AWA, Moser C, Krauspe R, Jansen SA. Autologous conditioned serum (Orthokine) is an effective treatment for knee osteoarthritis. Osteoarthr Cartil. 2009;17(2):152–60.

61. Barreto A, Braun TR. A new treatment for knee osteoarthritis: clinical evidence for the efficacy of ArthrokinexTM autologous conditioned serum. J Orthop. 2017;14(1):4–9.

62. Kon E, Engebretsen L, Verdonk P, Nehrer S, Filardo G. Clinical outcomes of knee osteoarthritis treated with an autologous protein solution injection: a 1-year pilot double-blinded randomized controlled trial. Am J Sports Med. 2018;46(1):171–80.

63. van Drumpt RA, van der Weegen W, King W, Toler K, Macenski MM. Safety and treatment effectiveness of a single autologous protein solution injection in patients with knee osteoarthritis. BioResearch. 2016;5(1):261–8.

64. King W, van der Weegen W, Van Drumpt R, Soons H, Toler K, et al. White blood cell concentration correlates with increased concentrations of IL-1ra and improvement in WOMAC pain scores in an open-label safety study of autologous protein solution. J Exp Orthop. 2016;3(1):9.

65. Multidisciplinary European Database. http://www.opengrey.eu/search/. Accessed 24 Nov 2019.

66. Papavasiliou AV, Isaac DL, Marimuthu R, Skyrme A, Armitage A. Infection in knee replacements after previous injection of intra-articular steroid. J Bone Jt Surg. 2006;88(3):321–3.

67. Charalambous C, Tryfonidis M, Sadiq S, Hirst P, Paul A. Septic arthritis following intra-articular steroid injection of the knee—a survey of current practice regarding antiseptic technique used during intra-articular steroid injection of the knee. Clin Rheumatol. 2003;22(6):386–90.

68. von Essen R, Savolainen HA. Bacterial infection following intra-articular injection: a brief review. Scand J Rheumatol. 1989;18(1):7–12.

69. Pal B, Morris J. Perceived risks of joint infection following intra-articular corticosteroid injections: a survey of rheumatologists. Clin Rheumatol. 1999;18(3):264–5.

70. Cawley P, Morris I. A study to compare the efficacy of two methods of skin preparation prior to joint injection. Rheumatology. 1992;31(12):847–8.

71. Pulido L, Ghanem E, Joshi A, Purtill JJ, Parvizi J. Periprosthetic joint infection: the incidence, timing, and predisposing factors. Clin Orthop Relat Res. 2008;466(7):1710–5.

72. Papalia R, Vespasiani-Gentilucci U, Longo UG, Esposito C, Zampogna B, et al. Advances in man-

agement of periprosthetic joint infections: an historical prospective study. Eur Rev Med Pharmacol Sci. 2019;23(2 Suppl):129–38.

73. Izakovicova P, Borens O, Trampuz A. Periprosthetic joint infection: current concepts and outlook. EFORT Open Rev. 2019;4(7):482–94.

74. Valle CD, Parvizi J, Bauer TW, DiCesare PE, Evans RP, et al. Diagnosis of periprosthetic joint infections of the hip and knee. J Am Acad Orthop Surg. 2010;18(12):760–70.

75. Wang Q, Jiang X, Tian W. Does previous intraarticular steroid injection increase the risk of joint infection following total hip arthroplasty or total knee arthroplasty? A meta-analysis. Med Sci Monit. 2014;20:1878–83.

76. Xing D, Yang Y, Ma X, Ma J, Ma B, et al. Dose intraarticular steroid injection increase the rate of infection in subsequent arthroplasty: grading the evidence through a meta-analysis. J Orthop Surg Res. 2014;9(1):107.

77. Alijanipour P, Parvizi J. Infection post-total knee replacement: current concepts. Curr Rev Musculoskelet Med. 2014;7(2):96–102.

78. Osmon DR, Berbari EF, Berendt AR, Lew D, Zimmerli W, et al. Diagnosis and management of prosthetic joint infection: clinical practice guidelines by the infectious diseases Society of America. Clin Infect Dis. 2012;56(1):e1–e25.

79. Desai A, Ramankutty S, Board T, Raut V. Does intraarticular steroid infiltration increase the rate of infection in subsequent total knee replacements? Knee. 2009;16(4):262–4.

80. Richardson SS, Schairer WW, Sculco TP, Sculco PK. Comparison of infection risk with corticosteroid or hyaluronic acid injection prior to total knee arthroplasty. JBJS. 2019;101(2):112–8.

81. Joshy S, Thomas B, Gogi N, Modi A, Singh BK. Effect of intra-articular steroids on deep infections following total knee arthroplasty. Int Orthop. 2006;30(2):91–3.

82. Kokubun BA, Manista GC, Courtney PM, Kearns SM, Levine BR. Intra-articular knee injections before total knee arthroplasty: outcomes and complication rates. J Arthroplasty. 2017;32(6):1798–802.

83. Evans CH, Chevalier X, Wehling P. Autologous conditioned serum. Phys Med Rehabil Clin. 2016;27(4):893–908.

84. Fox BA, Stephens MM. Treatment of knee osteoarthritis with Orthokine-derived autologous conditioned serum. Expert Rev Clin Immunol. 2010;6(3):335–45.

85. Vitale ND, Vandenbulcke F, Chisari E, Iacono F, Lovato L, et al. Innovative regenerative medicine in the management of knee OA: the role of autologous protein solution. J Clin Orthop Trauma. 2019;10(1):49–52.

86. Yang KA, Raijmakers N, Van Arkel E, Caron J, Rijk P, et al. Autologous interleukin-1 receptor antagonist improves function and symptoms in osteoarthritis when compared to placebo in a prospective randomized controlled trial. Osteoarthr Cartil. 2008;16(4):498–505.

87. Nguyen C, Rannou F. The safety of intra-articular injections for the treatment of knee osteoarthritis: a critical narrative review. Expert Opin Drug Saf. 2017;16(8):897–902.

88. Cancienne JM, Werner BC, Luetkemeyer LM, Browne JA. Does timing of previous intra-articular steroid injection affect the post-operative rate of infection in total knee arthroplasty? J Arthroplasty. 2015;30(11):1879–82.

89. Charlson ME, Pompei P, Ales KL, MacKenzie CR. A new method of classifying prognostic comorbidity in longitudinal studies: development and validation. J Chronic Dis. 1987;40(5):373–83.

90. Schairer WW, Nwachukwu BU, Mayman DJ, Lyman S, Jerabek SA. Preoperative hip injections increase the rate of periprosthetic infection after total hip arthroplasty. J Arthroplasty. 2016;31(9):166–169. e161.

91. Pereira L, Kerr J, Jolles B. Intra-articular steroid injection for osteoarthritis of the hip prior to total hip arthroplasty: is it safe? A systematic review. Bone Jt J. 2016;98(8):1027–35.

92. Chitre A, Fehily M, Bamford D. Total hip replacement after intra-articular injection of local anaesthetic and steroid. J Bone Jt Surg. 2007;89(2):166–8.

93. Charalambous CP, Prodromidis AD, Kwaees TA. Do intra-articular steroid injections increase infection rates in subsequent arthroplasty? A systematic review and meta-analysis of comparative studies. J Arthroplasty. 2014;29(11):2175–80.

94. Ucckay I, Hirose CB, Assal M. does intra-articular injection of the ankle with corticosteroids increase the risk of subsequent periprosthetic joint infection (PJI) following total ankle arthroplasty (TAA)? If so, how long after a prior intra-articular injection can TAA be safely performed? Foot Ankle Int. 2019;40(1_suppl):3S–4S.

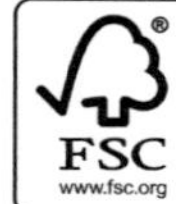